# MANAGEMENT OF DIABETIC NEPHROPATHY

# MANAGEMENT OF DIABETIC NEPHROPATHY

*Edited by*

**GEOFFREY BONER** MBBCh

*Institute of Hypertension and Kidney Disease*

*Rabin Medical Center*

*Beilinson Campus*

*Petah Tikva*

ISRAEL

**MARK E COOPER** MBBS PhD

*Department of Medicine*

*University of Melbourne*

*Melbourne*

AUSTRALIA

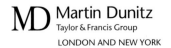 **Martin Dunitz**
Taylor & Francis Group
LONDON AND NEW YORK

© 2003 Martin Dunitz Ltd, an imprint of Taylor & Francis Group

First published in the United Kingdom in 2003
by Martin Dunitz Ltd, an imprint of Taylor and Francis Group, 11 New Fetter Lane, London EC4P 4EE

Tel.:      +44 (0) 20 7583 9855
Fax.:      +44 (0) 20 7842 2298
E-mail:   info@dunitz.co.uk
Website: http://www.dunitz.co.uk

Although every effort has been made to ensure that all owners of copyright material have been acknowledged in this publication, we would be glad to acknowledge in subsequent reprints or editions any omissions brought to our attention.

A CIP record for this book is available from the British Library.

ISBN 1 84184 076 9

Distributed in the USA by
Fulfilment Center
Taylor & Francis
10650 Toebben Drive
Independence, KY 41051, USA
Toll Free Tel.: +1 800 634 7064
E-mail: taylorandfrancis@thomsonlearning.com

Distributed in Canada by
Taylor & Francis
74 Rolark Drive
Scarborough, Ontario M1R 4G2, Canada
Toll Free Tel.: +1 877 226 2237
E-mail: tal_fran@istar.ca

Distributed in the rest of the world by
Thomson Publishing Services
Cheriton House
North Way
Andover, Hampshire SP10 5BE, UK
Tel.: +44 (0)1264 332424
E-mail: salesorder.tandf@thomsonpublishingservices.co.uk

Composition by Wearset Ltd, Boldon, Tyne and Wear

Printed and bound in Great Britain by TJ International Ltd, Padstow, Cornwall

# Contents

# Contributors

**Ruth Axer-Siegel**
Sackler Faculty of Medicine
Tel Aviv University and
Department of Ophthalmology
Rabin Medical Center
Beilinson Campus
Petah Tikva 49101
ISRAEL

**Peter H Bennett**
Phoenix Epidemiology & Clinical Research Branch
National Institute of Diabetes and Digestive and
Kidney Diseases
National Institutes of Health
Phoenix, AZ 85014
USA

**Rudolf Bilous**
Audrey Collins Teaching Unit
Education Centre
South Cleveland Hospital
Middlesbrough TS4 3BW
UK

**Geoffrey Boner**
Institute of Hypertension and Kidney Disease
Rabin Medical Center
Beilinson Campus
Petah Tikva
ISRAEL

**Fabrice Bonnet**
Senior Lecturer and
Consultant in Diabetology
Department of Endocrinology
Cardiovascular Hospital Lyon
University Claude Bernard
Lyon
FRANCE

**Riccardo Candido**
Division of Diabetes, Metabolism and Lipoproteins
Baker Heart Research Institute
Melbourne
Victoria
AUSTRALIA and
Department of Internal Medicine and Neurology
University of Trieste
Trieste
ITALY

**Mark E Cooper**
Department of Medicine
University of Melbourne
Melbourne
AUSTRALIA

**Gabriel Danovitch**
Kidney Transplant Program
UCLA Medical Center
UCLA School of Medicine
Los Angeles, CA 90095
USA

**An S De Vriese**
Department of Internal Medicine
Ghent University Hospital
Ghent
BELGIUM

**Gad Dotan**
Department of Ophthalmology
Rabin Medical Center
Beilinson Campus
Petah Tikva 49101
ISRAEL

**David Jonathan van Dijk**
Specialist in Internal Medicine and Nephrology
Director of the Diabetic Nephropathy Clinic
Institute of Hypertension and Kidney Diseases
Rabin Medical Center
Beilinson Campus
Petah Tikva
ISRAEL

**Claudia Ferrier**
Physician and Consultant Nephrologist
Clinica Moncucco
Lugano
SWITZERLAND

**Allan Flyvbjerg**
Medical Department M (Diabetes and
Endocrinology)
Medical Research Laboratories
Institute of Experimental Clinical Research
Aarhus University Hospital
8000 Aarhus
DENMARK

**Spiros Fourlanos**
Autoimmunity and Transplantation Division
The Walter and Eliza Hall Institute of Medical
Research
PO The Royal Melbourne Hospital
Victoria, 3050
AUSTRALIA

**Eli A Friedman**
Renal Diseases Division
Department of Medicine
State University of New York
Downstate Medical Center
Brooklyn, NY 11203
USA

**Philippe Froguel**
Endocrinologie
Hôpital Bichat – Claude Bernard
46 Rue Henry Huchard
Paris 75018
FRANCE

**Eileen Gallery**
Clinical Professor of Medicine, Clinical Professor of
Obstetrics and Gynaecology University of Sydney at
Royal North Shore Hospital
St Leonards, NSW
AUSTRALIA

**Richard Gilbert**
University of Melbourne
Department of Medicine
St Vincent's Hospital
41 Victoria Parade
AUSTRALIA

**Karin Jandeleit-Dahm**
Consultant Nephrologist and
Senior Research Fellow
Diabetic Complications
The Baker Heart Research Institute
Victoria
AUSTRALIA

**George Jerums**
Endocrinology Department
University of Melbourne
A & RMC – Austin Campus
Studley Road
Heidelberg, Victoria 3084
AUSTRALIA

**Steve Jones**
Audrey Collins Teaching Unit
Education Centre
South Cleveland Hospital
Middlesbrough TS4 3BW
UK

**Thomas WH Kay**
Autoimmunity and Transplantation Division
The Walter and Eliza Hall Institute of Medical
Research
PO The Royal Melbourne Hospital
Victoria, 3050
AUSTRALIA

**Darren J Kelly**
Senior Research Fellow
University of Melbourne
Department of Medicine
St Vincent's Hospital
Fitzroy, Vic
Australia

**Elizabeth Kendrick**
Kidney Transplant Program
UCLA Medical Center
UCLA School of Medicine
Los Angeles, CA
USA

**Mike Krimholtz**
UMDS Department of Endocrinology
Diabetes & Metabolic Medicine
5th Floor Tomas Guy House
UMDS Guy's Hospital
London SE1 9RT
UK

**Robyn G Langham**
Lecturer and Renal Physician
University of Melbourne
Department of Medicine
St Vincent's Hospital
Fitzroy, Victoria
AUSTRALIA

**Nick London MD FRCS**
University Department of Vascular Surgery
Leicester Royal Infirmary
Leicester LE1 5WW
UK

**Richard MacIsaac**
Endocrinology Department
University of Melbourne
A & RMC – Austin Campus
Studley Road
Heidelberg, Victoria 3084
AUSTRALIA

**Michel Marre**
Endocrinologie
Hôpital – Claude Bernard
46 Rue Henry Huchard
Paris 75018
FRANCE

**Robert G Nelson**
Staff Clinician
Phoenix Epidemiology and Clinical Research Branch
National Institute of Diabetes and Digestive and
Kidney Branches
National Institutes of Health
Phoenix
Arizona
USA

**Paul G McNally**
Department of Diabetes and Endocrinology
Leicester Royal infirmary
Leicester LE1 5WW
UK

**Sianna Panagiotopoulos**
Endocrinology Department
University of Melbourne
A & RMC – Austin Campus
Studley Road
Heidelberg, Victoria 3084
AUSTRALIA

**Carol A Pollock**
Professor of Medicine
Royal North Shore Hospital
University of Sydney
St Leonards, 2065 NSW
AUSTRALIA

**Rita Rachmani**
Department of Medicine
Meir Hospital and
Sackler Faculty of Medicine
Tel Aviv University
Tel Aviv
ISRAEL

**Mordechai Ravid**
Department of Medicine
Meir Hospital and
Sackler Faculty of Medicine
Tel Aviv University
Tel Aviv
ISRAEL

**Aileen Robertson**
Department of Dietetics
Aberdeen Royal Infirmary
Foresterhill
Aberdeen
UK

**Bieke F Schrijvers**
Departments of Internal Medicine
Ghent University Hospital
Ghent
BELGIUM and
Medical Department M (Diabetes and
Endocrinology)
Medical Research Laboratories
Institute of Experimental Clinical Research
Aarhus University Hospital
8000 Aarhus
DENMARK

**Piyush Srivastava**
Department of Cardiology
Austin and Repatriation Medical Centre
Heidelberg
Victoria
AUSTRALIA

**Merlin C Thomas**
NHRRC Biomedical Reserach Scholar
The Baker Medical Research Institute
Melbourne
AUSTRALIA

**Stephen Thomas**
UMDS Department of Endocrinology
Diabetes & Metabolic Medicine
5th Floor Tomas Guy House
UMDS Guy's Hospital
London SE1 9RT
UK

**Marianne Venegoor**
Specialist Renal Dietitian
Surrey
UK

**GianCarlo Viberti**
UMDS Department of Endocrinology
Diabetes & Metabolic Medicine
5th Floor Tomas Guy House
UMDS Guy's Hospital
London SE1 9RT
UK

**Norman R Waugh**
Professor, Department of Public Health
University of Aberdeen
Medical School Buildings
Foresterhill
Aberdeen AB25 2 ZD
UK

**Yalemzewd Woredekal**
Renal Diseases Division
Department of Medicine
State University of New York
Downstate Medical Center
450 Clarkson Avenue
Brooklyn, NY 11203
USA

# Preface

Geoffrey Boner and Mark E Cooper

Over the past half-century, it has become abundantly clear that one of the major medical problems facing the modern world is diabetes mellitus. This systemic disease, with a plethora of complications and comorbid conditions, is a major cause of mortality and morbidity and is associated with a large economic burden on the patients themselves, their families and the health-care systems of most countries.

Diabetic nephropathy is a major complication of diabetes and is today one of the major causes of end-stage renal failure in many developed and undeveloped nations. Moreover, diabetic nephropathy is associated with many of the other macro- and microvascular complications of diabetes. As diabetes and its complications are treated by general practitioners, family physicians and internists, as well as by many specialist physicians, the treatment is often fragmented and not coordinated. Coordination of treatment is especially important in those diabetic patients with renal involvement. The past few years have seen the emergence of several therapeutic regimens that may prevent the development of diabetic nephropathy and slow the progression of this disorder.

The time is thus opportune for publishing a book that contains a description of the development of diabetes mellitus, renal involvement and other comorbid conditions, and the latest therapeutic regimens. We are pleased that many senior investigators have contributed to this book, which should provide basic information on diabetes, diabetic nephropathy and some other complications, and at the same time provide data on recent therapeutic trials and accepted therapeutic regimens. The subject matter should be of interest to general practitioners, family physicians, internal physicians, endocrinologists and nephrologists as well as nurses and dietitians involved in the care of diabetic patients. We hope that the coming years will provide additional information in this important field and that there will be room for publishing more information on diabetic nephropathy.

# 1

# Introduction

Geoffrey Boner and Mark E Cooper

Chronic progressive degenerative diseases have emerged as the major medical problems of the new millennium. It has become clear that diabetes mellitus is one of the most important health hazards, especially in the developed nations. Type 1 diabetes mellitus, with reduced or absent secretion of insulin, presents mostly in childhood or early adulthood and is considered to be primarily immunologic in origin. The incidence of type 1 diabetes mellitus is increasing annually. This has been well demonstrated in a study of the incidence of childhood-onset diabetes in Europe.[1]

Type 2 diabetes mellitus, as manifested by resistance to the action of insulin, was always thought to be a disease of middle-aged to elderly adults. Over the last few years, it has become increasingly prevalent in young adults and even in children.[2] The incidence and prevalence vary among the different ethnic groups. However, there is a sharp increase in the number of patients with type 2 diabetes mellitus in all ethnic groups.[3–5] This rapid increase in the incidence and prevalence of the disease is associated with the exposure of large populations to the dietary habits and sedentary lifestyles of the developed nations. The increase in calorie intake, mainly derived from carbohydrates and animal fat, with a decrease in physical activity, has led to excessive obesity and increasing resistance to insulin action.[6,7] In fact, the increase in type 2 diabetes mellitus has been described as having reached epidemic proportions.[4–7]

Diabetes mellitus of type 1 and type 2 is associated with an increased risk of several comorbid conditions. These include localized or generalized atherosclerosis with eventual coronary heart disease and cardiac failure, hypertension, peripheral vascular disease, retinopathy and/or cerebrovascular disease.[8] Diabetes mellitus is also associated with renal involvement in a relatively high proportion of patients. Some 25–45% of both type 1 and type 2 diabetics have been shown to develop overt renal disease.[9,10] Diabetic nephropathy occurs as a result of both direct and indirect actions of glucose, which activates various pathways involved in the pathogenesis of diabetic nephropathy. These include oxidative stress, advanced glycation and activation of certain cytokines. Additional deleterious factors that need to be considered include hypertension, arteriosclerosis, and the toxic effects of the exposure of tubular cells to proteins.[11,12]

The involvement of the kidney in diabetes, known as diabetic nephropathy, is a progressive disease and is often associated with hypertension. Strict control of blood pressure, hyperglycemia and low-protein diet have all been shown to slow the progression of the renal disease. Guidelines that specifically address these modifiable factors have been established for the treatment of diabetic nephropathy.[13] In addition to the conventional methods of treatment, newer therapeutic modes have been proposed, but these are still in the early stages of clinical trials or preclinical investigation.[11]

Improved treatment of diabetes and its renal complications has enhanced the survival of these patients. However, this increase in survival has resulted in the appearance of other complications of the disease. For example, many of the patients with diabetic nephropathy develop cardiac disease, retinopathy and peripheral vascular disease. This demands a multidisciplinary approach in order to optimize the management of all the patients' problems.

Diabetic nephropathy eventually results in end-stage renal disease (ESRD) in a high proportion of patients. Over the past few years, more and more patients with diabetic nephropathy have been accepted onto renal replacement therapy (RRT) programs. Indeed, diabetic nephropathy has become the major cause of ESRD in most Western countries. Both the incidence and prevalence of diabetic nephropathy in patients on RRT continues to increase, with the majority of new patients entering end-stage renal failure programs now having the diagnosis of type II diabetes.[14,15]

The incidence of comorbid conditions in the patient on RRT is high, and this phenomenon may be even more prominent in the diabetic patient.[16] The mortality rate of the diabetic patient on RRT is greater than that of nondiabetic subjects, in spite of the recent improvement in survival of these patients over the past few years.[17] Diabetic patients on RRT are especially prone to develop additional complications and comorbid conditions, and they require intensive treatment not only to manage these specific conditions but also to improve their quality of life.

Many patients with diabetic nephropathy do not receive optimal treatment to slow progression of the renal disease and to prevent the development of comorbid conditions. The purpose of this book is to provide information on the pathogenesis and development of diabetic nephropathy to as wide a readership as possible in order to improve the care of the patient with this disorder. This should include family physicians, internal physicians, endocrinologists, nephrologists, cardiologists and other health-care professionals.

The first section of the book is devoted to general aspects of diabetes and diabetic nephropathy. It includes chapters describing diabetes mellitus and its epidemiology, the epidemiology of diabetic nephropathy, the genetic basis of diabetes and diabetic nephropathy, and factors influencing the progression of diabetic nephropathy. These chapters should provide a useful background to the physician looking for up-to-date, clinically relevant information on diabetic nephropathy.

The second section of the book is devoted to the treatment of diabetic nephropathy and its complications, starting with early changes in the diabetic kidney and progressing onto ESRD. This includes extensive discussion of the standard treatments of the patient with diabetic nephropathy. Chapters are devoted to the control of hyperglycemia, the treatment of hypertension, the use of low-protein diets, the treatment of hyperlipidemia, the management of cardiac complications and the treatment of acid–base disturbances. This is followed by a chapter describing the newer experimental approaches to the treatment of diabetic nephropathy. In order to develop a logical approach to treatment, we have included a

series of chapters summarizing the management of these patients at different levels of renal function. This is due to the fact that the emphasis may vary at different stages of nephropathy. We have divided the renal involvement into mild to moderate and advanced disease, followed by a chapter on the use of dialysis in the diabetic patient with end-stage renal failure. The dietary management of this type of patient is extremely difficult, since attention has to be paid to the regulation of carbohydrate intake and at the same time to the intake of protein; therefore, we have included a chapter on the approach of the dietitian to patients with diabetic nephropathy.

Special attention is given to three categories of patients with diabetic nephropathy. The approach to the pregnant female who has diabetic nephropathy is important to ensure the term delivery of a healthy infant. The pregnant diabetic patient with renal involvement is considered to be at high risk of complications affecting both the fetus and the mother. These patients should be followed by a team of physicians who have experience in treating this condition. The patient with diabetic nephropathy and, more often than not, hypertension is likely to have moderate to advanced retinopathy demanding a specific approach. The diabetic neuropathic foot and peripheral vascular disease are emerging as major problems of the patient with diabetic nephropathy. Most dialysis units treating diabetic patients have high rates of peripheral vascular disease, often requiring amputation of one or more limbs. The prevention of ischemia, infection and gangrene of the limbs requires very careful monitoring and treatment of the patient.

With the improvement in survival of transplanted patients following both living donor and cadaver donor transplants, diabetic patients have also been admitted to the waiting lists for renal transplantation. In fact, the survival rates of diabetic patients after transplantation are better than those in patients on dialysis.[18] Moreover, the simultaneous transplantation of a pancreas with a kidney in patients with type 1 diabetes results in increased survival of the transplanted kidney.[19] Indeed, successful transplantation of the pancreas in patients with type 1 diabetes and renal involvement has resulted in regression of the kidney damage.[20] An exciting new development has been the transplantation of isolated pancreatic islets, leading to specific treatment for type 1 diabetes.[21] A chapter has thus been devoted to the use of renal and pancreas transplantation in the diabetic patient with ESRD.

We hope that the contents of this book will provide guidelines for the treatment of patients with diabetic nephropathy and the various complications and comorbid conditions associated with this disease.

# REFERENCES

1. Green A, Patterson CC, on behalf of the EURODIAB TIGER study group, Trends in the incidence of childhood-onset diabetes in Europe 1989–1998, *Diabetologia* (2001) **44**(Suppl 3): B3–8.

2. Ludwig DS, Ebbeling CB, Type 2 diabetes mellitus in children. Primary care and public health considerations, *JAMA* (2001) **286:** 1427–30.

3. Burke JF, Williams K, Gaskill SP et al, Rapid rise in the incidence of type 2 diabetes from 1987 to 1996. Results from the San Antonio Heart Study, *Arch Intern Med* (1999) **159:** 1450–6.

4. Mokdad AH, Ford ES, Bowman BA et al, Diabetes trends in the US: 1990–1998, *Diabetes Care* (2000) **23:** 1278–83

5. Mokdad AH, Bowman BA, Ford ES et al, The continuing epidemics of obesity and diabetes in the United States, *JAMA* (2001) **286:** 1195–200.

6. Meyer KA, Jacobs DR, Kushi LH et al, Dietary fat and incidence of type 2 diabetes in older Iowa women, *Diabetes Care* (2001) **24:**1528–35.

7. Zimmet P, Alberti KG, Shaw J, Global and societal implications of the diabetes epidemic, *Nature* (2001) **414:** 782–7.

8. Clark CM, Lee DA, Prevention and treatment of the complications of diabetes mellitus, *N Engl J Med* (1995) **332:** 1210–17.

9. Parving HH, Hommel E, Mathiesen E et al, Prevalence of microalbuminuria, arterial hypertension, retinopathy and neuropathy in patients with insulin-dependent diabetes, *BMJ* (1988) **296:** 156–60.

10. Ismail N, Becker B, Strzelczyk P et al, Renal disease and hypertension in non-insulin-dependent diabetes mellitus, *Kidney Int* (1999) **55:** 1–28.

11. Cooper ME, Interaction of metabolic and haemodynamic factors in mediating experimental diabetic nephropathy, *Diabetologia* (2001) **44:** 1957–72.

12. Brownlee M, Biochemistry and molecular cell biology of diabetic complications, *Nature* (2001) **414:** 813–20.

13. Diabetic nephropathy. Position statement. American Diabetes Association, *Diabetes Care* (2002) **25**(Suppl 1): S85–9.

14. Incidence and prevalence (Chapter 1). Excerpts from the United States Renal Data System. 2001 Annual Data Report: Atlas of End-Stage Renal Disease in the United States, *Am J Kidney Dis* (2001) **38**(Suppl 3): S37–52.

15. International comparisons (Chapter 13). Excerpts from the United States Renal Data System. 2001 Annual Data Report: Atlas of End-Stage Renal Disease in the United States, *Am J Kidney Dis* (2001) **38**(Suppl 3): S195–203.

16. Morbidity and hospitalization (Chapter 5). Excerpts from the United States Renal Data System. 2001 Annual Data Report: Atlas of End-Stage Renal Disease in the United States, *Am J Kidney Dis* (2001) **38**(Suppl 3): S91–106.

17. Survival, mortality and causes of death (Chapter 8). Excerpts from the United States Renal Data System. 2001 Annual Data Report: Atlas of End-Stage Renal Disease in the United States, *Am J Kidney Dis* (2001) **38**(Suppl 3): S135–46.

18. Wolfe RA, Ashby VB, Milford EL et al, Comparison of mortality in all patients on dialysis, patients on dialysis awaiting transplantation, and recipients of a first cadaver transplant, *N Engl J Med* (1999) **341:** 1725–30.

19. Tyden G, Tollemar J, Bolinder J, Combined pancreas and kidney transplantation improves survival in patients with end-stage diabetic nephropathy, *Clin Transplant* (2000) **14:** 505–8.

20. Fioretto P, Steffes MW, Sutherland DE et al, Reversal of lesions of diabetic nephropathy after pancreas transplantation, *N Engl J Med* (1998) **339:** 69–75.

21. Shapiro AM, Lakey JR, Ryan EA et al, Islet transplantation in seven patients with type 1 diabetes mellitus using a glucocorticoid-free immunosuppressive regimen, *N Engl J Med* (2000) **343:** 230–8.

# I

## The pathogenesis and clinical description of diabetic nephropathy

# Type 2 diabetes: description and epidemiology

Peter H Bennett and Robert G Nelson

Type 2 diabetes, formerly known as non-insulin-dependent diabetes, is the most common form of diabetes. Its frequency is increasing throughout the world. In 2000, there were approximately 150 million individuals with the disease, and it is predicted that this number is likely to double by 2025.[1]

Diabetes is associated with excessive rates of coronary heart disease, stroke, renal disease and renal failure, retinopathy, and blindness, as well as peripheral vascular disease, neuropathy, and amputation. These complications give rise to most of the excess morbidity and mortality attributable to type 2 diabetes.

## CLASSIFICATION

Diabetes mellitus is a metabolic disorder of multiple etiologies and is characterized by chronic hyperglycemia with disturbances of carbohydrate, fat, and protein metabolism. These metabolic disturbances result from defects in insulin secretion, insulin action, or both. The current classification of diabetes mellitus, summarized below, is based on etiological characteristics. It was introduced by the American Diabetes Association (ADA) in 1997[2] and adopted in 1999 by the World Health Organization (WHO).[3]

Type 1 diabetes, accounting for 5–10% of cases of diabetes in populations of European origin, is associated with primary beta cell failure, commonly a result of autoimmune-associated destruction. In its initial stages, type 1 diabetes can be identified by the presence of circulating anti-glutamic acid dehydrogenase antibodies, islet cell autoantibodies, or insulin autoantibodies. In some subjects, particularly non-Caucasians with this clinical form of the disease, no evidence of an autoimmune disorder is demonstrable, and the causes of beta cell destruction remain obscure. Once the disease is established, patients with type 1 diabetes require insulin to prevent spontaneous ketosis and to permit survival.

Type 2 diabetes, the most common form of diabetes in all populations, is characterized by disordered insulin action and insulin secretion. Both defects are usually present at the time of clinical presentation, but the specific biochemical or genetic abnormalities giving rise to the defects in insulin resistance and insulin secretion are not yet known. Glycemic control may necessitate the use of insulin or oral antihyperglycemic agents, but dietary control may suffice in those with diabetes of recent onset.

Other specific types of diabetes are those forms in which the underlying disease process is known or can be identified in a relatively specific way. These include diabetes due to known genetic defects of beta cell function, such as several forms of maturity onset diabetes of the young, and diabetes resulting from mitochondrial mutations. In addition, other specific types of diabetes include those forms of the disease due to specific genetic defects in insulin action, diseases of the exocrine pancreas, those associated with other endocrinopathies, those associated with specific drugs or chemicals, and those due to some specific infections, as well as diabetes occurring in association with other well-defined genetic syndromes where the specific genetic defect may or may not be known.

Gestational diabetes mellitus (GDM) is diabetes or glucose intolerance that first appears during pregnancy. While any type of diabetes can first appear in pregnancy, in most women GDM is an early manifestation of type 2 diabetes. Women with GDM may revert to normal glucose tolerance after delivery, but they have an extremely high risk of developing type 2 diabetes within the next 5 years.[4]

Type 2 diabetes shows strong familial aggregation.[5,6] It has a genetic basis, although the specific genes involved are not yet well defined. Nevertheless, multiple genes, rather than a single major gene, usually contribute to its etiology.[7] While genetic susceptibility is almost certainly a prerequisite for the development of diabetes, exposures to environmental factors are responsible for the clinical expression of the disease.

Type 2 diabetes is characterized by insulin resistance in muscle, liver, and adipose tissue. There is also relative or absolute deficiency in insulin secretion, although the absolute insulin concentrations are often high or normal at the onset of the disease. In most instances, a progressive deterioration of beta cell function occurs with increasing duration of the disease, so that eventually subnormal insulin concentrations prevail. Type 2 diabetes may be associated with the classical symptoms of polydipsia, polyuria, and weight loss, but it is often asymptomatic. Indeed, the disease may be present for many years before symptoms or complications supervene. As a result, half of those with type 2 diabetes, and more in some populations, remain undiagnosed unless systematic screening for diabetes is carried out.

Patients with type 2 diabetes do not require exogenous insulin to prevent spontaneous ketonuria and ketoacidosis. However, these conditions may be precipitated by infection, trauma, or vascular events. In most instances, the diagnosis of type 2 diabetes is made during the adult years, but the disease does occur in adolescents and children.[8–11] The average age of diagnosis varies considerably in different ethnic groups. It develops typically in the later adult years in Caucasians, but in other ethnic groups such as Asian Indians, Chinese, Polynesians, and Micronesians, African-Americans, and Native Americans, the onset is more typically in 30–40-year-old individuals, although in any ethnic group the disease can occur at any age from childhood onwards.

## DIAGNOSIS

The diagnosis of type 2 diabetes may be made either because of symptomatic clinical presentation, or commonly as a result of opportunistic screening, as the disease is often asymptomatic for a number of years. Type 2 diabetes develops through several clinical stages that are delineated in the WHO and the ADA classifications[2,3] (Figure 2(i).1). Criteria for diagnosis have evolved over the past 30 years, but internationally standardized criteria have been in use since the 1980s.[12] The current diagnostic criteria for diabetes and the related stages of carbohydrate intolerance were published by the ADA in 1997 and the WHO in 1999 (Table 2(i).1). These criteria differ from earlier criteria insofar as the fasting glucose values considered diagnostic were lowered.

A clinical diagnosis of type 2 diabetes may be made in the presence of symptoms such as increased thirst, polyuria, unexplained weight loss, and a random or casual glucose determination of 11.1 mmol/l (200 mg/dl) or higher in capillary whole blood or in venous plasma, or 10 mmol/l (180 mg/dl) or higher in venous whole blood. Diabetes mellitus is unlikely if plasma glucose concentrations are less than 5.5 mmol/l (100 mg/dl) or less than 4.4 mmol/l (80 mg/dl) in whole blood. Concentrations of glucose between these ranges are indeterminate and cannot be used to exclude diabetes.

The fasting glucose concentrations for diagnosis of diabetes in the current ADA and WHO criteria are lower than those recommended previously. Venous or capillary fasting whole-blood glucose concentrations of $\geq 6.1$ mmol/l ($\geq 110$ mg/dl) or venous plasma glucose concentrations of $\geq 7$ mmol/l ($\geq 126$ mg/dl) are considered diagnostic of diabetes if such concentrations are confirmed by a subsequent test. Measurement of fasting glucose concentrations alone, however, detects only about one-third of those with undiagnosed diabetes.[13] Consequently, the WHO recommends that persons with fasting glucose concentrations in the range designated as impaired fasting glycemia (IFG) should receive an oral glucose tolerance test to confirm or exclude the diagnosis of diabetes.[3] During a 75-g oral glucose tolerance test, 2-hr glucose concentrations in capillary whole-blood or venous plasma samples of $\geq 11.1$ mmol/l ($\geq 200$ mg/dl) indicate diabetes regardless of the fasting concentrations. Because of the day-to-day variability in 2-hr and fasting glucose concentrations, a confirmatory diagnostic value, either fasting or 2-hr after a 75-g oral glucose load, should be obtained on a different occasion before a clinical diagnosis of diabetes is made. An oral glucose tolerance test also permits the recognition of impaired glucose tolerance (IGT), a condition entailing a high risk of the subsequent development of type 2 diabetes.[14,15] IGT cannot be identified if only fasting glucose measurements are made. Consequently, most epidemiological studies of type 2 diabetes are based on glucose concentrations measured before and during a 75-g oral glucose tolerance test.

## GEOGRAPHY

The prevalence of type 2 diabetes varies enormously

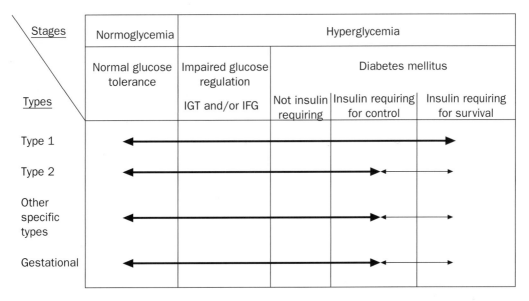

**Figure 2(i).1** Types and clinical stages of diabetes mellitus (adapted from references 2 and 3).

**Table 2(i).1  Diagnostic criteria for diabetes mellitus and related stages of glycemia. Glucose concentrations are expressed in mmol/l (mg/dl). The 2-hr post-glucose values are those measured after a 75-g oral glucose load. The glucose concentrations differ according to whether they are determined in venous or capillary samples, or measured in plasma or whole blood (adapted from references 2 and 3).**

| Diabetes mellitus | Venous whole blood | Capillary whole blood | Venous plasma |
|---|---|---|---|
| Fasting or | ≥6.1 (110) | ≥6.1 (110) | ≥7.0 (126) |
| 2-hr post-glucose Impaired glucose tolerance | ≥10.0 (180) | ≥11.1 (200) | ≥11.1 (200) |
| Fasting (if measured) and | <6.1 (110) | <6.1 (110) | <7.0 (126) |
| 2-hr post-glucose Impaired fasting glycemia | 6.7–9.9 (120–179) | 7.8–11.0 (140–199) | 7.8–11.0 (140–199) |
| Fasting (and if measured) | 5.6–6.0 (100–109) | 5.6–6.0 (100–109) | 6.1–6.9 (110–125) |
| 2-hr post-glucose | <6.7 (120) | <7.8 (140) | <7.8 (140) |

from population to population; in recent decades, dramatic increases in the prevalence and incidence of type 2 diabetes have been documented in many parts of the world, particularly in the newly industrialized and developing countries.[16] Rates differ in different ethnic groups in the same country and in migrants compared with people remaining in their country of origin.[17] These differences reflect the effect of changes in environment on the expression of the disease. Underprivileged people in the developed nations and those from rapidly developing countries are most likely to have high rates of diabetes. Yet,

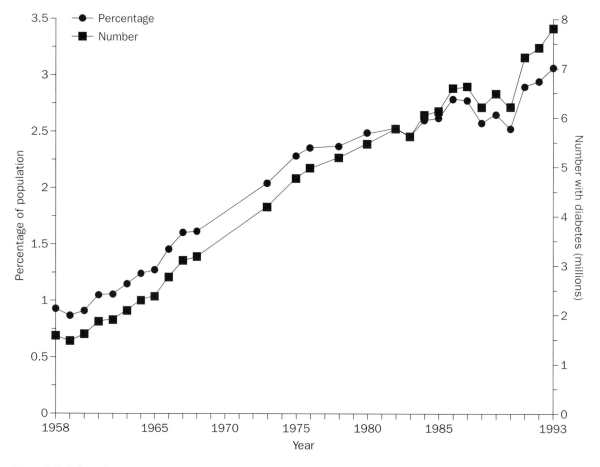

**Figure 2(i).2** Prevalence (percentage) and number of the US population with diagnosed diabetes between 1958 and 1993. The prevalence increased more than threefold between 1960 and 1991–93. Some of the increase is attributable to the aging of the population, but rates more than doubled in all age groups 45 years and over (data from US National Health Interview Surveys reproduced from Kenny et al[20]).

even in developed countries, such as the USA and Australia, the prevalence of type 2 diabetes has increased more then threefold during the past 30 years[18,19] (Figure 2(i).2). These increases in prevalence are related mainly to changing lifestyles and increasing degrees of obesity.

The USA has some of the most complete information on the prevalence of type 2 diabetes from the National Health and Nutrition Examination Surveys[20,21] (Figure 2(i).3). In the USA, the prevalence of diabetes in adults varies considerably by ethnicity. The prevalence in Mexican-Americans is higher than in the White or Black populations, and African-Americans have a greater prevalence than Whites.[22] Native American populations have prevalence rates of type 2 diabetes even higher than Mexican-

Americans, although the prevalence does vary from one Native American tribe to another.[23] Data from the US Health Examination Survey (NHANES III) conducted between 1988 and 1994 showed that almost 7% of the US adults aged 40–74 years had previously diagnosed diabetes.[21] By glucose tolerance testing and the 1985 WHO criteria,[12] a similar proportion were found to have undiagnosed diabetes, resulting in a total prevalence of 14.3%. This represents a 25% increase since the NHANES II survey a decade earlier.[24] The most recent estimates based on surveys of the prevalence of diagnosed diabetes in those 18 years and over have shown further increases of about 40% between 1991 and 1999, from 4.1% to 6% in men and from 5.6% to 7.6% in women.[25,26]

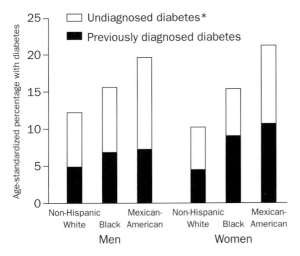

* by 1985 WHO criteria

**Figure 2(i).3** Prevalence of previously diagnosed and undiagnosed diabetes, according to 1985 WHO criteria,[12] in major ethnic groups among persons aged 40–74 years in the USA (data from the third US Nutrition and Health Examination Survey[21] conducted in 1988–94).

Increases in diabetes prevalence are occurring also in developing countries. In China, for example, the prevalence of type 2 diabetes has increased at least threefold during the past 20 years,[27] yet the rates are still far below those seen in populations of Chinese origin living in Singapore and Mauritius.[28,29] This suggests that with continuing economic development and the associated changes in lifestyle, diabetes prevalence in China is likely to increase considerably in the next decade. Similarly, rapid changes in the prevalence of type 2 diabetes are occurring in India.[30–32] In part, these changes are attributable to migration to urban areas, but even in rural areas, the prevalence has increased appreciably during the last decade. As a result of changing demographic characteristics and the predicted rural to urban migration, the worldwide prevalence of type 2 diabetes is expected to double between 2000 and 2025, with the greatest percentage change occurring in the developing nations.[1] By 2025, China and India will be the countries with the largest numbers of patients with type 2 diabetes.

## SEX AND AGE

The prevalence of type 2 diabetes varies to some extent between the sexes from one population to another. These differences are relatively small and can be accounted for by differences in other risk factors.

The prevalence of type 2 diabetes increases with age until the later decades of life, when a decrease in prevalence may be seen, due to excess mortality among persons with type 2 diabetes. In some populations with high frequencies of the disease and in many developing countries, the prevalence increases markedly in the younger adult years, whereas in developed countries major increases in prevalence occur in the age groups 45–70 years.[1] As the prevalence reflects the balance between the rate of development of new cases, the duration of the disease, and mortality, changes in incidence over time can have a large influence on the age patterns in the same population in different time periods.

Recent years have seen a number of reports of the occurrence of type 2 diabetes in childhood and adolescence.[8–11] As in adults, the disease in children and adolescents is frequently asymptomatic and is usually detected as a result of screening activities. In Japan, where a national screening program for schoolchildren has been in place since 1992, the number of schoolchildren recognized to have type 2 diabetes has increased progressively so that the prevalence of type 2 diabetes in children now greatly exceeds that of type 1 diabetes.[11] Similar increases in the prevalence of type 2 diabetes in children and adolescents have been observed among the Pima Indians,[9] but reports of type 2 diabetes in this age range have appeared from many ethnic groups including other Native American tribes, African-Americans, Mexican-Americans, Chinese, Polynesians, Asian Indians, and Arab children from the Gulf states.[33–35] The occurrence of type 2 diabetes in earlier age groups, especially in childhood and adolescence, portends the occurrence of the late complications of type 2 diabetes at earlier ages.

## FAMILIAL AGGREGATION

The risk of having type 2 diabetes is increased two- to sixfold in those with a parent or sibling with the disease. While familial aggregation may occur because of a shared environment, there is strong evidence that type 2 diabetes has major genetic determinants.

Concordance rates of type 2 diabetes are much higher in identical than in fraternal twins.[36] The high degree of concordance among twins, however, does not indicate that the majority of individuals who carry susceptibility genes will develop the disease, as twins often share a similar environment. Further evidence of the importance of genetic factors comes from the distribution of type 2 diabetes in admixed populations. Among people of mixed racial background, differences in prevalence from the parent populations are indicative of the importance of genetic factors in susceptibility. Studies of persons of mixed heritage indicate that their risk is intermediate between those of their parent populations.[37,38]

Type 2 diabetes is a complex genetic disorder. Genes that entail specific risks of its development have been identified only to a limited extent, and most of those identified so far do not appear to be major susceptibility genes. Some significant associations with type 2 diabetes and common variants of several genes have been found, such as PPAR gamma,[39] FABP2,[40] PPP1R3,[41] and adiponectin.[42] Genome-wide scans have shown evidence of a number of genetic loci that almost certainly contain major type 2 diabetes susceptibility genes. These loci appear to vary from population to population, although a number of genome scans in different ethnic groups indicate an important locus on chromosome 1q23–24 in several populations.[43–46] The specific gene(s) and variants contributing to susceptibility at this locus remain to be defined.

The complex nature of the susceptibility to type 2 diabetes is illustrated by its relationships with the Calpain 10 gene.[47,48] This gene appears to be a major susceptibility gene in the Mexican-American population of Star County, Texas, but the specific haplotypes associated with diabetes susceptibility appear to vary in different populations. Some genes associated with type 2 diabetes appear to show evidence of gene–gene interaction—for example, Calpain 10 and Calpain 15.[44] Given the importance of environmental determinants in the expression of type 2 diabetes, it can be predicted that many of the type 2 diabetes susceptibility genes will show evidence of gene–environment interaction and gene–gene interactions.[49]

Differences in genetic susceptibility almost certainly account for some of the differences in the prevalence rates of diabetes found among different ethnic groups living in the same environments. For example, in Singapore in 1992, the frequency of diabetes varied from 7.7% in the Chinese aged 18–69 years to 12% and 13% among the Malays and Asian Indians, respectively.[28] High prevalence rates have also been found among Asian Indians compared with the indigenous populations in the UK, Fiji, South Africa, Mauritius, and the Caribbean.[29,50–53] In New Zealand, the prevalence of diabetes in the Maori and Pacific Island immigrants of Polynesian origin is higher than in persons of European extraction. Although environmental factors may account for some of these differences, it is likely that they also reflect differences in inherent susceptibility to the disease among different ethnic and racial groups.

## ENVIRONMENTAL RISK FACTORS

The importance of environmental and lifestyle factors in the development of type 2 diabetes can be inferred from several lines of evidence. The rapid increases in the prevalence and incidence of the disease seen in the past 30 years can be attributed only to changes in exposure to the precipitating environmental factors. Changes in inherent genetic susceptibility, especially for a multigenic disease, cannot possibly account for the several-fold changes in prevalence and incidence documented over this short period of time. The development of high prevalences of the disease in migrant populations over the course of one or two decades likewise can be attributed only to environmental exposures that promote expression of the disease.[54] Furthermore, the strong associations of diabetes with risk factors that are largely determined by differences in lifestyle within populations, such as obesity and physical inactivity, further emphasize the importance of environmental factors as precipitants of type 2 diabetes.

Some factors that predispose to the development of type 2 diabetes are determined in early life. Infants of low birth weight have an excessive risk of developing the disease in adulthood.[55–58] While the specific reasons are still under investigation, it has been suggested that malnutrition *in utero*, leading to low birth weight, followed by exposure to a relatively affluent environment, leading to obesity, are some of the factors that predispose to the disease in infants of low birth weight.[59] Offspring of diabetic pregnancies are also at extremely high risk of developing the disease. While some of this risk is attributable to inherent susceptibility from the diabetic mother, offspring born after the development of diabetes have a much greater risk of developing type 2 diabetes than offspring born to the same mother before she developed diabetes.[60] This difference demonstrates the importance of the intrauterine environment as a determinant of the disease many years later. Exposure to other factors in early life may well represent important determinants of the future risk. For example, people breast-fed as infants have a lower risk than those who were bottle-fed, thus suggesting that nutrition in infancy determines subsequent risk.[34,61]

Obesity and physical inactivity are major risk factors for type 2 diabetes. The incidence of type 2 diabetes is strongly related to the body-mass index. Indeed, there is an interaction between obesity and inherent susceptibility to the disease. If one or both parents have type 2 diabetes, the risk to obese offspring is much higher than if neither parent has the disease.[62] Not only the presence of obesity, but also its distribution influences the risk of developing type 2 diabetes. Upper body or central obesity is associated with a greater risk than more generalized obesity.[63] Central obesity is also associated with an increased incidence of coronary heart disease, hyperinsulinemia, hypertriglyceridemia, and reduced high-density lipoprotein cholesterol concentrations, as well as hypertension and disturbances in sex-hormone patterns.[64] Insulin resistance, and the associated hyperinsulinemia, appears to be a central feature of this cluster of abnormalities. Furthermore, insulin resistance is a characteristic of patients with type 2 diabetes, and precedes and predicts its development.[65,66]

The level of physical activity is an important determinant of type 2 diabetes. Numerous prospective studies have shown that individuals who are relatively inactive have a much higher risk of developing type 2 diabetes than those who maintain a more active lifestyle.[67–69] However, in part because of the difficulty of assessing physical activity, the dose-response relationship between level of physical activity and risk of type 2 diabetes is relatively unclear.

Direct proof of the importance of obesity and physical inactivity as determinants of diabetes has emerged recently from a number of diabetes-prevention studies. Individuals at high risk of developing diabetes, identified by the presence of impaired glucose tolerance, have been exposed to lifestyle interventions to increase activity and weight loss. These studies have shown a major reduction in the risk of developing type 2 diabetes in response to lifestyle interventions[70–72] (Figure 2(i).4).

Diet is another environmental factor which may contribute to the development of type 2 diabetes.[73–77] Diets characterized by a high percentage of calories from fat, low fiber content, and high refined carbohydrate content are associated with high prevalence rates of the disease.[78] While there is clear evidence that the total caloric content of the diet is important, the question of which nutrients predispose to type 2 diabetes is less certain. There is, however, evidence from short-term studies that the amount and quality of dietary fat can modify glucose tolerance and insulin sensitivity.[73] The fatty acid composition of the diet affects tissue phospholipid composition, which has been shown to be related to insulin sensitivity.[79] Populations with a high prevalence of type 2 diabetes in general consume a diet that contains more fat, particularly saturated fat, than when they followed a more traditional way of life.[80] This pattern of dietary change is characteristic of the transition that

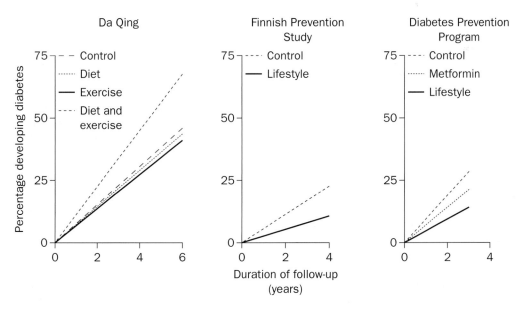

**Figure 2(i).4** Effect of interventions in people with impaired glucose tolerance in China (Da Qing),[70] Finland[71] and the USA (Diabetes Prevention Program[72]). Significant reductions in the incidence of type 2 diabetes were seen in the lifestyle intervention groups in each of these three randomized, controlled clinical trials.

occurs when populations move to a Western environment,[81] but it also occurs when they move from a rural to an urban environment.

Several studies have suggested that moderate alcohol intake may be associated with a reduced incidence of type 2 diabetes.[82] For example, among 20 000 male physicians in the USA, those consuming more than 2–4 drinks/week had a lower incidence of type 2 diabetes over the subsequent 12 years than nondrinkers, and these relationships persisted after adjustment for body-mass index and other diabetes risk factors.[83]

Other risk factors are associated with the development of type 2 diabetes. Several recent studies report a relationship between inflammatory markers—in particular, C-reactive protein, IL-6, TNF-alpha, and gamma globulin—and the risk of developing type 2 diabetes and, most recently, an inverse relationship between adiponectin and that risk.[84,85] Many of these inflammatory markers are secretory products of the adipocyte, and understanding the relationship of these markers to adiposity and glucose tolerance may shed important light on the mechanisms by which obesity relates to the development of type 2 diabetes.

## STAGES IN DEVELOPMENT OF TYPE 2 DIABETES

In most individuals, type 2 diabetes is preceded by a prolonged phase of insulin resistance during which normal glucose tolerance is present, but fasting insulin concentration is elevated due to the presence of insulin resistance (Figure 2(i).5). Insulin resistance is also characteristic of populations with a high risk of developing type 2 diabetes and is found in the nondiabetic siblings and offspring of patients with type 2 diabetes.[86–88] Such individuals are at high risk of later developing the disease, as discussed earlier. Insulin resistance has genetic determinants,[89] and is also characteristic of certain high-risk individuals such as infants of low birth weight and obese individuals.[64,90] Increasing obesity leads to worsening insulin resistance.[91] During the phase of normal glucose tolerance, many who later develop type 2 diabetes have subtle abnormalities of insulin secretion.[66] Nondiabetic offspring of diabetic pregnancies also show evidence of an insulin secretory defect.[92] Thus, in persons with normal glucose tolerance, defects in both insulin action and insulin secretion predict the development of type 2 diabetes.

Abnormalities of insulin action are the most consistent finding in individuals who subsequently

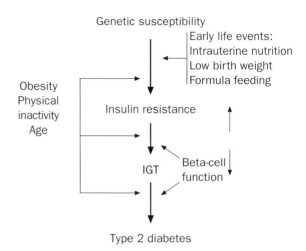

**Figure 2(i).5** Stages in the natural history and pathophysiology of type 2 diabetes and established risk factors. IGT: impaired glucose tolerance.

develop type 2 diabetes. Such abnormalities of insulin action are predominantly due to defects in insulin-mediated glucose clearance in skeletal muscle.[93] Investigations using hyperinsulinemic-euglycemic clamp techniques have shown that insulin resistance worsens before the development of definable abnormalities of glucose homeostasis, as reflected by impaired glucose tolerance or impaired fasting glycemia.[94]

Insulin resistance is also associated with other clinical phenomena such as increased blood pressure, microalbuminuria, hypertriglyceridemia, and lower high-density lipoprotein cholesterol concentrations as well as obesity.[95] States of insulin resistance are characterized by elevated fasting insulin concentrations relative to the degree of glycemia. Insulin resistance is also associated with increased atherosclerosis and with an increased incidence of coronary artery disease. Such a constellation of abnormalities, with or without the presence of impaired glucose tolerance or diabetes, is termed the insulin resistance, metabolic, or dysmetabolic syndrome.

Populations with a high risk of type 2 diabetes such as Australian Aborigines, Asian Indians, Mexican-Americans, and North American Indians have higher circulating fasting insulin concentrations even when they have normal glucose tolerance than populations in which the risk of type 2 diabetes is lower.[86,96,97] Insulin resistance shows familial aggregation and is associated with other risk factors such as obesity and physical inactivity. Consequently, insulin resistance is a phase during the development of type 2 diabetes not normally detected by clinical means. It is a mechanism by which many of the other risk factors for type 2 diabetes exert their pathophysiological effects. As insulin resistance worsens, glucose homeostasis becomes impaired and glucose intolerance develops.

Impaired glucose tolerance (IGT) is a clinical stage associated with a high risk of developing type 2 diabetes.[15,98] Persons with IGT are insulin resistant and typically have a relatively high body-mass index, central obesity, hyperinsulinemia, and various other features of the metabolic syndrome.[99] A high proportion of individuals with IGT progress to type 2 diabetes over the period of a few years.[15] Progression from IGT is usually associated with worsening beta cell function in the face of insulin resistance, which, with an inability of insulin secretion to compensate for the degree of insulin resistance, leads to relative insulin deficiency, even though the absolute concentrations of insulin secretion may be quite high.[100] IGT is also associated with increased risks of cardiovascular disease, both heart disease and stroke, and possibly cancer.[101] The risks of cardiovascular disease are intermediate between those seen in persons with normal glucose tolerance and those with diabetes.

Impaired fasting glycemia (IFG) is a clinical stage in the development of diabetes defined and introduced in the recent ADA and WHO classifications of carbohydrate intolerance.[2,3] IFG carries as high a risk of progression to type 2 diabetes as does IGT, but IFG and IGT often do not affect the same individual at the same time. In population samples, only about one-third of individuals with IFG or IGT have concomitant IFG and IGT.[13] Much less is known about the development of IFG than IGT, but IFG appears to be associated with a relatively greater deficit in insulin secretion than IGT.[102] The presence of IFG alone appears to be associated with a lower risk of the development of cardiovascular disease than IGT alone.[101]

Progression to type 2 diabetes from IFG or IGT may be the result of increasing insulin resistance, declining insulin secretion, or both. Once the circulating insulin concentrations after meals or in the fasting state are insufficient to compensate for the prevailing degree of insulin resistance, glucose homeostasis worsens.[103] Approximately 50% of patients with IFG or IGT develop diabetes within 5 years.[104–106] Although the risk is influenced to some extent by the degree of obesity, age, and ethnicity, the rates of progression are extremely high in all.

Because of the high risk of developing type 2 diabetes, a number of intervention studies have been performed among persons with IGT in order to reduce the rate of progression to type 2 diabetes. These studies, such as the Da Qing Study,[70] the Finnish Diabetes Prevention Study,[71] and the Diabetes Prevention Program,[72] have each shown that the risk of progression to type 2 diabetes in persons with IGT can be reduced by lifestyle interventions. Interventions designed to reduce weight and increase physical activity are highly effective means of reducing the incidence of type 2 diabetes in such subjects. Rates of progression were reduced by about 60% during a 3-year period in both the Finnish Study and the Diabetes Prevention Program. Other interventions designed to reduce the incidence of type 2 diabetes in persons with IGT have included the use of the alpha-glucosidase inhibitor, acarbose,[107] and metformin.[72] In the Stop NIDDM trial and in the Diabetes Prevention Program, acarbose and metformin, respectively, were associated with about 30% reduction in the incidence of type 2 diabetes. While these results were less dramatic than those achieved with lifestyle intervention, the results do point to the utility of pharmacologic agents as well as lifestyle interventions in reducing the development of type 2 diabetes in high-risk individuals.

## COMPLICATIONS

Prevention of type 2 diabetes is of importance because once type 2 diabetes develops individuals become at high risk of developing the complications that are the major cause of morbidity and mortality associated with the disease. In particular, the incidence of coronary heart disease and other cardiovascular diseases, such as stroke, retinal disease, neuropathy, and renal disease, is increased in persons with type 2 diabetes, as compared to nondiabetic persons of similar age and sex. For diabetic retinopathy and nephropathy, the development is effectively limited to persons with diabetes. These complications develop in type 2 diabetes, and in most, if not all, other forms of the disease. For other complications, such as coronary artery disease and stroke, persons with type 2 diabetes have an incidence two to four times higher than nondiabetic individuals of similar age. Overall, persons with type 2 diabetes have 1.5–2-fold higher mortality rates than nondiabetic individuals of similar age and sex.[108–110]

A detailed description of the epidemiology of the complications of type 2 diabetes is beyond the scope of this chapter. However, as most of the morbidity and mortality associated with type 2 diabetes result from complications of the disease rather than from the symptoms of the disease itself, some information on factors associated with type 2 diabetes and the development of complications is appropriate.

A striking feature of diabetes is that some individuals with the disease can survive for many years without developing complications, whereas others develop complications within a few years of developing diabetes. Detailed information concerning the development of complications in type 2 diabetes has been difficult to obtain because in most circumstances patients who are recognized to have type 2 diabetes may have had the disease for an undefined, but often considerable period of time. As type 2 diabetes is frequently asymptomatic, such complications may be present at the time of clinical diagnosis. It has been suggested that, on average, the onset of type 2 diabetes occurs some 4–7 years before diabetes is diagnosed.[111] Thus, the most reliable information concerning risk factors relating to complications of type 2 diabetes has been derived from prospective longitudinal studies of populations in which glucose tolerance is assessed periodically in all subjects.[112]

Such studies have led to the observation that the risk factors for coronary heart disease, one of the most common complications, are present even before the onset of diabetes.[113] Such complications are less clearly related to the duration of diabetes than the specific complications which develop only after the development of type 2 diabetes. For example, the incidence of diabetic retinopathy and nephropathy is strongly related to diabetes duration.[114–116]

The impact of different complications of type 2 diabetes varies considerably from population to population. For example, in Caucasian populations, cardiovascular disease especially ischemic heart disease, is responsible for much of the excess mortality from diabetes,[117] whereas in other populations, such as the American Indians, diabetic renal disease and end-stage renal disease attributable to diabetes are major contributors to the excess mortality experience of those with diabetes.[118] In part, these differences may result from differences in genetic susceptibility to certain complications in different populations and in part to differences in the age at onset of type 2 diabetes in different populations and different ethnic groups.

For many complications, and especially for retinopathy and nephropathy, the severity of hyperglycemia, probably best reflected by glycosylated hemoglobin (HbA1c) concentrations, is a strong risk factor. Furthermore, the duration of diabetes is important, with the incidence of complications increasing markedly with longer duration of the disease. Other risk factors not directly related to glycemia are also important. For example, diabetic

renal disease shows strong familial aggregation. This appears to be due to susceptibility genes for nephropathy, which are unrelated to diabetes per se, but which determine susceptibility to the complication among those who have diabetes.[119–122] Other exposures, such as blood pressure before the onset and during the course of diabetes, also play an important role in influencing the development of complications such as coronary heart disease, stroke, retinopathy, and nephropathy.[123,124] The classical risk factors for atherosclerosis among nondiabetic persons—hypertension, smoking, and dyslipidemia—play an important role in the pathogenesis of vascular disease in those with type 2 diabetes, but the effect of these classical risk factors is amplified among persons with diabetes.[125] Furthermore, microalbuminuria, which may occur even before type 2 diabetes develops, is a strong risk factor both for the development of cardiovascular complications and for diabetic renal disease.[126]

The current global epidemic of type 2 diabetes is having and will continue to have major effects on the incidence of complications of diabetes in the coming years.[127] Complications of type 2 diabetes related to the duration of diabetes, and whose development often occurs 15–20 years after the initial appearance of diabetes, will continue to increase in frequency as the global epidemic of type 2 diabetes progresses. Even if the incidence of diabetes itself were to become constant, complications attributable to type 2 diabetes, and the proportion of diabetic patients with such complications, will continue to increase for many years after the epidemic ends (Figure 2(i).6). Direct evidence of this increasing burden of diabetic complications has been demonstrated in the Pima Indian population, among whom the epidemic of type 2 diabetes began in the 1950s, whereas an epidemic of diabetic renal disease began in the 1970s and has continued into the 1990s[128] (Figure 2(i).7). The increasing burden of end-stage renal disease and the increasing proportion attributable to diabetes, predominantly type 2 diabetes, in developed countries is yet a further reflection of the impact of the increasing incidence of type 2 diabetes in earlier years in these countries (Figure 2(i).8). Consequently, the public health burden attributable to the complications of diabetes will continue to increase for many years even if current efforts to prevent type 2 diabetes are successful.

Persons with type 2 diabetes have a higher mortality rate than persons without diabetes of similar age and sex. Patients with type 2 diabetes have overall a 1.5–2-fold increase in age-adjusted mortality. The relative risk of death is greater among younger

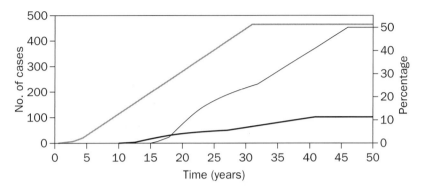

**Figure 2(i).6** Effect of an epidemic of diabetes on the future development of late complications. In this example, at a point in time, an additional 16 cases of diabetes are assumed to occur each year, and each patient dies 30 years after developing the disease. After having had diabetes for 15 years, 50% develop a late complication. The total number with diabetes (and its prevalence) in the population increases for 30 years after the onset of the epidemic, and stabilizes only when the number dying equals the number of new cases. However, the prevalence of the late complication and the number and proportion of diabetic patients affected by it continue to increase for 45 years after the onset of the epidemic. This hypothetical example reflects the likely and protracted effect that the current epidemic of type 2 diabetes will have on the increasing numbers and proportion of the diabetic population who will be affected by late complications in future years.

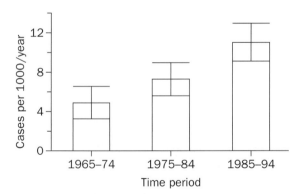

**Figure 2(i).7** Increasing incidence of renal failure in Pima Indians with diabetes over a 30-year period, expressed as cases/1000 per year ($\pm$95% confidence intervals). The increasing incidence of renal failure over the period is the result of the epidemic of type 2 diabetes among the Pima that probably began in the 1950s (unpublished data).

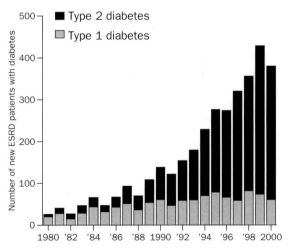

**Figure 2(i).8** Number of new patients with end-stage renal disease (ESRD) and diabetes mellitus in Australia in 1980–2000. The number of new cases with type 1 diabetes has increased modestly, whereas the numbers with type 2 diabetes, and the proportion of new ESRD patients with type 2 diabetes has increased dramatically in the past decade. (Reproduced by permission of Professor R. Atkins, adapted from the Australian and New Zealand Dialysis and Transplant Registry Report, 2001.)

subjects with type 2 diabetes. Type 2 diabetes in children and adolescents will lead to late complications and death at much earlier ages than in the past. Moreover, the earlier age of onset of type 2 diabetes in the ongoing epidemic, seen especially in the developing countries, indicates that the impact of type 2 diabetes on mortality will increase appreciably in the foreseeable future.

The global epidemic of type 2 diabetes represents perhaps the most important public health challenge of the twenty-first century in both the developed and the developing world. The rapid increases in incidence of type 2 diabetes that have occurred in many countries during the 1990s will result in enormous costs and burdens on the medical care systems for at least the next 20 years. The predicted doubling in the number of cases of type 2 diabetes worldwide between 2000 and 2025 may already be seen as an underestimate, as these predictions were based primarily upon predictable demographic variables. In fact, in a number of countries, such as the USA, Australia, and China, the more recent estimates of the prevalence of type 2 diabetes are appreciably higher than were used for those projections.[19,26,27] Type 2 diabetes has enormous social, economic, and political, as well as medical, consequences.

## REFERENCES

1. King H, Aubert RE, Herman WH, Global burden of diabetes, 1995–2025: prevalence, numerical estimates, and projections, *Diabetes Care* (1998) **21:**1414–31.
2. Gavin JR III, Alberti KGMM, Davidson MB, et al, Report of the Expert Committee on the Diagnosis and Classification of Diabetes Mellitus, *Diabetes Care* (1997) **20:**1183–97.
3. WHO Consultation Group, Definition, diagnosis and classification of diabetes mellitus and its complications. I. Diagnosis and classification of diabetes mellitus. In: *WHO/NCD/NCS/99,* 2nd edn (World Health Organization: Geneva, 1999) 1–59.
4. O'Sullivan JB, Diabetes mellitus after GDM, *Diabetes* (1991) **40** Suppl 2:131–5.
5. Newman B, Selby JV, King MC, et al, Concordance for type 2 (non-insulin-dependent) diabetes mellitus in male twins, *Diabetologia* (1987) **30:**763–8.
6. Sakul H, Pratley R, Cardon L, et al, Familiality of physical and metabolic characteristics that predict the development of non-insulin-dependent diabetes mellitus in Pima Indians, *Am J Hum Genet* (1997) **60:**651–6.
7. Elbein SC, Perspective: the search for genes for type 2 diabetes in the post-genome era, *Endocrinology* (2002) **143:**2012–18.
8. Fagot-Campagna A, Pettitt DJ, Engelgau MM, et al, Type 2 diabetes among North American children and adolescents: an epidemiologic review and a public health perspective, J Pediatr (2000) **136:**664–72.
9. Dabelea D, Hanson RL, Bennett PH, et al, Increasing prevalence of type II diabetes in American Indian children, *Diabetologia* (1998) **41:**904–10.
10. Dean HJ, Mundy RL, Moffatt M, Non-insulin-dependent diabetes mellitus in Indian children in Manitoba, *Can Med Assoc J* (1992) **147:**52–7.
11. Kitagawa T, Owada M, Urakami T, et al, Increased incidence of non-insulin dependent diabetes mellitus among Japanese schoolchildren correlates with an increased intake of animal protein and fat, *Clin Pediatr (Phila)* (1998) **37:**111–15.
12. WHO Study Group, *Diabetes Mellitus.* Technical Reports Series No. 727. (World Health Organization: Geneva, 1985).
13. Bennett PH, Impact of the new WHO classification and diagnostic criteria, *Diabetes Obes Metab* (1999) **1** Suppl 2:S1–S6.
14. Edelstein SL, Knowler WC, Bain RP, et al, Predictors of progression from impaired glucose tolerance to NIDDM: an analysis of six prospective studies, *Diabetes* (1997) **46:**701–10.
15. Saad MF, Knowler WC, Pettitt DJ, et al, The natural history of impaired glucose tolerance in the Pima Indians, *N Engl J Med* (1988) **319:**1500–6.
16. King H, Rewers M, *Diabetes in Adults is Now a Third World Problem, Bull World Health Organ* (1991) **69**.
17. Taylor R, Zimmet P, Migrant studies in diabetes epidemiology. In: Mann JI, Pyörälä K, Teuscher A, eds, *Diabetes in Epidemiological Perspective* (Churchill Livingstone: Edinburgh, 1983) 58–77.
18. Diabetes in America. In: Harris MI, Cowie CC, Stern MP, et al, eds. 2nd edn (National Institutes of Health) 1–782.
19. Dunstan DW, Zimmet PZ, Welborn TA, et al, The rising prevalence of diabetes and impaired glucose tolerance: the Australian Diabetes, Obesity and Lifestyle Study, *Diabetes Care* (2002) **25:**829–34.
20. Kenny SJ, Aubert RE, Geiss LS, Prevalence and incidence of non-insulin-dependent diabetes. In: Harris MI, Cowie CC, Stern MP, et al, eds, *Diabetes in America,* 2nd edn (National Institutes of Health: 1995) 47–65.
21. Harris MI, Flegal KM, Cowie CC, et al, Prevalence of diabetes, impaired fasting glucose, and impaired glucose tolerance in U.S. adults. The Third National Health and Nutrition Examination Survey, 1988–1994, *Diabetes Care* (1998) **21:**518–24.
22. Flegal KM, Ezzati TM, Harris MI, et al, Prevalence of diabetes in Mexican-Americans, Cubans, and Puerto Ricans from the Hispanic Health and Nutrition Examination Survey, 1982–1984, *Diabetes Care* (1991) **14:**628–38.
23. Gohdes D, Bennett PH, Diabetes in American Indians and Alaska Natives, *Diabetes Care* (1993) **16:**214–15.
24. Harris MI, Hadden WC, Knowler WC, et al, Prevalence of diabetes and impaired glucose tolerance and plasma glucose levels in U.S. population aged 20–74 yr, *Diabetes* (1987) **36:**523–34.
25. Mokdad AH, Ford ES, Bowman BA, et al, Diabetes trends in the U.S.: 1990–1998, *Diabetes Care* (2000) **23:**1278–83.
26. Mokdad AH, Bowman BA, Ford ES, et al, The continuing epidemics of obesity and diabetes in the United States, *JAMA* (2001) **286:**1195–200.
27. Pan XR, Yang WY, Li GW, et al, Prevalence of diabetes and its risk factors in China, 1994. National Diabetes Prevention and Control Cooperative Group, *Diabetes Care* (1997) **20:**1664–9.
28. Tan CE, Emmanuel SC, Tan BY, et al, Prevalence of diabetes and ethnic differences in cardiovascular risk factors. The 1992 Singapore National Health Survey, *Diabetes Care* (1999) **22:**241–7.
29. Dowse GK, Gareeboo H, Zimmet PZ, et al, High prevalence of NIDDM and impaired glucose tolerance in Indian, Creole, and Chinese Mauritians. Mauritius Noncommunicable Disease Study Group, *Diabetes* (1990) **39:**390–6.
30. Ramachandran A, Snehalatha C, Latha E, et al, Rising prevalence of NIDDM in an urban population in India, *Diabetologia* (1997) **40:**232–7.
31. Ramachandran A, Snehalatha C, Viswanathan V, et al, Risk of noninsulin dependent diabetes mellitus conferred by obesity

and central adiposity in different ethnic groups: a comparative analysis between Asian Indians, Mexican-Americans and Whites, *Diabetes Res Clin Pract* (1997) **36**:121–5.

32. Ramachandran A, Snehalatha C, Kapur A, et al, High prevalence of diabetes and impaired glucose tolerance in India: National Urban Diabetes Survey, *Diabetologia* (2001) **44**:1094–101.

33. Kaufman FR, Type 2 diabetes mellitus in children and youth: a new epidemic, *J Pediatr Endocrinol Metab* (2002) **15** Suppl 2:737–44.

34. Young TK, Martens PJ, Taback SP, et al, Type 2 diabetes mellitus in children: prenatal and early infancy risk factors among native Canadians. *Arch Pediatr Adolesc Med* (2002) **156**:651–5.

35. Arslanian S, Type 2 diabetes in children: clinical aspects and risk factors, *Horm Res* (2002) **57** Suppl 1:19–28.

36. Poulsen P, Kyvik KO, Vaag A, Beck-Nielsen H, Heritability of type II (non-insulin-dependent) diabetes mellitus and abnormal glucose tolerance – a population-based twin study, *Diabetologia* (1999) **42**:139–45.

37. Serjeantson SW, Owerbach D, Zimmet P, et al, Genetics of diabetes in Nauru: effect of foreign admixture. HLA antigens and the insulin-gene-linked polymorphism, *Diabetologia* (1984) **25**:13–17.

38. Knowler WC, Williams RC, Pettitt DJ, et al, Gm 3;5,13,14 and type 2 diabetes mellitus: an association in American Indians with genetic admixture, *Am J Hum Genet* (1988) **43**:520–6.

39. Altshuler D, Hirschhorn JN, Klannemark M, et al, The common PPARgamma Pro12Ala polymorphism is associated with decreased risk of type 2 diabetes, *Nat Genet* (2000) **26**:76–80.

40. Baier LJ, Sacchettini JC, Knowler WC, et al, An amino acid substitution in the human intestinal fatty acid binding protein is associated with increased fatty acid binding, increased fat oxidation, and insulin resistance, *J Clin Invest* (1995) **95**:1281–7.

41. Xia J, Scherer SW, Cohen PT, et al, A common variant in PPP1R3 associated with insulin resistance and type 2 diabetes, *Diabetes* (1998) **47**:1519–24.

42. Kondo H, Shimomura I, Matsukawa Y, et al, Association of adiponectin mutation with type 2 diabetes: a candidate gene for the insulin resistance syndrome, *Diabetes* (2002) **51**:2325–8.

43. Hanson RL, An autosomal genomic scan for loci linked to type II diabetes mellitus and body-mass index in Pima Indians, *Am J Hum Genet* (1998) **63**:1130–8.

44. Cox NJ, Frigge M, Nicolae DL, et al, Loci on chromosomes 2 (NIDDM1) and 15 interact to increase susceptibility to diabetes in Mexican-Americans, *Nat Genet* (1999) **21**:213–15.

45. Hanis CL, A genome-wide search for human non-insulin-dependent (type 2) diabetes genes reveals a major susceptibility locus on chromosome, *Nat Genet* (1996) **13**:161–6.

46. Wiltshire S, Hattersley AT, Hitman GA, et al, A genome-wide scan for loci predisposing to type 2 diabetes in a U.K. population (the Diabetes UK Warren 2 Repository): analysis of 573 pedigrees provides independent replication of a susceptibility locus on chromosome 1q, *Am J Hum Genet* (2001) **69**:553–69.

47. Horikawa Y, Oda N, Cox NJ, et al, Genetic variation in the gene encoding calpain-10 is associated with type 2 diabetes mellitus, *Nat Genet* (2000) **26**:163–75.

48. Baier LJ, Permana PA, Yang X, et al, A calpain-10 gene polymorphism is associated with reduced muscle mRNA levels and insulin resistance, *J Clin Invest* (2000) **106**:R69–R73.

49. Savage DB, Agostini M, Barroso I, et al, Digenic inheritance of severe insulin resistance in a human pedigree, *Nat Genet* (2002) **31**:379–84.

50. Mather HM, Chaturvedi N, Fuller JH, Mortality and morbidity from diabetes in South Asians and Europeans: 11-year follow-up of the Southall Diabetes Survey, London, UK, *Diabet Med* (1998) **15**:53–9.

51. Zimmet P, Taylor R, Ram P, et al, Prevalence of diabetes and impaired glucose tolerance in the biracial (Melanesian and Indian) population of Fiji: a rural–urban comparison, *Am J Epidemiol* (1983) **118**:673–88.

52. Omar MA, Seedat MA, Dyer RB, et al, The prevalence of diabetes mellitus in a large group of South African Indians, *S Afr Med J* (1985) **67**:924–6.

53. Miller GJ, Maude GH, Beckles GL, Incidence of hypertension and non-insulin-dependent diabetes mellitus and associated risk factors in a rapidly developing Caribbean community: the St James survey, Trinidad, *J Epidemiol Community Health* (1996) **50**:497–504.

54. Taylor R, Bennett P, Uili R, et al, Diabetes in Wallis Polynesians: a comparison of residents of Wallis Island and first generation migrants to Noumea, New Caledonia, *Diabetes Res Clin Pract* (1985) **1**:169–78.

55. Hales CN, Barker DJ, Type 2 (non-insulin-dependent) diabetes mellitus: the thrifty phenotype hypothesis, *Diabetologia* (1992) **35**:595–601.

56. McCance DR, Pettitt DJ, Hanson RL, et al, Birth weight and non-insulin dependent diabetes: thrifty genotype, thrifty phenotype, or surviving small baby genotype?, *BMJ* (1994) **308**:942–5.

57. Lithell HO, McKeigue PM, Berglund L, et al, Relation of size at birth to non-insulin dependent diabetes and insulin concentrations in men aged 50–60 years, *BMJ* (1996) **312**:406–10.

58. Lindsay RS, Bennett PH, Type 2 diabetes, the thrifty phenotype—an overview, *Br Med Bull* (2001) **60**:21–32.

59. Hales CN, Desai M, Ozanne SE, The thrifty phenotype hypothesis: how does it look after 5 years?, *Diabet Med* (1997) **14**:189–95.

60. Dabelea D, Hanson RL, Lindsay RS, et al, Intrauterine exposure to diabetes conveys risks for type 2 diabetes and obesity: a study of discordant sibships, *Diabetes* (2000) **49**:2208–11.

61. Pettitt DJ, Forman MR, Hanson RL, et al, Breastfeeding and incidence of non-insulin-dependent diabetes mellitus in Pima Indians, *Lancet* (1997) **350**:166–8.

62. Knowler WC, Pettitt DJ, Savage PJ, et al, Diabetes incidence in Pima Indians: contributions of obesity and parental diabetes, *Am J Epidemiol* (1981) **113**:144–56.

63. Boyko EJ, Fujimoto WY, Leonetti DL, et al, Visceral adiposity and risk of type 2 diabetes: a prospective study among Japanese-Americans, *Diabetes Care* (2000) **23**:465–71.

64. DeFronzo RA, Ferrannini E, Insulin resistance. A multifaceted syndrome responsible for NIDDM, obesity, hypertension, dyslipidemia, and atherosclerotic cardiovascular disease, *Diabetes Care* (1991) **14**:173–94.

65. Lillioja S, Bogardus C, Mott DM, et al, Relationship between insulin-mediated glucose disposal and lipid metabolism in man, *J Clin Invest* (1985) **75**:1106–15.

66. Weyer C, Bogardus C, Mott DM, et al, The natural history of insulin secretory dysfunction and insulin resistance in the pathogenesis of type 2 diabetes mellitus, *J Clin Invest* (1999) **104**:787–94.

67. Manson JE, Nathan DM, Krolewski AS, et al, A prospective study of exercise and incidence of diabetes among US male physicians, *JAMA* (1992) **268**:63–7.

68. Manson JE, Rimm EB, Stampfer MJ, et al, Physical activity and incidence of non-insulin-dependent diabetes mellitus in women, *Lancet* (1991) **338**:774–8.

69. Helmrich SP, Ragland DR, Leung RW, et al, Physical activity and reduced occurrence of non-insulin-dependent diabetes mellitus, *N Engl J Med* (1991) **325**:147–52.

70. Pan XR, Li GW, Hu YH, et al, Effects of diet and exercise in preventing NIDDM in people with impaired glucose tolerance. The Da Qing IGT and Diabetes Study, *Diabetes Care* (1997) **20**:537–44.

71. Tuomilehto J, Lindstrom J, Eriksson JG, et al, Prevention of type 2 diabetes mellitus by changes in lifestyle among subjects with impaired glucose tolerance, *N Engl J Med* (2001) **344:**1343–50.

72. Knowler WC, Barrett-Connor E, Fowler SE, et al, Reduction in the incidence of type 2 diabetes with lifestyle intervention or metformin, *N Engl J Med* (2002) **346:**393–403.

73. Feskens EJ, Virtanen SM, Rasanen L, et al, Dietary factors determining diabetes and impaired glucose tolerance. A 20-year follow-up of the Finnish and Dutch cohorts of the Seven Countries Study, *Diabetes Care* (1995) **18:**1104–12.

74. Salmeron J, Ascherio A, Rimm EB, et al, Dietary fiber, glycemic load, and risk of NIDDM in men, *Diabetes Care* (1997) **20:**545–50.

75. Salmeron J, Hu FB, Manson JE, et al, Dietary fat intake and risk of type 2 diabetes in women, *Am J Clin Nutr* (2001) **73:**1019–26.

76. Meyer KA, Kushi LH, Jacobs DR, Jr, et al, Dietary fat and incidence of type 2 diabetes in older Iowa women, *Diabetes Care* (2001) **24:**1528–35.

77. Hu FB, Manson JE, Stampfer MJ, et al, Diet, lifestyle, and the risk of type 2 diabetes mellitus in women, *N Engl J Med* (2001) **345:**790–7.

78. West KM, *Epidemiology of Diabetes and Its Vascular Complications* (Elsevier: New York, 1978).

79. Kriketos AD, Pan DA, Lillioja S, et al, Interrelationships between muscle morphology, insulin action, and adiposity, *Am J Physiol* (1996) **270:**R1332–9.

80. Reid JM, Fullmer SD, Pettigrew KD, et al, Nutrient intake of Pima Indian women: relationships to diabetes mellitus and gallbladder disease, *Am J Clin Nutr* (1971) **24:**1281–9.

81. Williams DE, Knowler WC, Smith CJ, et al, The effect of Indian or Anglo dietary preference on the incidence of diabetes in Pima Indians, *Diabetes Care* (2001) **24:**811–16.

82. Stampfer MJ, Colditz GA, Willett WC, et al, A prospective study of moderate alcohol drinking and risk of diabetes in women, *Am J Epidemiol* (1988) **128:**549–58.

83. Ajani UA, Hennekens CH, Spelsberg A, et al, Alcohol consumption and risk of type 2 diabetes mellitus among US male physicians, *Arch Intern Med* (2000) **160:**1025–30.

84. Pradhan AD, Manson JE, Rifai N, et al, C-reactive protein, interleukin 6, and risk of developing type 2 diabetes mellitus, *JAMA* (2001) **286:**327–34.

85. Lindsay RS, Krakoff J, Hanson RL, et al, Gamma globulin levels predict type 2 diabetes in the Pima Indian population, *Diabetes* (2001) **50:**1598–603.

86. Haffner SM, Stern MP, Hazuda HP, et al, Hyperinsulinemia in a population at high risk for non-insulin-dependent diabetes, *N Engl J Med* (1986) **315:**220–4.

87. Lillioja S, Mott DM, Zawadzki JK, et al, In vivo insulin action is familial characteristic in nondiabetic Pima Indians, *Diabetes* (1987) **36:**1329–35.

88. Forsblom CM, Eriksson JG, Ekstrand AV, et al, Insulin resistance and abnormal albumin excretion in non-diabetic first-degree relatives of patients with NIDDM, *Diabetologia* (1995) **38:**363–9.

89. Sakul H, Pratley R, Cardon L, et al, Familiality of physical and metabolic characteristics that predict the development of non-insulin-dependent diabetes mellitus in Pima Indians, *Am J Hum Genet* (1997) **60:**651–6.

90. Dabelea D, Pettitt DJ, Hanson RL, et al, Birth weight, type 2 diabetes, and insulin resistance in Pima Indian children and young adults, *Diabetes Care* (1999) **22:**944–50.

91. Lillioja S, Mott DM, Howard BV, et al, Impaired glucose tolerance as a disorder of insulin action: longitudinal and cross-sectional studies in Pima Indians, *N Engl J Med* (1988) **318:**1217–25.

92. Gautier JF, Wilson C, Weyer C, et al, Low acute insulin secretory responses in adult offspring of people with early onset type 2 diabetes, *Diabetes* (2001) **50:**1828–33.

93. Lillioja S, Mott DM, Zawadzki JK, et al, Glucose storage is a major determinant of in vivo 'insulin resistance' in subjects with normal glucose tolerance, *J Clin Endocrinol Metab* (1986) **62:**922–7.

94. Weyer C, Bogardus C, Mott DM, et al, The natural history of insulin secretory dysfunction and insulin resistance in the pathogenesis of type 2 diabetes mellitus, *J Clin Invest* (1999) **104:**787–94.

95. Groop LC, Insulin resistance: the fundamental trigger of type 2 diabetes, *Diabetes Obes Metab* (1999) **1** Suppl 1:S1–S7.

96. Mohan V, Sharp PS, Cloke HR, et al, Serum immunoreactive insulin responses to a glucose load in Asian Indian and European type 2 (non-insulin-dependent) diabetic patients and control subjects. *Diabetologia* (1986) **29:**235–7.

97. Aronoff SL, Bennett PH, Gorden P, et al, Unexplained hyperinsulinemia in normal and 'prediabetic' Pima Indians compared with normal Caucasians, *Diabetes* (1977) **26:**827–40.

98. Bennett PH, Knowler WC, Pettitt DJ, et al, Longitudinal studies of the development of diabetes in the Pima Indians. In: Eschwege E, ed., *Advances in Diabetes Epidemiology* (Elsevier Biomedical Press: Amsterdam, 1982) 65–74.

99. Hanley AJ, Karter AJ, Festa A, et al, Factor analysis of metabolic syndrome using directly measured insulin sensitivity: the Insulin Resistance Atherosclerosis Study, *Diabetes* (2002) **51:**2642–7.

100. Saad MF, Knowler WC, Pettitt DJ, et al, Sequential changes in serum insulin concentration during development of non-insulin-dependent diabetes, *Lancet* (1989) **i:**1356–9.

101. DECODE Study Group, Glucose tolerance and mortality: comparison of WHO and American Diabetes Association diagnostic criteria. The DECODE Study Group. European Diabetes Epidemiology Group. Diabetes Epidemiology: Collaborative Analysis of Diagnostic Criteria in Europe, *Lancet* (1999) **354:**617–21.

102. Weyer C, Bogardus C, Pratley RE, Metabolic characteristics of individuals with impaired fasting glucose and/or impaired glucose tolerance, *Diabetes* (1999) **48:**2197–203.

103. Saad MF, Knowler WC, Pettitt DJ, et al, A two-step model for development of non-insulin-dependent diabetes, *Am J Med* (1991) **90:**229–35.

104. Gabir MM, Hanson RL, Dabelea D, et al, The 1997 American Diabetes Association and 1999 World Health Organization criteria for hyperglycemia in the diagnosis and prediction of diabetes, *Diabetes Care* (2000) **23:**1108–12.

105. Shaw JE, Hodge AM, De Courten MP, et al, Isolated post-challenge hyperglycaemia confirmed as a risk factor for mortality, *Diabetologia* (1999) **42:**1050–4.

106. de Vegt F, Dekker JM, Jager A, et al, Relation of impaired fasting and postload glucose with incident type 2 diabetes in a Dutch population: the Hoorn Study, *JAMA* (2001) **285:**2109–13.

107. Chiasson JL, Josse RG, Gomis R, et al, Acarbose for prevention of type 2 diabetes mellitus: the STOP-NIDDM Randomised Trial, *Lancet* (2002) **359:**2072–7.

108. Kleinman JC, Donahue RP, Harris MI, et al, Mortality among diabetics in a national sample, *Am J Epidemiol* (1988) **128:**389–401.

109. Gu K, Cowie CC, Harris MI, Mortality in adults with and without diabetes in a national cohort of the U.S. population, 1971–1993, *Diabetes Care* (1998) **21:**1138–45.

110. Roper NA, Bilous RW, Kelly WF, et al, Excess mortality in a population with diabetes and the impact of material deprivation: longitudinal, population-based study, *BMJ* (2001) **322:**1389–93.

111. Harris MI, Klein R, Welborn TA, et al, Onset of NIDDM occurs at least 4–7 yr before clinical diagnosis, *Diabetes Care* (1992) **15**:815–19.

112. Knowler WC, Pettitt DJ, Saad MF, et al, Diabetes mellitus in the Pima Indians: incidence, risk factors and pathogenesis, *Diabetes Metab Rev* (1990) **6**:1–27.

113. Haffner SM, Stern MP, Hazuda HP, et al, Cardiovascular risk factors in confirmed prediabetic individuals. Does the clock for coronary heart disease start ticking before the onset of clinical diabetes?, *JAMA* (1990) **263**:2893–8.

114. Nelson RG, Wolfe JA, Horton MB, et al, Proliferative retinopathy in NIDDM. Incidence and risk factors in Pima Indians, *Diabetes* (1989) **38**:435–40.

115. Kunzelman CL, Knowler WC, Pettitt DJ, et al, Incidence of proteinuria in type 2 diabetes mellitus in the Pima Indians, *Kidney Int* (1989) **35**:681–7.

116. Nelson RG, Bennett PH, The development and course of renal disease among Pima Indians with non-insulin-dependent diabetes mellitus, *Diab Nutr Metab* (1995) **8**:149–58.

117. Fuller JH, Stevens LK, Wang SL, Risk factors for cardiovascular mortality and morbidity: the WHO Multinational Study of Vascular Disease in Diabetes, *Diabetologia* (2001) **44** (Suppl 2): S54–S64.

118. Sievers ML, Nelson RG, Bennett PH, Sequential trends in overall and cause-specific mortality in diabetic and nondiabetic Pima Indians, *Diabetes Care* (1996) **19**:107–11.

119. Pettitt DJ, Saad MF, Bennett PH, et al, Familial predisposition to renal disease in two generations of Pima Indians with type 2 (non-insulin-dependent) diabetes mellitus, *Diabetologia* (1990) **33**:438–43.

120. Imperatore G, Hanson RL, Pettitt DJ, et al, Sib-pair linkage analysis for susceptibility genes for microvascular complications among Pima Indians with type 2 diabetes. Pima Diabetes Genes Group, *Diabetes* (1998) **47**:821–30.

121. Imperatore G, Knowler WC, Nelson RG, et al, Genetics of diabetic nephropathy in the Pima Indians, *Curr Diabetes Rep* (2001) **1**:275–81.

122. Imperatore G, Knowler WC, Pettitt DJ, et al, Segregation analysis of diabetic nephropathy in Pima Indians, *Diabetes* (2000) **49**:1049–56.

123. Nelson RG, Pettitt DJ, Baird HR, et al, Pre-diabetic blood pressure predicts urinary albumin excretion after the onset of type 2 (non-insulin-dependent) diabetes mellitus in Pima Indians, *Diabetologia* (1993) **36**:998–1001.

124. Sievers ML, Bennett PH, Roumain J, et al, Effect of hypertension on mortality in Pima Indians, *Circulation* (1999) **100**:33–40.

125. Haffner SM, Lehto S, Ronnemaa T, et al, Mortality from coronary heart disease in subjects with type 2 diabetes and in nondiabetic subjects with and without prior myocardial infarction, *N Engl J Med* (1998) **339**:229–34.

126. Mogensen CE, Microalbuminuria predicts clinical proteinuria and early mortality in maturity-onset diabetes, *N Engl J Med* (1984) **310**:356–60.

127. Howard BV, Rodriguez BL, Bennett PH, et al, Prevention Conference VI: Diabetes and Cardiovascular Disease: Writing Group I: Epidemiology, *Circulation* (2002) **105**:e132–7.

128. Nelson RG, Diabetic renal disease in transitional and disadvantaged populations, *Nephrology* (2001) **6**:9–17.

# 2(ii)

# Type 1 diabetes: immunology, genetics, and epidemiology

Spiros Fourlanos and Thomas WH Kay

## INTRODUCTION

Type 1 diabetes, or insulin-dependent diabetes mellitus, is an organ-specific chronic autoimmune disease.[1] It is due to highly specific autoimmune-mediated destruction of β-cells in the pancreatic islets of Langerhans with consequent insulin deficiency and hyperglycaemia requiring life-long insulin therapy.[2,3] Type 1 diabetes accounts for about 10% of all primary diabetes and is one of the most common chronic diseases of childhood, with prevalence rates of 0.2–0.5% in many Caucasian populations.[4] The long-term microvascular and macrovascular complications in type 1 diabetes are responsible for the increased morbidity and mortality of individuals with type 1 diabetes compared with non-diabetic adults.

It was not until 1866 that Harley, a British physician, reported that there were 'at least two forms of the disease (diabetes) requiring diametrically opposing forms of treatment'.[5] Most children and some adults who developed diabetes died within months, whereas overweight adult patients survived for many years. When insulin became available for therapeutic use, it became apparent that there were two broad groups of patients, the insulin-sensitive and the insulin-resistant. Subsequently, bioassays for circulating insulin concentration confirmed insulin deficiency in thin, insulin-sensitive patients.[6] Further evidence for insulin deficiency was found in autopsy studies that showed almost undetectable insulin in the pancreata of people with diabetes who died before the age of 20 years.[7]

The clinical presentation of type 1 diabetes is based on clinical, metabolic and immunological criteria. It classically occurs in children or young adults with normal or low body weight and is characterized by rapid onset of symptoms secondary to hyperglycaemia, including polydipsia, polyuria, blurred vision and weight loss. In most populations, there is a slight peak of type 1 diabetes at puberty, and recent trends suggest that type 1 diabetes may occur at a younger age. It is also apparent that type 1 diabetes occurs in all age groups, and some estimate that approximately 40% of type 1 diabetes occurs after age 20.[8] The clinical features of type 1 diabetes compared with type 2 diabetes are outlined in Table 2(ii).1. The key distinctions are that insulin deficiency results in lower body weight and the risk of diabetic ketoacidosis. Insulin deficiency may be confirmed by low plasma insulin levels and reduced plasma C-peptide that is produced in an equimolar ratio with insulin by the β-cell. In contrast, in type 2 diabetes, insulin resistance is present with variable and relatively milder insulin deficiency. Insulin and C-peptide levels are higher than in type 1 diabetes, although β-cell dysfunction also plays an important role in type 2 diabetes. The presence of overt hyperglycaemia in type 1 diabetes is indicative of extensive β-cell destruction. At the time of diagnosis, up to 15% residual β-cell function may remain, but ongoing autoimmune destruction eventually results in complete loss of β-cell function over a period of up to 10–15 years. Conventional treatment in type 1 diabetes consists of exogenous insulin replacement in the form of subcutaneous injections.

## AUTOIMMUNITY IN TYPE 1 DIABETES

The presence of circulating islet autoantibodies can be used to identify β-cell autoimmunity and therefore confirm the diagnosis of type 1 diabetes. Diabetes was originally hypothesized to be an autoimmune disease for a number of reasons, including familial clustering with other organ-specific

**Table 2(ii).1   Clinical features of type 1 compared with type 2 diabetes.**

|  | Type 1 diabetes | Type 2 diabetes |
|---|---|---|
| Age at diagnosis | Usually <30 years | Usually >30 years |
| Weight | Normal/thin | Overweight |
| Ketoacidosis | Susceptible | Not susceptible |
| Plasma insulin/C-peptide | Decreased | Normal/increased |
| Islet autoantibodies | Present | Absent |

diseases such as thyroid autoimmunity. Autopsy studies showed that lymphocytic infiltration was evident in the pancreatic islets of patients with type 1 diabetes.[9] The concept of type 1 diabetes as an autoimmune disease emerged in the mid-1970s with the identification of islet cell antibodies (ICA) in 1974 by Botazzo et al[10] and Nerup et al,[11] establishing HLA associations for genetic susceptibility to the disease.

Not all β-cell loss is due to demonstrable autoimmunity, a fact which has led to the subclassification of type 1 diabetes into *type 1a*, related to autoimmune disease, and *type 1b*, which constitutes non-immune-mediated disease. A minority of people, usually of African or Asian descent, are believed to have type 1b diabetes. This entity displays strong inheritance, but no HLA association, unlike type 1a diabetes, and is clinically characterized by episodic ketoacidosis, variable insulin deficiency and a lack of islet autoantibodies.

## Histology

The endocrine pancreas consists of about 1 million microscopic clusters of cells, the islets of Langerhans, weighing approximately 1–1.5 g.[12] β-Cells produce insulin and constitute about 70% of islet cells and the other predominant cell types are α (glucagon-secreting), δ (somatostatin-secreting) and PP (pancreatic polypeptide-secreting).[13] Autopsy studies identified a lymphocyte-rich inflammatory infiltrate in the islets of patients with early diabetes, and this was termed 'insulitis'.[9,14] Insulitis has also been observed in animal models of autoimmune diabetes. The infiltrate consists mainly of CD8+ T cells and variable numbers of CD4+ T cells and macrophages.[15,16] The insulitis is associated with increased expression of class I major histocompatability complex (MHC) molecules and other inflammatory markers of possible pathological significance, including adhesion molecules, interferon-alpha and Fas (CD95).[17] Insulitis detected in type 1 diabetes is direct evidence for the immunopathogenesis of the disease. Interestingly, the pancreata from normal individuals donated to their identical twins with diabetes have also been histologically analysed when type 1 diabetes recurred in the recipients.[18] These data also support the immunological basis of type 1 diabetes. The limited availability of pancreatic tissue specimens has made further research in this area difficult.

## T cells

Although autoantibodies are the best available markers of the presence of β-cell autoimmunity, it is believed that they play no role in the pathogenesis of the disease. There is *in vitro* evidence for T-cell reactivity to islet antigens, and it is believed that T cells are the major determinant of β-cell destruction. Very direct evidence for this exists in rodent models of type 1 diabetes.[19] Adoptive transfer of T cells causes diabetes, and diabetes can be prevented with anti-T-cell antibodies directed against either the CD4+ or CD8+ T-cell subsets. In contrast, diabetes has not been transferred with antibodies, and there is no evidence that ICA have transplacental effects on the fetus. There has been a recent report of a patient with X-linked agammaglobulinaemia who presented with diabetes,[20] consistent with progression to diabetes not requiring antibody production. B cells may, however, have a role as antigen-presenting cells. Diabetes can also be transferred with bone-marrow transplantation.[21] T-cell responses to islet antigens have been difficult to standardize and are not yet used in routine clinical practice.[22]

## Islet autoantibodies

Since the discovery of ICA in the sera of people with

type 1 diabetes,[10] they have become established as markers of a β-cell autoimmune response, but there is good evidence that autoantibodies are not directly involved in β-cell destruction. ICA are traditionally measured by indirect immunofluorescence with frozen sections of human blood group O pancreas. The sensitivity of ICA is 85% at diagnosis of type 1 diabetes, and the specificity is over 90%.[23,24] Sensitivity declines with increasing duration of disease so that many patients with type 1 diabetes for several years are ICA negative.[25,26] The ICA assay is well known for technical problems with interlaboratory variation and poor reproducibility. In part to develop better assays but also to clarify the disease process, the antigenic targets of ICA were studied and molecularly defined. The ICA reaction is attributed to autoantibodies against the β-cell proteins, glutamic acid decarboxylase (GAD) and IA-2. Insulin autoantibodies (IAA) are also important markers of disease but are not thought to contribute to the ICA reaction. Used in combination, multiple autoantibodies improve the sensitivity and specificity of autoantibody testing in type 1 diabetes.[27] Almost all (>95%) patients with type 1 diabetes have one of these autoantibodies, and hardly any (<1%) normal subjects have all three (Figure 2(ii).1).

GADAb is the most sensitive autoantibody in new-onset type 1 diabetes.[26] Unlike ICA, it can be detected many years after diagnosis. GAD was identified as an autoantigen by studies that showed that antibodies from ICA-positive patients immunoprecipitated a 64-kDa protein of unknown identity from islet cells. Subsequently, patients with stiff-man syndrome, a rare neurological disorder, were found to have autoantibodies to a 64-kDa protein in brain that was identified as GAD. These patients also had ICA, and 30% of them developed diabetes. These observations led to the identification of GAD as a molecular target of ICA.[28] GAD is a rate-limiting enzyme in the biosynthesis of γ-amino butyric acid (GABA), which is abundant in both β-cells and the central nervous system. GAD occurs in two isoforms, GAD65 and GAD67, GAD65 being more abundant in human islets. The function of GABA in islets is not fully understood, but it appears to inhibit glucagon secretion by α-cells and may have a role in cellular mitochondrial function.[29] The expression of GAD is associated with insulin release,[30] and glucose may stimulate its expression.[31] IAA are present in type 1 diabetes prior to insulin treatment. The sensitivity of IAA in people with newly diagnosed diabetes is approximately 40%[32] and is age dependent, with IAA being more prevalent in young children diagnosed with type 1 diabetes than in adults. Insulin is the only major autoantigen that is β-cell specific. The sensitivity of IA-2Ab in type 1 diabetes is approximately 50%.[33] IA-2 and its reactivity with autoantibodies was discovered by screening β-cell cDNA expression libraries with patient serum.[34] IA-2 accounts for a 38-kDa protein previously found in immunoprecipitation studies. IA-2 is a transmembrane molecule that belongs to the family of protein tyrosine phosphatases and is expressed in pancreatic islets and the central nervous system.[1,35] IA-2Ab are present more frequently in younger subjects.

The identification of the molecular targets of

**Islet cell autoantibodies**

**GAD**
GABA biosynthesis
2 forms
not β-cell specific
sensitivity 72%
specificity 99.3%

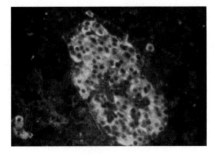

**IA-2**
tyrosine phosphatase
2 forms
not β-cell specific
sensitivity 62% (57%)
specificity 96% (99.5%)

**(pro-) insulin**
β-cell specific
sensitivity 40%
specificity 90%

**Figure 2(ii).1** Islet cell autoantibodies in type 1 diabetes.

autoantibodies enabled the establishment of more satisfactory assays for diabetes-related autoantibodies that have gradually replaced ICA and allowed the routine testing of large numbers of subjects. In general, molecular characterization has not led to rapid or dramatic insights into how autoimmunity develops in diabetes or other autoimmune diseases. All three of these autoantigens are intracellular; therefore, antibodies against them do not bind to the surface of living β-cells. Thus, they cannot directly mediate β-cell destruction. The identification of autoantigenic targets has paved the way for the development of antigen-specific therapies for type 1 diabetes.

## CLINICAL APPLICATION OF ISLET AUTOANTIBODIES

### Preclinical diabetes

Prior to the discovery of ICA, it had been believed that type 1 diabetes is an acute illness with a sudden onset, but it is now recognized that acute metabolic decompensation is the final stage in a relatively slow disease process that erodes the reserve of insulin secretory capacity in the pancreas. This was revealed by a landmark sequential study of ICA over a 15-year period in monozygotic twins and triplets. It was found that the natural history of type 1 diabetes is characterized by a long preclinical period when immunological markers of diabetes are present but blood glucose is normal.[36] ICA were detected in two triplets 5 and 8 years, respectively, before the onset of clinical diabetes. The third triplet had no detectable antibodies and did not develop diabetes in 17 years of observation after the development of diabetes in the index triplet. There also appeared to be a correlation between the development of ICA and insulin secretion. Another small prospective study of relatives with type 1 diabetes showed that ICA were present up to 30 months before any biochemical abnormality suggestive of β-cell failure.[37]

### Autoantibodies in disease prediction

Because islet autoantibodies are often found many years before the onset of clinical diabetes, they have been used to investigate the natural history of type 1 diabetes and to develop ways of predicting its onset. Studies have been carried out in first-degree relatives of patients who have a 10-fold increased risk of diabetes and in the general population. In the Melbourne Pre-Diabetes Study, 2.6% of first-degree

relatives had elevated ICA levels, 1.3% had elevated IAA levels and 0.3% had both.[38] Over 3000 relatives were tested in an 8-year period, and 33 relatives developed diabetes. High ICA levels were detected in 58% of people before they developed clinical diabetes.

The factors that predict progression to diabetes in ICA-positive first-degree relatives are age, insulin response, ICA titre, the presence of IAA and the number of autoantibodies. The first-phase insulin response (FPIR) to glucose in an intravenous glucose tolerance test (IVGTT) is the sum of the plasma insulin concentration 1 and 3 min after glucose injection.[39] Loss of the first-phase insulin response in people with high levels of islet autoantibodies is highly predictive of the development of type 1 diabetes. The 5-year risk of diabetes in ICA-positive relatives of people with type 1 diabetes is 85% if the FPIR is <50 mU/l, 48% if the FPIR is 50–100 mU/l and 17% if the FPIR is >100 mU/l;[40] hence, the FPIR is very strongly associated with progression to diabetes. An impaired FPIR is the first metabolic defect detectable, with β-cell destruction followed by impaired glucose tolerance (IGT) and/or impaired fasting glycaemia prior to overt diabetes.

### Onset of β-cell autoimmunity

Islet autoantibodies can be detected in early childhood and are presumed to be a guide to when β-cell autoimmunity begins. When autoantibodies were measured from birth in children of parents with type 1 diabetes, 11% were positive by 2 years of age for an islet autoantibody on at least one occasion,[41] and 2.8% were persistently positive for two or more antibodies.[42] Importantly, the latter group had a higher frequency of the 'at-risk' HLA DR4 and DR3 alleles.[43] When present, maternal autoantibodies were not detected in infants after 6–9 months of age, and autoantibodies began to develop after 18 months. How accurately this indicates the time of onset of autoimmune disorder within the pancreas is unknown. Most commonly, but not always, IAA are the first autoantibody detected. These studies continue in several countries to follow children through to the development of clinical diabetes. Another study reported that approximately 13% of children of first-degree relatives initially had markers of β-cell autoimmunity (ICA or IAA), but the prevalence decreased to 6–7% at ages 5–9 years.[44] The cumulative incidence of type 1 diabetes in this population was 2–3% by the age of 10 years. It has therefore been hypothesized that some children may progress very slowly or may even recover from autoimmunity.

## Latent autoimmune diabetes in adults

Screening patients clinically diagnosed with type 2 diabetes who are not treated with insulin has identified a significant subgroup with evidence of β-cell autoimmunity.[45,46] They appear to have a slowly progressive form of type 1 diabetes that has been termed latent autoimmune diabetes in adults (LADA).[47] A substudy of the UKPDS identified that LADA has a frequency of approximately 10% of all adult-onset diabetes,[48] and 94% of patients aged <45 years with ICA required insulin 6 years after diagnosis, compared with 14% of the antibody-negative patients.

The diagnosis of LADA is based on a combination of clinical and immunological features. The key features are gradual onset diabetes in adult life and detectable islet autoantibodies, most commonly GADAb. The presence of GADAb has been associated with a slightly lower body-mass index (BMI) than typically seen in type 2 diabetes patients,[48] although it is not possible to specify a cut-off point BMI for the diagnosis of LADA. In contrast to patients with classical type 2 diabetes, those with LADA display an early requirement for insulin treatment because they are primarily insulin deficient rather than insulin resistant and therefore do not respond as well to diet and oral hypoglycaemic treatment.[49]

Previously, type 1 diabetes had been referred to as juvenile-onset diabetes. However, it is apparent that this condition is more heterogeneous than suggested by its original description 50 years ago, and the number of patients with type 1 diabetes across all age groups is likely to be much higher than previously thought.[1]

## GENETICS OF TYPE 1 DIABETES

The concordance of type 1 diabetes in monozygotic twins is 30–40%, compared with 5% in siblings. This indicates the importance of genetic factors in the development of the disease,[50] (Table 2(ii).2) but at the some time this intermediate level of concordance shows that non-genetic or environmental factors must also be involved. Transmission of type 1 diabetes is considered to be polygenic, meaning that several genetic loci are associated with an increased risk of diabetes. Non-Mendelian or polygenic inheritance and the probable heterogeneity of type 1 diabetes have contributed to the complexity of type 1 diabetes genetics.

**Table 2(ii).2 Lifetime risks of type 1 diabetes in first-degree relatives (proband diagnosed before 20 years of age).**

| | |
|---|---|
| Parents | 2.2 ± 0.6% |
| Children | 5.6 ± 2.8% |
| Siblings | 6.9 ± 1.3% |
| Siblings | |
| HLA Nonidentical sib | 1.2% |
| HLA Haploidentical | 4.9% |
| HLA Identical sib | 15.9% |
| Identical twin | 30–40% |

## Association with the HLA locus

The most clearly established genetic association with type 1 diabetes is the major histocompatibility complex (MHC) that in man is also known as the human leucocyte antigen (HLA) locus and is located on the short arm of chromosome 6.[51] The MHC or HLA region accounts for at least 35% and up to 50% of familial clustering in type 1 diabetes and is therefore the major susceptibility locus identified currently.[52]

MHC class II proteins function as peptide-binding proteins. MHC class II molecules are assembled in the endoplasmic reticulum and then transported through the Golgi apparatus to the cytosol, where they take up peptide fragments of degraded protein. The molecules are then transported to the cell surface, where they present the peptides as antigen to CD4+ T cells, including autoreactive T cells involved in autoimmune disease as well as those involved in adaptive immune responses to infectious microorganisms. Polymorphisms within MHC molecules affect which antigenic peptides are bound and presented. Pancreatic β-cells do not express class II MHC proteins; therefore, presentation to CD4+ T cells of autoantigens derived from β-cells is likely to occur on professional antigen-presenting cells such as dendritic cells.

DQ alleles, which encode one of the three class II molecules, are most closely associated with diabetes. The HLA region tends to be inherited en bloc, so that particular class I and II alleles are closely linked; for example, DQ and DR alleles are tightly linked. HLA-DR3 (closely linked to DQ2), HLA-DR4 (closely linked to DQ8) or both alleles are present in 95% of Caucasians with type 1 diabetes. The DR3/4, DQB1*0302 haplotype (HLA DR3-DQ2 and HLA DR4-DQ8) carries the highest relative risk, 19–25 times, compared with the general population.[53] It is present in 30–40% of Caucasians with type I diabetes compared with 2–3% of controls and is associated with an earlier age at diagnosis.[54] This HLA type is used to define neonates with a high risk of diabetes who may be candidates for primary prevention therapy prior to the detection of autoantibodies. The positive predictive value of the HLA DR3/4, DQB1*0302 genotype is 6.3% for the onset of type 1 diabetes by age 20.[54] In some cases, the non-HLA loci appear to be more strongly linked to diabetes in the absence of the highest risk HLA genotype.[55]

Genetic studies have revealed an even stronger association between the HLA-DQ locus and disease susceptibility than described for HLA-DR.[56,57] Molecular analysis of human HLA-DQ genes has shown that position 57 of the DQβ-chain is strongly associated with type 1 diabetes incidence; a negatively charged aspartic acid at position 57 (Asp-57) correlates with protection against type 1 diabetes, whereas alleles with a neutral amino acid, such as alanine, valine or serine (Non-Asp-57), correlate with increased susceptibility to the disease.[58,59] An explanation for the changes in disease susceptibility is that small structural changes in HLA-encoded class II molecules may result in large functional changes in the antigen-presenting ability of these molecules.

HLA class I alleles were the first HLA alleles associated with insulin-dependent diabetes mellitus (IDDM) susceptibility[11] and are still believed to contribute independently of class II. In studies of unrelated diabetes patients, the HLA class I alleles B15, B8 and B18 have been demonstrated to have increased frequency. The frequency of B7 has been shown to be decreased compared with a non-diabetes control population.[60] HLA A24 has been associated with rapidly progressive β-cell destruction, independently of class II genes.[61]

Apart from identifying HLA alleles associated with increased risk of developing type 1 diabetes, certain alleles are protective. The haplotype with the least susceptibility to diabetes is DR2-DQ6(32). Individuals with HLA DR2-DQ6 have a considerably reduced relative risk at 0.12.

## Associations with non-HLA loci

The significant difference between the concordance rate for type 1 diabetes in monozygotic twins (30–40%) and the concordance rate in MHC-identical siblings (12–16%) suggests that genetic factors outside the MHC also have an important role in the development of diabetes (Table 2(ii).2). It is thought that non-MHC genes may account for approximately 50% of genetic susceptibility to the disease.[54] These include the IDDM2 locus defined by polymorphisms in the promoter region of the insulin gene on

**Table 2(ii).3  Type 1 diabetes susceptibility genetic loci.**

| Association | Locus | Chromosome |
|---|---|---|
| Confirmed (gene polymorphism demonstrated) | IDDM1 *(HLA)* | 6p21 |
| | IDDM2 *(insulin)* | 11p15.5 |
| Confirmed (linkage analysis demonstrated) | IDDM4 | 11q13 |
| | IDDM5 | 6q25 |
| | IDDM6 | 18q21 |
| | IDDM8 | 6q27 |
| | IDDM12 *(CTLA-4)* | 2q33 |
| Suggestive (less evidence) | IDDM3 | 15q26 |
| | IDDM7 | 2q31 |
| | IDDM10 | 10p11.2–q11.2 |
| | IDDM11 | 14q24.3–q31 |
| | IDDM13 | 2q34 |
| | IDDM18 | 5q33–34 |

chromosome 11 (Table 2(ii).3), and recently defined polymorphisms in the interleukin-12 p40 gene and polymorphisms in the CTLA4 gene that have also been associated with other autoimmune diseases. There are also many other loci with less well-established candidate genes.

## Gender

Type 1 diabetes is distinct from other major organ-specific autoimmune disorders, such as Graves' disease, Hashimoto's thyroiditis, rheumatoid arthritis, pernicious anaemia and multiple sclerosis, because these other diseases are much more common in women[62] (Table 2(ii).4). The risk of developing type 1 diabetes is similar for human males and females.[63] Conversely, in the non-obese diabetic mouse model of type 1 diabetes, diabetes is several times more common in females than males.[64] In most mouse colonies, the frequency of diabetes is 75–85% for females and 15–25% for males.

The overall sex ratio is believed to be equal in children diagnosed under the age of 15 years. In many populations with a high incidence of diabetes greater than 23/100 000, a male excess has been observed, whereas in populations with an incidence below 4.5/100 000, a female excess has been noted. The significance of these observations is unclear. A slight male excess (1.5:1) has been seen in type 1 diabetes diagnosed at 15–40 years,[64] and male excess may begin at the time of puberty.[65] The gender distribution after the age of 40 years is unclear due to the lack of epidemiological data that is related to difficulties with phenotypic characterization of type 1 diabetes in this age group.

## Parental inheritance

Different risk for diabetes inheritance depends on which parent has diabetes. It has been found that children with type 1 diabetes have a higher prevalence of type 1 diabetes in fathers than mothers in caucasoid populations.[66,67] The offspring of fathers with type 1 diabetes are estimated to have a risk of about 1 in 40 compared with 1 in 66 for offspring of mothers with type 1 diabetes. A recent study in Finland also suggests that the risk of type 1 diabetes in offspring may depend in part on the sex of the offspring.[67] If the parent with diabetes shares the same sex as the offspring, the offspring is less likely to develop diabetes. One could conclude that in a given population the susceptibility to type 1 diabetes may be transferred more often through the father, who would then more often transmit the disease to a daughter than a son. A possible explanation for the higher prevalence of diabetes in fathers is that men with type 1 diabetes might have been more able to reproduce than women with type 1 diabetes, who are more prone to significant complications in pregnancy, and some studies have shown a relative increase in mortality in females with type 1 diabetes.

## EPIDEMIOLOGY OF TYPE 1 DIABETES

### Worldwide increase in frequency

The current prevalence of type 1 diabetes in Western nations is estimated to be 0.2–0.5%. There has been intense interest recently in studying global trends in diabetes incidence. Up until the early 1980s, data on the incidence of type 1 diabetes were available only for a few populations with high or intermediate risk of the disease.[68] Since the mid-1980s, a large number of registries have been established worldwide;[69] however, the lack of standardized data has meant that variation in incidence and trends over time should be studied with caution. The Diabetes Epidemiology Research International Group (DERI) collects aggregate data on incidence of type 1

| Table 2(ii).4    Gender and autoimmune disease.[62] | |
|---|---|
| **Diseases** | **% Females** |
| Childhood | |
| • Systemic lupus erythematosus (SLE) | 70 |
| • Dermatomyositis | 70 |
| • Rheumatoid arthritis | 65 |
| • Type 1 diabetes | 50 |
| Adulthood | |
| • Sjögren's syndrome | 95 |
| • Primary biliary cirrhosis | 90 |
| • SLE | 90 |
| • Hashimoto's thyroiditis | 85 |
| • Myasthenia gravis | 75 |
| • Multiple sclerosis | 60 |
| • Ulcerative colitis | 50 |
| • Type 1 diabetes | 50 |

diabetes from many registries worldwide,[70] including the World Health Organization Project on Childhood Diabetes (DIAbetes MONdiale).[71] The collaborative research project EURODIAB ACE was established also in the late 1980s to obtain information on type 1 diabetes in Europe.[72]

A recent pooled analysis of data from 1960 to 1996, involving 37 studies in 27 countries, showed that the incidence of type 1 diabetes is increasing worldwide in both high- and low-risk populations[68] at a rate of approximately 3–4% per year. Type 1 diabetes appears to be developing at an earlier age, with the age group 5–10 years having the largest proportional increase. The overall increase was 3.0% per year, and the relative increase was steeper in the populations with lower incidence. According to this estimate, the incidence of type 1 diabetes will be 40% higher in 2010 than 1998. In Finland in 1953, the incidence in children was 13 per 100 000; by 2010, it is estimated to reach 50 per 100 000. The reason for the worldwide increasing incidence is unclear, but it is likely to be related to non-genetic factors, given that the genetic pool is essentially unchanged. These factors might include changes in diet or childhood infections leading to altered development of the immune system.

## Geographical variation

A key epidemiological feature of type 1 diabetes is its impressive geographical variability. There is a 60-fold difference between Finland, the country with the highest rate, and Japan, which has the lowest recorded rate of diabetes worldwide (Figure 2(ii).2). The highest reported incidence rates are in Finland and Sardinia (approximately 30/100 000 per year), with most other European, American and Australian populations having a moderate incidence rate (3–19 /100 000 per year). The lowest rates are in Asia (China, Japan, Korea) and Latin America (Mexico, Chile, Peru).

### North–south gradient
It has been suggested that the incidence of diabetes increases with distance from the equator, so that people living near the equator have a risk of disease one-tenth or less that of populations bordering the Arctic and Antarctic Circles. Epidemiological data indicate that the geographical relationship is not as straightforward as initially reported, as genetic differences of populations are emerging as a likely factor in the geographical variation. The largest intracontinental variation is in Europe between Finland and Greece,

the southernmost European country, with the lowest incidence of 5 per 1000.[63] Evidence against the north–south gradient theory is offered by Iceland, the northernmost nation in Europe, which has a lower incidence than Finland, yet Sardinia has an incidence comparable with that of Finland. Iceland is an interesting example, as it has a twofold lower risk of type 1 diabetes than Norway, yet the racial origins of both populations are similar, suggesting that environmental factors may be important.[73] Significant variations within countries have been noted, including the Scandinavian nations, the UK and the USA, with Italy showing the greatest within-country variation in Europe[73,74] probably because of its genetically heterogeneous population. The north–south gradient phenomenon has not been consistently reported within countries. On the basis of these geographical observations, one can conclude that there is no simple correlation between incidence of type 1 diabetes and latitude or climate.

### Migration studies
Potentially, it should be possible to analyse the influence of genetic background in comparison with environment by studying populations that have migrated. Studies of migration to explore the importance of environment relative to genetics can be done in two ways; one may compare either the genetically different ethnic groups living in the same environment or genetically identical individuals living in different environments. Both epidemiological designs have been adopted in studies of migrants across the world.

A recent Italian migration study compared children with Sardinian ancestry living in Lazio, a low-incidence region for type 1 diabetes in Italy, and children living in Sardinia.[75,76] Sardinians are a homogeneous population and are genetically distinct from other European populations, including Italians. Next to Finns, Sardinians have the highest incidence of type 1 diabetes as well as the highest population frequency (39%) of the HLA DR3 phenotype (43). Children from the indigenous population of Lazio had an annual incidence of 7.9 per 100 000 compared with 34.4 for Sardinians. Children of Sardinian migrants to Lazio retained the same high incidence of diabetes, 33 per 100 000. Children with one Sardinian parent had a rate half that of Sardinians (15.9) and double that of the native population of Lazio. This study showed that the higher incidence of diabetes was attributable to genetic factors. Further evidence which may support genetics as a relatively more significant factor than environment is that the Anglo-Celtic populations of the British Isles

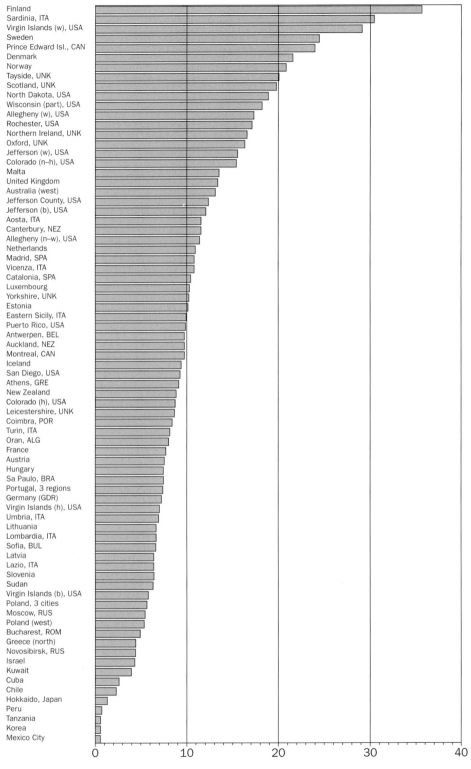

**Figure 2(ii).2**
Incidence of type 1 diabetes mellitus worldwide. Age-specific incidence (per 100 000 population) of type 1 diabetes in age group under 15 years. Data for boys and girls have been pooled. The populations are arranged in an ascending order according to the incidence. AUS, Australia; BEL, Belgium; BRA, Brazil; BUL, Bulgaria; GRE, Greece; ITA, Italy; JPN, Japan; NEZ, New Zealand; POL, Poland; POR, Portugal; SPA, Spain; UNK, United Kingdom; USA, United States of America; w, White; n-w, non-White; b, Black; h, Hispanic; n-h, non-Hispanic.

share a similar incidence of type 1 diabetes when compared with similar populations in Australia and New Zealand.[63]

An example of studying different genetic populations in the same environment was the comparison of diabetes incidence between native Estonians and an immigrant group, consisting predominantly of Russians who had emigrated to Estonia in the previous 50 years.[77] There had been little intermarriage between Estonians and non-Estonians; therefore, it was felt that this time period was too short for significant genetic admixture. The incidence was expected to be higher in native Estonians because their ethnic background is similar to that of Finns, who have a high incidence of type 1 diabetes. The average annual incidence was significantly higher in Estonians (11.8 per 100 000 children aged <15 years) than in non-Estonians (7.6 per 100 000 children aged <15 years). It was therefore concluded that immigrant populations need not acquire the same risk of type 1 diabetes as the native population. Another study showed that French children in Canada have an incidence of 7.4 per 100 000 compared with 4.7 per 100 000 for children in France.[78] The French-Canadian incidence is lower than that of the rest of the Canadian population. Possible explanations for the difference are unidentified environmental factors or genetic admixture of the descendants of immigrants from France, given that French immigration to Canada occurred several hundred years ago. On the basis of epidemiological data on migration, it is possible to conclude that both genetics and the environment are factors in the evolution of type 1 diabetes, genetics appearing to have a more dominant role.

## Environmental triggers

The most important pieces of evidence for the role of non-genetic factors in the pathogenesis of type 1 diabetes are the low concordance of type 1 diabetes in identical twins (Table 2(ii).2) and the increasing frequency of type 1 diabetes in genetically stable populations. Environmental factors may either trigger or exacerbate progression to diabetes; alternatively, they may retard the development of β-cell autoimmunity in individuals genetically at risk. There are many proposed candidates for environmental triggers (Table 2(ii).5).

### Viral infection

It has been hypothesized that viral infection may initiate β-cell autoimmunity as well as precipitate clinical diabetes in people who have developed

---

**Table 2(ii).5    Environmental trigger candidates in man.**

**Viral**
- Rubella (congenital)
- Coxsackie B4
- Rotavirus

**Nutritional**
- Cow's milk infant feeding

**Seasonal**
- Sunlight exposure
- Ambient temperature

**Chemotoxins**
- Vacor (rodenticide *N*-3-pyriylmethyl-*N-P*-nitrophenyl urea)

---

autoimmunity. Candidate viruses for causing β-cell autoimmunity include picornavirus[67] and rubella virus,[79] as well as herpesvirus, rotavirus, influenza virus, measles virus, mumps virus, and retrovirus.[79] Currently, the viral group with the strongest evidence for a role in the pathogenesis of type 1 diabetes is the picornaviruses, particularly enterovirus and rhinovirus. A case-control study of GAD autoantibodies found that 54% of subjects with high titres of IgM against Coxsackievirus B had GAD autoantibodies compared with 35% GAD Ab in those with low IgM titre.[80] The difference appeared to be stronger in controls than in patients with type 1 diabetes. An explanation proposed by some is the possibility of 'molecular mimicry' due to homology between the PC-2 protein of Coxsackievirus and GAD protein.[81,82] Congenital rubella was the first infection shown to have a definite association with type 1 diabetes.[16] Of patients with congenital rubella syndrome, 70% have been found to be ICA positive.[79] Approximately 20% of people with congenital rubella develop diabetes in their lifetime, particularly those with HLA risk alleles. They are also recognized to have a higher incidence of other immunological disorders including thyroiditis. The mechanism for induction of diabetes by this agent is unkown.

The immune response to a viral antigen is likely to be dependent on the age of the host at the time of antigen presentation; for example, neonates and infants are more likely to develop chronic infection due to immaturity of the immune system. Some have hypothesized that an 'age-window' model exists for candidate viruses and the development of autoimmunity, but so far no definite evidence has been discovered to support this belief. It is important to note that studies conducted at the time of diagnosis of type 1 diabetes may well be of limited value, given that the clinical phase of this disease is preceded by a long preclinical phase of β-cell autoimmunity. With the availability of β-cell autoantibodies that identify individuals with preclinical diabetes, more effort is being concentrated on investigating viral infection and serology at the onset of β-cell autoimmunity.

## Nutrition

An inverse relationship was initially reported between breastfeeding and type 1 diabetes incidence. Subsequent retrospective case-control studies revealed a significantly shorter duration of breast-feeding, less than 3 months on average, and a younger exposure to cow's milk for type 1 diabetes cases than controls.[83] The significance of these associations is uncertain, as their magnitude was relatively low, with odds ratios of approximately 2.0, and the presence of confounding factors such as socio-economic status and ethnic origin. It has been hypothesized that exposure to milk proteins may result in cross-reaction to islet cell antigens, as in the 'molecular mimicry' theory of viruses; however, currently, this remains controversial.

## Seasonality

A distinct seasonal variation in the onset of type 1 diabetes has been reported in many countries,[84] although the magnitude of the variation is not large. There is a slight decrease in incidence during the summer when compared with the colder months. The seasonal changes in the diagnosis of the disease are more noticeable in regions where the seasons are well demarcated. Some studies suggest that the variation is most apparent in children of peripubertal age and less pronounced in the younger age group.[85] Possibly, certain seasons result in a delayed diagnosis or lack of prompt medical attention; [86] however, it has been observed that seasonality is associated with both time of diagnosis of diabetes and onset of symptoms.[84]

Given the long preclinical course of type 1 diabetes, it is most likely that seasonality is not an aetiological factor but rather a trigger which may be associated with expression of symptoms in people who are already at an advanced stage of disease. Seasonality has been argued by some as further evidence for the role of infection in diabetes, as some viral infections exhibit strong seasonal trends.[87] Several viruses, including Coxsackievirus, echovirus and rotavirus,[75] have been implicated in diabetes, but

without conclusive evidence. Another hypothesis to account for the seasonal variation is that certain seasons coincide with a return to school. The start of school may result in increased exposure to viruses, as well as psychological stress, which may then have effects on immunoregulatory function. Ambient temperature associated with the different seasons has been thought to be implicated in the pathogenesis of type 1 diabetes, but there is a lack of biological evidence to support this. A possible explanation for seasonal variation is varying vitamin D metabolism related to sunlight. Vitamin D has been shown to have immune effects and may modulate the pathogenesis of type 1 diabetes.[88]

## CONCLUSION AND PROSPECTS FOR THERAPY

The treatment of type 1 diabetes is entering an exciting period in which a variety of candidate immune-based therapies and definitive treatment by β-cell replacement are now entering clinical trial and clinical practice. Preventative therapy trials include antigen-specific therapies with insulin, GAD or heat shock protein 70 delivered in various ways designed to reduce endogenous pathological autoimmune reactions. The Diabetes Prevention Trial 1 (DPT-1), the first major trial using antigen-specific prevention in preclinical subjects (that is, before diagnosis of diabetes) was reported in 2001.[89] While the treatment did not prevent diabetes, this will be only the first of many such trials, and one should not be too discouraged by the lack of immediate success. Treatment of early type 1 diabetes (that is, post-diagnosis) is also being trialled with anti-CD3 monoclonal antibody, showing some promise. A large trial of nicotinamide to protect β-cells from destruction will also be reported in the near future.

Islet allotransplantation has been dramatically improved in the protocol used in Edmonton, Alberta, and further confirmatory studies are planned. While the limited numbers of available organs and the generalized immunosuppression required mean that this will never be the solution to diabetes, it is an important breakthrough. It is likely to be followed by other forms of β-cell replacement technologies, including differentiated stem cells, genetically engineered cells or xenotransplantation of pig islets.

This wide range of innovative therapies for type 1 diabetes should lead to as many changes in managing diabetes in the next 25 years as have occurred in understanding type 1 diabetes over the last 25 years.

# REFERENCES

1. Notkins AL, Lernmark A, Autoimmune type 1 diabetes: resolved and unresolved issues, *J Clin Invest* (2001) **108**:1247–52.
2. Harrison LC, Campbell IL, Colman PG, et al, Type 1 diabetes: immunopathology and immunotherapy, *Adv Endocrinol Metab* (1990) **1**:35–94.
3. Bach JF, Insulin-dependent diabetes mellitus as an autoimmune diabetes. *Endocr Rev* (1994) **15**:516–42.
4. LaPorte RE, Matsushima M, Chang YF, *Prevalence and Incidence of Insulin-Dependent Diabetes* (National Institutes of Health: Bethesda, MD, 1995).
5. Gale EA, The discovery of type 1 diabetes, *Diabetes* (2001) **50**:217–26.
6. Lister J, Nash J, Ledingham U, Constitution and insulin sensitivity in diabetes mellitus, *Br Med J* (1951) **i**:376–9.
7. Wrenshall GA, Ritchie R, Extractable insulin of pancreas, *Diabetes* (1952) **1**:87–107.
8. Laakso M, Pyorala K, Age of onset and type of diabetes, *Diabetes Care* (1985) **8**:114–17.
9. Gepts W, Pathologic anatomy of the pancreas in juvenile diabetes mellitus, *Diabetes* (1965) **14**:619–33.
10. Bottazzo GF, Florin-Christensen A, Doniach D, Islet-cell antibodies in diabetes mellitus with autoimmune polyendocrine deficiencies, *Lancet* (1974) **ii**:1280–3.
11. Nerup J, Platz P, et al, HL-A antigens and diabetes mellitus, *Lancet* (1974) **ii** (7885):864–6.
12. Ogilvie RF, A quantitative study of the pancreatic islet tissue, *Q J Med* (1937) **6**:287–300.
13. Foulis AK, Frier BM, Pancreatic endocrine-exocrine function in diabetes: an old alliance disturbed, *Diabet Med* (1984) **1**:263–6.
14. Bottazzo, GF, Dean BM, et al, In situ characterization of autoimmune phenomena and expression of HLA molecules in the pancreas in diabetic insulitis, *N Engl J Med* (1985) **313**:353–60.
15. Foulis AK, The pathology of the endocrine pancreas in type 1 (insulin-dependent) diabetes mellitus, *APMIS* (1996) **104**:161–7.
16. Itoh N, Hanafusa T, et al, Mononuclear cell infiltration and its relation to the expression of major histocompatibility complex antigens and adhesion molecules in pancreas biopsy specimens from newly diagnosed insulin-dependent diabetes mellitus patients *J Clin Invest* (1993) **92**:2313–22.
17. Hanafusa T, Miyazaki A, et al, Examination of islets in the pancreas biopsy specimens from newly diagnosed type 1 (insulin-dependent) diabetic patients, *Diabetologia* (1990) **33**:105–11.
18. Sutherland DE, Goetz FC, et al, Pancreas transplants from related donors, *Transplantation* (1984) **38**:625–33.
19. Kay TW, Thomas HE, et al, The beta cell in autoimmune diabetes: many mechanisms and pathways of loss, *Trends Endocrinol Metab* (2000) **11**:11–15.
20. Martin S, Wolf-Eichbaum D, et al, Development of type 1 diabetes despite severe hereditary B-lymphocyte deficiency, *N Engl J Med* (2001) **345**:1036–40.
21. Lampeter EF, McCann SR, et al, Transfer of diabetes type 1 by bone-marrow transplantation, *Lancet* (1998) **351** (9102):568–9.
22. Roep BO, Standardization of T-cell assays in type I diabetes. Immunology of Diabetes Society T-cell Committee, *Diabetologia* (1999) **42**:636–7.
23. Landin-Olsson M, Palmer JP, et al, Predictive value of islet cell and insulin autoantibodies for type 1 (insulin-dependent) diabetes mellitus in a population-based study of newly-diagnosed diabetic and matched control children, *Diabetologia* (1992) **35**:1068–73.
24. Harrison L, Risk assessment, prediction and prevention of type 1 diabetes *Pediatr Diabetes* (2001) **2**:71–82.
25. Lendrum R, Walker G, Cudworth AG, et al, Islet cell antibodies in diabetes mellitus, *Lancet* (1976) **ii**:1097–102.
26. Borg H, Marcus C, et al, Islet cell antibody frequency differs from that of glutamic acid decarboxylase antibodies/IA2 antibodies after diagnosis of diabetes, *Acta Paediatr* (2000) **89**:46–51.
27. Verge CF, Stenger D, Bonifacio E, et al, Combined use of autoantibodies (IA2-autoantibody, GAD autoantibody, insulin autoantibody, cytoplasmic islet cell antibodies in type 1 diabetes. Combinatorial Islet Autoantibody Workshop, *Diabetes* (1998) **47**:1857–66.
28. Lernmark A, Glutamic acid decarboxylase—gene to antigen to disease, *J Intern Med* (1996) **240**:259–77.
29. Degli Esposti M, Mackay IR, The GABA network and the pathogenesis of IDDM, *Diabetologia* (1997) **40**:352–6.
30. Bjork E, Kampe O, et al, Expression of the 64 kDa/glutamic acid decarboxylase rat islet cell autoantigen is influenced by the rate of insulin secretion, *Diabetologia* (1992) **35**:490–3.
31. Bjork E, Kampe O, et al, Glucose regulation of the autoantigen GAD65 in human pancreatic islets, *J Clin Endocrinol Metab* (1992) **75**:1574–6.
32. Palmer JP, Asplin CM, et al, Insulin antibodies in insulin-dependent diabetics before insulin treatment, *Science* (1983) **222** (4630):1337–9.
33. Rabin DU, Pleasic SM, et al, Islet cell antigen 512 is a diabetes-specific islet autoantigen related to protein tyrosine phosphatases, *J Immunol* (1994) **152**:3183–8.
34. Payton MA, Hawkes CJ, et al, Relationship of the 37,000– and 40,000-M(r) tryptic fragments of islet antigens in insulin-dependent diabetes to the protein tyrosine phosphatase-like molecule IA-2 (ICA512), *J Clin Invest* (1995) **96**:1506–11.
35. Lan MS, Lu J, et al, Molecular cloning and identification of a receptor-type protein tyrosine phosphatase, IA-2, from human insulinoma, *DNA Cell Biol* (1994) **13**:505–14.
36. Srikanta S, Ganda OP, et al, Islet-cell antibodies and beta-cell function in monozygotic triplets and twins initially discordant for type I diabetes mellitus, *N Engl J Med* (1983) **308**:322–5.
37. Gorsuch AN, Spencer KM, et al, Evidence for a long prediabetic period in type I (insulin-dependent) diabetes mellitus, *Lancet* (1981) **2** (8260–1):1363–5.
38. Colman PG, McNair P, et al, The Melbourne Pre-Diabetes Study: prediction of type 1 diabetes mellitus using antibody and metabolic testing, *Med J Aust* (1998) **169**:81–4.
39. Bingley PJ, Christie MR, et al, Combined analysis of autoantibodies improves prediction of IDDM in islet cell antibody-positive relatives, *Diabetes* (1994) **43**:1304–10.
40. Bingley PJ, Interactions of age, islet cell antibodies, insulin autoantibodies, and first-phase insulin response in predicting risk of progression to IDDM in ICA+ relatives: the ICARUS data set. Islet Cell Antibody Register Users Study, *Diabetes* (1996) **45**:1720–8.
41. Ziegler AG, Hummel M, et al, Autoantibody appearance and risk for development of childhood diabetes in offspring of parents with type 1 diabetes: the 2-year analysis of the German BABYDIAB Study, *Diabetes* (1999) **48**:460–8.
42. Colman PG, Steele C, et al, Islet autoimmunity in infants with a type I diabetic relative is common but is frequently restricted to one autoantibody, *Diabetologia* (2000) **43**:203–9.
43. Schenker M, Hummel M, et al, Early expression and high prevalence of islet autoantibodies for DR3/4 heterozygous and DR4/4 homozygous offspring of parents with type I diabetes: the German BABYDIAB study, *Diabetologia* (1999) **42**:671–7.
44. Tuomilehto J, Rewers M, et al, Increasing trend in type 1 (insulin-dependent) diabetes mellitus in childhood in Finland. Analysis of age, calendar time and birth cohort effects during 1965 to 1984, *Diabetologia* (1991) **34**:282–7.
45. Gottsater A, Landin-Olsson M, et al, Glutamate decarboxylase antibody levels predict rate of beta-cell decline in adult-onset diabetes, *Diabetes Res Clin Pract* (1995) **27**:133–40.

46. Humphrey AR, McCarty DJ, Mackay IR, et al, Autoantibodies to glutamic acid decarboxylase and phenotypic features associated with Early insulin treatment in individuals with adult-onset diabetes mellitus, *Diabet Med* (1998) **15:**113–19.

47. Tuomi T, Groop LC, et al, Antibodies to glutamic acid decarboxylase reveal latent autoimmune diabetes mellitus in adults with a non-insulin-dependent onset of disease, *Diabetes* (1993) **42:**359–62.

48. Turner R, Stratton I, et al, UKPDS 25: autoantibodies to islet-cell cytoplasm and glutamic acid decarboxylase for prediction of insulin requirement in type 2 diabetes. UK Prospective Diabetes Study Group, *Lancet* (1997) **350** (9087):1288–93.

49. Juneja R, Palmer JP, Type 1 1/2 diabetes: myth or reality?, *Autoimmunity* (1999) **29:**65–83.

52. Todd JA, Genetic analysis of type 1 diabetes using whole genome approaches, *Proc Natl Acad Sci USA* (1995) **92:**8560–5.

53. Merriman RTJ, Genetics of autoimmune disease, *Curr Opin Immunol* (1995) **7:**786–92.

54. Lucassen AM, Bell J, *Genetics of Insulin-Dependent Diabetes* (Cambridge University Press: Cambridge, 1995).

55. Morahan G, Huang D, et al, Markers on distal chromosome 2q linked to insulin-dependent diabetes mellitus, *Science* (1996) **272** (5269):1811–13.

56. Schreuder GM, Tilanus MG, et al, HLA-DO polymorphism associated with resistance to type I diabetes detected with monoclonal antibodies, isoelectric point differences, and restriction fragment length polymorphism, *J Exp Med* (1986) **164:**938–43.

57. Owerbach D, Gunn S, et al, Oligonucleotide probes for HLA-DQA and DQB genes define susceptibility to type 1 (insulin-dependent) diabetes mellitus, *Diabetologia* (1988) **31:**751–7.

58. Todd JA, Bell JI, et al, HLA-DQ beta gene contributes to susceptibility and resistance to insulin-dependent diabetes mellitus, *Nature* (1987) **329** (6140):599–604.

59. Horn GT, Bugawan TL, et al, Allelic sequence variation of the HLA-DQ loci: relationship to serology and to insulin-dependent diabetes susceptibility *Proc Natl Acad Sci USA* (1988) **85:**6012–16.

60. Cudworth AG, Woodrow JC, Evidence for HL-A-linked genes in 'juvenile' diabetes mellitus, *Br Med J* (1975) **3:**133–5.

61. Tait BD, Harrison LC, et al, HLA antigens and age at diagnosis of insulin-dependent diabetes mellitus, *Hum Immunol* (1995) **42:**116–22.

62. Beeson PB, Age and sex associations of 40 autoimmune diseases, *Am J Med* (1994) **96:**457–62.

63. Karvonen M, Tuomilehto J, et al, A review of the recent epidemiological data on the worldwide incidence of type 1 (insulin-dependent) diabetes mellitus. World Health Organization DIAMOND Project Group, *Diabetologia* (1993) **36:**883–92.

64. Gale EA, Gillespie KM, Diabetes and gender, *Diabetologia* (2001) **44:**3–15.

65. Nystrom L, Dahlquist G, et al, Risk of developing insulin-dependent diabetes mellitus (IDDM) before 35 years of age: indications of climatological determinants for age at onset, *Int J Epidemiol* (1992) **21:**352–8.

66. Warram JH, Krolewski AS, et al, Determinants of IDDM and perinatal mortality in children of diabetic mothers, *Diabetes* (1988) **37:**1328–34.

67. Tuomilehto J, Podar T, et al, Evidence for importance of gender and birth cohort for risk of IDDM in offspring of IDDM parents, *Diabetologia* (1995) **38:**975–82.

68. Onkamo P, Vaananen S, et al, Worldwide increase in incidence of type I diabetes—the analysis of the data on published incidence trends, *Diabetologia* (1999) **42:**1395–403.

69. LaPorte RE, Tajima N, et al, Geographic differences in the risk of insulin-dependent diabetes mellitus: the importance of registries, *Diabetes Care* (1985) **8** Suppl 1:101–7.

70. Rewers M, LaPorte RE, et al, Trends in the prevalence and incidence of diabetes: insulin-dependent diabetes mellitus in childhood, *World Health Stat Q* (1988) **41:**179–89.

71. World Health Organization Project on Childhood Diabetes, Childhood diabetes, epidemics, and epidemiology: an approach for controlling diabetes, *Am J Epidemiol* (1992) **135:**803–16.

72. Green A, Gale EA, et al, Incidence of childhood-onset insulin-dependent diabetes mellitus: the EURODIAB ACE Study, *Lancet* (1992) **339** (8798):905–9.

73. Green A, Prevention of IDDM: the genetic epidemiologic perspective, *Diabetes Res Clin Pract* (1996) **34** Suppl:101–6.

74. Bruno G, Merletti F, Vuolo A, The registry of IDDM in the province of Turin, Italy. Report on a 5 year (1984–1988) incidence survey in the age group 0–29 years, *Diabetes Care* (1990) **13:**1051–7.

75. Wagenknecht LE, Roseman JM, et al, Increased incidence of insulin-dependent diabetes mellitus following an epidemic of Coxsackievirus B5, *Am J Epidemiol* (1991) **133:**1024–31.

76. Muntoni S, New insights into the epidemiology of type 1 diabetes in Mediterranean countries, *Diabetes Metab Res Rev* (1999) **15:**133–40.

77. Podar T, Tuomilehto-Wolf E, et al, Insulin-dependent diabetes mellitus in native Estonians and immigrants to Estonia, *Am J Epidemiol* (1992) **135:**1231–6.

78. Colle E, Siemiatycki J, et al, Incidence of juvenile onset diabetes in Montreal—demonstration of ethnic differences and socioeconomic class differences, *J Chronic Dis* (1981) **34:**611–16.

79. Ginsberg-Fellner F, Witt ME, et al, Congenital rubella syndrome as a model for type 1 (insulin-dependent) diabetes mellitus: increased prevalence of islet cell surface antibodies, *Diabetologia* (1984) **27** Suppl:87–9.

80. Hagopian WA, Kaliappan SB, Karlsen AE, et al, Recent Coxsackie B virus infection associates with glutamic acid decarboxylase autoantibodies (GAD65 Ab) regardless of insulin-dependent diabetes mellitus (DDM) status. American Diabetes Association 12th International Immunology and Diabetes Workshop, Orlando, Florida (1993).

81. Gerling I, Nejman C, et al, Effect of Coxsackievirus B4 infection in mice on expression of 64,000-Mr autoantigen and glucose sensitivity of islets before development of hyperglycemia, *Diabetes* (1988) **37:**1419–25.

82. Clare-Salzler MJ, Tobin AJ, et al, Glutamate decarboxylase: an autoantigen in IDDM, *Diabetes Care* (1992) **15:**132–5.

83. Kostraba JN, Dorman JS, et al, Early infant diet and risk of IDDM in blacks and whites. A matched case-control study, *Diabetes Care* (1992) **15:**626–31.

84. Ludvigsson J, Afoke AO, Seasonality of type 1 (insulin-dependent) diabetes mellitus: values of C-peptide, insulin antibodies and haemoglobin A1c show evidence of a more rapid loss of insulin secretion in epidemic patients, *Diabetologia* (1989) **32:**84–91.

85. Joner G, Sovik O, Increasing incidence of diabetes mellitus in Norwegian children 0–14 years of age 1973–1982, *Diabetologia* (1989) **32:**79–83.

86. Christau B, Kromann H, et al, Incidence, seasonal and geographical patterns of juvenile-onset insulin-dependent diabetes mellitus in Denmark, *Diabetologia* (1977) **13:**281–4.

87. Gamble DR, The epidemiology of insulin dependent diabetes with particular reference to the relationship of virus infection to its etiology, *Epidemiol Rev* (1980) **2:**49–70.

88. EURODIAB Substudy 2 Study Group, Vitamin D supplement in early childhood and risk for type I (insulin-dependent) diabetes mellitus, *Diabetologia* (1999) **42:**51–4.

89. Diabetes Prevention Trial – Type 1 Diabetes Study Group, Effects of insulin in relatives of patients with type 1 diabetes mellitus, *N Engl J Med* (2002) **346:**1685–91

# 3

# Diabetic nephropathy: epidemiology and clinical description

George Jerums, Sianna Panagiotopoulos and Richard J MacIsaac

## INTRODUCTION

Approximately one-third of patients with type 1 diabetes mellitus (DM)[1,2] and one-sixth of patients with type 2 DM develop overt diabetic nephropathy (DN).[3] Once DN is present, the interval to the onset of end-stage renal disease (ESRD) varies from 4 years in earlier studies[4] to over 10 years in recent studies[5] and is similar in type 1 and type 2 diabetes. Although type 2 diabetes is now the most common cause of ESRD in Western countries, many people with renal disease and type 2 diabetes do not reach ESRD because cardiovascular mortality is increased twofold and four- to eightfold in the presence of microalbuminuria or overt nephropathy, respectively.[6] The modifiable risk factors for DN include glycaemic control, blood pressure, dyslipidaemia and smoking. Unmodifiable risk factors include male sex; duration of diabetes; and familial, genetic and ethnic factors. In type 1 diabetes, the incidence of DN rises to 2–3% per year 10–13 years after the onset of diabetes, but then falls to 0.5–1% per year after 20 years of diabetes.[7,8]

## DEFINITION OF DIABETIC NEPHROPATHY (DN)

The structural features of DN were described originally by Kimmelstiel and Wilson in 1936 as a glomerulopathy with diffuse and/or nodular intercapillary glomerulosclerosis.[9] The nodular changes are still considered specific for diabetes, although the diffuse lesions are also seen in other renal diseases. It was recognized that these ultrastructural changes were accompanied by increases in proteinuria. However, progress in the field was slow until the development of sensitive immunoassays for urinary albumin[10] and the demonstration that increases in albuminuria are detectable several years before changes occur in total proteinuria.[11–13]

Although DN may be defined by both functional and structural criteria, functional criteria alone are generally used in clinical practice. The major functional parameter of DN is albumin excretion rate (AER), which may increase more than 100-fold during the evolution of DN (for example from 10 to 1000 µg/min). Biphasic changes in glomerular filtration rate (GFR), consisting of an initial increase followed by progressive decline, also occur in DN, but are not routinely used to define early stages of DN. Initial increases in AER and GFR, although very sensitive, are not always sufficiently specific to diagnose DN, and should be regarded as surrogate markers for the 'hard' clinical end point of a progressive decline in GFR, which occurs 10–15 years later. In unusual clinical circumstances or for research purposes, changes in AER and GFR need to be correlated with renal ultrastructural changes. Renal biopsy is particularly useful in distinguishing three entities occurring in older people with type 2 diabetes: non-diabetic renal disease, typical DN defined according to the original Kimmelstiel–Wilson criteria and atypical DN with a focus on renal interstitial and vascular changes (Figure 3.1).[14,15]

The five studies summarized in Figure 3.1 emphasize the heterogeneity of renal ultrastructural morphology in type 2 diabetes and demonstrate differences in classification of renal disease among different investigators. Two studies have related renal ultrastructural changes to the course of diabetic nephropathy in patients with type 2 diabetes. Ruggenenti et al[16] showed that the rate of decline of GFR is more closely related to the level of albuminuria than to renal ultrastructural category. Christensen et al[17] also showed that the level of

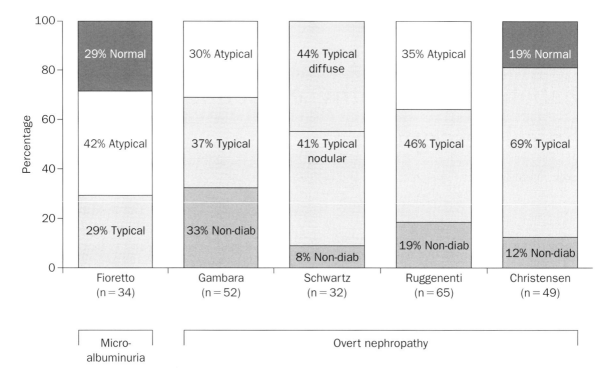

**Figure 3.1** Renal ultrastructure in patients with type 2 diabetes (data from Fioretto et al,[204] Gambara et al,[205] Ruggenenti et al[16] and Schwartz et al[206]). Note that the rate of decline in renal function correlated with degree of proteinuria rather than the histological type in the study by Ruggenenti et al.[16] Typical refers to the classical glomerular changes described for diabetic nephropathy.

albuminuria is related to the level of GFR loss but, in addition, demonstrated a faster rate of decline in GFR in patients with diabetic glomerulopathy than in patients with glomerulonephritis or normal glomerular structure.

Clinically, overt DN is characterized by a persistent increase in AER above 300 mg/24 hr (>200 µg/min) in timed samples or an albumin:creatinine ratio (ACR) of >30 mg/mmol (>300 mg/g) in spot urine samples. This is equivalent to total proteinuria exceeding 0.5 g/24 hr and is detectable by conventional dipstick tests. Overt DN is usually associated with hypertension and a decline in GFR, and is the late stage of a process that is difficult to arrest or reverse. It is now possible to diagnose nephropathy several years before progression to overt DN, by serial measurements of AER or ACR, which can monitor the transition from normoalbuminuria to microalbuminuria (AER of >20 µg/min, or ACR of >2.5 mg/mmol (>25 mg/g) for males—ACR of >3.5 mg/mmol (>35 mg/g) for females). This microalbuminuric stage is also called 'incipient nephropathy' in patients with type 1 diabetes. It should be appreciated that incipient and overt DN is

part of a continuum and that sequential measurement of AER in individual patients may show variable results and may not necessarily progress from one stage to the next.

## NATURAL HISTORY OF DN

The concept of the 'natural' history of DN implies the existence of a process leading to progressive renal damage, which eventually reaches ESRD. However, longitudinal studies of DN in patients with type 1 diabetes over the last 30 years strongly suggest that there has been an amelioration of the rate of progression of DN. Several studies have shown that the rate of progression of both early and late nephropathy in patients with type 1 diabetes and to a lesser extent in type 2 diabetes can be attenuated by intensive multifactorial intervention (Table 3.1). Interventions consisting of intensive glycaemic control for prevention of overt DN, and intensive blood-pressure control in patients with existing DN, have been the main contributors to the improved prognosis of DN in patients treated at specialized centres.[18] Arrest or

**Table 3.1 Potential contributors to the changing natural history of diabetic nephropathy.**

| Decade | Microalbuminuria | Glycaemic control | Blood pressure | Dyslipidaemia |
|---|---|---|---|---|
| 1980s | **1982–4** Concept of microalbuminuria predicting overt DN<br><br>**1988** Renoprotection by ACE inhibitors in normotensive microalbuminuric subjects with type 1 DM[194] | | **1984** Hypertension defined as 160/90 (WHO)[195] | **1985–90** Statins introduced for treatment of hypercholesterolaemia |
| 1990s | **1994** Reduction in AER predicts slowing of GFR decline during antihypertensive treatment[196]<br><br>**1995** Concept of microalbuminuria as incipient DN and independent target of therapy[49] | **1993** Intensive glycaemic control (HbA$_{1c}$ 7.2%) attenuates microvascular complications of type 1 diabetes (DCCT)[69]<br><br>**1998** Intensive glycaemic control (HbA$_{1c}$ 7.0%) attenuates microvascular complications of type 2 diabetes (UKPDS)[137] | **1993** Renoprotection by ACE inhibitors based on antihypertensive therapy in DN due to type 1 diabetes[197]<br><br>**1994** Hypertension defined as 140/90 (JNC-V)[156]<br><br>**1997–8** Recommendation to commence treatment at BP of 130/85 (JNC-VI and WHO–ISH)[157,158] | **1993–1998** Suggestion that lipid-lowering therapy reported to decrease microalbuminuria in type 2 diabetes,[198–200] although not a consistent finding[201] |
| 2000s | 'High-normal' AER predicts nephropathy[31,74,75] | | **2000** NKF recommends target BP of 130/80 in patients with type 2 diabetes[146]<br><br>**2001** Renoprotection by ARB-based therapy in DN due to type 2 diabetes (IDNT and RENAAL)[202,203] | |

DN = diabetic nephropathy, BP = blood pressure, ACE = angiotensin-converting enzyme, ARB = angiotensin receptor binder, DM = diabetes mellitus, GFR = glomerular filtration rate, HbA$_{1c}$ = glycosylated haemoglobin, WHO = World Health Organization, JNC = Joint National Committee, IDNT = Irbesartan Diabetic Nephropathy Trial, RENAAL = Reduction in Endpoints in NIDDM with the angiotensin-II antagonist losartan, UKPDS = United Kingdom Prospective Diabetes Study, NKF = National Kidney Foundation, WHO–ISH = World Health Organization–International Society of Hypertension.

**Table 3.2 Potential promoters of progression of diabetic nephropathy.**

| Reversible | Irreversible |
| --- | --- |
| Glycaemic control | Age |
| Blood pressure | Gender |
| Smoking | Race |
| Albuminuria | Ethnicity |
| Dyslipidaemia | Family history |
| | Duration of diabetes |

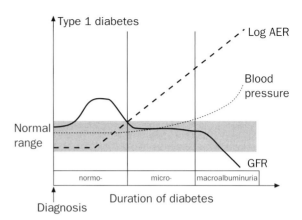

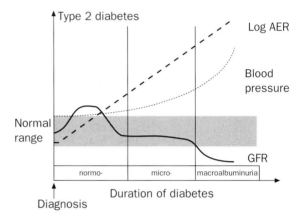

**Figure 3.2** The natural history of DN in type 1 and type 2 diabetes. The three stages, normo-, micro- and macroalbuminuria, last 5–10 years. Note that a rise in blood pressure generally precedes the onset of microalbuminuria in type 2 diabetes.

even reversal of overt DN has been documented in a small group of patients treated with intensive antihypertensive therapy based on inhibition of the renin-angiotensin system.[19,20] Other potential contributors to an improved prognosis of DN include a focus on new targets of therapy such as AER itself, dyslipidaemia and antismoking advice (Table 3.2). There is also emerging evidence of the potential benefits accruing from the treatment of endothelial dysfunction with ACE inhibitors, glitazones and aspirin.[21] Despite the potential for changing the natural history of DN with correct application of existing therapies, DN has become the main cause of ESRD in Western countries. This paradox may be explained by the dramatic increase in the incidence of type 2 diabetes associated with an affluent lifestyle as well as the failure of health-care systems to deliver intensive multifactorial intervention as a reasonable cost to people at risk of DN.[6] This failure of health-care delivery applies in particular to the early identification of patients at risk of DN by regular surveillance of AER or ACR.

## STAGES OF DN

The simplest classification of DN consists of three stages: microalbuminuria (incipient DN), lasting 5–15 years; macroalbuminuria (overt DN), lasting 5–10 years; and ESRD, lasting 3–6 years without renal replacement therapy (Figure 3.2). Mogensen has suggested a five-stage classification, with two additional stages preceding microalbuminuria, for patients with type 1 diabetes. These are (stage 1) renal enlargement associated with hyperfiltration and (stage 2) a silent stage with normal AER but glomerular ultrastructural changes including mesangial expansion and basement membrane thickening[22,23] (Table 3.3). Stage 1 may be present at

diagnosis while stage 2 may occur within 5 years of diagnosis and persist for many years. Transient microalbuminuria may be found in both of these early stages. Stages 1 and 2 are usually clinically 'silent' since estimation of GFR and renal biopsy are not performed routinely. However, early mesangial and basement membrane abnormalities are often found on renal biopsy in stage 1 or 2, if this is performed.

## HYPERFILTRATION AND DN

Enlargement of the kidneys (nephromegaly) and increase in GFR (hyperfiltration) occur frequently in untreated patients with type 1 diabetes, and both can be normalized by insulin treatment.[23] Patients with

**Table 3.3 Stages in diabetic renal disease (modified from Mogensen).[26]**

| Stage | Characteristics | Diabetes | Duration (years) | AER (µg/min) | BP (mmHg) | GFR (ml/min) | Treatment effects |
|---|---|---|---|---|---|---|---|
| 1. | Hyperfiltration and nephromegaly | Type 1 | 0–5 | ↑ then <20 | N | ↑ | |
| | | Type 2 | Not clearly defined | | ↑ | ↑ or N | Reversed by strict glycaemic control |
| 2. | Normoalbuminuria and ↑ GBMT and mesangial expansion | Type 1 | 5–15 | <20 | N | ↑ | Effects of BP control not documented |
| | | Type 2 | Not clearly defined | ↑130 10–20%/year | ↑ | N | |
| 3. | Microalbuminuria (incipient DN) | Type 1 | 10–20 | 20–200 | N then ↑ | N | Attenuated by strict glycaemic control; attenuated, arrested or reversed by strict BP control based on RAS inhibition |
| | | Type 2 | 0–15 | ↑20–40%/year | ↑ (↑Δ 3 mmHg/year) | ↓ 3–5/year | |
| 4. | Overt DN (macroalbuminuria) | Type 1 | 15–25 | > 200 | ↑ (↑Δ 5 mmHg/year) | ↓Δ 8–12/year* | Faster progression with poor glycaemic control (observational studies only) |
| | | Type 2 | 5–20† | | | ↓Δ 4–12/year* | |
| 5. | ESRD | Type 1 | 20–30 | > 200 | ↑ | ↓(< 20) | Attenuated by strict BP control based on RAS inhibition |
| | | Type 2 | 10–20† | | | | |

DN = diabetic nephropathy; in type 2 diabetes, this may include hypertensive, ischaemic, atherosclerotic and non-diabetic glomerular disease as well as DN, N = normal, GBMT = glomerular basement membrane thickening, BP = blood pressure, including isolated systolic BP in elderly people with type 2 diabetes, RAS = renin-angiotensin system. *Rise in serum creatinine is a late and insensitive index of progression of overt DN and indicates loss of 50% or more of renal function, †Many people with type 2 diabetes do not reach stage 4 or 5 because of increased cardiovascular mortality associated with stages 3 and 4.

particularly large kidneys have been shown to be at greater risk of the development of overt DN.[24]

In an 8-year study of 75 Swedish adolescents with type 1 diabetes, a high GFR after more than 8 years of diabetes predicted the development of DN, independently of glycaemic control.[25] The glomerular hyperfiltration preceded the onset of persistent microalbuminuria, and it was suggested that an elevated GFR takes part in the pathogenetic process heading to overt DN. Therefore, hyperfiltration was considered to represent the first stage in the development of DN.[26] However, 21 of the 45 patients with initial hyperfiltration (>125 ml/min per 1.73 m$^2$) were still normoalbuminuric after 8 years of follow-up, suggesting that a high GFR is a necessary, but not a sufficient, prerequisite for the development of DN. This concept is supported by earlier retrospective studies.[12] Although hyperfiltration has also been demonstrated in type 2 diabetes,[27] its possible link with the development of overt DN has not been explored in longitudinal studies.

Two difficulties remain in understanding the role of hyperfiltration in DN. Firstly, GFR may be increased transiently in association with hyperglycaemia[28] and, secondly, no prospective studies have been long enough to document a decrease in GFR in patients with hyperfiltration at baseline. Despite the above evidence linking hyperfiltration and nephromegaly with the subsequent development of DN, most diabetes centres do not include assessments of either parameter as part of routine clinical practice. This is partly because measurements of GFR and renal size are more time-consuming and expensive than measurement of AER.

## CONCEPT OF MICROALBUMINURIA

In the early 1980s three studies in type 1 diabetic patients linked the presence of increased amounts of albumin in the urine, as measured by immunoassay, to the subsequent development of overt DN 10–14 years later.[12,13,29,30] By consensus, this 'minimally raised' albumin excretion rate (AER of 30–300 mg/24 hr or 20–200 µg/min) has been termed 'microalbuminuria', because it cannot be detected by standard bedside tests, and overt nephropathy has been termed 'macroalbuminuria' (AER of >300 mg/24 hr or >200 µg/min). The terms 'normoalbuminuria', 'microalbuminuria' (incipient DN) and 'macroalbuminuria' do not refer to discrete, qualitatively different aspects of DN. They are part of a continuum, and serial measurements of AER in individual patients frequently transgress the boundaries between these

zones. Nevertheless, categorization of AER has facilitated communication between researchers and has simplified analysis of new therapeutic approaches. It is important to note that the lower limit of microalbuminuria exceeds the upper limit of AER in normal subjects, and recent studies have shown that AER levels in the range of 10–20 µg/min also predict progression to overt DN.[31]

The presence of microalbuminuria in patients with type 2 diabetes who are young and non-Caucasian is more likely to be associated with the development of renal disease,[32,33] whereas in elderly Caucasians it is more closely linked to cardiovascular disease.[34,35] In patients with type 2 diabetes and microalbuminuria, the rate of progression of AER over 7 years was found to be a powerful independent predictor of death from coronary heart disease.[36] Microalbuminuria is also associated with an increased risk of cardiovascular disease in subjects without diabetes.[37] In subjects at high risk of cardiovascular events enrolled in the Heart Outcomes Prevention Evaluation Study,[38] microalbuminuria was detected in 32.6% of subjects with diabetes and 14.8% of subjects without diabetes. Furthermore, the increase in risk of a further cardiovascular event was similar in non-diabetic subjects with microalbuminuria (approximately 1.5-fold) and diabetic subjects with microalbuminuria (approximately twofold).[39] Why microalbuminuria predicts cardiovascular events is not clear, but it may be a reflection of widespread vascular disease, as outlined in the Steno hypothesis.[40] Furthermore, endothelial dysfunction as evidenced by increased circulating levels of von Willebrand factor has been shown to precede the development of microalbuminuria in patients with type 1 diabetes.[41]

## CHOICE OF SCREENING MODALITY FOR ALBUMINURIA

A timed urine collection, either 24 hr or overnight, is the reference standard for microalbuminuria assessment. Because of high intraindividual variability,[42] transient elevations of AER into the microalbuminuric range occur frequently, and clinical assessment should therefore be based on at least three measurements taken over 3–6 months. Persistent microalbuminuria is confirmed when at least two out of three consecutive, timed urine collections are in the range 20–200 µg/min.[43] Expert committees recommend annual screening for microalbuminuria, usually with an albumin-to-creatinine ratio (ACR) on an early-morning urine sample,[44,45] a random sample[45,46] or a timed urine collection.[47] The use of a semiquantitative urine-testing strip is an alternative to laboratory testing by immunoassay.[48] If a screening test is positive, confirmation of microalbuminuria with a timed urine collection is generally recommended.[44,45,47] Albumin concentration alone, in a timed or spot urine collection, is prone to inaccuracies due to variation in urine volumes and is therefore not recommended. The choice of screening modality will depend upon physician preference, patient convenience, and the compliance and availability of laboratory services.

Screening is recommended from the time of diagnosis in all patients with type 2 diabetes and for all with type 1 diabetes of greater than 5 years' duration.[46] Several factors can confound the assessment of microalbuminuria, including urinary tract infection, heavy exercise, high dietary protein intake, congestive cardiac failure, acute febrile illness, metabolic decompensation, water loading and menstruation/vaginal discharge.[49] For accurate evaluation, testing should be postponed if these factors are present. Once microalbuminuria has been confirmed, ongoing monitoring may be done with either a timed urine collection or ACR measurement.[49,50]

ACR is considered a very good screening test for microalbuminuria, its sensitivity ranging from 88% to 100%.[51–57] The significant influence of sex on the relationship between the ACR and AER has been recognized,[53] and current guidelines for screening for microalbuminuria with the ACR reflect this, with recommended cutoffs of >2.5 and >3.5 mg/mmol (>25 and >35 mg/g) in males and females, respectively.[49] Previously, age has not been widely recognized as an important determinant in the interpretation of ACR. However, there is now some evidence to suggest that age-adjusted cutoffs for ACR may be appropriate.[58] Moreover, a recent study has investigated the effects of age and sex on the ability of a spot ACR to predict AER accurately. The spot ACR false-positive rate increased with age from 15.9% (40–65 years) to 31.8% (>65 years) in males and from 10.5% (45–65 years) to 28.3% (>65 years) in females. It was concluded that spot ACR is a good screening test for microalbuminuria, but a poor predictor of quantitative AER. The increase in spot ACR with age, relative to 24-hr AER, supports the use of sex- and age-adjusted ACR cutoff values.[59]

Despite the prognostic significance of microalbuminuria and hence the recommendation of annual testing, the frequency of annual screening for microalbuminuria in diabetes clinics remains low (<20%). Furthermore, patients are often not started on inhibitors of the renin-angiotensin system even when microalbuminuria is detected. Although there is good evidence that treating microalbuminuria prevents the progression to overt nephropathy, no controlled trials have been performed to assess the effectiveness of screening for microalbuminuria in preventing this outcome.[60,61]

## PREVALENCE AND INCIDENCE OF MICROALBUMINURIA IN PEOPLE WITH DIABETES

In adults with type 1 diabetes, the prevalence of microalbuminuria in clinic-based studies is of the order of 10–20%[62] and 15–30% in patients with type 2 diabetes,[62–64] being higher in clinic-based than in community-based studies. The prevalence of overt DN is about 10–20% in type 1 diabetes but varies in type 2 diabetes from 5% to 50% in different populations.[64–68] Microalbuminuria is uncommon in patients with less than 5 years' duration of type 1 diabetes. It reaches a peak incidence after 15–20 years' duration of type 1 diabetes and then falls progressively.[1] Estimates for the annual incidence rate of microalbuminuria in type 1 diabetes range from 2.5% to 5.0% per year.[62] In the Diabetes Control and Complications Trial, which was performed over 9 years in newly diagnosed patients with type 1 diabetes aged less than 35 years, the incidence of microalbuminuria varied from 4.5% per year in the control group given conventional therapy to 2.9% per year in the intensive glycaemic therapy group.[69]

In a nationwide cross-sectional study of overnight AER in 957 Danish children with type 1 diabetes aged 2–19 years with a mean diabetes duration of 6 years, persistent microalbuminuria was found in 4.3%.[70] The fact that a significant proportion of the study population was prepubertal may explain this low prevalence. Microalbuminuria occurs extremely rarely before puberty, and, in the same study, the prevalence of microalbuminuria was 2–4% before the age of 16 years and 12–13% in patients over 16 years. Other studies in paediatric clinics have reported a higher prevalence of microalbuminuria of approximately 20%.[71,72] It is likely that estimates of microalbuminuria prevalence in different studies reflect variations in age, diabetes duration, pubertal status, blood-glucose control and ethnicity, as well as variations in urine-collection protocols.

## PREDICTIVE VALUE OF AER BELOW THE MICROALBUMINURIC RANGE

A longitudinal study over 5 years was the first to suggest that incipient nephropathy begins below the accepted cutoff value for microalbuminuria. The 95th percentile for AER in non-diabetic subjects was 7.6 μg/min. Type 1 diabetic subjects with baseline AER between 7.6 and 20 μg/min showed a higher rate of progression from normoalbuminuria to microalbuminuria than type 1 diabetic subjects with baseline AER of <7.6 μg/min.[73]

Three recent studies have also suggested that DN may be predicted by AER levels that are above normal but below the microalbuminuric range. One study of 511 children with type 1 diabetes compared those who developed microalbuminuria over a 6-year period with those who did not progress. Children who developed microalbuminuria showed a higher baseline albumin:creatinine ratio, although it remained well within the normal range (progressors [n = 33] 1.0 mg/mmol [95% CI 0.6–2.1] versus non-progressors [n = 303] 0.8 mg/mmol [95% CI 0.6–1.2]).[74] A second study was performed in 1201 normoalbuminuric type 1 diabetic patients, of whom 4% developed overt DN over 5 years.[75] Patients with baseline AER in the range 7.4–19.1 mg/l had a relative risk of the development of DN nine times that of patients with lower baseline AER. Unfortunately, only a single early-morning urine sample was available at baseline, and albumin concentrations, rather than AER, were used. A third study was performed in 599 normoalbuminuric Israeli patients with type 2 diabetes over 8 years.[31] The patients were divided into three groups according to baseline AER (0–10, 10–20 and 20–30 mg/24 hr). In comparison to the 0–10 mg/24 hr group the risk ratio for progression to microalbuminuria over an 8-year follow-up was 2.34 (CI 1.32–4.43) in the middle group, and 12.36 (CI 8.9–16.5) in the upper group. There was also a significant increase in the rate of decline of GFR in the middle and upper baseline AER groups compared with the 0–10 mg/24 hr group. In addition, there was a highly significant relationship between baseline AER and cardiovascular events (death and non-fatal myocardial infarction), with higher rates of cardiovascular events in the two groups with AER of >10 mg/24 hour. All three of these recent studies are consistent with the concept that albuminuria is a continuous variable and that patients with AER of >10 mg/24 hr have an increased risk of progression to microalbuminuria, on the one hand, and cardiovascular disease, on the other hand, as originally suggested by Chase et al.[73]

The above studies support the concept that any rise in AER above normal should be considered evidence of an increased risk of progression to overt DN. These data suggest that clinically important increases in AER and ACR occur up to 5 years before the appearance of microalbuminuria. They also imply that measurements of AER/ACR should be performed in all patients more frequently than the current recommendation for yearly tests, that semi-quantitative categorical tests for the presence or absence of microalbuminuria are not optimal, and that patients with small, submicroalbuminuric increases in AER are at increased risk of progression to DN and macrovascular disease.

In contrast to the above results, a study from the University of Michigan has questioned the predictive power of microalbuminuria for the development of DN in a cohort of type 1 and type 2 diabetic patients.[76] Twenty-three diabetic patients with microalbuminuria in at least two separate urine specimens and 209 subjects without microalbuminuria were followed for 7 years. AER regressed to normal in 56% of patients with baseline microalbuminuria, whereas new microalbuminuria developed in 16% of patients without baseline microalbuminuria. Only 6% of patients with microalbuminuria at baseline progressed to DN, whereas 7% of normoalbuminuric patients matched for age, sex, duration of diabetes and diabetes type progressed to DN. The above results are in contrast to earlier reports showing that approximately 80% of patients with type 1 diabetes and microalbuminuria progress to DN[12,29] and have been criticized for lack of statistical power.[77]

Other studies from the USA have pointed out that the initial estimates of an 80% rate of progression from microalbuminuria to proteinuria in type 1 diabetes may have been an overestimate. Recent studies have observed a 30–45% risk of progression from microalbuminuria to proteinuria over 10 years, while about 30% of type 1 diabetic patients with microalbuminuria become normoalbuminuric and the rest remain microalbuminuric.[78] Furthermore, some normoalbuminuric, long-standing type 1 diabetic patients have well-established lesions of diabetic nephropathy on biopsy, and approximately 40% of all patients destined to progress to proteinuria are normoalbuminuric at initial screening despite many years of diabetes.[78] Other studies have documented regression of microalbuminuria, a finding which may indicate a calendar effect leading to a lower cumulative incidence of DN in type 1 diabetes.[79–81] A similar scenario is emerging in type 2 diabetic patients, although this has not been fully defined. It is unclear why there has been an apparent change in the predictive value of microalbuminuria for progression to overt nephropathy in the last 20 years. It is possible that this is due to changes in the natural history of DN resulting from improved glycaemic and blood-pressure control, or that the original studies overestimated the risk because of small sample sizes, post hoc analyses and/or variable definitions of microalbuminuria.[78] These data suggest that AER or ACR measurements may be unable to define patients who are safe from or at risk of DN with an accuracy that is adequate for optimal clinical decision making. However, further studies are needed to confirm or refute this new evidence. These results emphasize that 'persistent microalbuminuria' should not be defined on the basis of only one or two AER measurements, because the intraindividual variability of AER is over 30%.[42] It is advisable to perform more than two, and perhaps four, measurements in order to achieve confidence intervals within approximately 20% of the true mean for AER.[82]

## PREVALENCE OF MICROALBUMINURIA IN NORMAL SUBJECTS

The prevalence of microalbuminuria in the community depends on the characteristics of the study population. In healthy adults, mean AER is 5 µg/min and rarely exceeds 15 µg/min.[83] In another study in normal adults, median AER was 4 µg/min during the day (90th percentile 15 µg/min) and 3 µg/min overnight (90th percentile 10 µg/min).[84]

In 223 people aged 60–74 years selected as control subjects during systematic screening for diabetes in the municipality of Federicia, Denmark, median AER was 7.5 µg/min. During a mean follow-up of 6 years, 31 of the 223 people died, and the median AER in those who died was 15.0 µg/min. A baseline AER above the median value was associated with 23 deaths, while a baseline AER below the median value was associated with eight deaths.[34] Thus, an AER above the median value conferred about a threefold increase in risk of mortality in these elderly non-diabetic subjects. The above studies also demonstrated an association between an increased AER and risk factors for macrovascular disease such as age, male sex, hypertension and dyslipidaemia. By contrast, these factors did not influence albuminuria in paediatric populations. In normal children, the upper 95% confidence limit for overnight AER was 12.2 µg/min[85] and another study in normal children reported an upper 95% confidence limit of 10 µg/min per 1.73 m².[86]

## MICROALBUMINURIA AND CARDIOVASCULAR DISEASE

Although the prevalence of microalbuminuria is similar in type 1 and type 2 diabetes,[64] the rate of progression to overt DN is slower in elderly Caucasian patients with type 2 diabetes, being of the order of 20% over a decade, compared with approximately 80% within a decade for patients with type 1 diabetes in the original studies published in the early 1980s.[87] The cumulative risk of ESRD is also less in patients with type 2 diabetes, with one early study showing a cumulative risk of ESRD of 11%.[88] The main reason for this disparity is that most Caucasian patients with type 2 diabetes die from cardiovascular disease before developing DN,[89,90] therefore leading to survivor bias in published studies (Figure 3.3). Microalbuminuria has been identified as a predictor of increased mortality from cardiovascular disease in both type 1[91] and type 2 diabetes[13,35,92] and also in non-diabetic subjects.[37] In some but not all of these studies, microalbuminuria predicted mortality independently of other conventional cardiovascular risk factors such as dyslipidaemia, hypertension and smoking.

Two studies from the Steno Diabetes Centre in Denmark have described predictors of total mortality in patients with type 1 and type 2 diabetes. In the first study of 328 patients with type 2 diabetes over 5 years, the median AER at baseline was 8 mg/24 hr, and subjects with AER above the median value had a relative risk of all-cause mortality of 2.7. After 5 years of follow-up, 8% of patients with normoalbuminuria, 20% with microalbuminuria and 35% with macroalbuminuria had died (predominantly from cardiovascular causes). Predictors of all-cause mortality when examined by multivariate regression were pre-existing coronary heart disease (relative risk [RR] 2.9, 95% CI 1.6–5.1), AER (RR 1.9, 95% CI 1.4–2.6), HbA$_{1c}$ (RR 1.2, 95% CI 1.0–1.4) and age (RR 1.08, 95% CI 1.03–1.13). Predictors of cardiovascular mortality were pre-existing coronary heart disease (RR 6.1, 95% CI 2.8–13.5), macroalbuminuria (RR 2.5, 95% CI 1.1–5.8), 1% increase in HbA$_{1c}$ (RR 1.3, 95% CI 1.1–1.6) and a 10 mmHg rise in systolic blood pressure (RR 1.2, 95% CI 1.0–1.4).[93]

The second study from the Steno Diabetes Centre involved a 10-year follow-up in 1984–94 of 939 patients with 5 or more years' duration of type 1 diabetes.[94] Total mortality increased according to baseline level of AER. Ten-year total mortality was 15% in patients with normoalbuminuria, 25% in patients with microalbuminuria and 44% in macroalbuminuric patients. The median survival after onset of

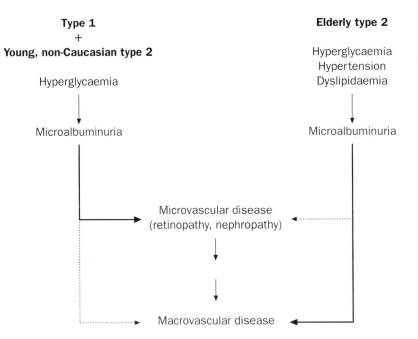

**Figure 3.3** Differing relationships of microalbuminuria to vascular disease in patients with type 1 diabetes and non-Caucasian type 2 diabetes compared with elderly patients with type 2 diabetes (modified from Jerums and Chattington[207]).

overt DN was 17.2 years. Multivariate regression analysis showed that the relative risk of all-cause mortality was 2.03 for male sex, 1.07 for age, 0.96 for height, 1.51 for smoking, 1.70 for lower social class, 1.45 for AER category, 1.63 for hypertension, 8.96 for serum creatinine and 1.11 for $HbA_{1c}$. Age, smoking, AER category and hypertension were also significant predictors of cardiovascular mortality. These results indicate that similar risk factors predict mortality in type 1 and type 2 diabetes.

The relationship of DN and cardiovascular mortality in patients with type 1 diabetes has been studied extensively by Borch-Johnsen in Denmark. Studies between 1933 and 1981 in a cohort of 1030 patients with type 1 diabetes showed a markedly increased relative risk of death in patients with overt DN compared to patients without DN.[95–97] Recent studies in some ethnic groups have suggested that the prognostic importance of proteinuria for cardiovascular disease in type 2 diabetes is considerably less than in type 1 diabetes. For instance, in studies in Pima Indians, proteinuria was shown to entail a 3.5-fold higher risk of death, and proteinuria combined with hypertension was associated with a sevenfold higher risk of death.[98] This compares with a 40-fold increase in risk of death entailed by proteinuria in patients with type 1 diabetes studied before 1952.[95]

## INCIDENCE OF DN

The incidence of DN is about 1–2% per year in patients with type 1 diabetes.[1,99] In younger patients of non-Caucasian origin with type 2 diabetes, such as the Pima Indians,[98] Japanese[66] and African Americans[100] the incidence of DN is similar to that in type 1 diabetes. By contrast, the incidence of overt DN is much lower in elderly Caucasian patients with type 2 diabetes.[101,102]

The cumulative incidence of overt DN after a 25–30-year duration of type 1 diabetes was 40–50% before 1942, but it decreased to 25–30% in patients diagnosed after 1953.[1,95] In the last 50 years, studies from specialized clinics indicate that there has been a significant decline in the incidence of DN in type 1 diabetes. There has been an opposite trend in the incidence of DN in type 2 diabetes, so that about half of patients presenting to ESRD management centres now have type 2 diabetes.[103]

## SECULAR TRENDS IN DN

Over the last 50 years, there have been opposite calendar effects on the incidence of DN in the two types of diabetes. In patients with type 1 diabetes, there has been a marked decrease in the incidence of DN as reported from specialized clinics.[1,5,104] By contrast, the incidence of DN associated with type 2 diabetes mellitus has increased over the last 50 years, so that in the USA about half of all patients now entering ESRD replacement programmes have diabetes (mostly type 2) compared with 25–50% in Europe and about 25% in Australia.[105] Earlier estimates suggested that only 5% of patients with type 2 diabetes developed ESRD.[106]

In patients with type 1 diabetes, it has been possible to assess the evolution of DN over intervals of 30 years or more. Early studies from the Joslin Clinic showed that the cumulative incidence of microalbuminuria was about 50%, and reached a plateau after 20 years of postpubertal duration of diabetes.[1] The cumulative incidence of overt DN (macroalbuminuria) in type 1 diabetes was about 30%, and that of ESRD was about 20% in early studies from the Joslin Clinic[1] and Denmark.[2] The median survival after diagnosis of persistent proteinuria was about 10 years, whereas recent studies from Denmark have documented a median survival of 17 years.[5] A similar pattern is seen in young, non-Caucasian patients with type 2 diabetes. This type of analysis assumes that patients must first pass through the stages of microalbuminuria and macroalbuminuria before developing ESRD. This concept has been challenged by studies that have shown that some patients develop impaired renal function[107] and also renal ultrastructural change of DN[78,108] without corresponding increases in AER.

There has been a progressive increase in median survival after diagnosis of overt DN over the last 50 years. The median survival in 45 type 1 diabetic patients after onset of nephropathy was reported as 5 years in 1971.[109] In a study of 360 patients with type 1 diabetes published in 1983, survival after diagnosis of DN was 7 years,[110] and in a study published in 1985, survival in 67 patients with type 1 diabetes was 10 years after onset of DN.[1] These survival times are much lower than the median survival of over 17.2 years after onset of DN in a study from the Steno Diabetes Centre published in 1996.[94] The improved survival in the later studies was attributed to aggressive, long-term antihypertensive treatment.

## ASSESSMENT OF RATE OF PROGRESSION OF DN

The rate of progression of early DN is most accurately assessed as a percentage rate of increase in AER per year. In patients with type 1 diabetes, the increase in AER within the microalbuminuric range is generally not associated with a decrease in GFR.[22] Once overt nephropathy develops, there is a progressive decline in GFR that can be assessed as an absolute decline in ml/min per year. In most patients with overt nephropathy and type 1 diabetes, the decrease in GFR approaches linearity and is of the order of 11 ml/min per year.[111] The most accurate method for measurement of GFR is the direct isotopic technique. Alternative and simpler approaches to assessment of changes in GFR include the reciprocal of serum creatinine, the time to doubling of serum creatinine, and calculation of glomerular filtration rate by the Cockcroft–Gault technique, which takes into account age, sex, height, weight and serum creatinine levels.[112] A more recent method of calculating GFR has been derived by the Modification of Diet in Renal Disease Group[113] and is based on age, creatinine, urea, serum albumin (Alb), sex and race:

$$\text{GFR} = 170 \times [P_{cr}]^{-0.999} \times [\text{age}]^{-0.176} \times [0.762 \text{ if patient is female}] \times [1.180 \text{ if patient is black}] \times [\text{SUN}]^{-0.170} \times [\text{Alb}]^{+0.318}$$

$P_{cr}$ = serum creatinine concentration (mg/dl);
SUN = serum urea nitrogen concentration (mg/dl)

Timed creatinine clearance measurements, which are often used as a surrogate for GFR, underestimate hyperfiltration and overestimate low GFR,[114] and they are subject to urine-collection error.

In a study from the Joslin Clinic published in 1985, 10 years after the onset of proteinuria, 50% of type 1 diabetic patients progressed to ESRD.[1] By contrast, 3–11% of patients with type 2 diabetes progressed to ESRD 10 years after the onset of proteinuria in an analysis of several studies published in 1988.[115] However, in studies in Pima Indians, 65% of patients with type 2 diabetes progressed to ESRD 10 years after onset of proteinuria.[116] These marked differences in progression of DN to ESRD are likely to be explained by a relative resistance to cardiovascular disease in the younger Pima Indians. A further analysis in Pima Indians with type 2 diabetes showed that 97% of the excess mortality in these subjects was associated with proteinuria, 16% of the deaths being related to ESRD and 22% to cardiovascular disease.[117]

## PROGRESSION PROMOTERS OF DN

In patients with overt DN and in the absence of intensive glycaemic and blood-pressure control, AER increases at 20–40% per year and GFR declines at approximately 11 ml/min per year.[118,119] Since there is an exponential relationship between GFR and serum creatinine, the rate of decline in renal function, which is in the order of 10 ml/min per year, is not easily recognizable, while serum creatinine levels remain within the normal range. Yearly increments in serum creatinine are small until levels exceed 90 µmol/l in females and 110 µmol/l in males. Timed creatinine-clearance measurements or GFR calculated by the Cockcroft–Gault[112] or Modification of Diet in Renal Disease (MDRD) formula[113] are other options for more accurate assessment of early changes in GFR.

There are several potential progression promoters of DN, both reversible and irreversible, the most important being glycaemic control and blood pressure (Table 3.3). The relative importance of individual progression promoters of DN has been examined by multivariate analysis. In the Wisconsin study, odds ratios were calculated for the development of overt proteinuria in patients with type 2 diabetes.[120] The odds ratios were 2.5 (95% CI 1.5–4.0) for systolic blood pressure, 2.4 (95% CI 1.3–4.3) for total pack years smoked and 2.17 (95% CI 1.2–3.8) for $HbA_{1c}$ of ≥8.7%. In a UK study, the odds ratios for the development of microalbuminuria were 3.7 (95% CI 1.2–11.3) for current smoking and 2.3 (95% CI 1.3–3.9) for fasting plasma glucose in patients with type 2 diabetes.[121] Dyslipidaemia has also been reported as a progression promoter for DN, although the evidence is not as strong as for glycaemic control, blood pressure and smoking.[92,122] Studies in patients with type 1 diabetes have shown similar results.[123]

## GLYCAEMIC CONTROL AND DN

DN does not occur in the absence of hyperglycaemia, and glycaemic control is the main determinant of the onset of DN in both type 1 and type 2 diabetes. However, glycaemic control may interact with other risk factors such as hypertension, dyslipidaemia and smoking to promote the development and progression of DN. Incipient nephropathy (microalbuminuria) is closely associated with $HbA_{1c}$ levels over 8.0% in type 1[124–126] and also in type 2 diabetic patients.[127,128] In an observational, clinic-based study in type 1 and type 2 diabetic patients, the per cent rate of increase in AER was closely related to mean $HbA_{1c}$ levels over 9 years.[129] Observational studies in type 1 patients with overt nephropathy have shown that the rate of decline of GFR is related to glycaemic control.[130] The Diabetes Control and Complications Trial (DCCT)[69] in type 1 diabetes and the UK Prospective Diabetes Study (UKPDS)[131] in type 2 diabetes have shown that there is a strong relationship

between $HbA_{1c}$ and diabetic microvascular disease, both retinal and renal, without a clear-cut $HbA_{1c}$ threshold. In addition, the DCCT data suggest that the relationship is curvilinear in type 1 diabetic patients; that is, the tendency to develop microvascular disease per unit increase in $HbA_{1c}$ is greater at higher $HbA_{1c}$ levels than at lower levels.[69] By contrast, in type 2 diabetes, there was a linear relationship between systolic blood pressure and the incidence of microvascular endpoints (Figure 3.4) over the range of 120–160 mmHg.[132]

The aetiological role of hyperglycaemia in the development and progression of DN is supported by the effects of pancreas transplantation on the morphological changes of both transplanted and native kidneys. In patients who have already received a renal transplant, a subsequent pancreatic transplant prevents any progression of the morphological changes associated with DN over a follow-up period of approximately 2 years.[133] Furthermore, the structural changes of DN can even be reversed in native kidneys after pancreatic transplantation, but it takes 10 years of normoglycaemia to demonstrate this effect.[14] By contrast, the use of intensive insulin therapy after the onset of overt DN has not been shown to improve its course in a controlled trial.[134,135] In patients with existing microalbuminuria, the DCCT and a meta-analysis of seven other studies in type 1 diabetic patients[136] showed that intensive glycaemic control reduced the progression to overt DN. In type 2 diabetic patients, tight glycaemic control reduced the development of overt DN in the UKPDS.[137]

In summary, hyperglycaemia is a prerequisite for the development of DN, and two large studies have shown that intensive glycaemic control attenuates the development of DN in patients with type 1 diabetes and type 2 diabetes. However, the UKPDS was not sufficiently powered to show whether the rate of development of overt DN was attenuated in type 2 diabetic patients with existing microalbuminuria. In patients with type 2 diabetes and microalbuminuria, intensive glycaemic control is associated with a decreased rate of progression of AER, but not renal function as measured by creatinine clearance.[138]

## THE RELATIONSHIP OF BLOOD PRESSURE TO DN

In early observational studies of the natural history of DN, about 80% of patients with type 1 diabetes and persistent microalbuminuria showed progressive increases in AER of 10–30% per year to the stage of overt DN over 10–15 years.[139] In a later study,

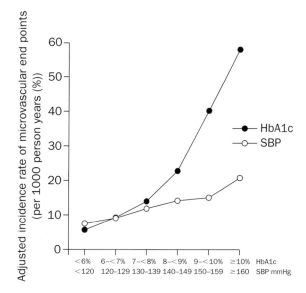

**Figure 3.4** Observational analysis from the UK Prospective Diabetes Study of the relationship between microvascular end points and HbA$_{1c}$[131] and systolic blood pressure[132] in patients with type 2 diabetes. Note the exponential increase in the risk of microvascular end points at higher levels of HbA$_{1c}$, compared with the linear relationship with blood pressure.

18.6% of type 1 diabetic patients with microalbuminuria developed overt DN over a period of 5 years, compared to 1.8% of normoalbuminuric patients.[79]

The terms 'incipient' and 'overt' nephropathy have also been applied to patients with increased AER and type 2 diabetes. This presents few problems in younger patients, in whom the prognostic implications of persistent microalbuminuria are similar to those in type 1 diabetes. However, an increase in AER to the microalbuminuric range does not necessarily equate with 'incipient nephropathy' in elderly patients with type 2 diabetes. In this group of elderly patients, approximately 20% progress to overt nephropathy over 10–14 years. Microalbuminuria in the elderly is also associated with large vessel disease and may lead to fatal cardiovascular events.[13,34,35] This lowers the predictive value of microalbuminuria for overt DN due to survival bias. At present, there is no simple test to determine whether microalbuminuria is a predictor of cardiovascular disease whether it represents a stage in the development of overt diabetic nephropathy or whether it predicts both cardiovascular and renal disease in a particular patient. The presence of microalbuminuria in association with retinopathy would suggest that a renal association is most likely.

A high rate of increase in AER in patients with type 2 diabetes and microalbuminuria has usually been interpreted to indicate a renal association signifying a progression towards overt DN. Although this association may be present, a recent study has demonstrated that the rate of progression of AER over 7 years in patients with type 2 diabetes is also a powerful independent predictor of death from coronary heart disease.[36] Patients with type 2 diabetes, macroalbuminuria and retinopathy are more likely to have the typical renal ultrastructural features of DN than similar patients without retinopathy.[140]

In type 1 diabetes, the evolution of micro- to macroalbuminuria is usually accompanied by an increase in blood pressure. Some studies show that an increase in blood pressure follows the onset of microalbuminuria in patients with type 1 diabetes,[141,142] while others suggest either a close association or that a rise in blood pressure precedes the onset of microalbuminuria.[143] By contrast, in elderly patients with type 2 diabetes, a rise in blood pressure usually precedes the onset of microalbuminuria.[64,143] Regardless of the sequence, the combination of hypertension and microalbuminuria promotes an accelerated increase in AER and a decline in GFR. This is likely to be mediated by dilatation of the afferent glomerular arteriole, which allows transmission of elevated systemic blood pressure to the glomerulus.[144] Conversely, the development of DN is attenuated by renal artery stenosis, which reduces the transmission of systemic blood pressure to the glomerulus.[145]

Mogensen was the first to show that the presence of hypertension accelerates the development of renal failure in patients with overt DN.[111] Although there is general agreement that raised blood pressure, even within what was traditionally considered the normal range, accelerates DN, it is less clear which component of blood pressure (systolic, diastolic, pulse or mean) is the mediator of renal damage. An overview of ten clinical studies of antihypertensive therapy has shown that the rate of fall of GFR in established DN increases in proportion to the level of mean arterial pressure (MAP).[146] The rate of decline in GFR approaches zero when MAP is reduced to less than 90 mmHg, equivalent to 120/75 mmHg. One study in elderly Danish patients with type 2 diabetes and an Australian study have suggested that systolic blood pressure relates to the rate of progression of albuminuria.[147,148] However, definitive comparisons of the relative roles of systolic, diastolic, pulse pressure and MAP in promoting renal injury have not been performed. By contrast, systolic blood pressure and pulse pressure were more closely related to macrovascular events than diastolic blood pressure in a reanalysis of the Framingham Study.[149]

The increase in blood pressure during the evolution of DN is detected more sensitively by 24-hr ambulatory blood-pressure monitoring than by office blood-pressure measurements. In patients with type 1 diabetes, abnormalities in 24-hr blood pressure and autonomic function have been related to small increases in AER below the microalbuminuric range[150] and are also seen in overt DN.[151,152] Furthermore, loss of the normal nocturnal drop in blood pressure in evolving DN may contribute to an increase in overall blood-pressure load without detection by office blood-pressure readings.[153,154]

In type 2 diabetes, the relation between blood pressure and DN differs from that in type 1 diabetes. Hypertension may precede the diagnosis of type 2 diabetes and microalbuminuria in elderly Caucasian people and in Pima Indians. In addition, microalbuminuria may precede the diagnosis of type 2 diabetes.[128] Furthermore, progressive changes in the definition of hypertension in diabetic patients have required a reappraisal of the prevalence of hypertension, especially in type 2 DM. The threshold for diagnosis of hypertension in people with diabetes has fallen from 160/95 in 1969[155] to 140/90 in 1993.[156] Two recent consensus statements (1997–9) recommend that antihypertensive therapy should be considered if blood pressure exceeds 130/85.[157,158] The prevalence of hypertension in type 2 diabetes mellitus has been estimated at approximately 80% in a clinic-based study using JNC-V guidelines,[143] and the community-based AusDiab study has estimated that 70% of Australian people with type 2 diabetes are hypertensive.[159] By contrast, less than 5% of normoalbuminuric type 1 diabetic patients are hypertensive, this rate rising to above 20% in microalbuminuric patients and above 80% in overt DN.[160]

The natural history is for blood pressure to increase by 3–4 mmHg per year in type 1 diabetic patients with microalbuminuria and approximately 6 mmHg per year in overt DN.[22] Similar changes in blood pressure occur in type 2 diabetic patients during the evolution of DN, but are more difficult to define because most patients are already on antihypertensive treatment. Two early studies from Germany and Austria have shown similar rates of development of DN and similar rates of progression to ESRD in patients with type 1 or type 2 diabetes. In the German study, 312 patients with type 1 diabetes and 464 patients with type 2 diabetes were followed for at least 2 years. There was a similar risk of development of overt nephropathy of 10–15% and raised serum creatinine levels (>123 mmol/l) occurred with a cumulative risk of 60–70% over 3 years in patients with type 1 or type 2 diabetes.[161]

In the Austrian study, the rate of progression from clinically overt nephropathy with baseline creatinine clearance of >70 ml/min per 1.73 m$^2$ to the start of dialysis was compared in 16 people with type 1 and 16 people with type 2 diabetes.[162] There was a similar rate of progression of nephropathy in patients with either type of diabetes, with a mean rate of decline of creatinine clearance of about 0.9 ml/min per month. Dialysis was started after a mean interval of 81 (40–124) months in patients with type 2 diabetes and 77 (44–133) months in patients with type 1 diabetes. Higher blood-pressure levels during the study were associated with a more rapid progression to dialysis in both type 1 and type 2 diabetes. However, the similar rate of progression of DN in its later stages in type 1 and type 2 diabetic patients documented in the above studies is at variance with similar studies of early DN, which have shown a slower rate of progression from microalbuminuria to macroalbuminuria in type 2 diabetes. The main characteristics of diabetic nephropathy in patients with type 1 and type 2 diabetes are summarized in Table 3.4.

## DYSLIPIDAEMIA AND DN

Type 2 diabetes is one component of the metabolic syndrome which includes impaired glucose tolerance, insulin resistance, central obesity, hypertension, combined dyslipidaemia, impaired fibrinolysis and hyperuricaemia.[163] Microalbuminuria has also been linked to this pattern of metabolic disturbances.[164] In the Third National Health and Nutrition Examination Survey from the USA, unadjusted and age-adjusted prevalences of the metabolic syndrome were 21.8% and 23.7%, respectively.[165] This indicates that dyslipidaemia often coexists with microalbuminuria in patients with impaired glucose tolerance or type 2 diabetes. A cross-sectional study of type 2 diabetic patients from the UK showed that microalbuminuria was associated with hypertriglyceridaemia and also low high-density lipoprotein (HDL) cholesterol.[166] In a longitudinal study of 574 Israeli patients followed for 8 years, high baseline total cholesterol and low baseline HDL cholesterol predicted the development of microalbuminuria in univariate analyses, with odds ratios of 20.6 (CI 12.7–33.5) for cholesterol and 7.8 (CI 5.2–11.6) for HDL. A multiple logistic-regression analysis showed that total cholesterol was a major determinant of the subsequent decline in renal function.[122]

**Table 3.4  Diabetic nephropathy in patients with type 1 or type 2 diabetes.**

|  | Type 1 diabetes | Type 2 diabetes (elderly Caucasian or young non-Caucasian) |
|---|---|---|
| Percentage developing diabetic nephropathy | ~30% | 15–45% |
| Prevalence of: |  |  |
| microalbuminuria | 10–20% | 15–30% |
| macroalbuminuria | 10–20% | 5–50% |
| Percentage progressing: |  |  |
| incipient → overt nephropathy | 80% | 50–80% |
| overt nephropathy → ESRD | 50% | 10–50% |
| Rate of progression from onset of overt DN to ESRD* | 5–20 years | 5–25 years |
| Hypertension | Accompanies progression of micro- to macroalbumuria | Precedes microalbuminuria |
| Histological characteristics | Kimmelstiel–Wilson diffuse and nodular glomerulosclerosis, and interstitial fibrosis | Three patterns: typical DN, atypical DN, non-diabetic renal disease |

*In general, the rate of progression from micro- to macroalbuminuria is slower in elderly patients with type 2 diabetes than in type 2 diabetes. However, once overt nephropathy is present, the rate of progression to ESRD is similar in type 1 and type 2 diabetes.

In type 1 diabetes, microalbuminuria is associated with a high prevalence of dyslipidaemia,[35] which is more pronounced in overt nephropathy.[167] In longitudinal studies, the determinants of progression of microalbuminuria to overt DN include serum cholesterol in type 1 diabetes[168] and serum triglycerides in type 2 diabetes.[169] The relationship between DN and dyslipidaemia, as well as between DN and blood pressure, is complicated by the fact that DN may be causally related to both parameters. Therefore, to distinguish cause and effect, it is necessary to perform longitudinal studies. In an Australian study involving 666 patients with type 2 diabetes over 7 years, baseline serum triglyceride levels were significantly associated with urine albumin concentration over 30 mg/l after logarithmic transformation of triglycerides and adjustment for other risk factors.[92] In an Israeli study of 574 patients with type 2 diabetes over 7.8 years, total cholesterol predicted the risk of development of microalbuminuria and total cholesterol also predicted a decline in renal function.[122] By contrast, serum cholesterol and triglycerides were not related to the development of microalbuminuria in a UK study.[121]

Some small studies (Table 3.1) have suggested that cholesterol-lowering therapy may lower AER. However, this has not been confirmed by other studies, and large, long-term, multicentre studies will need to be performed to resolve this question.

## ASSOCIATION OF RETINOPATHY WITH NEPHROPATHY

Although clinically recognized diabetic retinopathy is more common than DN, it is likely that DN would be diagnosed more frequently if morphological criteria, based on renal biopsy, were used.[22] In patients with type 1 diabetes, microalbuminuria has been shown to predict proliferative retinopathy,[170] and early nephropathy has been shown to predict vision-threatening retinal disease.[171]

Patients with DN usually have diabetic retinopathy. Both complications share the risk factors of poor glycaemic control, raised blood pressure and long duration of diabetes.[172,173] However, while nearly all patients with type 1 diabetes eventually develop retinopathy, only about a third develop clinically

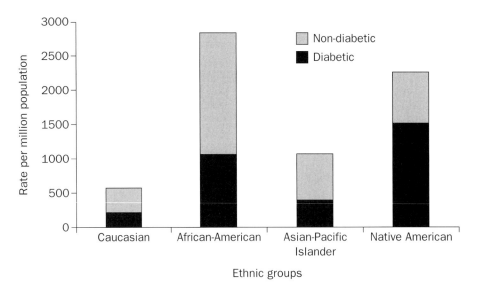

**Figure 3.5** The prevalence of end-stage renal disease (ESRD) as the result of diabetic and non-diabetic causes in the USA in 1994–7 (modified from Agodoa[179]).

overt DN (macroalbuminuria).[174] The EURODIAB study showed that the prevalence of retinopathy in type 1 diabetes was positively correlated with blood pressure, in those with and without DN, but the increase in prevalence of retinopathy with higher blood-pressure levels was more marked in those with DN than those without.[175] Furthermore, in people with retinopathy, AER increased exponentially with increasing blood-pressure, whereas in people without retinopathy there was no rise in AER with increasing blood pressure.[176] In type 2 diabetes, retinopathy correlates with glomerular ultra-structural changes, but some patients have protein-uria without overt retinopathy.[177] Preliminary unpublished data from the Irbesartan Diabetic Nephropathy Trial (IDNT) suggests that the presence of retinopathy in patients with type 2 diabetes and nephropathy increases the risk of progressive renal disease. Conversely, in the absence of retinopathy, the prevalence of non-diabetic renal disease in patients with macroalbuminuria has been estimated to be approximately 30%.[178]

## ETHNIC AND RACIAL DIFFERENCES IN THE INCIDENCE OF DIABETIC RENAL DISEASE

Several large population studies[6,179,180] have established that substantial ethnic and racial differences exist in the incidence rates of ESRD attributable to type 2 diabetes (Figure 3.5).[179] Even after accounting

for the higher prevalence of type 2 diabetes in some populations, we find that variations in the incidence of diabetic ESRD still persist. This suggests that some ethnic groups have an inherent susceptibility to diabetic renal disease. High rates of diabetic ESRD have been reported in Native Americans, African-Americans, Hispanics, Asians, Australian and Canadian aborigines, Pacific Islanders and New Zealand Maoris than in whites. These differences in the prevalence of diabetic renal disease are also associated with variations in rates of hypertension, coronary artery disease and other metabolic abnormalities.

Ethnic and racial differences in the incidence of DN have their origins in a complex interplay between genetic and environmental factors. Recently, the susceptibility factors associated with the development of DN in transitional and disadvantaged populations have been reviewed.[181] Familial clustering of DN has been reported in Pima Indians, black Americans, Brazilian patients and Caucasians.[182] At present, the genes responsible for the presumed inheritance of susceptibility have not been identified. Candidate genes include the angiotensin-I-converting enzyme and the Na/H anti-porter genes, which may predispose to hypertension. In Pima Indians, segregation analysis has suggested that there is a major gene, inherited in a codominant fashion, that is associated with an increased risk of the development of DN.[183] In utero programming may also be an important factor. Fetal malnutrition possibly results in impaired nephron development, as infants of low birth weight have fewer glomeruli than those of normal birth weight. In support of this concept, it has been shown that adult Australian aborigines who had a low birth weight have a higher prevalence of microalbuminuria compared with those of normal birth weight. There is also evidence to suggest that high glucose levels may damage the developing nephron. Pima Indians exposed in utero to diabetes have a four times greater chance of having an elevated albumin excretion rate than infants born as a result of a pregnancy not complicated by diabetes.[184] The relatively early onset of diabetes, poor glycaemic control, hypertension, dyslipidaemia and the effects of poor nutrition, coupled with limited access to health care, are all possible factors that may promote the development of DN in disadvantaged populations.

Pima Indians have the world's highest reported incidence and prevalence of type 2 diabetes, and the development of diabetic complications has been studied extensively in this population. Pima Indians under the age of 25 years frequently develop type 2 diabetes, and the prevalence of diabetes after 45 years of age is approximately 60%, which is almost 13 times greater than in Caucasians. In this population, ESRD as a result of DN is the leading cause of death. The cumulative incidence of ESRD in Pima Indians after the onset of clinically detectable proteinuria has been reported to be 40% at 10 years and 61% at 15 years. In contrast, ESRD develops in only 11% of Caucasians after 10 years of proteinuria and in 17% after 15 years.[33] The relatively young age of onset of diabetes and the low rate of coronary artery disease partly explain the high incidence of ESRD. High blood pressure has also been found to contribute to the development of diabetic renal disease in Pima Indians. However, once clinical proteinuria has occurred in this population, blood pressure does not appear to be a significant promoter in the progression of ESRD.[33] This contrasts with studies involving other populations that suggest that hypertension is an important promoter of the progression of diabetes-related ESRD.[6,100]

It is well known that the prevalence of ESRD is greater in African-Americans than whites. Although diabetes has accounted for this increase to some extent, blacks having a 2.6-fold increased risk of developing diabetic ESRD compared to Caucasians,[100] primary hypertension has often been reported to be the most common cause. This high incidence of ESRD as a result of hypertension may in part be due to a classification error, as a recent UK study has suggested that the incidence of ESRD attributable to hypertension in blacks has been overestimated. This study was a retrospective case review, which validated the underlying cause of renal failure for blacks admitted to three large London hospitals. After validation, the percentage of cases of ESRD with a diagnosis of diabetes increased to 38% and those with hypertension decreased to 10%. In contrast, there was no significant change in the diagnosis given to white patients.[185] Black patients with type 2 diabetes have also been reported to have a relatively high prevalence of microalbuminuria despite a short duration of diabetes. In a study of 1044 blacks with type 2 diabetes attending an outpatient clinic in Atlanta, USA, with a mean duration of diabetes of 5 months, microalbuminuria was detected in 23% and macroalbuminuria in 3.8% of patients. Risk factors identified for the presence of microalbuminuria included male sex, poor glycaemic control, endogenous hyperinsulinaemia, high blood pressure, high triglyceride levels and obesity.[186]

A high incidence of DN has been reported for Hispanics. The prevalence of microalbuminuria is approximately 31% and there is a sixfold increase in the incidence of diabetic ESRD when compared to non-Hispanic whites.[187] This population also has a significantly increased risk (odds ratio 2.13, CI 1.34, 95% 3.37, $P = 0.0013$) of retinopathy when compared to non-Hispanic whites, even after controlling for the severity and duration of diabetes. There is also accumulating evidence that patients with type 2 diabetes in India, Japan and Korea have a high prevalence of microalbuminuria and diabetes-related ESRD[188–191] compared with Caucasians.

Dyck has explored the factors associated with the 'epidemic' of diabetic ESRD among Canada's indigenous population.[192] The major contributing factors were a dramatic increase in the incidence of type 2 diabetes over the last half century and the higher rates of ESRD per se among aboriginal people with diabetes. Indeed, after accounting for differences in the rates of diabetes between aboriginal and non-aboriginal people of Saskatchewan, the risk ratio for diabetic ESRD was still 7.0 (95% CI 4.9–9.9) times greater for the aboriginal population. The reasons for these differences are most likely multifactorial in origin, involving both genetic and environmental factors. Possible factors include a younger age of onset of diabetes and diabetic nephropathy among aboriginal people, as in the Pima Indians, leading to a greater likelihood of survival to the stage of ESRD.

An epidemic of ESRD had also been reported in aboriginal communities in the Northern Territory of Australia. Incidence rates are 21 times higher than in non-aboriginal Australians. Although multiple factors, including post-streptococcal glomerulonephritis, have been implicated, an increased prevalence of

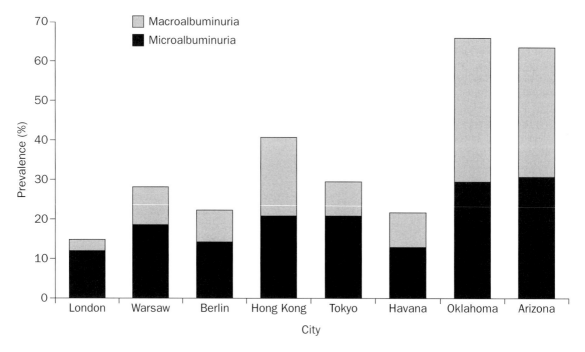

**Figure 3.6** The prevalence (percentage) of microalbuminuria and macroalbuminuria recorded at eight different diabetes centres (modified from Bennett et al[180]).

diabetes remains an important contributing factor. Indeed, diabetic nephropathy is the leading cause of ESRD in aboriginal Australians, accounting for approximately 42% of cases.[193] In aboriginal communities in the Northern Territory, microalbuminuria has been detected in 34% and macroalbuminuria in 30% of the adult population. There is a high incidence of overt albuminuria at every age in aboriginal persons with diabetes compared to those without diabetes. Diabetic nephropathy has also been reported to be the primary cause of ESRD in New Zealand Maoris and in Pacific Islanders, accounting for 61% and 49% of cases, respectively.[6]

The prevalence of microalbuminuria, overt DN and diabetes-related ESRD varies widely around the world. Although not a population-based study, the prevalence of microalbuminuria for diabetic patients attending eight centres in seven different countries has been reported to vary between 12% and 31% (mean 19.7%), the prevalence of macroalbuminuria varying between 3% and 37% (mean 15.6%).[180] The prevalence of increased albumin excretion rate was highest for Native Americans followed by Asians (Figure 3.6). Much of the variation in the prevalence of abnormal albumin excretion remains unexplained. However, regardless of the genetic background of patients attending the different centres, the associa-

tion between a raised albumin excretion and risk factors, such as hypertension, smoking and vascular complications, was similar at all centres.

Although a worldwide increase in the incidence of type 2 diabetes is contributing to an epidemic of diabetes-related ESRD, disadvantaged and transitional populations are disproportionately affected. Factors contributing to the high incidence rates of diabetic renal disease in these groups include a complex interplay between genetic susceptibility, age of onset of diabetes, glycaemic control, hypertension, obesity, smoking, socio-economic factors and access to health care.

## REFERENCES

1. Krolewski AS, Warram JH, Christlieb AR et al, The changing natural history of nephropathy in type I diabetes, *Am J Med* (1985) **78**: 785–94.
2. Andersen AR, Christiansen JS, Andersen JK et al, Diabetic nephropathy in type 1 (insulin-dependent) diabetes: an epidemiological study, *Diabetologia* (1983) **25**: 496–501.
3. ADA, American Diabetes Association Clinical Practice Recommendations 2001, *Diabetes Care* (2001) **24**(Suppl 1): S69–72.
4. Fabre J, Balant LP, Dayer PG et al, The kidney in maturity onset diabetes mellitus: a clinical study of 510 patients, *Kidney Int* (1982) **21**: 730–8.
5. Parving HH, Jacobsen P, Rossing K et al, Benefits of long-term

antihypertensive treatment on prognosis in diabetic nephropathy, *Kidney Int* (1996) **49:** 1778–82.

6. Ritz E, Rychlik I, Locatelli F et al, End-stage renal failure in type 2 diabetes: a medical catastrophe of worldwide dimensions, *Am J Kidney Dis* (1999) **34:** 795–808.

7. Forsblom CM, Groop PH, Ekstrand A et al, Predictive value of microalbuminuria in patients with insulin-dependent diabetes of long duration, *BMJ* (1992) **305:** 1051–3.

8. Krolewski AS, Warram JH, Rand LI et al, Epidemiologic approach to the etiology of type I diabetes mellitus and its complications, *N Engl J Med* (1987) **317:** 1390–8.

9. Kimmelstiel P, Wilson C, Intercapillary lesions in the glomeruli in the kidney, *Am J Pathol* (1936) **12:** 83–97.

10. Keen H, Chlouverakis C, An immunoassay method for urinary albumin at low concentrations, *Lancet* (1963) **2:** 913–14.

11. Mogensen CE, Christensen CK, Vittinghus E, The stages in diabetic renal disease. With emphasis on the stage of incipient diabetic nephropathy, *Diabetes* (1983) **32**(Suppl 2): 64–78.

12. Mogensen CE, Christensen CK, Predicting diabetic nephropathy in insulin-dependent patients, *N Engl J Med* (1984) **311:** 89–93.

13. Mogensen CE, Microalbuminuria predicts clinical proteinuria and early mortality in maturity-onset diabetes, *N Engl J Med* (1984) **310:** 356–60.

14. Fioretto P, Steffes MW, Sutherland DE et al, Reversal of lesions of diabetic nephropathy after pancreas transplantation, *N Engl J Med* (1998) **339:** 69–75.

15. Fioretto P, Stehouwer CD, Mauer M et al, Heterogeneous nature of microalbuminuria in NIDDM: studies of endothelial function and renal structure, *Diabetologia* (1998) **41:** 233–6.

16. Ruggenenti P, Gambara V, Perna A et al, The nephropathy of non-insulin-dependent diabetes: predictors of outcome relative to diverse patterns of renal injury, *J Am Soc Nephrol* (1998) **9:** 2336–43.

17. Christensen PK, Larsen S, Horn T et al, Renal function and structure in albuminuric type 2 diabetic patients without retinopathy, *Nephrol Dial Transplant* (2001) **16:** 2337–47.

18. Gaede P, Vedel P, Parving HH et al, Intensified multifactorial intervention in patients with type 2 diabetes mellitus and microalbuminuria: the Steno type 2 randomised study, *Lancet* (1999) **353:** 617–22.

19. Rodby RA, Firth LM, Lewis EJ, An economic analysis of captopril in the treatment of diabetic nephropathy. The Collaborative Study Group, *Diabetes Care* (1996) **19:** 1051–61.

20. Rodby RA, Firanek CA, Cheng YG et al, Reproducibility of studies of peritoneal dialysis adequacy, *Kidney Int* (1996) **50:** 267–71.

21. Calles-Escandon J, Cipolla M, Diabetes and endothelial dysfunction: a clinical perspective, *Endocr Rev* (2001) **22:** 36–52.

22. Mogensen CE, Microalbuminuria, blood pressure and diabetic renal disease: origin and development of ideas, *Diabetologia* (1999) **42:** 263–85.

23. Mogensen CE, Andersen MJ, Increased kidney size and glomerular filtration rate in untreated juvenile diabetes: normalization by insulin-treatment, *Diabetologia* (1975) **11:** 221–4.

24. Baumgartl HJ, Sigl G, Banholzer P et al, On the prognosis of IDDM patients with large kidneys, *Nephrol Dial Transplant* (1998) **13:** 630–4.

25. Rudberg S, Persson B, Dahlquist G, Increased glomerular filtration rate as a predictor of diabetic nephropathy—an 8-year prospective study, *Kidney Int* (1992) **41:** 822–8.

26. Mogensen CE, Definition of diabetic renal disease in insulin dependent diabetes mellitus based on renal function tests. In: Mogensen C, *The Kidney and Hypertension in Diabetes Mellitus*, 5th edn (Kluwer Academic: Boston, MA, 2000) 13–28.

27. Vora JP, Dolben J, Dean JD et al, Renal hemodynamics in newly presenting non-insulin dependent diabetes mellitus, *Kidney Int* (1992) **41:** 829–35.

28. Wiseman MJ, Viberti GC, Keen H, Threshold effect of plasma glucose in the glomerular hyperfiltration of diabetes, *Nephron* (1984) **38:** 257–60.

29. Viberti GC, Jarrett RJ, Mahmud U et al, Microalbuminuria as a predictor of clinical nephropathy in insulin-dependent diabetes mellitus, *Lancet* (1982) **1:** 1430–2.

30. Mathiesen ER, Oxenboll B, Johansen K et al, Incipient nephropathy in type 1 (insulin-dependent) diabetes, *Diabetologia* (1984) **26:** 406–10.

31. Rachmani R, Levi Z, Lidar M et al, Considerations about the threshold value of microalbuminuria in patients with diabetes mellitus: lessons from an 8-year follow-up study of 599 patients, *Diabetes Res Clin Pract* (2000) **49:** 187–94.

32. Nelson RG, Knowler WC, Pettitt DJ et al, Diabetic kidney disease in Pima Indians, *Diabetes Care* (1993) **16:** 335–41.

33. Nelson RG, Knowler WC, McCance DR et al, Determinants of end-stage renal disease in Pima Indians with type 2 (non-insulin-dependent) diabetes mellitus and proteinuria, *Diabetologia* (1993) **36:** 1087–93.

34. Damsgaard EM, Froland A, Jorgensen OD et al, Microalbuminuria as predictor of increased mortality in elderly people, *BMJ* (1990) **300:** 297–300.

35. Jarrett RJ, Viberti GC, Argyropoulos A et al, Microalbuminuria predicts mortality in non-insulin-dependent diabetics, *Diabet Med* (1984) **1:** 17–19.

36. Spoelstra-de Man AM, Brouwer CB, Stehouwer CD et al, Rapid progression of albumin excretion is an independent predictor of cardiovascular mortality in patients with type 2 diabetes and microalbuminuria, *Diabetes Care* (2001) **24:** 2097–101.

37. Yudkin JS, Forrest RD, Jackson CA, Microalbuminuria as predictor of vascular disease in non-diabetic subjects. Islington Diabetes Survey, *Lancet* (1988) **2:** 530–3.

38. Effects of ramipril on cardiovascular and microvascular outcomes in people with diabetes mellitus: results of the HOPE study and MICRO-HOPE substudy. Heart Outcomes Prevention Evaluation Study Investigators, *Lancet* (2000) **355:** 253–9.

39. Gerstein HC, Mann JF, Yi Q et al, Albuminuria and risk of cardiovascular events, death, and heart failure in diabetic and nondiabetic individuals, *JAMA* (2001) **286:** 421–6.

40. Deckert T, Feldt-Rasmussen B, Borch-Johnsen K et al, Albuminuria reflects widespread vascular damage. The Steno hypothesis, *Diabetologia* (1989) **32:** 219–26.

41. Stehouwer CD, Fischer HR, van Kuijk AW et al, Endothelial dysfunction precedes development of microalbuminuria in IDDM, *Diabetes* (1995) **44:** 561–4.

42. Feldt-Rasmussen B, Dinesen B, Deckert M, Enzyme immunoassay: an improved determination of urinary albumin in diabetics with incipient nephropathy, *Scand J Clin Lab Invest* (1985) **45:** 539–44.

43. Mogensen CE, Chachati A, Christensen CK et al, Microalbuminuria: an early marker of renal involvement in diabetes, *Uremia Invest* (1985) **9:** 85–95.

44. Viberti G, Mogensen C, Passa P et al, St Vincent Declaration, 1994: guidelines for the prevention of diabetic renal failure, In: Mogensen C, *The Kidney and Hypertension in Diabetes Mellitus* 2nd edn (Kluwer Academic: Boston, MA, 1994) 515–27.

45. Bennett PH, Haffner S, Kasiske BL et al, Screening and management of microalbuminuria in patients with diabetes mellitus: recommendations to the Scientific Advisory Board of the National Kidney Foundation from an ad hoc committee of the Council on Diabetes Mellitus of the National Kidney Foundation, *Am J Kidney Dis* (1995) **25:** 107–12.

46. Consensus Development Conference on the Diagnosis and

Management of Nephropathy in Patients with Diabetes Mellitus. American Diabetes Association and the National Kidney Foundation, *Diabetes Care* (1994) **17:** 1357–61.

47. Jerums G, Cooper M, Gilbert R et al, Microalbuminuria in diabetes, *Med J Aust* (1994) **161:** 265–8.

48. Gilbert RE, Akdeniz A, Jerums G, Semi-quantitative determination of microalbuminuria by urinary dipstick, *Aust N Z J Med* (1992) **22:** 334–7.

49. Mogensen CE, Keane WF, Bennett PH et al, Prevention of diabetic renal disease with special reference to microalbuminuria, *Lancet* (1995) **346:** 1080–4.

50. Warram J, Krolewski A, Use of the albumin/creatinine ratio in patient care and clinical studies. In: Mogensen C, *The Kidney and Hypertension in Diabetes Mellitus* 4th edn (Kluwer Academic: Boston, MA, 1998) 85–96.

51. Marshall SM, Alberti KG, Screening for early diabetic nephropathy, *Ann Clin Biochem* (1986) **23:** 195–7.

52. Cohen DL, Close CF, Viberti GC, The variability of overnight urinary albumin excretion in insulin-dependent diabetic and normal subjects, *Diabet Med* (1987) **4:** 437–40.

53. Connell SJ, Hollis S, Tieszen KL et al, Gender and the clinical usefulness of the albumin: creatinine ratio, *Diabet Med* (1994) **11:** 32–6.

54. Eshoj O, Feldt-Rasmussen B, Larsen ML et al, Comparison of overnight, morning and 24-hour urine collections in the assessment of diabetic microalbuminuria, *Diabet Med* (1987) **4:** 531–3.

55. Shield JP, Hunt LP, Baum JD et al, Screening for diabetic microalbuminuria in routine clinical care: which method?, *Arch Dis Child* (1995) **72:** 524–5.

56. Wiegmann TB, Chonko AM, Barnard MJ et al, Comparison of albumin excretion rate obtained with different times of collection, *Diabetes Care* (1990) **13:** 864–71.

57. Zelmanovitz T, Gross JL, Oliveira JR et al, The receiver operating characteristics curve in the evaluation of a random urine specimen as a screening test for diabetic nephropathy, *Diabetes Care* (1997) **20:** 516–19.

58. Bakker AJ, Detection of microalbuminuria. Receiver operating characteristic curve analysis favors albumin-to-creatinine ratio over albumin concentration, *Diabetes Care* (1999) **22:** 307–13.

59. Houlihan C, Tsalamandris C, Akdeniz A et al, Albumin to creatinine ratio: a screening test with limitations, *Am J Kidney Dis* (2002) **39:** 1183–9.

60. Scheid DC, McCarthy LH, Lawler FH et al, Screening for microalbuminuria to prevent nephropathy in patients with diabetes: a systematic review of the evidence, *J Fam Pract* (2001) **50:** 661–8.

61. Peterson KA, Screening for microalbuminuria, *J Fam Pract* (2001) **50:** 674–5.

62. Mogensen CE, Poulsen PL, Epidemiology of microalbuminuria in diabetes and in the background population, *Curr Opin Nephrol Hypertens* (1994) **3:** 248–56.

63. Dinneen SF, Gerstein HC, The association of microalbuminuria and mortality in non-insulin-dependent diabetes mellitus. A systematic overview of the literature, *Arch Intern Med* (1997) **157:** 1413–18.

64. Gall MA, Rossing P, Skott P et al, Prevalence of micro- and macroalbuminuria, arterial hypertension, retinopathy and large vessel disease in European type 2 (non-insulin-dependent) diabetic patients, *Diabetologia* (1991) **34:** 655–61.

65. Rolfe M, Diabetic renal disease in central Africa, *Diabet Med* (1988) **5:** 630–3.

66. Ishihara M, Yukimura Y, Yamada T et al, Diabetic complications and their relationships to risk factors in a Japanese population, *Diabetes Care* (1984) **7:** 533–8.

67. Haffner SM, Mitchell BD, Pugh JA et al, Proteinuria in Mexican Americans and non-Hispanic whites with NIDDM, *Diabetes Care* (1989) **12:** 530–6.

68. Klein R, Klein BE, Moss S et al, Proteinuria in diabetes, *Arch Intern Med* (1988) **148:** 181–6.

69. DCCT, The effect of intensive treatment of diabetes on the development and progression of long-term complications in insulin-dependent diabetes mellitus. The Diabetes Control and Complications Trial Research Group, *N Engl J Med* (1993) **329:** 977–86.

70. Mortensen HB, Marinelli K, Norgaard K et al, A nation-wide cross-sectional study of urinary albumin excretion rate, arterial blood pressure and blood glucose control in Danish children with type 1 diabetes mellitus. Danish Study Group of Diabetes in Childhood, *Diabet Med* (1990) **7:** 887–97.

71. D'Antonio JA, Ellis D, Doft BH et al, Diabetes complications and glycemic control. The Pittsburgh Prospective Insulin-Dependent Diabetes Cohort Study Status Report after 5 yr of IDDM, *Diabetes Care* (1989) **12:** 694–70.

72. Mathiesen ER, Saurbrey N, Hommel E et al, Prevalence of microalbuminuria in children with type 1 (insulin-dependent) diabetes mellitus, *Diabetologia* (1986) **29:** 640–3.

73. Chase HP, Marshall G, Garg SK et al, Borderline increases in albumin excretion rate and the relation to glycemic control in subjects with type I diabetes, *Clin Chem* (1991) **37:** 2048–52.

74. Schultz CJ, Neil HA, Dalton RN et al, Risk of nephropathy can be detected before the onset of microalbuminuria during the early years after diagnosis of type 1 diabetes, *Diabetes Care* (2000) **23:** 1811–15.

75. Royal College of Physicians of Edinburgh Diabetes Register Group, Near-normal urinary albumin concentrations predict progression to diabetic nephropathy in type 1, *Diabetic Med* (2000) **17:** 782–91.

76. Tabaei BP, Al-Kassab AS, Ilag LL et al, Does microalbuminuria predict diabetic nephropathy? *Diabetes Care* (2001) **24:** 1560–6.

77. Parving HH, Chaturvedi N, Viberti G et al, Does microalbuminuria predict diabetic nephropathy? *Diabetes Care* (2002) **25:** 406–7.

78. Caramori ML, Fioretto P, Mauer M, The need for early predictors of diabetic nephropathy risk: is albumin excretion rate sufficient? *Diabetes* (2000) **49:** 1399–408.

79. Almdal T, Norgaard K, Feldt-Rasmussen B et al, The predictive value of microalbuminuria in IDDM. A five-year follow-up study, *Diabetes Care* (1994) **17:** 120–5.

80. Bojestig M, Arnqvist HJ, Karlberg BE et al, Glycemic control and prognosis in type I diabetic patients with microalbuminuria, *Diabetes Care* (1996) **19:** 313–17.

81. Ellis D, Lloyd C, Becker DJ et al, The changing course of diabetic nephropathy: low-density lipoprotein cholesterol and blood pressure correlate with regression of proteinuria, *Am J Kidney Dis* (1996) **27:** 809–18.

82. Tsalamandris C, Panagiotopoulos S, Allen TJ et al, Long-term intraindividual variability of serum lipids in patients with type I and type II diabetes, *J Diabetes Complications* (1998) **12:** 208–14.

83. Viberti GC, Wiseman MJ, The kidney in diabetes: significance of the early abnormalities, *Clin Endocrinol Metab* (1986) **15:** 753–82.

84. Damsgaard EM, Mogensen CE, Microalbuminuria in elderly hyperglycaemic patients and controls, *Diabet Med* (1986) **3:** 430–5.

85. Rowe DJ, Hayward M, Bagga H et al, Effect of glycaemic control and duration of disease on overnight albumin excretion in diabetic children, *BMJ (Clin Res Edn)* (1984) **289:** 957–9.

86. Davies AG, Postlethwaite RJ, Price DA et al, Urinary albumin excretion in schoolchildren, *Arch Dis Child* (1984) **59:** 625–30.

87. Mogensen CE, Microalbuminuria as a predictor of clinical diabetic nephropathy, *Kidney Int* (1987) **31:** 673–89.

88. Humphrey LL, Ballard DJ, Frohnert PP et al, Chronic renal failure in non-insulin-dependent diabetes mellitus. A population-

based study in Rochester, Minnesota, *Ann Intern Med* (1989) **111:** 788–96.

89. Schmitz A, Vaeth M, Microalbuminuria: a major risk factor in non-insulin-dependent diabetes. A 10-year follow-up study of 503 patients, *Diabet Med* (1988) **5:** 126–34.

90. Levey AS, Beto JA, Coronado BE et al, Controlling the epidemic of cardiovascular disease in chronic renal disease: what do we know? What do we need to learn? Where do we go from here? National Kidney Foundation Task Force on Cardiovascular Disease, *Am J Kidney Dis* (1998) **32:** 853–906.

91. Messent JW, Elliott TG, Hill RD et al, Prognostic significance of microalbuminuria in insulin-dependent diabetes mellitus: a twenty-three year follow-up study, *Kidney Int* (1992) **41:** 836–9.

92. Beilin J, Stanton KG, McCann VJ et al, Microalbuminuria in type 2 diabetes: an independent predictor of cardiovascular mortality, *Aust N Z J Med* (1996) **26:** 519–25.

93. Gall MA, Borch-Johnsen K, Hougaard P et al, Albuminuria and poor glycemic control predict mortality in NIDDM, *Diabetes* (1995) **44:** 1303–9.

94. Rossing P, Hougaard P, Borch-Johnsen K et al, Predictors of mortality in insulin dependent diabetes: 10 year observational follow up study, *BMJ* (1996) **313:** 779–84.

95. Borch-Johnsen K, Kreiner S, Deckert T, Mortality of type 1 (insulin-dependent) diabetes mellitus in Denmark: a study of relative mortality in 2930 Danish type 1 diabetic patients diagnosed from 1933 to 1972, *Diabetologia* (1986) **29:** 767–72.

96. Borch-Johnsen K, Kreiner S, Proteinuria: value as predictor of cardiovascular mortality in insulin dependent diabetes mellitus, *BMJ (Clin Res Edn)* (1987) **294:** 1651–4.

97. Borch-Johnsen K, The prognosis of insulin-dependent diabetes mellitus. An epidemiological approach, *Dan Med Bull* (1989) **36:** 336–48.

98. Nelson RG, Newman JM, Knowler WC et al, Incidence of end-stage renal disease in type 2 (non-insulin-dependent) diabetes mellitus in Pima Indians, *Diabetologia* (1988) **31:** 730–6.

99. Breyer JA, Diabetic nephropathy in insulin-dependent patients, *Am J Kidney Dis* (1992) **20:** 533–47.

100. Cowie CC, Port FK, Wolfe RA et al, Disparities in incidence of diabetic end-stage renal disease according to race and type of diabetes, *N Engl J Med* (1989) **321:** 1074–9.

101. Ballard DJ, Humphrey LL, Melton LJ 3rd et al, Epidemiology of persistent proteinuria in type II diabetes mellitus. Population-based study in Rochester, Minnesota, *Diabetes* (1988) **37:** 405–12.

102. Schmitz A, The kidney in non-insulin-dependent diabetes, *Acta Diabetol* (1992) **29:** 47–69.

103. Ismail N, Becker B, Strzelczyk P et al, Renal disease and hypertension in non-insulin-dependent diabetes mellitus, *Kidney Int* (1999) **55:** 1–28.

104. Bojestig M, Arnqvist HJ, Hermansson G et al, Declining incidence of nephropathy in insulin-dependent diabetes mellitus, *N Engl J Med* (1994) **330:** 15–18.

105. Disney APS, Twenty-third report of the Australia and New Zealand Dialysis and Transplant Registry, Adelaide (2000).

106. Tung P, Levin SR. Nephropathy in non-insulin-dependent diabetes mellitus, *Am J Med* (1988) **85:** 131–6.

107. Tsalamandris C, Allen TJ, Gilbert RE et al, Progressive decline in renal function in diabetic patients with and without albuminuria, *Diabetes* (1994) **43:** 649–55.

108. Lane PH, Steffes MW, Mauer SM, Glomerular structure in IDDM women with low glomerular filtration rate and normal urinary albumin excretion, *Diabetes* (1992) **41:** 581–6.

109. Knowles HC Jr, Long-term juvenile diabetes treated with unmeasured diet, *Trans Assoc Am Physicians* (1971) **84:** 95–101.

110. Andersen AR, Andersen JK, Christiansen JS et al, Prognosis for juvenile diabetics with nephropathy and failing renal function, *Acta Med Scand* (1978) **203:** 131–4.

111. Mogensen CE, Progression of nephropathy in long-term diabetics with proteinuria and effect of initial anti-hypertensive treatment, *Scand J Clin Lab Invest* (1976) **36:** 383–8.

112. Cockcroft DW, Gault MH, Prediction of creatinine clearance from serum creatinine, *Nephron* (1976) **16:** 31–41.

113. Levey AS, Bosch JP, Lewis JB et al, A more accurate method to estimate glomerular filtration rate from serum creatinine: a new prediction equation. Modification of Diet in Renal Disease Study Group, *Ann Intern Med* (1999) **130:** 461–70.

114. Shemesh O, Golbetz H, Kriss JP et al, Limitations of creatinine as a filtration marker in glomerulopathic patients, *Kidney Int* (1985) **28:** 830–8.

115. Mogensen CE, Schmitz A, Christensen CK, Comparative renal pathophysiology relevant to IDDM and NIDDM patients, *Diabetes Metab Rev* (1988) **4:** 453–83.

116. Kunzelman CL, Nelson RG, Knowler WC et al, Proteinuria determines prognosis in type 2 (non-insulin-dependent) diabetes, *Kidney Int* (1988) **33:** 197[Abstract].

117. Nelson RG, Pettitt DJ, Carraher MJ et al, Effect of proteinuria on mortality in NIDDM, *Diabetes* (1988) **37:** 1499–504.

118. Parving HH, Andersen AR, Smidt UM et al, Early aggressive antihypertensive treatment reduces rate of decline in kidney function in diabetic nephropathy, *Lancet* (1983) **1:** 1175–9.

119. Cooper ME, Frauman A, O'Brien RC et al, Progression of proteinuria in type 1 and type 2 diabetes, *Diabet Med* (1988) **5:** 361–8.

120. Klein R, Klein BE, Moss SE et al, Ten-year incidence of gross proteinuria in people with diabetes, *Diabetes* (1995) **44:** 916–23.

121. Mattock MB, Barnes DJ, Viberti G et al, Microalbuminuria and coronary heart disease in NIDDM: an incidence study, *Diabetes* (1998) **47:** 1786–92.

122. Ravid M, Brosh D, Ravid-Safran D et al, Main risk factors for nephropathy in type 2 diabetes mellitus are plasma cholesterol levels, mean blood pressure, and hyperglycemia, *Arch Intern Med* (1998) **158:** 998–1004.

123. Chaturvedi N, Bandinelli S, Mangili R et al, Microalbuminuria in type 1 diabetes: rates, risk factors and glycemic threshold, *Kidney Int* (2001) **60:** 219–27.

124. Viberti G, Recent advances in understanding mechanisms and natural history of diabetic renal disease, *Diabetes Care* (1988) **11**(Suppl 1): 3–9.

125. Mogensen CE, Prediction of clinical diabetic nephropathy in IDDM patients. Alternatives to microalbuminuria?, *Diabetes* (1990) **39:** 761–7.

126. Krolewski AS, Laffel LM, Krolewski M et al, Glycosylated hemoglobin and the risk of microalbuminuria in patients with insulin-dependent diabetes mellitus, *N Engl J Med* (1995) **332:** 1251–5.

127. Torffvit O, Agardh E, Agardh CD, Albuminuria and associated medical risk factors: a cross-sectional study in 451 type II (non-insulin-dependent) diabetic patients. Part II, *J Diabet Complications* (1991) **5:** 29–34.

128. Nelson RG, Bennett PH, Beck GJ et al, Development and progression of renal disease in Pima Indians with non-insulin-dependent diabetes mellitus. Diabetic Renal Disease Study Group, *N Engl J Med* (1996) **335:** 1636–42.

129. Gilbert RE, Tsalamandris C, Bach LA et al, Long-term glycemic control and the rate of progression of early diabetic kidney disease, *Kidney Int* (1993) **44:** 855–9.

130. Nyberg G, Blohme G, Norden G, Impact of metabolic control in progression of clinical diabetic nephropathy, *Diabetologia* (1987) **30:** 82–6.

131. Stratton IM, Adler AI, Neil HA et al, Association of glycaemia with macrovascular and microvascular complications of type 2 diabetes (UKPDS 35): prospective observational study, *BMJ* (2000) **321:** 405–12.

132. Adler AI, Stratton IM, Neil HA et al, Association of systolic blood pressure with macrovascular and microvascular complications of type 2 diabetes (UKPDS 36): prospective observational study, *BMJ* (2000) **321:** 412–19.

133. Bilous RW, Mauer SM, Sutherland DE et al, The effects of pancreas transplantation on the glomerular structure of renal allografts in patients with insulin-dependent diabetes, *N Engl J Med* (1989) **321:** 80–5.

134. Drury PL, Watkins PJ, Viberti GC et al, Diabetic nephropathy, *Br Med Bull* (1989) **45:** 127–47.

135. Tuttle KR, DeFronzo RA, Stein JH, Treatment of diabetic nephropathy: a rational approach based on its pathophysiology, *Semin Nephrol* (1991) **11:** 220–35.

136. Wang PH, Lau J, Chalmers TC, Meta-analysis of effects of intensive blood-glucose control on late complications of type I diabetes, *Lancet* (1993) **341:** 1306–9.

137. UKPDS 33, Intensive blood-glucose control with sulphonylureas or insulin compared with conventional treatment and risk of complications in patients with type 2 diabetes (UKPDS 33). UK Prospective Diabetes Study (UKPDS) Group, *Lancet* (1998) **352:** 837–53.

138. Levin SR, Coburn JW, Abraira C et al, Effect of intensive glycemic control on microalbuminuria in type 2 diabetes. Veterans Affairs Cooperative Study on Glycemic Control and Complications in Type 2 Diabetes Feasibility Trial Investigators, *Diabetes Care* (2000) **23:** 1478–85.

139. Defronzo RA, Diabetic nephropathy: etiologic and therapeutic considerations, *Diabetes Rev* (1995) **3:** 510–64.

140. Schwartz MM, Lewis EJ, Leonard-Martin T et al, Renal pathology patterns in type II diabetes mellitus: relationship with retinopathy. Collaborative Study Group, *Nephrol Dial Transplant* (1998) **13:** 2547–52.

141. Mathiesen ER, Ronn B, Jensen T et al, Relationship between blood pressure and urinary albumin excretion in development of microalbuminuria, *Diabetes* (1990) **39:** 245–9.

142. Schultz CJ, Neil HA, Dalton RN et al, Blood pressure does not rise before the onset of microalbuminuria in children followed from diagnosis of type 1 diabetes. Oxford Regional Prospective Study Group, *Diabetes Care* (2001) **24:** 555–60.

143. Tarnow L, Rossing P, Gall MA et al, Prevalence of arterial hypertension in diabetic patients before and after the JNC-V, *Diabetes Care* (1994) **17:** 1247–51.

144. Hostetter TH, Troy JL, Brenner BM, Glomerular hemodynamics in experimental diabetes mellitus, *Kidney Int* (1981) **19:** 410–15.

145. Berkman J, Rifkin H, Unilateral nodular diabetic glomerulosclerosis (Kimmelstiel–Wilson): report of a case, *Metabolism* (1973) **22:** 715–22.

146. Bakris GL, Williams M, Dworkin L et al, Preserving renal function in adults with hypertension and diabetes: a consensus approach. National Kidney Foundation Hypertension and Diabetes Executive Committees Working Group, *Am J Kidney Dis* (2000) **36:** 646–61.

147. Jerums G, Cooper ME, Seeman E et al, Comparison of early renal dysfunction in type I and type II diabetes: differing associations with blood pressure and glycaemic control, *Diabetes Res Clin Pract* (1988) **4:** 133–41.

148. Schmitz A, Vaeth M, Mogensen CE, Systolic blood pressure relates to the rate of progression of albuminuria in NIDDM, *Diabetologia* (1994) **37:** 1251–8.

149. Franklin SS, Khan SA, Wong ND et al, Is pulse pressure useful in predicting risk for coronary heart disease? The Framingham Heart Study, *Circulation* (1999) **100:** 354–60.

150. Poulsen PL, Ebbehoj E, Hansen KW et al, 24-h blood pressure and autonomic function is related to albumin excretion within the normoalbuminuric range in IDDM patients, *Diabetologia* (1997) **40:** 718–25.

151. Torffvit O, Agardh CD, Day and night variation in ambulatory blood pressure in type 1 diabetes mellitus with nephropathy and autonomic neuropathy, *J Intern Med* (1993) **233:** 131–7.

152. Monteagudo PT, Nobrega JC, Cezarini PR et al, Altered blood pressure profile, autonomic neuropathy and nephropathy in insulin-dependent diabetic patients, *Eur J Endocrinol* (1996) **135:** 683–8.

153. Gilbert R, Phillips P, Clarke C et al, Day–night blood pressure variation in normotensive, normoalbuminuric type I diabetic subjects. Dippers and non-dippers, *Diabetes Care* (1994) **17:** 824–7.

154. Hansen KW, Sorensen K, Christensen PD et al, Night blood pressure: relation to organ lesions in microalbuminuric type 1 diabetic patients, *Diabet Med* (1995) **12:** 42–5.

155. Kannel WB, Schwartz MJ, McNamara PM, Blood pressure and risk of coronary heart disease: the Framingham Study, *Dis Chest* (1969) **56:** 43–52.

156. JNC-V, The Fifth Report of the Joint National Committee on Detection, Evaluation, and Treatment of High Blood Pressure, *Arch Intern Med* (1993) **153:** 154–83.

157. JNC-VI, The Sixth Report of the Joint National Committee on Prevention, Detection, Evaluation, and Treatment of High Blood Pressure, *Arch Intern Med* (1997) **157:** 2413–46.

158. WHO-ISH, 1999 World Health Organization–International Society of Hypertension Guidelines for the Management of Hypertension. Guidelines Subcommittee, *J Hypertens* (1999) **17:** 151–83.

159. Gan SK, Chisholm DJ, The type 2 diabetes epidemic: a hidden menace, *Med J Aust* (2001) **175:** 65–6.

160. Norgaard K, Feldt-Rasmussen B, Borch-Johnsen K et al, Prevalence of hypertension in type 1 (insulin-dependent) diabetes mellitus, *Diabetologia* (1990) **33:** 407–10.

161. Hasslacher C, Ritz E, Wahl P et al, Similar risks of nephropathy in patients with type I or type II diabetes mellitus, *Nephrol Dial Transplant* (1989) **4:** 859–63.

162. Biesenbach G, Janko O, Zazgornik J, Similar rate of progression in the predialysis phase in type I and type II diabetes mellitus, *Nephrol Dial Transplant* (1994) **9:** 1097–102.

163. Reaven GM, Role of insulin resistance in human disease, *Diabetes* (1988) **37:** 1595–607.

164. Nosadini R, Cipollina MR, Solini A et al, Close relationship between microalbuminuria and insulin resistance in essential hypertension and non-insulin dependent diabetes mellitus, *J Am Soc Nephrol* (1992) **3:** S56–63.

165. Ford ES, Giles WH, Dietz WH, Prevalence of the metabolic syndrome among US adults: findings from the Third National Health and Nutrition Examination Survey, *JAMA* (2002) **287:** 356–9.

166. UKPDS X, UK Prospective Diabetes Study (UKPDS). X. Urinary albumin excretion over 3 years in diet-treated type 2 (non-insulin-dependent), diabetic patients, and association with hypertension, hyperglycaemia and hypertriglyceridaemia, *Diabetologia* (1993) **36:** 1021–9.

167. Groop PH, Elliott T, Ekstrand A et al, Multiple lipoprotein abnormalities in type I diabetic patients with renal disease, *Diabetes* (1996) **45:** 974–9.

168. Mulec H, Johnson SA, Bjorck S, Relation between serum cholesterol and diabetic nephropathy, *Lancet* (1990) **335:** 1537–8.

169. Smulders YM, Rakic M, Stehouwer CD et al, Determinants of progression of microalbuminuria in patients with NIDDM. A prospective study, *Diabetes Care* (1997) **20:** 999–1005.

170. Vigstrup J, Mogensen CE, Proliferative diabetic retinopathy: at risk patients identified by early detection of microalbuminuria, *Acta Ophthalmol (Copenh)* (1985) **63:** 530–4.

171. Gilbert RE, Tsalamandris C, Allen TJ et al, Early nephropathy predicts vision-threatening retinal disease in patients with type I diabetes mellitus, *J Am Soc Nephrol* (1998) **9:** 85–9.

172. Watts GF, Harris R, Shaw KM, The determinants of early nephropathy in insulin-dependent diabetes mellitus: a prospective study based on the urinary excretion of albumin, *Q J Med* (1991) **79:** 365–78.

173. Knuiman MW, Welborn TA, McCann VJ et al, Prevalence of diabetic complications in relation to risk factors, *Diabetes* (1986) **35:** 1332–9.

174. Chavers BM, Mauer SM, Ramsay RC et al, Relationship between retinal and glomerular lesions in IDDM patients, *Diabetes* (1994) **43:** 441–6.

175. Stephenson JM, Fuller JH, Viberti GC et al, Blood pressure, retinopathy and urinary albumin excretion in IDDM: the EURODIAB IDDM Complications Study, *Diabetologia* (1995) **38:** 599–603.

176. Chaturvedi N, Fuller J, Retinopathy in relation to albuminuria and blood pressure in IDDM. In: Mogensen C, *The Kidney and Hypertension in Diabetes Mellitus,* 5th edn (Kluwer Academic: Boston, MA, 2000) 29–38.

177. Osterby R, Gall MA, Schmitz A et al, Glomerular structure and function in proteinuric type 2 (non-insulin-dependent) diabetic patients, *Diabetologia* (1993) **36:** 1064–70.

178. Christensen PK, Larsen S, Horn T et al, Causes of albuminuria in patients with type 2 diabetes without diabetic retinopathy, *Kidney Int* (2000) **58:** 1719–31.

179. Agodoa L, Hypertensive kidney disease in African Americans, *Nephrology* (2001) **6:** 25–31.

180. Bennett PH, Lee ET, Lu M et al, Increased urinary albumin excretion and its associations in the WHO Multinational Study of Vascular Disease in Diabetes, *Diabetologia* (2001) **44**(Suppl 2): S37–45.

181. Nelson RG. Diabetic renal disease in transitional and disadvantaged populations, *Nephrology* (2001) **6:** 9–17.

182. Seaquist ER, Goetz FC, Rich S et al, Familial clustering of diabetic kidney disease: evidence for genetic susceptibility to diabetic nephropathy, *N Engl J Med* (1989) **320:** 1161–5.

183. Imperatore G, Hanson RL, Pettitt DJ et al, Sib-pair linkage analysis for susceptibility genes for microvascular complications among Pima Indians with type 2 diabetes. Pima Diabetes Genes Group, *Diabetes* (1998) **47:** 821–30.

184. Nelson RG, Morgenstern H, Bennett PH, Intrauterine diabetes exposure and the risk of renal disease in diabetic Pima Indians, *Diabetes* (1998) **47:** 1489–93.

185. Frassinetti Fernandes P, Ellis PA, Roderick PJ et al, Causes of end-stage renal failure in black patients starting renal replacement therapy, *Am J Kidney Dis* (2000) **36:** 301–9.

186. Kohler KA, McClellan WM, Ziemer DC et al, Risk factors for microalbuminuria in black Americans with newly diagnosed type 2 diabetes, *Am J Kidney Dis* (2000) **36:** 903–13.

187. Pugh JA, Stern MP, Haffner SM et al, Excess incidence of treatment of end-stage renal disease in Mexican-Americans, *Am J Epidemiol* (1988) **127:** 135–44.

188. Varghese A, Deepa R, Rema M et al, Prevalence of microalbuminuria in type 2 diabetes mellitus at a diabetes centre in southern India, *Postgrad Med J* (2001) **77:** 399–402.

189. Park JY, Kim HK, Chung YE et al, Incidence and determinants of microalbuminuria in Koreans with type 2 diabetes, *Diabetes Care* (1998) **21:** 530–4.

190. Allawi J, Rao PV, Gilbert R et al, Microalbuminuria in non-insulin-dependent diabetes: its prevalence in Indian compared with Europid patients, *BMJ (Clin Res Edn)* (1988) **296:** 462–4.

191. Yokoyama H, Okudaira M, Otani T et al, High incidence of diabetic nephropathy in early-onset Japanese NIDDM patients. Risk analysis, *Diabetes Care* (1998) **21:** 1080–5.

192. Dyck R, Mechanisms of renal disease in indigenous populations: influences at work in Canadian indigenous peoples, *Nephrology* (2001) **6:** 3–7.

193. Hoy WE, Mathews JD, McCredie DA et al, The multidimensional nature of renal disease: rates and associations of albuminuria in an Australian Aboriginal community, *Kidney Int* (1998) **54:** 1296–304.

194. Marre M, Chatellier G, Leblanc H et al, Prevention of diabetic nephropathy with enalapril in normotensive diabetics with microalbuminuria, *BMJ* (1988) **297:** 1092–5.

195. 1989 Guidelines for the Management of Mild Hypertension: Memorandum from a WHO/ISH meeting, *Clin Exp Hypertens—Theory Pract* (1989) **A11:** 1203–16.

196. Rossing P, Hommel E, Smidt UM et al, Reduction in albuminuria predicts a beneficial effect on diminishing the progression of human diabetic nephropathy during antihypertensive treatment, *Diabetologia* (1994) **37:** 511–16.

197. Lewis EJ, Hunsicker LG, Bain RP et al, The effect of angiotensin-converting-enzyme inhibition on diabetic nephropathy. The Collaborative Study Group, *N Engl J Med* (1993) **329:** 1456–62.

198. Smulders YM, van Eeden AE, Stehouwer CD et al, Can reduction in hypertriglyceridaemia slow progression of microalbuminuria in patients with non-insulin-dependent diabetes mellitus? *Eur J Clin Invest* (1997) **27:** 997–1002.

199. Lam KS, Cheng IK, Janus ED, Pang RW. Cholesterol-lowering therapy may retard the progression of diabetic nephropathy. *Diabetologia* (1995) **38:** 604–9.

200. Tonolo G, Ciccarese M, Brizzi P et al, Reduction of albumin excretion rate in normotensive microalbuminuric type 2 diabetic patients during long-term simvastatin treatment, *Diabetes Care* (1997) **20:** 1891–5.

201. Nielsen S, Schmitz O, Moller N et al, Renal function and insulin sensitivity during simvastatin treatment in type 2 (non-insulin-dependent) diabetic patients with microalbuminuria, *Diabetologia* (1993) **36:** 1079–86.

202. Brenner BM, Cooper ME, de Zeeuw D et al, Effects of losartan on renal and cardiovascular outcomes in patients with type 2 diabetes and nephropathy, *N Engl J Med* (2001) **345:** 861–9.

203. Lewis EJ, Hunsicker LG, Clarke WR et al, Renoprotective effect of the angiotensin-receptor antagonist irbesartan in patients with nephropathy due to type 2 diabetes, *N Engl J Med* (2001) **345:** 851–60.

204. Fioretto P, Mauer M, Brocco E et al, Patterns of renal injury in NIDDM patients with microalbuminuria, *Diabetologia* (1996) **39:** 1569–76.

205. Gambara V, Mecca G, Remuzzi G et al, Heterogeneous nature of renal lesions in type II diabetes, *J Am Soc Nephrol* (1993) **3:** 1458–66.

206. Schwartz M, Lewis E, Leonard-Martin T, Renal clinicopathology of type II diabetes mellitus, *J Am Soc Nephrol* (1996) **7:** 1364.

207. Jerums G, Chattington PD, Management of hypertension in patients with diabetes. In: McNally P, ed., *Diabetes and Cardiovascular Complications* (Science Press: London, 1999) 59–71.

# 4

# Inherited susceptibility to diabetic nephropathy

Merlin C Thomas

## BACKGROUND

Nephropathy is a common complication of diabetes. However, unlike retinopathy, its occurrence is by no means inevitable. Only a subset of patients with diabetes may be susceptible to the development of diabetic renal disease. After 15 years of diabetes, 30–50% of patients with type 1 diabetes and around 50% of all patients with type 2 diabetes show evidence of clinical nephropathy.[1,2] Subsequently, the prevalence of diabetic nephropathy declines, with additional cases falling to less than 0.5% per year after 30 years of diabetes,[3] although this may underestimate the true incidence, as patients with nephropathy have an increased risk of premature mortality.[4]

Nonetheless, there remain patients who, despite prolonged hyperglycaemia and poor blood-pressure control, appear resistant to the development of diabetic renal disease. Similarly, there are patients who, despite optimal glycaemic control, seem to spiral inexorably toward renal failure and a premature death. While it is not currently possible to predict which patients will develop diabetic nephropathy, there is increasing evidence for the role of genetic modifiers in determining at least some of the susceptibility to diabetic nephropathy.

This chapter will review the possible role of 'susceptibility' genes in the development and progression of diabetic nephropathy (Table 4.1). Although a genetic predisposition to diabetes per se may be important to the initial development of both type 1 and type 2 diabetes (and therein nephropathy), the role of such genes has been reviewed elsewhere[5,6] and will not be further considered. It should be noted, however, that some forms of genetic diabetes (in particular, maturity-onset diabetes of the young) may be associated with an increased prevalence of nephropathy.

**Table 4.1. Some candidate genes implicated in the susceptibility to diabetic nephropathy.**

Angiotensin-converting enzyme (ACE)

Aldose reductase

Angiotensin II receptor (type 1)

Angiotensinogen

Apolipoprotein E

Atrial natriuretic peptide (ANP)

Decorin

Geterotrimeric G-protein

Glucokinase (MODY 2)

GLUT-1 transporter

Heparan sulphate

Hepatocyte nuclear factor-1 beta (MODY 5)

11B hydroxysteroid dehydrogenase type 2

Intercellular adhesion molecule-1 (ICAM-1)

Leukocyte-endothelial cell adhesion molecule 1 (LECAM-1)

Lipoprotein lipase (LPL)

Matrix metalloproteinase-9 (MMP-9)

Methylene-tetrahydrofolate reductase

Na/H exchanger

Nitric oxide synthase (especially endothelial NOS-3)

Plasminogen activator inhibitor-1 (PAI-1)

Peroxisome proliferator-activated receptor (PPAR)

T-cell receptor b-chain (TCRBC)

Vitamin D receptor

Vascular endothelial growth factor (VEGF)

## FAMILIAL AGGREGATION OF DIABETIC NEPHROPATHY

The strongest evidence for an inherited susceptibility to diabetic nephropathy comes from studies showing that some families in particular have an increased risk of renal disease. A family history of nephropathy (or premature cardiovascular disease as its surrogate) continues to be the most accurate and available marker for identifying patients most at risk, with familial aggregation now described for nephropathy in both type 1[7,8] and type 2 diabetes.[9,10] The diabetic offspring of parents with diabetes and proteinuria have three to four times the prevalence of nephropathy compared to the siblings of diabetic parents without renal disease.[7,8] The risk appears to be further increased if both parents have diabetic nephropathy, as opposed to only one parent with albuminuria (Figure 4.1).[9] This has led to the suggestion that the predisposition to diabetic nephropathy may be inherited as a dominant trait.[7,11] In addition to proteinuria, familial aggregation has also been demonstrated in the severity and pattern of diabetic glomerular structural lesions, independently of glycaemic control.[12]

As yet, it is unclear exactly what this 'susceptibility' trait represents. It is conceivable that any number of shared environmental factors may contribute independently to the development of disease with or without the interaction of any shared genes. It is also possible that clustering of other traits in the family of patients with nephropathy contributes to the development and severity of diabetes rather than renal disease directly. Such factors include hypertension, glucose tolerance, insulin resistance and body habitus. However, even after adjusting for a family record of hypertension and poor glycaemic control, a family history of albuminuria remains strongly linked to a risk of nephropathy in patients both with type 1[13] and type 2 diabetes.[14]

An inherited susceptibility to nephropathy may not even be specific to diabetic renal disease. The risk of albuminuria may be inherited independently of diabetes. The non-diabetic offspring of parents with diabetic nephropathy have a higher albumin excretion rate[14] and an exaggerated albuminuric response to physical exercise (at least in type 2 diabetes) than patients with no family history of nephropathy.[15] It has been suggested that a genetic predisposition may exist to renal disease of any cause. Non-diabetic renal disease also exhibits familial aggregation.[16] Thompson et al,[17] in a two-by-two factorial study of proteinuria in Polynesians, examined 90 people with a first-degree relative with end-stage renal disease (ESRD) and diabetes. They were compared with 90 people with a relative having non-diabetic ESRD, 90 people with a relative with diabetes but no known nephropathy, and a further 90 people with no known relatives with either diabetes or nephropathy (Figure 4.2). Subjects with a family history of ESRD had an increased mean albumin creatinine ratio ($P = 0.01$), particularly in the presence of diabetes. However, a family history of diabetes per se was not an independent factor associated with albuminuria ($P = 0.09$). Similar data have been described in African-American patients with type II diabetes and ESRD, who are nearly twice as likely to have a relative with ESRD as patients without nephropathy.[10,18]

The identification and early management of albuminuric patients with diabetes is a comparatively recent phenomenon. Historically, the earliest manifestation of nephropathy was a premature cardiovascular event. Diabetic nephropathy is associated with an increased risk of cardiovascular disease compared to diabetes of similar duration but without nephropathy.[19] As a result, parental history of cardiovascular disease appears to provide an appropriate surrogate for identifying patients at increased risk of diabetic nephropathy. This has now been demonstrated in studies of patients with type 1 and type 2 diabetes.[20-22] While the association between a familial history of cardiovascular disease and diabetic nephropathy may reflect undiagnosed nephropathy parents, the cosegregation of other traits, including hypertension, dyslipidaemia and activity of the renin-angiotensin system, may also be an important contributor.

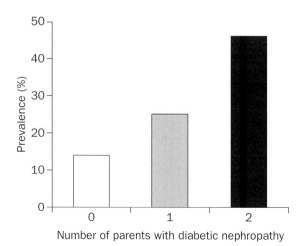

**Figure 4.1** Increased prevalence of nephropathy with increasing number of family members with known nephropathy. Adapted with permission from Pettitt 1990.

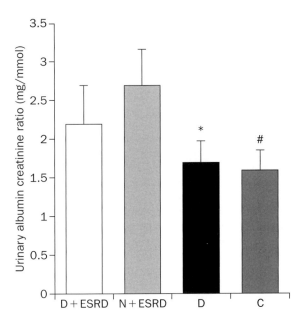

**Figure 4.2** Increased prevalence of nephropathy in Polynesian patients with a family history of end-stage renal disease (ESRD) rather than diabetes. D + ESRD: people with a first-degree relative with ESRD and diabetes; N + ESRD: people with a relative having non-diabetic ESRD; D: people with a relative with diabetes but no known nephropathy; C: people with no known relatives with either diabetes or nephropathy (*D-ESRD vs D, p = 0.01, #D vs C, p = 0.2). Adapted from *Diabetic Medicine* with permission.[17]

## ETHNIC VARIABILITY IN DIABETIC NEPHROPATHY

The prevalence of diabetic nephropathy varies significantly among different ethnic groups For example, African-American, Indo-Asian and Polynesian patients have a much greater risk of nephropathy than matched Caucasian patients.[23] Among Jews developing type 1 diabetes, the non-Ashkenazi ethnic group are at a higher risk of the development of nephropathy.[24] One of the highest rates of nephropathy is described in Pima Indians, who have a cumulative incidence of persistent proteinuria of 80% after 25 years of diabetes. In addition, Pima Indians have a 61% cumulative incidence of ESRD 15 years after the onset of proteinuria, in contrast to only 17% in a comparable Caucasian population.[4]

Like familial clustering, it has also been proposed that the increased risk of diabetic nephropathy in African-Americans is a marker of an inherited susceptibility to the development of renal disease of any cause, independently of any predisposition to devel-

oping diabetes mellitus.[18] This may also be manifested in the high rates of HIV-associated nephropathy in African-American men.[25]

While candidate genes predisposing to nephropathy may exist at different rates in different ethnic groups, the exact nature of the ethnic predisposition to diabetes is again unclear. Some of these differences may result from the lead-time bias associated with the earlier onset of diabetes in high-risk populations. Competing causes of death may also bias interracial differences. For example, Pima Indians have a lower rate of cardiovascular mortality than Caucasian patients.[26] Ethnic clustering of other risk factors for nephropathy may also contribute to the perceived increased risk of some populations. For instance, patients of African-Caribbean origin have, in general, higher systolic blood pressure, greater insulin resistance, increased body-mass index and higher circulating markers of oxidative stress.[27] Differences in affluence, diet, activity and health behaviour may also contribute to the racial dissimilarities in the prevalence of nephropathy, without invoking genetic factors. Race/ethnicity and socioeconomic status influence the availability and quality of health and prevention services that directly impinge on risk factors such as blood glucose, lipid and blood-pressure control. Any number (or indeed all) of these differences could contribute to racial disparity in the prevalence of nephropathy.

## THE ROLE OF GENDER

Gender-specific differences in both the prevalence[28,29] and progression[30] of diabetic nephropathy have also been found, with women being at significantly greater risk. There also appears to be a gender dimorphism in age of onset of nephropathy. This may be especially apparent in type 1 diabetes, where nephropathy generally develops after puberty but before menopause, after which many gender differences may be reduced. Nonetheless, recent studies have demonstrated an excess of diabetic nephropathy in African-American women with predominantly type 2 diabetes.[31] However, an excess of cardiovascular mortality in men may bias this kind of survey.

Gender-specific differences in renal mass, blood pressure, and lipids may modify the development and progression of diabetic complications in men and women. These factors would seem to influence the progression of all renal disease, rather than diabetic nephropathy per se. However, it should be noted that, unlike diabetes, the progression of non-diabetic renal disease is significantly slower in women.[30] Nonetheless, excessive albumin excretion (of any cause) is two to three times more common in girls than boys.[32]

Sex hormones may also directly influence nephropathy. In humans, puberty is associated with accelerated microvascular complications of diabetes mellitus, including nephropathy.[33] In animal models of experimental renal injury, sex hormones modify the development of renal hypertrophy and glomerulosclerosis.[34] Nephropathy in the Cohen diabetic rat (genetically selected, sucrose-fed) is significantly attenuated by gonadectomy in both sexes.[35,36] However, testosterone administration to the ovariectomized animals results in a significantly increased incidence of nephropathy.[35] Hyperandrogenicity in women with type 1 diabetes may also be linked to an increased albumin excretion rate.[37] Against this, there is no evidence that the excess of sex hormones associated with pregnancy or polycystic ovary syndrome influence the subsequent risk of development of albuminuria.

Iron stores also represent another important gender difference implicated in the development of diabetic nephropathy. From the time of menarche, women have consistently lower iron stores than men. Increased proximal tubular iron concentration has been observed in patients with early diabetic nephropathy, possibly contributing to tubular injury through the induction of oxidative stress.[38] An early development and accelerated course of diabetic nephropathy has been observed in iron-loaded patients with β-thalassemia.[39] In addition, mutations for the haemochromatosis allele H63D (associated with elevated iron stores) appear to predict the development of diabetic nephropathy in patients without haemochromatosis.[40] While patients with elevated iron stores may have an earlier onset of type 2 diabetes,[38] there is currently insufficient evidence to define a precise role for iron in the development of nephropathy.

## THE ROLE OF GENETIC HYPERTENSION

As discussed elsewhere in this text, hypertension is one of the most important predictors of the onset and progression of nephropathy in patients with diabetes. While there are many environmental influences on blood pressure, hypertension also comes under significant genetic control. A number of studies have demonstrated that blood-pressure traits appear to segregate with the risk of nephropathy in patients with diabetes.[41,42] The concept that genetic hypertension may predispose to accelerated nephropathy is clearly demonstrated in the spontaneously hypertensive rat, a model of polygenetic (essential) hypertension. When compared to normotensive diabetic rats, hypertensive diabetic rats have an earlier and more rapid rise in urinary albumin excretion and increased glomerular basement-membrane thickness.[43]

However, the evidence for the role of human genetic hypertension in determining the susceptibility to diabetic nephropathy is less clear. Some studies have suggested that parental hypertension increases the risk of nephropathy in both type 1 and type 2 diabetes.[21,22,44] Diabetic patients with a positive family history of hypertension are also more likely to develop nephropathy than patients without familial hypertension.[42] Seen another way, systolic and diastolic blood pressures are greater in the parents of diabetic patients with nephropathy than in the parents of diabetic subjects without proteinuria. These data could suggest that inherited traits that contribute to the development of hypertension also influence the development of nephropathy in the setting of hyperglycaemia. However, it is more likely that the traits that determine hypertension (and subsequent risk of nephropathy) are multifactorial. Moreover, at least in type I diabetes, the susceptibility trait appears to be related to the subsequent development of hypertension in offspring rather than nephropathy in itself.[44]

## LIPIDS AND DIABETIC NEPHROPATHY

Dyslipidaemia is also an important component of the development of diabetic complications such as nephropathy.[45] Triglycerides, intermediate-density lipoproteins, remnant-like particles and postprandial lipaemia are all increased in patients with albuminuria.[46] In addition, low-density lipoprotein size is decreased in diabetic nephropathy. These changes may be apparent before the development of albuminuria.[47] Several studies have correlated the presence of an abnormal lipid profile with the onset and progression of diabetic nephropathy.[48,49] Research in atherosclerosis disease has long established the importance of the genetic influences on lipid metabolism. It is therefore plausible that some of these modifiers may also contribute to the development and progression of diabetic renal disease.

An example of the risk associated with inherited dyslipidaemia may be demonstrated in experimental studies using mice in whom the gene for apolipoprotein E (Apo E) has been 'knocked out'. These animals have dyslipidaemia, accelerated vascular disease[50] and nephropathy in the setting of experimental diabetes (unpublished data) (Figure 4.3). In humans,

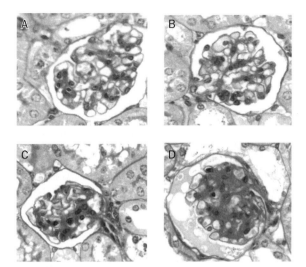

**Figure 4.3** Increased diabetic glomerulosclerosis in the Apo E 'knock-out' mouse [D] compared to control (c57/bl6) mouse without diabetes [C]. Normal glomerular architecture in the Apo E knockout [B] and control mice [A] without diabetes is shown by comparison.
(Pictures Courtesy of Dr Karin Jandeliet-Dahm, unpublished data.) [Stained with periodic acid Schiff reagent (PAS), 400x magnification.]

there are three common polymorphisms of the Apo E gene (E2, E3 and E4). Individuals homozygous for the Apo E2 allele have impaired very-low-density lipoprotein remnant clearance and type 3 dyslipidaemia. Recent studies have suggested an association between the Apo E polymorphisms and nephropathy in both type 1[51,52] and type 2 diabetes.[53–55] For example, in one study, patients with type 1 diabetes and nephropathy were three times more likely to be a carrier of the Apo E2 allele than normoalbuminuric patients.[52] In another study, the frequency of nephropathy was significantly greater in Apo E2 patients with type 2 diabetes (59.1%) than in Apo E3/3 (34.3%) or Apo E4 patients (8.8%).[55] While the E2 allele may be associated with an increased risk, the E4 allele may also be protective.[56] For example, there is research showing that 67.6% of patients with diabetes homozygous for the Apo E4 allele were normoalbuminuric, compared to 34.3% with the Apo E3/3 and only 4.5% of patients homozygous for the Apo E2 allele.[55] While these findings seem robust, it should be noted that other studies have shown no association between Apo E polymorphisms in type 1 diabetes[57] or even protection conferred by Apo E2 polymorphisms in type 2 diabetes[58]

## INSULIN AND NEPHROPATHY

Insulin sensitivity, while contributing to glycaemic control, is also a strong independent predictor of the development of diabetic nephropathy. This effect is not confined to patients with type 2 diabetes. There are now data describing the role of insulin sensitivity in the development of complications in type 1 diabetes.[59] An association between insulin sensitivity and diabetic nephropathy may be inferred from the strong link between insulin sensitivity and cardiovascular mortality. In addition, markers of insulin resistance, such as triglyceride levels and waist to hip ratio, are also risk factors for albuminuria.

Insulin sensitivity may also be genetically determined. Yip et al[59] described familial clustering of insulin sensitivity in type 1 diabetes. Insulin resistance is also more common in the relatives of patients with nephropathy than in the relatives of patients with diabetes and normoalbuminuria. Similar findings have been reported in type 2 diabetes.[60] In this context, insulin sensitivity is associated with reduced risk of nephropathy.[61] However, although it has been shown that insulin resistance may develop prior to the appearance of hypertension and albuminuria,[62] the HOORN study found no association between either impaired glucose tolerance, hyperinsulinaemia, or insulin sensitivity and the prevalence of microalbuminuria.[63]

Specific genetic influences on insulin sensitivity may also influence the presentation of nephropathy. For example, polymorphisms of GLUT transporter genes may contribute both to glycaemic control and independently to the development of nephropathy. In particular, GLUT1 activity has been implicated in renal hypertrophy and extracellular matrix formation in mesangial cells. The Xba1 polymorphisms of the GLUT1 gene may be associated with an increased prevalence of nephropathy in some ethnic groups.[64] In addition, maturity onset diabetes of the young (MODY) has been associated with an accelerated progression of diabetic complications, including nephropathy.[65] While this may reflect difficulties in glycaemic control in this group of patients,[66] genes associated with MODY have also been associated with the development and progression of diabetic renal disease. While mutations associated with the hepatocyte nuclear factor-1 alpha and beta (MODY 3 and 5) loci have been linked with nephropathy in some patients,[67] larger population-based studies have failed to demonstrate this association.

## THE RENIN-ANGIOTENSIN SYSTEM (RAS) AND DIABETIC NEPHROPATHY

The pivotal role of the RAS in the pathogenesis of diabetic nephropathy has long been recognized. This is perhaps best manifested by the unique protective effects conferred by inhibitors of the RAS in diabetic renal disease.[68] In experimental models, upregulation of the RAS in the setting of diabetes is associated with accelerated nephropathy. In the transgenic (mRen-2)27 rat, a mouse Ren-2 gene is inserted into the genome of a Sprague-Dawley rat, resulting in the overexpression of renin at sites of normal physiological expression[69] and activation of the intrarenal RAS.[70] The induction of diabetes in this model results in progressive renal pathology with features similar to human diabetic nephropathy (Figure 4.4). Similarly, insertion of multiple copies of the human angiotensin-converting enzyme (ACE) gene into transgenic mice results in increased proteinuria in response to diabetes, correlating with plasma ACE activity.[71] These studies suggest that genetic modifications in the RAS may have a significant potential to influence the predisposition and development of diabetic nephropathy.

In humans, activity of the RAS can be modified by a number of genetic factors. For example, circulating ACE activity is strongly associated with polymorphisms in the ACE gene.[72] The best characterized of these is the biallelic polymorphism defined by the presence of an extra 287-base-pair sequence in intron 16 of the ACE gene (the so-called insertion, or I, genotype) or its absence (the so-called D, or deletion, genotype). Although the ACE insertion/deletion (I/D) polymorphism involves the intronic region of the ACE gene, this polymorphism accounts for at least half of the phenotypic variance in serum ACE activity.[72] It has been suggested that the insertion fragment may have a silencing function, as the sequence is similar to other suppressor genes.[73] Patients homozygous for deletion (DD) allele display the highest ACE values (126% of average). Those homozygous for insertion allele (II) show the lowest ACE values (76%), and those heterozygous (I/D) have intermediate values (arbitrarily 100%).[71]

Initial studies suggested that the D allele was associated with an increased prevalence of nephropathy and premature death in patients, in both type 1 and type 2 diabetes. For example, the GENEDIAB study of 449 patients with type 1 diabetes found that the D allele was associated with increased incidence and severity of diabetic nephropathy (with an odds ratio of 1.9) independent of hypertension or glycaemic control.[74] In a similar study in type 2 diabetes, Jeffers[75] also found the DD genotype to be an independent risk factor for diabetic nephropathy with an odds ratio of 2.8. Further studies along the same lines have now been conducted in many populations with many ethnic groups. However, as with virtually all of the candidate genes associated with nephropathy, a number of these studies have failed to replicate earlier findings.[76,77] While this may, to some extent, reflect ethnic differences in the frequency of the D allele, even within individual ethnic groups the results of studies remain conflicting. Nonetheless, pooled meta-analyses incorporating many disparate studies confirm a significant odds ratio in individuals (OR = 1.32; $P < 0.0001$) with the DD genotype for diabetic renal disease.[78]

While one consequence of the ACE I/D polymorphism is the modification of circulating ACE activity, it is not clear whether the predisposition to nephropathy is mediated through this mechanism. It is possible that the polymorphism is closely linked with another variant around the ACE gene rather than being the quantitative trait locus. For example, Freire et al[79] showed that type 1 diabetic patients homozygous at the PstI site (intron 7) of the ACE gene were at a greater risk of developing nephropathy. One suggestion is that the ACE polymorphism may identify subgroups of patients who fail to benefit from standard ACE inhibition, rather than directly influence the progression of diabetic renal disease.[80] For example, Jacobsen et al demonstrated that ACE polymorphisms independently influenced the decline in albuminuria after initiation of ACE inhibition in patients with type 1 diabetes.[81] Patients with the DD genotype were three times less likely to

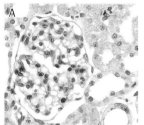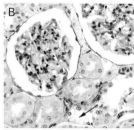

**Figure 4.4** Augmented diabetic glomerulosclerosis in the mREN-2 rat (renin over-expressing).
A: Untreated nondiabetic Ren-2 rat showing minimal glomerulosclerosis and normal tubules.
B: Untreated diabetic Ren-2 rat exhibiting glomerular damage and degenerated tubules (arrow).
[Stained with periodic acid Schiff reagent (PAS), 350x magnification.]

respond than patients with the II genotype.[81] Against this, Ha et al[82] described an augmented reduction of proteinuria in patients with type 2 diabetes and the DD genotype. The interpretation of these studies is complicated by survival bias due to the increased risk of premature death in patients possessing the D allele and racial differences in allele frequencies. At present, there are insufficient data to make a firm conclusion either way.

Genes coding for other components of the RAS have also been variably associated with nephropathy.[83] For example, polymorphisms of the angiotensinogen gene encoding threonine instead of methionine (M235T), or substituting methionine for threonine (T174M), have been associated with increased plasma angiotensinogen concentration, hypertension and nephropathy in some studies,[84] but not all.[85] Similarly, polymorphisms of the type 1 angiotensin II receptor have been associated with nephropathy in case-control studies.[83] Again, larger family-based studies have failed to replicate this association.[20]

## ALDOSE REDUCTASE AND DIABETIC NEPHROPATHY

Aldose reductase is a key enzyme of the polyol pathway, involved in the metabolism of glucose and the NADPH-dependent reduction of a broad range of carbonyl compounds. In particular, the downstream accumulation of sorbitol and activation of the hexose kinase pathway have been implicated in the pathogenesis of a number of diabetic complications, including nephropathy.[86,87] Recent studies have shown that polymorphisms in the aldose reductase gene may be associated with susceptibility to nephropathy in patients with both type 1[88] and type 2 diabetes.[89] In particular, the polymorphism in the (A-C)n microsatellite repeat sequence (located upstream of the transcription start site) may modulate expression of the aldose reductase gene. Among the eight different alleles at this site, the Z-2 allele is associated with upregulated expression of the aldose reductase gene in the presence of hyperglycaemia[90] and increased prevalence of the nephropathy.[91] Segregation of the Z-2 allele has also been demonstrated from diabetic parent to affected sibling with nephropathy.[92] However, individuals with the Z+2 allele are more than seven times less likely to develop diabetic renal disease than those without this marker (although this may reflect the absence of the Z-2 allele rather than a specific protective trait). Again, not all studies support this association.[89,93,94]

In a recent large study, Fanelli et al[95] failed to demonstrate that microsatellite polymorphisms contributed significantly to nephropathy in the combined GENEDIAB and SURGENE populations. Moreover, it is not clear that the putative risk associated with these polymorphisms is related to aldose reductase. Recent work suggests that the gene coding for endothelial nitric oxide synthase may be localized to the same chromosomal region as aldose reductase.[96] In addition, other polymorphisms in the aldose reductase gene (specifically the 106 polymorphism) may better correlate with the development of nephropathy than the microsatellite polymorphisms.[89]

## SODIUM/HYDROGEN EXCHANGER (NHE) ACTIVITY AND NEPHROPATHY

Overactivity of the amiloride-sensitive $Na^+/H^+$ exchanger (NHE) has been described in patients with type 1 diabetes who develop nephropathy. As its name suggests, the NHE mediates excretion of intracellular $H^+$ in exchange for extracellular sodium. It is therefore important in the regulation of intracellular pH and cell volume, and stimulus-response coupling, as well as matrix synthesis and cell proliferation. Exchanger activity and expression are modulated by a large variety of stimuli, including growth promoters, hormones, changes in cell volume and extracellular pH. In addition, some NHE activity may be genetically determined. For example, Trevisan et al[97] demonstrated concordance for NHE activity in cultured skin fibroblasts from siblings with type 1 diabetes. Matteucci and Giampietro[98] demonstrated that NHE activity was also altered in non-diabetic siblings of patients with nephropathy.

There is evidence that the traits that determine NHE activity may segregate with the predisposition to diabetic nephropathy rather than hypertension or other influencing traits.[97] In prospective studies, the activity of the red-cell NHE has been found to predict the development of proteinuria in patients with diabetes.[99,100] However, once more, the data appear to conflict with other studies that have found little or no significant relationship between the NHE and albuminuria.[101] The role of genetic polymorphisms in determining NHE activity, particularly for tissue-specific isoforms, remains to be addressed.

## ERYTHROCYTE NA/LI COUNTERTRANSPORT

Erythrocyte Na/Li countertransport is also increased in patients with diabetes and nephropathy.[102–104] Like

NHE, most of the variability in the activity of this transport system is thought to be genetic in origin. This is supported by the close concordance of sodium–lithium countertransport activity in identical twins discordant for type 1 diabetes.[105] In a recent study by Mead et al, first-degree relatives of diabetic patients with nephropathy were found to have similar abnormalities in their Na/Li countertransport kinetics to the patients themselves.[102] Notably, the relatives had no clinically detectable abnormality, suggesting that the changes were not a direct result of diabetes or hypertension. This suggests an association between abnormal Na/Li countertransport and an inherited susceptibility to nephropathy. Some data suggest that Na/Li countertransport may be a reasonable marker for the susceptibility to nephropathy. For example, in adolescents with type 1 diabetes, an elevated baseline erythrocyte $Na^+/Li^+$ countertransport was associated with an adjusted odds ratio of 4.5 (95% CI of 2.1–11.4) for the development of microalbuminuria.[103] However, like NHE, the evidence for this link is also in dispute. While a number of studies have since demonstrated correlation between the Na/Li countertransport flux rate in diabetic patients with nephropathy, other studies have suggested that Na/Li countertransport was increased in all diabetic patients and unconnected with nephropathy.[106,107] Furthermore, the increase in Na/Li countertransport activity seen in patients with diabetes may not parallel the onset of glomerular hyperfiltration.[108]

Finally, the physiological significance of the linkage trait is also uncertain. Countertransport represents a derived *in vitro* measure of the rate of lithium efflux. This has no functional correlate in vivo. The increase in Na/Li countertransport is not associated with changes in endothelial function, degree of metabolic control, blood pressure or renal haemodynamics.[109] It is possible that Na/Li countertransport activity may be a marker of changes in the composition of the cell membrane or alterations in intracellular ion-exchanger or signalling systems, manifested as the predisposition to nephropathy. Another suggestion is that erythrocyte sodium–lithium countertransport may parallel NHE activity.[110]

## RENAL STRUCTURAL PARAMETERS AS RISK FACTORS FOR DIABETIC NEPHROPATHY

While a number of phenotypes may be associated with the development of diabetic nephropathy, there is evidence that at least some of these traits may be intrinsic to the kidney. That is, certain renal structural or physiological traits appear to be associated with nephropathy.[111] For example, mesangial cells from diabetic mice that progress to nephropathy are characterized by a sclerosing phenotype.[112] The concept may be further demonstrated in transplantation studies, where the development and progression of diabetic lesions in the allograft are independent of the historical rate and progression of nephropathy in the recipient despite the presence of a similar diabetic environment.[113] In addition, a number of studies have now demonstrated familial segregation of glomerular lesions associated with the development of nephropathy in diabetes.[114] For example, Fioretto et al[12] demonstrated a strong correlation between glomerular basement-membrane width, mesangial expansion and nephropathy risk in patients with type 1 diabetes.

Hyperfiltration is also thought to be a key determinant in early renal injury in diabetes. This is supported by studies showing accelerated nephropathy following subtotal nephrectomy in experimental models.[115] Glomerular volumes are significantly higher in patients with nephropathy than in those who remain normoalbuminuric.[116] Glomerular pressure and volume may also be influenced by genetic factors though a variety of mechanisms. One that has received recent attention has been the strong association between nephron endowment and mean glomerular volume. In humans, no further nephronogenesis occurs after birth. At the time of birth, infants possess all the glomeruli that they will ever develop. Nephronogenesis is linked to a number of factors, including intrauterine nutrition as well as genetic influences such as maternal body mass. There is a strong correlation between glomerular size and nephron number, so that fewer glomeruli result in an increase in mean glomerular volume.[117] This may be seen as an adaptive response appropriate to the optimization of glomerular surface filtration area.

However, in the setting of hyperglycaemia, this may become maladaptive, resulting in glomerular hypertension, protein leakage and accelerated 'nephron' dropout. This hypothesis suggests that diabetic patients born with fewer glomeruli could be more prone to develop renal impairment when exposed to hyperglycaemia.[118] To support this hypothesis, Rossing et al[119] demonstrated that patients without proteinuria had a greater birth weight than those with microalbuminuria or proteinuria. Similarly, small-statured patients with diabetes (as a proxy measure of nephron endowment) appear to have an increased prevalence of nephropathy in both type 1[120] and type 2 diabetes.[121] Microalbuminuria may also be more common in nondiabetic patients of small stature.[122] Low birth weight is also a strong predictor of albuminuria and premature mortality in aboriginal Australians.[123] However, not all studies have found this association.[124,125] The difficulty in interpreting these data rests in the many factors that contribute to birth weight. For example, studies may be confounded by intrauterine hyperglycaemia acting to increase birth weight.[126] The association may also be less clear in populations with higher birth weights and fewer renal disease risk factors.[127] At present, there is no reliable way to predict nephron numbers. Even within birth-weight cohorts, it is apparent that glomerular numbers are extremely variable.[117,128,129] While the concept of nephron endowment is appealing, further research is required to determine its role in the development of nephropathy in diabetes.

## PROGRESSION OF MICROALBUMINURIA

The development of microalbuminuria is the most important risk factor and an obligatory precursor for the development of overt nephropathy. However overt nephropathy is not its inevitable consequence. While many patients who manifest microalbuminuria go on to develop overt nephropathy, a subset of patients remain microalbuminuric or even regress to a normoalbuminuric state.[130] This variability in rate of progression casts a shadow over the interpretation of many of the studies above, particularly those that use the development of microalbuminuria as their sole end point. It may well be that some of the associations demonstrated may be weakened by the inclusion of 'non-progressors' in the nephropathy cohorts. In addition, it is possible that the determinants of disease progression may be significantly different from those which predispose to albuminuria in the first place. For example, glycaemic control is only a weak predictor of progression to overt nephropathy once a patient becomes albuminuric.[131] Abnormalities in the albumin excretion rate in type 2 diabetes may also be the expression of different phenotypes reflecting a heterogeneity in renal lesions.[132] As it is not possible to predict which patients will progress to overt nephropathy, intensive treatment must be applied to all patients with microalbuminuria. Future genetic studies must, first and foremost, be able to obtain accurate phenotypes of diabetic nephropathy to ensure the predictive validity of any putative inherited marker.

## DEVELOPMENT OF SUSCEPTIBILITY GENES TO NEPHROPATHY

If an inherited susceptibility to diabetic nephropathy exists, it raises a number of questions about how such a trait came to be and why it should continue to be present in at least a third of patients with diabetes. Since the trait is so commonplace, it suggests primeval origins. Moreover, it must have been propagated widely because, in the absence of hyperglycaemia, it is not deleterious. It may even be that a theoretical survival advantage exists in a predisposition to diabetic nephropathy in the absence of hyperglycaemia.[11] For example, genes which benefited preagriculturalist hunter-gatherers, adapted to life in a variety of habitats, may be counterproductive in sedentary people whose Westernized diet is characterized by high amounts of fat, refined carbohydrates, and salt, as well as being poor in fibre, nutrients and vitamins. It is also worth considering that genes which protect against perinatal mortality (the main cause of prereproductive death) also predispose to nephropathy. These genes may range from those behind the development of an aggressive and sustained inflammatory response to noxious stimuli[133] to a thrifty phenotype in response to undernutrition.[134] It seems likely that this survivor bias continues to influence our genetic response to environmental stimuli in ways that have not been established.

## CONCLUSIONS

Hyperglycaemia, though critical for the development of diabetic renal disease, is insufficient alone to account for it. It is clear that there are many other mediators that determine why one individual may be susceptible to nephropathy while another remains unscathed despite inadequate glycaemic or blood-pressure control. While there is strong evidence for an inherited predisposition contributing to diabetic nephropathy, the precise role of genetic influences in determining the development of clinical disease remains to be established. None of the candidate genes described in this chapter can, on their own, account for more than 5% of all variability in the prevalence of nephropathy.[11] In addition, it seems unlikely that any single gene, as yet undiscovered, can significantly determine the risk of diabetic nephropathy in any given population. It is conceivable that the influence of genetic factors is obscured by the overriding influence of phenotypic risk factors, such as glycaemic, lipid and blood-pressure control, to which these genes contribute in a multifactorial way. However, it is more likely that a number of genes, as well as environmental factors, predispose to diabetic renal disease. This does not mean that the search for susceptibility genes is a meaningless endeavour. Specific genetic polymorphisms may significantly contribute to the risk of nephropathy in an individual or family with diabetes while they have little effect in a population of patients where diabetes appears multifactorial in origin. In addition, the mere existence of specific genetic risk factors can provide pivotal understanding to the pathogenesis of disease. For example, the gene for familial hypercholesterolaemia (FH) is an uncommon cause of cardiovascular disease, yet the understanding of FH leads directly to lipid-lowering therapy in the general population. It is anticipated that new approaches using family-based strategies and large genome-scan analyses will yield novel targets for therapeutic intervention for both the prevention and treatment of diabetic nephropathy.

## REFERENCES

1. Hasslacher C, Ritz E, Wahl P et al, Similar risks of nephropathy in patients with type I or type II diabetes mellitus, *Nephrol Dial Transplant* (1989) **4:** 859–63.
2. Ritz E, Orth SR, Nephropathy in patients with type 2 diabetes mellitus, *N Engl J Med* (1999) **341:** 1127–33.
3. Borch-Johnsen K, The incidence of nephropathy in IDDM as related to mortality. Costs and benefits of early intervention. In: Mogensen CE, ed., *The Kidney and Hypertension in Diabetes Mellitus*, 5th edn (Kluwer Academic: Dordrecht, The Netherlands, 2000) 169–78.
4. Nelson RG, Pettitt DJ, Carraher MJ et al, Effect of proteinuria on mortality in NIDDM, *Diabetes* (1988) **37:** 1499–504.
5. Friday RP, Trucco M, Pietropaolo M, Genetics of type 1 diabetes mellitus, *Diabetes Nutr Metab* (1999) **12:** 3–26.
6. McIntyre EA, Walker M, Genetics of type 2 diabetes and insulin resistance: knowledge from human studies, *Clin Endocrinol (Oxf)* (2002) **57:** 303–11.
7. Seaquist ER, Goetz FC, Rich S et al, Familial clustering of diabetic kidney disease: evidence for genetic susceptibility to diabetic nephropathy, *N Engl J Med* (1989) **320:** 1161–5.
8. Quinn M, Angelico MC, Warram JH et al, Familial factors determine the development of diabetic nephropathy in patients with IDDM, *Diabetologia* (1996) **39:** 940–5.
9. Pettitt DJ, Saad MF, Bennett PH et al, Familial predisposition to renal disease in two generations of Pima Indians with type II (non-insulin dependent) diabetes mellitus, *Diabetologia* (1990) **33:** 438–43.
10. Freedman BI, Tuttle AB, Spray BJ, Familial predisposition to nephropathy in African-Americans with non-insulin dependent diabetes mellitus, *Am J Kidney Dis* (1999) **5:** 710–13.
11. Krolewski AS, Genetics of diabetic nephropathy: evidence for major and minor gene effects, *Kidney Int* (1999) **55:** 1582–96.
12. Fioretto P, Steffes MW, Barbosa J et al, Is diabetic nephropathy inherited? Studies of glomerular structure in type I diabetic sibling pairs, *Diabetes* (1999) **48:** 865–9.
13. Borch-Johnsen K, Norgaard K, Hommel E et al, Is diabetic nephropathy an inherited complication? *Kidney Int* (1992) **41:** 719–22.
14. Forsblom CM, Kanninen T, Lehtovirta M et al, Heritability of albumin excretion rate in families of patients with type II diabetes, *Diabetologia* (1999) **42:** 1359–66.
15. Strojek K, Grzeszczak W, Morawin E et al, Nephropathy of type II diabetes: evidence for hereditary factors?, *Kidney Int* (1997) **51:** 1602–7.
16. Lei HH, Perneger TV, Klag MJ et al, Familial aggregation of renal disease in a population-based case-control study, *J Am Soc Nephrol* (1998) **9:** 1270–6.
17. Thompson CF, Simmons D, Collins JF et al, Predisposition to nephropathy in Polynesians is associated with family history of renal disease, not diabetes mellitus, *Diabet Med* (2001) **18:** 40–6.
18. Satko SG, Langefeld CD, Daeihagh P et al, Nephropathy in siblings of African Americans with overt type II diabetic nephropathy, *Am J Kidney Dis* (2002) **40:** 489–94.
19. Rossing P, Hougaard P, Borch-Johnsen K et al, Predictors of mortality in insulin dependent diabetes: 10-year observational follow-up study, *BMJ* (1996) **313:** 779–84.
20. Tarnow L, Cambien F, Rossing P et al, Angiotensin-II type 1 receptor gene polymorphism and diabetic microangiopathy, *Nephrol Dial Transplant* (1996) **11:** 1019–23.
21. Roglic G, Colhoun HM, Stevens LK et al, EURODIAB IDDM Complications Study Group. Parental history of hypertension and parental history of diabetes and microvascular complications in insulin-dependent diabetes mellitus: EURODIAB IDDM Complications Study, *Diabetes Med* (1998) **15:** 418–26.
22. Canini LH, Gerchman F, Gross JL, Increased familial history of arterial hypertension, coronary heart disease, and renal disease in Brazilian type II diabetic patients with diabetic nephropathy, *Diabetes Care* (1998) **21:** 1545–50.
23. Earle KK, Porter KA, Ostberg J et al, Variation in the progression of diabetic nephropathy according to racial origin, *Nephrol Dial Transplant* (2001) **16:** 286–90.
24. Kalter-Leibovici O, Van Dyk DJ, Leibovici L et al, Risk factors for development of diabetic nephropathy and retinopathy in Jewish IDDM patients, *Diabetes* (1991) **40:** 204–10.
25. Martins D, Tareen N, Norris KC, The epidemiology of end-stage renal disease among African Americans, *Am J Med Sci* (2002) **323:** 65–71.
26. Nelson RG, Knowler WC, McCance DR et al, Determinants of end-stage renal disease in Pima Indians with type II (non-insulin-dependent) diabetes mellitus and proteinuria, *Diabetologia* (1993) **36:** 1087–93.
27. Mehrotra S, Ling KL, Bekele Y et al, Lipid hydroperoxide and markers of renal disease susceptibility in African-Caribbean and Caucasian patients with type 2 diabetes mellitus, *Diabet Med* (2001) **18:** 109–15.
28. Schultz CJ, Konopelska-Bahu T, Dalton RN et al, Microalbuminuria prevalence varies with age, sex, and puberty in children with type 1 diabetes followed from diagnosis in a longitudinal study. Oxford Regional Prospective Study Group, *Diabetes Care* (1999) **22:** 495–502.
29. Holl RW, Grabert M, Thon A et al, Urinary excretion of albumin in adolescents with type 1 diabetes: persistent versus intermittent microalbuminuria and relationship to duration of diabetes, sex, and metabolic control, *Diabetes Care* (1999) **22:** 1555–60.
30. Seliger SL, Davis C, Stehman-Breen C, Gender and the progression of renal disease, *Curr Opin Nephrol Hypertens* (2001) **10:** 219–25.
31. Crook ED, Diabetic nephropathy in African Americans, *Am J Hypertens* (2001) **14**(6 Pt 2):132S–8S.
32. Mueller PW, Caudill SP, Urinary albumin excretion in children:

factors related to elevated excretion in the United States population, *Ren Fail* (1999) **21:** 293–302.

33. Lane PH. Diabetic kidney disease: impact of puberty, *Am J Physiol Renal Physiol* (2002) **283:** F589–600.

34. Sakemi T, Ohtsuka N, Tomiyosi Y et al, Attenuating effect of castration on glomerular injury is age-dependent in unilaterally nephrectomized male Sprague-Dawley rats, *Nephron* (1997) **75:** 342–9.

35. Cohen AM, Rosenmann E, Male sex hormone and nephropathy in Cohen diabetic rat (genetically selected sucrose fed), *Diabete Metab* (1984) **10:** 199–205.

36. Weksler-Zangen S, Yagil C, Zangen DH et al, The newly inbred Cohen diabetic rat: a nonobese normolipidemic genetic model of diet-induced type II diabetes expressing sex differences, *Diabetes* (2001) **50:** 2521–9.

37. Rudberg S, Persson B, Serum leptin levels in young females with insulin-dependent diabetes and the relationship to hyperandrogenicity and microalbuminuria, *Horm Res* (1998a) **50:** 297–302.

38. Fernandez-Real JM, Lopez-Bermejo A, Ricart W, Cross-talk between iron metabolism and diabetes, *Diabetes* (2002) **51:** 2348–54.

39. Loebstein R, Lehotay DC, Luo X et al, Diabetic nephropathy in hypertransfused patients with beta-thalassemia. The role of oxidative stress, *Diabetes Care* (1998) **21:** 1306–9.

40. Moczulski DK, Grzeszczak W, Gawlik B, Role of hemochromatosis C282Y and H63D mutations in HFE gene in development of type 2 diabetes and diabetic nephropathy, *Diabetes Care* (2001) **24:** 1187–91.

41. Barzilay J, Warram JH, Bak M et al, Predisposition to hypertension: risk factor for nephropathy and hypertension in IDDM, *Kidney Int* (1992) **41:** 723–30.

42. Fogarty DG, Krolewski AS, Genetic susceptibility and the role of hypertension in diabetic nephropathy, *Curr Opin Nephrol Hypertens* (1997) **6:** 184–91.

43. Cooper ME, Allen TJ, Macmillan P et al, Genetic hypertension accelerates nephropathy in the streptozotocin diabetic rat, *Am J Hypertens* (1988) **1:** 5–10.

44. Rudberg S, Stattin EL, Dahlquist G, Familial and perinatal risk factors for micro- and macroalbuminuria in young IDDM patients, *Diabetes* (1998b) **47:** 1121–6.

45. Bonnet F, Cooper ME. Potential influence of lipids in diabetic nephropathy: insights from experimental data and clinical studies, *Diabetes Metab* (2000) **26:** 254–64.

46. Yoshino G, Hirano T, Kazumi T, Dyslipidaemia in diabetes mellitus, *Diabetes Res Clin Pract* (1996) **33:** 1–14.

47. Myrup B, Mathiesen ER, Ronn B et al, Endothelial function and serum lipids in the course of developing microalbuminuria in insulin-dependent diabetes mellitus, *Diabetes Res* (1994) **26:** 33–9.

48. Ravid M, Brosh D, Ravid-Safran D et al, Main risk factors for nephropathy in type 2 diabetes mellitus are plasma cholesterol levels, mean blood pressure, and hyperglycemia, *Arch Intern Med* (1998) **158:** 998–1004.

49. Gall MA, Hougaard P, Borch-Johnsen K et al, Risk factors for development of incipient and overt diabetic nephropathy in patients with non-insulin dependent diabetes mellitus: prospective, observational study, *BMJ* (1997) **314:** 783–8.

50. Candido R, Jandeleit-Dahm KA, Cao Z et al, Prevention of accelerated atherosclerosis by angiotensin-converting enzyme inhibition in diabetic apolipoprotein E-deficient mice, *Circulation* (2002) **106:** 246–53.

51. Chowdhury TA, Dyer PH, Kumar S et al, Association of apolipoprotein 2 allele with diabetic nephropathy in Caucasian subjects with IDDM, *Diabetes* (1998) **47:** 278–80.

52. Araki S, Moczulski DK, Hanna L et al, Apo E polymorphism and the development of diabetic nephropathy in type I diabetes. Results of case-control and family-based studies, *Diabetes* (2000) **49:** 2190–5.

53. Ha SK, Park HS, Kim KW et al, Association between apolipoprotein E polymorphism and macroalbuminuria in patients with non-insulin dependent diabetes mellitus, *Nephrol Dial Transplant* (1999) **14:** 2144–9.

54. Werle E, Fiehn W, Hasslacher C, Apolipoprotein E polymorphism and renal function in German type I and type II diabetic patients, *Diabetes Care* (1998) **21:** 994–8.

55. Eto M, Saito M, Okada M et al, Apolipoprotein E genetic polymorphism, remnant lipoproteins, and nephropathy in type II diabetic patients, *Am J Kidney Dis* (2002) **40:** 243–51.

56. Kimura H, Suzuki Y, Gejyo F et al, Apolipoprotein E4 reduces risk of diabetic nephropathy in patients with NIDDM, *Am J Kidney Dis* (1998) **31:** 666–73.

57. Onuma T, Laffel LM, Angelico MC et al, Apolipoprotein E genotypes and risk of diabetic nephropathy. *J Am Soc Nephrol* (1996) **7:**1075–8.

58. Ukkola O, Kervinen K, Salmela PI et al, Apolipoprotein E phenotype is related to macro- and microangiopathy in patients with non-insulin dependent diabetes mellitus, *Atherosclerosis* (1993) **101:** 9–15.

59. Yip J, Mattock MB, Morocutti A, Insulin resistance in insulin dependent diabetic patients with microalbuminuria, *Lancet* (1993) **342:** 883–7.

60. Forsblom CM, Eriksson JG, Ekstrand AV et al, Insulin resistance and abnormal albumin excretion in non-diabetic first-degree relatives of patients with NIDDM, *Diabetologia* (1995) **38:** 363–9.

61. Orchard TJ, Chang YF, Ferrell RE et al, Nephropathy in type I diabetes: a manifestation of insulin resistance and multiple genetic susceptibilities? Further evidence from the Pittsburgh Epidemiology of Diabetes Complication Study, *Kidney Int* (2002) **62:** 963–70.

62. Fujikawa R, Okubo M, Egusa G et al, Insulin resistance precedes the appearance of albuminuria in non-diabetic subjects: 6 year follow-up study, *Diabetes Res Clin Pract* (2001) **53:** 99–106.

63. Jager A, Kostense PJ, Nijpels G et al, Microalbuminuria is strongly associated with NIDDM and hypertension, but not with the insulin resistance syndrome: the Hoorn Study, *Diabetologia* (1998) **41:** 694–700.

64. Hodgkinson AD, Millward BA, Demaine AG. Polymorphisms of the glucose transporter (GLUT1) gene are associated with diabetic nephropathy, *Kidney Int* (2001b) **59:** 985–9.

65. Stride A, Hattersley AT, Different genes, different diabetes: lessons from maturity-onset diabetes of the young, *Ann Med* (2002) **34:** 207–16.

66. Isomaa B, Henricsson M, Lehto M et al, Chronic diabetic complications in patients with MODY3 diabetes, *Diabetologia* (1998) **41:** 467–73.

67. Velho G, Vaxillaire M, Boccio V et al, Diabetes complications in NIDDM kindreds linked to the MODY3 locus on chromosome 12q, *Diabetes Care* (1996) **19:** 915–19.

68. Cooper ME. Pathogenesis, prevention, and treatment of diabetic nephropathy, *Lancet* (1998) **352:** 213–19.

69. Mullins JJ, Peters J, Ganten D, Fulminant hypertension in transgenic rats harbouring the mouse Ren-2 gene, *Nature* (1990) **344:** 541–4.

70. Kelly DJ, Wilkinson-Berka JL, Cooper ATJ et al, A new model of progressive diabetic renal impairment in the transgenic (mRen-2)27 rat. *Kidney Int* (1998) **54:** 343–52.

71. Huang W, Gallois Y, Bouby N et al, Genetically increased angiotensin I-converting enzyme level and renal complications in the diabetic mouse, *Proc Natl Acad Sci USA* (2001) **98:** 13330–4.

72. Rigat B, Hubert C, Alhenc-Gelas F et al, An insertion/deletion polymorphism in the angiotensin I-converting enzyme gene accounting for half the variance of serum enzyme levels, *J Clin Invest* (1990) **86:** 1343–6.

73. Hunley TE, Julian BA, Phillips JA 3rd et al, Angiotensin converting enzyme gene polymorphism: potential silencer motif and impact on progression in IgA nephropathy, *Kidney Int* (1996) **49:** 571–7.

74. Marre M, Jeunemaitre X, Gallois Y et al, Contribution of genetic polymorphism in the renin-angiotensin system to the development of renal complications in insulin-dependent diabetes: Génétique de la Nephropathie Diabetique (GENEDIAB) Study Group, *J Clin Invest* (1997) **99:** 1585–95.

75. Jeffers BW, Estacio RO, Raynolds MV et al, Angiotensin-converting enzyme gene polymorphism in non-insulin dependent diabetes mellitus and its relationship with diabetic nephropathy, *Kidney Int* (1997) **52:** 473–7.

76. Schmidt S, Schone N, Ritz E, Association of ACE gene polymorphism and diabetic nephropathy? The Diabetic Nephropathy Study Group, *Kidney Int* (1995) **47:** 1176–81.

77. Chowdhury TA, Dronsfield MJ, Kumar S et al, Examination of two genetic polymorphisms within the renin-angiotensin system: no evidence for an association with nephropathy in IDDM, *Diabetologia* (1996) **39:** 1108–14.

78. Fujisawa T, Ikegami H, Kawaguchi Y et al, Meta-analysis of association of insertion/deletion polymorphism of angiotensin I-converting enzyme gene with diabetic nephropathy and retinopathy, *Diabetologia* (1998) **41:** 47–53.

79. Freire MB, van Dijk DJ, Erman A et al, DNA polymorphisms in the ACE gene, serum ACE activity and the risk of nephropathy in insulin-dependent diabetes mellitus, *Nephrol Dial Transplant* (1998) **13:** 2553–8

80. Parving HH, Jacobsen P, Tarnow L et al, Effect of deletion polymorphism of angiotensin converting enzyme gene on progression of diabetic nephropathy during inhibition of angiotensin converting enzyme: observational follow up study, *BMJ* (1996) **313:** 591–4.

81. Jacobsen P, Rossing K, Rossing P et al, Angiotensin converting enzyme gene polymorphism and ACE inhibition in diabetic nephropathy, *Kidney Int* (1998) **53:** 1002–6.

82. Ha SK, Yong Lee S, Su Park H et al, ACE DD genotype is more susceptible than ACE II and ID genotypes to the antiproteinuric effect of ACE inhibitors in patients with proteinuric non-insulin-dependent diabetes mellitus, *Nephrol Dial Transplant* (2000) **15:** 1617–23.

83. Fradin S, Goulet-Salmon B, Chantepie M et al, Relationship between polymorphisms in the renin-angiotensin system and nephropathy in type II diabetic patients, *Diabete Metab* (2002) **28:** 27–32.

84. Fogarty DG, Harron JC, Hughes AE et al, A molecular variant of angiotensinogen is associated with diabetic nephropathy in IDDM, *Diabetes* (1996) **45:** 1204–8.

85. Kinoshita JH, Nishimura C. The involvement of aldose reductase in diabetic complications. *Diabetes Metab Rev* (1988) **4:** 323–37.

86. Zychma MJ, Zukowska-Szczechowska E, Lacka BI et al, Angiotensinogen M235T and chymase gene CMA/B polymorphisms are not associated with nephropathy in type II diabetes, *Nephrol Dial Transplant* (2000) **15:** 1965–70.

87. Park HK, Ahn CW, Lee GT et al, (AC)(n) polymorphism of aldose reductase gene and diabetic microvascular complications in type II diabetes mellitus, *Diabetes Res Clin Pract* (2002) **55:** 151–7.

88. Liu YF, Wat NM, Chung SS et al, Diabetic nephropathy is associated with the 5'-end dinucleotide repeat polymorphism of the aldose reductase gene in Chinese subjects with type II diabetes, *Diabet Med* (2002) **19:** 113–18.

89. Neamat-Allah M, Feeney SA, Savage DA et al, Analysis of the association between diabetic nephropathy and polymorphisms in the aldose reductase gene in type I and type II diabetes mellitus, *Diabet Med* (2001) **18:** 906–14.

90. Hodgkinson AD, Sondergaard KL, Yang B et al, Aldose reductase expression is induced by hyperglycemia in diabetic nephropathy, *Kidney Int* (2001a) **60:** 211–18.

91. Shah VO, Scavini M, Nikolic J et al, Z-2 microsatellite allele is linked to increased expression of the aldose reductase gene in diabetic nephropathy, *J Clin Endocrinol Metab* (1998) **83:** 2886–91.

92. Moczulski DK, Scott L, Antonellis A et al, Aldose reductase gene polymorphisms and susceptibility to diabetic nephropathy in type I diabetes mellitus, *Diabet Med* (2000) **17:** 111–18.

93. Dyer PH, Chowdhury TA, Dronsfield MJ et al, The 5'-end polymorphism of the aldose reductase gene is not associated with diabetic nephropathy in Caucasian type in diabetic patients, *Diabetologia* (1999) **42:** 1030–1.

94. Maeda S, Haneda M, Yasuda H et al, Diabetic nephropathy is not associated with the dinucleotide repeat polymorphism upstream of the aldose reductase (alr2) gene but with erythrocyte aldose reductase content in Japanese subjects with type II diabetes, *Diabetes* (1999) **48:** 420–2.

95. Fanelli A, Hadjadj S, Gallois Y et al, [Polymorphism of aldose reductase gene and susceptibility to retinopathy and nephropathy in Caucasians with type I diabetes], *Arch Mal Coeur Vaiss* (2002) **95:** 701–8.

96. Patel A, Hibberd ML, Millward BA et al, Chromosome 7q35 and susceptibility to diabetic microvascular complications, *J Diabetes Complications* (1996) **10:** 62–7.

97. Trevisan R, Fioretto P, Barbosa J et al, Insulin-dependent diabetic sibling pairs are concordant for sodium-hydrogen antiport activity, *Kidney Int* (1999) **55:** 2383–9.

98. Matteucci E, Giampietro O, Erythrocyte sodium/hydrogen exchange activity and albuminuria in type 1 diabetic families, *Diabetes Care* (2000) **23:** 418–20.

99. Koren W, Koldanov R, Pronin VS et al, Enhanced erythrocyte Na$^+$/H$^+$ exchange predicts diabetic nephropathy in patients with IDDM, *Diabetologia* (1998) **41:** 201–5.

100. Matteucci E, Giampietro O, Sodium/hydrogen exchange activity in type I diabetes mellitus: the never-ending story, *Diabetes Nutr Metab* (2001) **14:** 225–33.

101. Jensen JS, Mathiesen ER, Norgaard K et al, Increased blood pressure and erythrocyte sodium/lithium countertransport activity are not inherited in diabetic nephropathy, *Diabetologia* (1990) **33:** 619–24.

102. Mead PA, Wilkinson R, Thomas TH, Na/Li countertransport abnormalities in type I diabetes with and without nephropathy are familial, *Diabetes Care* (2001) **24:** 527–32.

103. Chiarelli F, Catino M, Tumini S et al, Increased Na$^+$/Li$^+$ countertransport activity may help to identify type I diabetic adolescents and young adults at risk for developing persistent microalbuminuria, *Diabetes Care* (1999) **22:** 1158–64.

104. Van Norren K, Thien T, Berden JH et al, Relevance of erythrocyte Na$^+$/Li$^+$ countertransport measurement in essential hypertension, hyperlipidaemia and diabetic nephropathy: a critical review, *Eur J Clin Invest* (1998) **28:** 339–52.

105. Hardman TC, Dubrey SW, Leslie RD et al, Kinetic behavior of the erythrocyte sodium-lithium countertransporter in non-nephropathic diabetic twins, *Metabolism* (1996) **45:** 1203–7.

106. Rutherford PA, Thomas TH, Carr SJ et al, Changes in erythrocyte sodium–lithium countertransport kinetics in diabetic nephropathy, *Clin Sci (Lond)* (1992) **82:** 301–7.

107. West IC, Rutherford PA, Thomas TH, Sodium–lithium counter transport: physiology and function, *J Hypertens* (1998) **16:** 3–13.

108. Rota R, Timsit J, Hannedouche T et al, Erythrocyte Na$^+$/Li$^+$

countertransport and glomerular hyperfiltration in insulin-dependent diabetics, *Am J Hypertens* (1993) **6:** 534–7.

109. Vervoort G, Elving LD, Wetzels JF et al, Sodium-lithium countertransport is increased in normoalbuminuric type 1 diabetes but is not related to other risk factors for microangiopathy, *Eur J Clin Invest* (2002) **32:** 93–9.

110. Ng LL, Quinn PA, Baker F et al, Red cell $Na^+/Li^+$ countertransport and $Na^+/H^+$ exchanger isoforms in human proximal tubules, *Kidney Int* (2000) **58:** 229–35.

111. Siperstein MD, Unger RH, Madison LL, Studies of muscle capillary basement membranes in normal subjects, diabetic, and prediabetic patients, *J Clin Invest* (1968) **47:** 1973–99.

112. Fornoni A, Striker LJ, Zheng F et al, Reversibility of glucose-induced changes in mesangial cell extracellular matrix depends on the genetic background, *Diabetes* (2002) **51:** 499–505.

113. Mauer SM, Goetz FC, McHugh LE et al, Long-term study of normal kidneys transplanted into patients with type I diabetes, *Diabetes* (1989) **38:** 516–23.

114. Hannedouche TP, Marques LP, Natov S et al, Renal abnormalities in normotensive insulin-dependent diabetic offspring of hypertensive parents, *Hypertension* (1992) **19:** 378–84.

115. Yokozawa T, Nakagawa T, Wakaki K et al, Animal model of diabetic nephropathy, *Exp Toxicol Pathol* (2001) **53:** 359–63.

116. Ellis EN, Steffes MW, Goetz FC et al, Relationship of renal size to nephropathy in type I (insulin-dependent) diabetes, *Diabetologia* (1985) **28:** 12–15.

117. Manalich R, Reyes L, Herrera M et al, Relationship between weight at birth and the number and size of renal glomeruli in humans: a histomorphometric study, *Kidney Int* (2000) **58:** 770–4.

118. Bilous RW, Mauer SM, Sutherland DE et al, Mean glomerular volume and rate of development of diabetic nephropathy, *Diabetes* (1989) **38:** 1142–7.

119. Rossing P, Tarnow L, Nielsen FS et al, Low birth weight. A risk factor for development of diabetic nephropathy? *Diabetes* (1995) **44:** 1405–7.

120. Rossing P, Tarnow L, Nielsen FS et al, Short stature and diabetic nephropathy, *BMJ* (1995) **310:** 296–7.

121. Fava S, Azzopardi J, Watkins PJ et al, Adult height and proteinuria in type II diabetes, *Nephrol Dial Transplant* (2001) **16:** 525–8.

122. Gould MM, Mohamed-Ali V, Goubet SA. Microalbuminuria: associations with height and sex in non-diabetic subjects, *BMJ* (1993) **306:** 240–2.

123. Hoy WE, Wang Z, Van Buynder P et al, The natural history of renal disease in Australian Aborigines. II. Albuminuria predicts natural death and renal failure, *Kidney Int* (2001) **60:** 249–56.

124. Eshoj O, Vaag A, Borch-Johnsen K et al, Is low birth weight a risk factor for the development of diabetic nephropathy in patients with type 1 diabetes? A population-based case-control study, *J Intern Med* (2002) **252:** 524–8.

125. Nyengaard JR, Bendtsen TF, Mogensen CE, Low birth weight—is it associated with few and small glomeruli in normal subjects and NIDDM patients? *Diabetologia* (1996) **39:** 1634–7.

126. Nelson RG, Morgenstern H, Bennett PH, Birth weight and renal disease in Pima Indians with type II diabetes mellitus, *Am J Epidemiol* (1998) **148:** 650–6.

127. Hoy WE, Rees M, Kile E et al, A new dimension to the Barker hypothesis: low birthweight and susceptibility to renal disease, *Kidney Int* (1999) **56:** 1072–7.

128. Jones SE, Nyengaard JR, Flyvbjerg A et al, Birth weight has no influence on glomerular number and volume, *Pediatr Nephrol* (2001) **16:** 340–5.

129. Merlet-Benichou C, Gilbert T, Vilar J et al, Nephron number: variability is the rule. Causes and consequences, *Lab Invest* (1999) **79:** 515–27.

130. Caramori ML, Fioretto P, Mauer M. The need for early predictors of diabetic nephropathy risk: is albumin excretion rate sufficient? *Diabetes* (2000) **49:** 1399–408.

131. Rossing P, Hougaard P, Parving HH, Risk factors for development of incipient and overt diabetic nephropathy in type 1 diabetic patients: a 10-year prospective observational study, *Diabetes Care* (2002) **25:** 859–64.

132. Christensen PK, Larsen S, Horn T et al, Renal function and structure in albuminuric type II diabetic patients without retinopathy, *Nephrol Dial Transplant* (2001) **16:** 2337–47.

133. Fernandez-Real JM, Ricart W, Insulin resistance and inflammation in an evolutionary perspective: the contribution of cytokine genotype/phenotype to thriftiness, *Diabetologia* (1999) **42:** 1367–74.

134. Kagawa Y, Yanagisawa Y, Hasegawa K et al, Single nucleotide polymorphisms of thrifty genes for energy metabolism: evolutionary origins and prospects for intervention to prevent obesity-related diseases, *Biochem Biophys Res Commun* (2002) **295:** 207–22.

# 5

# Factors influencing the progression of diabetic nephropathy

Bieke F Schrijvers, An S De Vriese and Allan Flyvbjerg

## INTRODUCTION

The most important cause of increased mortality and morbidity in diabetic patients is micro- and macrovascular complications. Diabetic microangiopathy consists of diabetic nephropathy, retinopathy, and possibly neuropathy.[1] Diabetic kidney disease is associated with well-known morphological and functional renal alterations. The early stage is characterized by induction of growth factors and cytokines along with kidney growth, glomerular hyperfiltration and increased synthesis of extracellular matrix (ECM), leading to albuminuria and proteinuria in later diabetic nephropathy.[2,3] The Diabetes Control and Complications Trial showed that hyperglycaemia is a major factor in the development of diabetic microvascular complications.[1] Several biochemical pathways have been proposed to be involved, and to explain in part the adverse effects of hyperglycaemia. First, metabolic factors such as non-enzymatic glycation, polyol pathway activation, and diacylglycerol (DAG)-protein kinase C (PKC) activation will be discussed. Second, growth factors and cytokines, the most important being growth hormone (GH), insulin-like growth factors (IGFs), transforming growth factor β (TGF-β), and vascular endothelial growth factor (VEGF), will be discussed. Of the different vasoactive factors that play a role, mainly the renin-angiotensin system (RAS) and angiotensin II (Ang II) have been reported, and recent data on the importance of endothelin (ET) will be discussed. Other factors influencing diabetic kidney disease will be mentioned in brief. An introduction to each system will be given, followed by the changes found in the diabetic kidney, supported by evidence from both *in vitro*, and *in vivo* (animal and clinical) studies. The known interactions and links between different pathways will be mentioned, as well as potential treatment strategies targeting the specific pathways.

## METABOLIC FACTORS

The leading metabolic factor involved in the development and progression of diabetic complications is undoubtedly hyperglycaemia.[1] The mechanisms involved are not completely understood, but hyperglycaemia may exert direct effects as well as *in*direct effects by activating other pathways. Three pathways have been proposed: advanced glycation end-product formation, the aldose reductase pathway, and the activation of PKC isoforms.

### Advanced glycation end-products (AGEs)

Non-enzymatic glycation occurs through a series of biochemical reactions between glucose and other reactive carbonyl compounds, on the one hand, and proteins, lipids or nucleic acids, on the other hand (Table 5.1).[4] Early formed and reversible products of these reactions are Schiff bases and Amadori products (e.g., haemoglobin $A_{1c}$). Further rearrangement and modification lead to the formation and accumulation of a heterogeneous group of AGEs, such as[3,4] $N^\epsilon$-(carboxymethyl)-lysine (CML) and pentosidine, both of which are glycoxidation products;[5] imidazolone;[6] and pyrraline.[5] AGEs interact with specific receptors, the best characterized being the receptor for AGEs (RAGE).[7] Other identified AGE-binding proteins include the components of the AGE-receptor complex *p60*, *p90*, galectin-3,[8] and the macrophage scavenger receptor types I and II.[9] AGEs can also act in a direct non-receptor-mediated way by cross-linking proteins.[10] By both mechanisms,

**Table 5.1 Metabolic factors that have been implicated in the pathogenesis of diabetic kidney disease: list of different components of advanced glycation end-products (AGEs), aldose reductase (AR)/polyol pathway, and diacylglycerol-protein kinase C (DAG-PKC) pathway and known or potential inhibitors of these systems.**

| Metabolic factors | Components | Inhibitors |
|---|---|---|
| AGEs | *Early glycation products:* Schiff bases, Amadori products | *Inhibitors of AGE formation:* Aminoguanidine, pyridorin, 2,3 diamino-phenazine, OPB-9195, ALT-946 |
| | *Glycoxidation products:* CML, pentosidine | |
| | *Others:* imidazolone, pyrraline | |
| | *Cross-linking* | *AGE-cross-link breakers:* N-phenacylthiazolium bromide, ALT-711 |
| | *Receptors:* RAGE, AGE RI, RII, RIII | *RAGE-blockers:* Anti-RAGE antibodies, soluble RAGE |
| | | *Others:* aldose reductase inhibitors |
| AR/polyol pathway | *Enzymes:* aldose reductase, sorbitol dehydrogenase | *Aldose reductase inhibitors:* HOE-843 (ponalrestat, sorbinil, tolrestat) |
| | *Accumulation* of sorbitol, fructose | |
| | *Reduction* of myo-inositol | |
| | Changes in $NADPH/NADP^+$ and $NADG/NAD^+$ | *Others:* vanadate |
| DAG–PKC pathway | *10 isoforms:* classical PKCs ($\alpha$, $\beta_I$, $\beta_{II}$, $\gamma$), novel PKCs ($\delta$, $\epsilon$, $\eta$, $\theta$, $\mu$) and atypical ($\zeta$, $\iota$, $\lambda$) | *PKC inhibitors:* bisindolylmaleimide compounds, e.g., LY333531 |
| | *Diacylglycerol* | *Vitamin E* |
| | *Receptors:* RACKs (receptors for activated C-kinase) | *RACK antagonists* |
| | | *Others:* aminoguanidine, ramipril |

For further explanation and references, please see text.

AGEs may activate signal transduction pathways that involve cytokines and growth factors.[11] Another important pathogenetic effect of AGEs and AGE–RAGE interaction is the induction of oxidative stress.[12] In the normal kidney, AGE staining is absent in humans,[13] but present in rodent glomeruli and tubulointerstitium.[14] RAGE is constitutively expressed in renal interstitial cells and vascular smooth muscle cells (VSMC).[15]

## Evidence for a role of AGEs in diabetic kidney disease

In cultured glomerular endothelial and mesangial cells *in vitro*, glycated albumin and AGE-rich proteins have been shown to enhance the expression of type IV collagen[16] and TGF-β1,[16] and increase PKC activity,[16,17] more specifically that of PKCβ_{II}.[17] When carried out under physiological glucose conditions, *in vitro* studies provide evidence that early glycation products may contribute to the pathogenesis of diabetic glomerulopathy independently of glucose.[16] Furthermore, hyperglycaemia and glycated albumin exert an additive effect.[16] In cultured kidney epithelial cells, CML reduces proteoglycan expression,[18] suggesting that AGEs might be involved in changes in the glomerular basement membrane (GBM) filter in diabetes. Cross-link formation, induced by AGEs such as pentosidine, leads to increased stiffness of the protein matrix in advanced diabetes, and is potentially linked to vascular leakiness and hyper-permeability.[19] *In vivo* evidence for a role of AGEs in the development and progression of diabetic kidney disease comes mainly from studies in streptozotocin (STZ)-induced diabetic rats. AGEs react with mesangial matrix and GBM, and do this in a more intense way in renal tissue from diabetic rats.[20] AGE staining increases with age, and increases further by diabetes.[21] Renal AGE levels are increased after 3 weeks of diabetes,[22] and over a period of 32 weeks,[14,23] confirming that *in vivo* generation of AGEs in the kidney is time-dependent and closely linked to the development of experimental diabetic glomerulopathy. The co-localization of AGEs and RAGE in renal glomeruli and other sites of diabetic microvascular injury suggests that this ligand-receptor interaction may represent an important mechanism in the genesis of diabetic complications.[21] A significant increase in [125]I-labelled AGE binding is found in diabetic rat kidney and appears to be modulated by endogenous AGE levels.[22] Further, in the absence of hyperglycaemia, exogenously administered AGEs induce ECM genes specific for early diabetic kidney disease in non-diabetic mice,[24] and mimic the long-term effects of diabetes, such as increased mesangial expansion, in non-diabetic rats,[25] which is accompanied in both mice and rats by upregulation of TGF-β1.[24,25]

Recently, diabetic transgenic mice overexpressing human RAGE have been shown to develop renal and glomerular hypertrophy, increased albuminuria, mesangial expansion, advanced glomerulosclerosis, and increased serum creatinine compared with diabetic littermates lacking the RAGE transgene.[26] This study provides the first direct *in vivo* evidence that interactions between AGEs and RAGE lead to diabetic vascular derangement.[26] In type 1 diabetic patients, increased circulating AGEs precede the development of micro- and macrovascular complications,[27] and predict the progression of the early morphological renal changes in basement membrane thickness and matrix/glomerular volume fraction.[28] In type 2 diabetic patients, increased cross-line serum levels have been shown to be associated with the presence of nephropathy.[29] Amadori products, pentosidine,[30] CML,[30] pyrraline, and imidazolone are demonstrated in renal tissue of diabetic patients.[6,13,30] Immunohistochemically, AGEs, and more specifically CML and pentosidine, accumulate in expanded mesangial matrix and nodular lesions in patients with diabetic kidney disease.[30,31] Their co-localization with malondialdehyde-lysine (MDA-lysine), a lipoxidation product, suggests a local oxidative stress and increased protein carbonyl modification in diabetic glomerular lesions.[32] The importance of MDA in diabetes has recently been reviewed.[33] RAGE accumulation in the kidney is not specific for diabetic nephropathy, as patients with various non-diabetic renal diseases display a similar pattern of RAGE expression.[15]

## Treatments targeting AGEs

### Inhibitors of AGE formation

Aminoguanidine (AG), a hydrazine-like compound, reacts with early glycation products and inhibits further AGE formation.[34] *In vitro*, both fructose-induced fluorescence and protein oxidation are almost completely suppressed in the presence of AG.[35] *In vivo*, AG has been shown to retard the development of diabetic nephropathy in long-term experimental diabetes in rats.[14,23,36] It appears that the renoprotective effects of AG in diabetes are related to the duration, and not the timing, of treatment,[14,37] and are mediated by a decrease of AGE formation.[21,22,38] In addition, AG restores the diabetes-induced changes in lysosomal processing,[39] and glomerular PKC activity[37,40] in STZ-diabetic rats. Pimagedine, the generic form of AG, lowers total urinary protein and slows progression of overt diabetic nephropathy in optimally treated type 1 diabetic patients compared with placebo-treated subjects,[41] providing preliminary clinical evidence for a beneficial effect of AG in diabetic kidney disease. Pyridorin (pyridoxamine dihydrochloride) (PM) inhibits the conversion of Amadori intermediates to AGEs. In an *in vitro* study in human erythrocytes, PM inhibited superoxide radicals and prevented high glucose-induced AGE formation,[42] lipid peroxidation, and reduction of $Na^+K^+$ ATPase activity, all mechanisms which may delay or inhibit the development of complications in diabetes.[42] In rats injected chronically with glycated albumin, PM ameliorates diabetic-like changes in glomerular heparan sulphate and glomerular deposition of glycated albumin.[43] Further, PM inhibits AGE formation and retards the development of nephropathy in STZ-diabetic rats.[44] The therapeutic potential of PM is currently being investigated in clinical trials. *In vitro* studies clearly document inhibition of AGE formation by 2,3 diamino-phenazine (2,3 DAP).[38] In addition, 2,3 DAP treatment inhibits AGE accumulation *in vivo* in the kidney and blood vessels of STZ-diabetic rats,[38] and significantly ameliorates collagen solubility,[45] but has no effect on increased urinary albumin excretion (UAE).[45] OPB-9195, a thiazolidine derivative, effectively inhibits both AGE formation and AG-derived cross-linking *in vitro*.[46] In Otsuka-Long-Evans-Tokushima-Fatty (OLETF) rats, an experimental model of type 2 diabetes, the administration of OPB-9195 lowers elevated serum AGE levels and UAE, attenuates AGE deposition in glomeruli, and thereby prevents the progression of diabetic glomerular sclerosis.[46] Furthermore, administering OPB-9195 in a RAGE transgenic mouse model prevents the phenotypes of advanced diabetic nephropathy, thus establishing the AGE-RAGE system as a promising therapeutic target.[26,47] ALT-946 is a potent inhibitor of AGE accumulation *in vitro* and reproduces the renoprotective effects of AG *in vivo*.[48] Recently, a new compound (EXO-226) inhibiting albumin glycation has proven to ameliorate diabetic nephropathy in the db/db mouse.[49]

### AGE-cross-link breakers

*N*-Phenacylthiazolium bromide (PTB) reacts with and cleaves covalent, glucose-derived protein cross-links *in vitro* and *in vivo*.[50] In STZ-diabetic rats, PTB treatment prevents the diabetes-associated increase in vascular AGE accumulation and mesenteric vascular hypertrophy, thereby suggesting that PTB may have a potential role in the treatment of diabetic vascular complications.[51] However, in STZ-diabetic rats, decreased tail collagen pepsin solubility, reflecting the formation of AGE cross-linking, was not affected by PTB treatment.[45] In the years to come, the use of AGE-cross-link breakers, such as ALT-711,[52] in diabetic settings[47,53] may provide new strategies in the treatment of diabetic kidney disease.

### RAGE blockers

In cultured endothelial cells, the incubation with antisense RAGE oligonucleotides suppresses RAGE transcription and the AGE-induced translocation of nuclear factor κB (NF-κB).[54] In VSMCs, AGEs induce RAGE-dependent induction of a p21 (ras)-dependent mitogen-activated protein kinase (MAPK) pathway, an effect that can be blocked by anti-RAGE antibodies or soluble RAGE (sRAGE), a truncated form of RAGE.[55] In cultured mesangial cells, anti-*p60* antibodies prevent AGE-induced increases in IGF-I, TGF-β1, and ECM production or gene expression, suggesting that AGE-induced growth factor and ECM synthesis is AGE-receptor dependent and participates in the pathogenesis of hyperglycaemia-induced mesangial expansion.[56] In an STZ-diabetic rat model, blockade of RAGE by sRAGE largely prevents the increased vascular permeability/albumin leakage found in kidney and other organs.[57] At present, more studies in rodent models of diabetic complications employing RAGE blockade are under way.[19]

### Aldose reductase inhibitors (ARIs)

Erythrocyte fructose 3-phosphate and AGEs are significantly elevated in diabetic patients compared to non-diabetic individuals.[58] The ARI epalrestat significantly decreases erythrocyte fructose 3-phosphate, and erythrocyte AGEs after 1 or 2 months of treatment, respectively.[58] These results show that the polyol pathway is likely to play a substantial role in the non-enzymatic glycation of proteins.[58] A link between the polyol pathway and advanced glycation has also been suggested elsewhere.[59]

## Aldose reductase/polyol pathway

Aldose reductase (AR) is the rate-limiting enzyme of the polyol pathway, and facilitates the reduction of glucose to sorbitol. Sorbitol dehydrogenase (SDH) converts sorbitol to fructose using $NAD^+$.[60] The physiological role of this pathway remains unknown, although sorbitol is thought to be involved in osmotic regulation.[61] In the kidney, AR is located in tubular epithelial cells, interstitial cells in the inner medulla, podocytes, and mesangial cell.[62] AR is found mainly in the medulla, while aldehyde reductase is primarily localized in the cortex.[63] Both enzymes have been demonstrated to produce kidney polyols, and thereby it is suggested that aldehyde reductase contributes to polyol production in the kidney cortex, which is the predominant site of diabetic kidney lesions.[64]

## Evidence for a role of the AR/polyol pathway in diabetic kidney disease

During diabetic hyperglycaemia, cellular glucose levels rapidly increase in tissues, such as the kidney, that are independent of insulin for glucose uptake. It is only in hyperglycaemic conditions when the enzyme hexokinase, which converts glucose to glucose-6-phosphate, is saturated that excess glucose enters the polyol pathway and AR is activated.[60] Since the activity of SDH is not increased to the same extent, sorbitol accordingly accumulates.[60] Concerning the role of the polyol pathway in the onset of diabetic microvascular complications, different mechanisms have been implicated: cellular accumulation of sorbitol or fructose,[64–66] reduction of myo-inositol,[67] or alterations in the $NADPH/NADP^+$ and $NADH/NAD^+$ ratios.[68] In an *in vitro* experiment in mesangial cells, increased expression of glucose transporter 1 leads to increased AR expression and activity along with polyol accumulation, and increased PKCα protein levels, which leads to detrimental stimulation of matrix protein synthesis.[69] In STZ-diabetic rats, increased levels of renal sorbitol and fructose are seen, with reduction to below control levels by insulin treatment.[65] In addition, myo-inositol levels increase in the kidney. These changes are accompanied by elevated renal AR mRNA levels, but STZ-diabetes has no influence on renal SDH mRNA levels or SDH activities, nor does insulin treatment.[65] Myo-inositol depletion and reduction of $Na^+K^+$-ATPase activity owing to sorbitol accumulation have been demonstrated in glomeruli of diabetic animal models.[70] In diabetic patients, sorbinil treatment reduces the elevated erythrocyte sorbitol levels to normal or slightly below normal, but does not affect the erythrocyte myo-inositol concentration.[71] The AR/polyol pathway is linked to reductive and oxidative stress, glycolytic metabolism, lipid metabolism and PKC activation, as well as to intracellular glycation and AGEs, growth factors and ECM secretion, pathways which have all been implicated in the development of diabetic complications.[72]

## Treatments targeting the AR/polyol pathway

### Aldose reductase inhibitors

Aldose reductase inhibitors (ARI) block the flux of glucose through the polyol pathway, have no effect on plasma glucose levels and hence do not pose the risk of hypoglycaemia.[73] Addition of HOE 843, a specific ARI, to glomerular explants *in vitro* prevents the high-glucose-induced increases in flux of glucose through the pentose phosphate pathway, DAG synthesis, membrane PKC activity, $PLA_2$ activity, and $PGE_2$ production. These *in vitro* data suggest a link between increased polyol pathway activity and increased prostaglandin production, as observed in diabetes of recent onset.[74] Orally administered HOE 483 has been evaluated in a double-blind, placebo-controlled, clinical trial. HOE 483 is well tolerated and decreases red blood cell sorbitol concentrations, a biochemical marker of pharmacologic activity, in a dose-related fashion in diabetic patients.[75]

Numerous experimental and clinical studies with different ARI have implicated the diabetes-induced increased flux of glucose through the polyol pathway in the development of diabetic retinopathy and neuropathy; however, only a few studies have investigated the influence of ARI in diabetic kidney. Sorbinil, tolrestat and ponalrestat have been withdrawn from clinical trials due to toxicity or a lack of efficacy in human diabetic neuropathy,[76] although ponalrestat has a positive effect on renal hyperfiltration in type 1 diabetic patients.[77]

### Others

Oral administration of vanadate, a nutritional trace element, to alloxan diabetic rats prevents the increase

in kidney growth and restores the renal changes in AR and SDH activities and sorbitol content.[78] This may be partially due to the normalization of blood and renal glucose by vanadate. The vanadium level of kidney is much higher than the plasma level, probably due to greater accumulation in the kidney during administration.[78]

## Diacylglycerol (DAG)–protein kinase C (PKC) pathway

PKC, a family of serine-threonine kinases, consists of at least 10 structurally related isoforms, which can be divided into three categories by their cofactor requirements.[79] The classical PKCs ($\alpha$, $\beta_I$, $\beta_{II}$, and $\gamma$) require $Ca^{2+}$ and DAG to become activated; the novel PKCs ($\delta$, $\epsilon$, $\eta$, $\theta$ and $\mu$) require only DAG; and the atypical PKCs, namely, $\zeta$, $\iota$ and $\lambda$ (the mouse homologue of human PKC$\iota$), require neither $Ca^{2+}$ nor DAG.[79] PKCs participate in intracellular signal transduction in response to specific hormonal, neuronal and growth factor stimuli.[80] DAG, the major cellular mediator of PKC activation, can be derived from the hydrolysis of phosphoinositol biphosphate to inositol triphosphate,[80] or can be formed *de novo* from glycolytic intermediates.[81] PKC activation involves translocation of the isoform by isozyme-specific anchoring proteins, named receptors for activated C-kinase (RACKs).[82] PKC activation can increase vascular permeability, ECM synthesis, contractility, leucocyte attachment, cell growth and angiogenesis, all vascular functions that have been reported to be abnormal in the diabetic state.[80,83–85] The $\beta_I$-, $\beta_{II}$-, and $\gamma$-isoforms of PKC are associated with cellular events such as mitogenesis, matrix production and differentiation.[86] PKC$\beta$ ($\beta_I$ and $\beta_{II}$) are most frequently associated with alterations in mesangial cell phenotypic behaviour such as proliferation and matrix deposition.[87] The expression and distribution of PKC isoforms varies markedly between cells and tissues. In normal kidney, expression of the PKC$\alpha$, -$\beta_I$, -$\beta_{II}$, -$\delta$, -$\epsilon$, -$\zeta$, -$\mu$ isoforms is found on protein and/or mRNA level, whereas the expression of PKC$\gamma$ is absent and the expression of the $\eta$-, $\theta$-, $\lambda/\iota$-isoforms is unknown.[79]

## Evidence for the role of PKC in diabetic kidney disease

*In vitro* studies have shown that PKC is activated in cultured vascular cells,[88] glomerular mesangial cells,[89] and explants of rat glomeruli,[74,90] exposed to elevated glucose concentrations. At the same time, some of these studies reported a concomitant increase in total cellular DAG levels.[74,90] Hyperglycaemia-induced PKC activation increases arachidonic acid release, and production of prostaglandins PGE$_2$ and PGI$_2$, probably by activation of phospholipase A$_2$[89] and decreases Na$^+$, K$^+$-ATPase activity.[91,92] These changes might contribute to the development of diabetic glomerulopathy, since prostaglandins have been implicated in glomerular hyperfiltration and growth,[91] and Na$^+$, K$^+$-ATPase is important in the regulation of cellular contractility, growth, and differentiation.[93] Glucose-induced increases in TGF-β1, fibronectin, and α$_1$-type IV collagen mRNA are likewise PKC-dependent.[89] High glucose stimulates mesangial cell proliferation through the PKC/NF-κB pathway.[94] Increases in total DAG have been reported in tissues from diabetic animals and humans,[81] including glomeruli.[95–97] PKC activity is increased in glomeruli of STZ-induced diabetic rats.[89,90,95,97] Further, in diabetic db/db mice at 25 weeks of age, glomerular PKC activity is 180% relative to that observed in non-diabetic db/+ mice.[96] In addition, hyperglycaemia preferentially leads to the activation of the PKCα, -β$_1$, and -δ isoforms in glomerular cells.[81]

## Treatments targeting DAG-PKC pathway

### PKC inhibitors

Recently, the available pharmacological compounds that inhibit PKC have been reviewed.[98] Due to in vivo toxicity and non-specificity, in vivo studies have not been feasible with staurosporine and several of its indolocarbazole derivatives.[98,99] The bisindolylmaleimide PKC inhibitors are less potent than staurosporine but show greater selectivity for PKC isoforms. As PKCβ is shown to be preferentially activated in kidney in the diabetic state,[89] one of the most promising isoform-selective inhibitors developed to date is the bisindolylmaleimide compound, LY333531,[98] a highly specific PKCβ$_1$/β$_{II}$ inhibitor, effective in vitro and in vivo.[89,95,100] In STZ-induced diabetic rats, treatment with LY333531 prevents early diabetes-induced glomerular hyperfiltration, albuminuria, and enhanced mRNA expression of TGF-β1 and ECM components, demonstrating that PKCβ plays a role in these glucose-induced changes.[89] Recently, it has been demonstrated that long-term inhibition of PKC by treatment with LY333531 prevents not only a rise in UAE, but also glomerular histological changes in an animal model of type 2 diabetes, the db/db mouse.[96] LY333531 normalizes

the increased glomerular PKC activity, prevents mesangial expansion, and reduces the overexpression of TGF-β and ECM components such as fibronectin and type IV collagen, providing evidence that overexpression of fibronectin and type IV collagen might occur through glomerular PKCβ activation, although the role of other PKC isoforms cannot be excluded.[96] In a recent study in STZ-diabetic rats, LY333531 shows renoprotective effects without effect on any components of the intrarenal TGF-β system.[101] These data suggest that diabetes- or high-glucose-induced PKC activation may promote ECM overproduction independently of TGF-β or that TGF-β acts upstream to PKC. Pretreatment of rat mesangial cells with Ro320432, a selective PKC inhibitor, inhibits the proliferation stimulated by thrombin, ET-1, phorbol 12,13-dibutyrate or EFG, suggesting that all these mitogens mediate their effect through a PKC-dependent pathway.[102]

### Vitamin E

In vitro, vitamin E (d-α-tocopherol), a well-known antioxidant, suppresses the DAG level in thrombin-stimulated endothelial cells,[103] and prevents the hyperglycaemia-induced activation of the DAG–PKC pathway in VSMC,[104] by increasing the activity of DAG kinase,[103,104] which lowers intracellular DAG levels by converting DAG to phosphatidic acid. d-α-Tocopherol does not affect purified PKCα and -β isoforms, indicating that vitamin E may act upstream to PKC.[105] In experimental diabetes, vitamin E prevents the hyperglycaemia-induced increases of DAG and PKC levels in rat glomeruli, normalizes glomerular hyperfiltration, and improves UAE in STZ-induced diabetic rats.[106] Furthermore, vitamin E has been shown to reduce the diabetes-associated increases in glomerular TGF-β immunoreactivity, and glomerular volume, but vitamin E has no effect on albumin clearance.[107] In type 1 diabetic patients of short disease duration, oral vitamin E treatment normalizes elevated baseline creatinine clearance without inducing a significant change in glycaemic control.[108] These results suggest that vitamin E supplementation may be beneficial for the prevention of renal injury in diabetes.

### RACK antagonists

These isozyme-selective inhibitors of PKC are peptide fragments that act by blocking the association of activated isozymes with their corresponding RACKs.[82,109] Three such peptides inhibit the translocation and function of PKCβ in vitro and in vivo.[110] These peptide inhibitors can help to elucidate the role of individual PKC isoforms, and identify candidate PKC isozymes to target for drug development in a variety of diseases including diabetes.

### Others

Interestingly, AG and ramipril, both therapeutic interventions that reduce proteinuria and slow the progression of diabetic nephropathy, prevent diabetes-associated increases in glomerular PKC activity, suggesting that the PKC pathway plays a role in disease progression.[40]

## GROWTH HORMONES AND CYTOKINES

Due to their growth-promoting and proliferative effects, various growth factors and cytokines have been supposed to be important in the development of diabetic kidney disease.[111] In particular, growth hormone (GH)/insulin-like growth factors (IGFs), TGF-βs, and vascular endothelial growth factor (VEGF) have measurable effects on the development of experimental diabetic kidney disease. Some of these effects are not mediated by their action as hormones, but directly through paracrine/autocrine mechanisms (Table 5.2).

## Growth hormone (GH) and insulin-like growth factors (IGFs)

The GH/IGF system constitutes a complex system of peptides in the circulation, extracellular space and most tissues. Pituitary-secreted GH classically induces IGF-I synthesis in various organs through activation of specific growth hormone receptors (GHRs). The effects of IGF-I and IGF-II are mediated through two specific IGF receptors, the IGF-I receptor (IGF-IR), or type 1 IGF receptor, and the IGF-II/mannose-6-phosphate receptor (IGF-II/man-6-PR), or type 2 IGF receptor, the latter playing a role in the trafficking of lysosomal enzymes.[112,113] IGFs are bound to specific IGF-binding proteins (IGFBPs), of which six high-affinity (IGFBP-1 to IGFBP-6)[114,115] and several low-affinity IGFBP-related proteins (IGFBP-rP)[116] have been characterized. Circulating IGFBPs are believed to prolong the half-life and regulate the endocrine effects of IGFs, whereas cellular IGFBPs are believed to inhibit or stimulate local actions of IGFs. The GH/IGF system is expressed in normal kidney, i.e., GHR and GHBP,[117,118] IGF-I and IGF-II,[119–121] the respective IGF-IR and IGF-II/man-6-PR,[112,113,122] and all six specific IGFBPs.[114–116]

---

**Table 5.2 Growth hormones and cytokines that have been implicated in the pathogenesis of diabetic kidney disease: list of different components of the growth hormone-insulin-like growth factor (GH-IGF) axis, transforming growth factor β (TGF-β) system, and vascular endothelial growth factor (VEGF) system and known or potential inhibitors of these systems.**

| Growth factors and cytokines | Components | Inhibitors |
|---|---|---|
| GH/IGF-axis | *Hormones:* GH, IGF-I, IGF-II | *Long-acting somatostatin analogues:* octreotide, lanreotide |
| | *Receptors:* GHRs, IGF-RI, IGF-RII | *GHR antagonists:* pegvisomant |
| | *Binding proteins:* GHBP, IGFBP-1 to -6 (high-affinity), IGFBPs-rP (low-affinity) | *IGF-I receptor antagonists:* JB3 |
| | | *Others:* AGE inhibition, ACE inhibition |
| TGF-β | TGF-β1, TGF-β2, TGF-β3, activins, inhibins, bone morphogenic proteins | *Neutralizing antibodies* |
| | *Receptors:* TGF-β type RI and TGF-β type RII | *Others:* ACE inhibition, PKCβ inhibition, AGE inhibition |
| VEGF | *5 VEGF-isoforms* | *Neutralizing antibodies* |
| | *Receptors:* VEGFR-1, VEGFR-2 | *Others:* AGE inhibition |

For further explanation and references, please see text.

## Evidence for a role of GH/IGFs in diabetic kidney disease

In mesangial cells, IGF-I stimulates cell growth,[123] and proteoglycan production,[124] and contributes to altered ECM accumulation.[125] These data provide *in vitro* evidence for IGF-I being an important player in the development of diabetic glomerulopathy. Experimental evidence concerning the role of GH/IGFs in development of diabetic kidney disease is quite extended.[111] It is well known that serum GHBP concentrations are decreased in experimental diabetes.[126,127] Renal GHBP mRNA expression, on the contrary, is increased in both short-term and long-term diabetic rats, but is not accompanied by a change in GHR mRNA expression.[118] STZ-diabetic dwarf rats with isolated GH and IGF-I deficiency show less renal and glomerular hypertrophy than diabetic control rats with intact pituitary.[128] In addition, long-term diabetic dwarf rats display a smaller rise in UAE, indicating that GH and IGF-I may be involved in the development of specific diabetic renal changes.[129] The initial increase in renal growth and function in experimental diabetes is preceded by a rise in renal IGF-I,[120,130–132] IGFBPs[112,133,134] and IGF-II/man-6-P receptor concentration.[135] Furthermore, specific changes occur in the renal GHBP mRNA, IGF-I receptor mRNA and IGFBP mRNA expression in long-term experimental diabetes.[136] Recently, two cross-sectional clinical studies have been published, dealing with possible correlations between serum or urinary GH/IGF-I levels and kidney function in patients with type 1 diabetes.[137,138] At puberty, serum IGF-I has a positive correlation to glomerular filtration rate (GFR), but not to UAE.[138] In adult normo- and microalbuminuric patients, urinary IGF-I is strongly correlated to kidney volume, and both urinary IGF-I and GH are positively correlated to microalbuminuria.[137] In contrast, another study concluded that under physiological conditions in normoalbuminuric type 1 diabetic patients, IGF-I has no role as a mediator of glomerular hyperfiltration.[139] Finally, in a recent study, increasing IGFBP-3 proteolysis with increasing renal impairment was reported in the urines from type 1 and type 2 diabetic subjects.[140] Induction of IGFBP-3 proteolysis may contribute to diabetes-induced renal structural changes, as it is believed to increase IGF bioavailability.[140]

## Treatments targeting the GH/IGF axis

### Long-acting somatostatin analogues

In short-term experimental diabetes, treatment with octreotide or lanreotide from diabetes onset completely inhibits initial renal hypertrophy and kidney IGF-I accumulation,[141,142] whereas postponing treatment results in only a partial inhibition of the early diabetic renal hypertrophy.[143] In long-term experimental diabetes, 6 months of octreotide treatment from the induction of diabetes results in a significant reduction of increase in kidney weight, kidney IGF-I levels and UAE when compared with untreated rats.[144] Three weeks' treatment with octreotide alone and in combination with captopril following 3 months of untreated diabetes has been shown to reduce kidney weight significantly compared with placebo-treated animals.[145] Further, the combined treatment of octreotide and captopril significantly reduces UAE compared with placebo-treated diabetic rats.[145] Taken together, these results suggest a beneficial effect of somatostatin analogues on early and late renal changes in experimental diabetes. In clinical studies, acute infusion of octreotide to type 1 diabetic patients induces a reduction in RPF and GFR, along with decreases in plasma GH and glucagon levels.[146] Octreotide administration for 12 weeks in type 1 diabetic patients significantly reduces elevated GFR and kidney volume.[147]

### GHR antagonists

*In vitro*, GH antagonists bind to the GHR with the same affinity as native GH, but *in vivo* a phenotypic dwarf animal with low circulating IGF-I levels develops when the GH antagonist is expressed in transgenic mice. Recently, renoprotective effects have been reported in long-term diabetic transgenic mice expressing these GH antagonists.[148–150] Further, in STZ-diabetic mice, subcutaneous injection of a GHR antagonist (G120K-PEG) normalizes the diabetes-associated increase in kidney weight and glomerular volume and partially attenuates the rise in UAE.[130] No clinical studies have yet appeared on the effects of this new group of GHR antagonists on metabolism or diabetic complications in patients.

### IGF-I receptor antagonists

Treatment with JB3, a peptide analogue of IGF-I, in short-term diabetic rats normalizes the diabetes-induced increase in kidney size, kidney protein and DNA.[151] The effects of long-term JB3 treatment in experimental models of diabetes are not known.

## AGE inhibition

A recent study in long-term STZ-diabetic rats shows the classic changes in the intrarenal IGF axis, with decreased IGF-I mRNA and IGFBP-4 mRNA and increased IGFBP-1 mRNA expression.[152] Administration of AG (see also above) reduces renal IGFBP-1 mRNA expression to normal, along with partial restoration to normal of diabetes-associated changes in IGFBP-4 and IGF-I mRNA.[152]

## ACE inhibition

Recently, an interaction between the RAS and GH/IGF-I axis in renal development has been demonstrated, with suppression of the medullary IGF-I mRNA expression, and it altered the local distribution of both IGF-I and GHR by neonatal ACE inhibition.[153] The possible effects of ACEi on the GH/IGF axis in diabetic kidney disease have not been examined extensively. In a short-term experimental study in STZ-diabetic rats, trandolapril treatment for 1 week had no effect on renal IGF-I accumulation or renal changes, despite a pronounced reduction in renal ACE activity.[154] As mentioned above, monotherapy with an ACEi or octreotide has no effects on renal IGF-I concentrations or functional parameters, although the attenuating effects of these drugs are seen when given in combination.[145]

## TGF-β

The TGF-β system includes three mammalian TGF-β isoforms (TGF-β1, TGF-β2, and TGF-β3), activins, inhibins and bone morphogenic proteins. The TGF-β isoforms are unique among growth factors in their broad effects on ECM. It is believed that the TGF-βs are synthesized as inactive precursor proteins that are activated proteolytically.[155] TGF-β isoforms induce intracellular signalling through a complex cascade of receptor binding involving two different types of TGF-β receptors, the TGF-β type II receptor (TGF-β type RII) and the TGF-β type I receptor (TGF-β type RI).[156] The kidney is a site of TGF-β production and a target of TGF-β action, as both mRNA for TGF-β isoforms and receptors and the active TGF-β proteins have been shown in the glomerulus and proximal tubular cells (PTCs).[156–159]

## Evidence for a role of TGF-β in diabetic kidney disease

*In vitro*, TGF-β modulates ECM production in glomerular mesangial and epithelial cells.[160,161] In addition, TGF-β inhibits the synthesis of collagenases and stimulates the production of metalloproteinase inhibitors, an effect which could lead to reduced degradation of ECM and hence ECM accumulation.[162,163] Furthermore, high glucose concentrations increase TGF-β1 mRNA expression in renal cells,[157,159] and stimulate TGF-β mRNA expression and bioactivity, cellular hypertrophy, and collagen transcription in proximal tubules,[159] providing *in vitro* evidence for a role of TGF-β in the development of diabetic kidney disease. In different models of experimental type 1 diabetes, increased glomerular TGF-β1 mRNA has been found early in the course of diabetes-induced renal growth.[164,165] In addition, in long-term STZ-diabetic rats, a sustained increase in glomerular TGF-β1 mRNA has been described.[157] Recently, changes in the whole TGF-β system (i.e., TGF-β1, TGF-β2, TGF-β3 isoforms and TGF-β type RI, RII, and TGF-β type III receptors) have been studied rigorously in acute and chronic diabetes.[158] The TGF-β1 and TGF-β2 isoforms and the TGF-β type RII were the most responsive elements within the glomerulus and the tubules in response to diabetes induction.[158] The changes in TGF-β1 in diabetes seem to be compartmentalized in the kidney, whereas glomerular TGF-β2 and TGF-β type RII are both upregulated in diabetes, suggesting that fibrogenic signalling is increased.[158] In diabetic subjects with nephropathy, an increased TGF-β immunostaining has been described both in glomeruli[166,167] and in tubulointerstitium,[166] but this finding has also been reported in other renal diseases characterized by accumulation of ECM.[166] Further, a positive correlation between TGF-β, fibronectin and plasminogen activator inhibitor-1 levels in glomeruli and tubulointerstitium was found.[166] By measuring the renal arteriovenous TGF-β1 gradient in type 2 diabetic patients, an increased renal production of TGF-β1 has been shown.[168] Type 2 diabetic subjects also present with increased urinary TGF-β1 levels[168,169] which correlate with UAE.[169] Taken together, these experimental and clinical studies indicate that the glucose-induced rise in renal TGF-β is responsible for some of the renal changes that precede the development of diabetic kidney disease.

## Treatment targeting TGF-β

### Neutralizing antibodies

*In vitro*, the glucose-mediated increase in type IV collagen synthesis[170] and glycated albumin-induced increase in fibronectin gene expression[171] in mesangial cells depends on the autocrine action of TGF-β1, as neutralizing antibodies to TGF-β attenuate the rise. Further, short-term treatment with anti-TGF-β antibodies in STZ-diabetic mice attenuates the increased renal TGF-β1 and TGF-β type RII mRNA levels, and reduces both the diabetes-associated renal/glomerular growth and enhanced renal expression of collagen IV and fibronectin.[172] In addition, chronic inhibition of the biological actions of TGF-β with a neutralizing antibody in db/db mice substantially attenuates the increase in renal collagen IV and fibronectin mRNAs, and thus prevents glomerulosclerosis resulting from type 2 diabetes.[173] Interestingly, this study has found no effect of TGF-β antibodies on UAE.[173]

### ACE inhibition

It has been suggested from *in vitro* studies that renal TGF-β activation in diabetes may be mediated through activation of the renin-angiotensin system (RAS).[174] The ACEi captopril reduces the high-glucose-induced increases in TGF-β RI and RII expression and in cellular hypertrophy in LLC-PK$_1$ cells, but has no effect on TGF-β mRNA.[175] Recently, the effect of ACE inhibition on intrarenal changes in all three TGF-β isoforms and receptors has been examined in experimental diabetes *in vivo*.[176] Enalapril reduces diabetes-associated renal hypertrophy, prevents increased UAE, and has pronounced inhibitory effects on the increased concentrations of the TGF-β receptors, but not on the glomerular expression of the TGF-β isoforms.[176] Finally, in a recent clinical study, captopril treatment for 6 months in type 1 diabetic patients lowered serum TGF-β1 levels, and this fall in serum TGF-β1 correlated with the ACEi-induced stabilization of GFR over a 2-year period in patients with overt nephropathy.[177] These findings suggest a possible new mechanism of action for ACEi through regulation of a pathophysiologically enhanced circulating and renal TGF-β system.

### PKCβ inhibition

The antioxidant α-tocopherol blocks the high-glucose-induced increase in PKC, TGF-β and matrix accumulation *in vitro* in mesangial cells.[178] In addition, α-tocopherol administered to STZ-diabetic rats prevents the increase in glomerular TGF-β immunoreactivity and reduces glomerular size, but it has no effect on albumin clearance.[107] LY333531, a specific PKCβ isoform inhibitor, abolishes the diabetes-associated increase in glomerular TGF-β mRNA, matrix accumulation and renal vascular dysfunctions[89] when given to STZ-diabetic rats for 3 months.[89,95] In a long-term study in diabetic db/db mice, PKCβ inhibition results in the reduction of long-term renal changes, including the increase in glomerular TGF-β1 immunostaining.[96] In contrast,

LY333531 has been shown to be renoprotective in STZ-diabetic rats without effect on any components of the intrarenal TGF-β system.[101]

### AGE inhibition

Oral treatment with a new AGE-inhibitor (OPB-9195) for up to 68 weeks in OLETF rats reduces the diabetes-associated increased renal expressions of TGF-β1 mRNA and protein levels to normal, along with restoring the diabetes-associated renal collagen IV accumulation to normal and diminishing the increased UAE.[179]

## Vascular endothelial growth factor (VEGF)

The group of VEGFs consists of at least five different isoforms of homodimeric glycoproteins,[180,181] with angiogenic actions and effects on vascular permeability.[182] VEGF has an important role in physiological and pathological angiogenesis[183] and has potent mitogenic actions in endothelial cells.[181] The two best-described VEGF receptors (VEGFR-1 and VEGFR-2), also known as the fms-like tyrosine kinase and fetal liver kinase 1 (Flk-1), are high-affinity transmembrane tyrosine kinase receptors.[180] The VEGFs and their receptors are crucial for embryologic development, as shown in knockout animals.[184,185] Both VEGF and the two VEGFRs are expressed in the glomeruli and tubules of normal kidney.[186–188]

## Evidence for a role of VEGF in diabetic kidney disease

*In vitro* mesangial cells, glomerular endothelial cells, VSMCs, and proximal and distal tubular cells are capable of producing VEGF.[189–191] Ang II can stimulate VEGF production in mesangial cells,[189–191] and high glucose-induced VEGF production in VSMCs seems to be PKC-dependent.[192] Further, various growth factors and cytokines have been shown to stimulate VEGF production in non-renal cells.[111] Finally, VEGF stimulates NF-κB concentrations in endothelial cells *in vitro*.[193] The recent study in OLETF rats described above reported renal VEGF mRNA and glomerular immunoreactivity to be increased.[179] Changes in renal VEGF and VEGF receptor concentrations have also been described in STZ-diabetic rats.[186] In a clinical study in children and adolescents with type 1 diabetes, serum VEGF levels are similar to the levels in non-diabetic controls.[194] However, another clinical study, describing

VEGF expression in renal biopsy specimens from patients with different kidney diseases, included a small number of five patients with diabetic nephropathy.[195] These preliminary data indicate that glomerular VEGF expression is highest in the patients with mildest sclerotic changes, and decreases with increasing sclerosis.[195]

## Treatments targeting VEGF

### Neutralizing antibodies

Only two studies have been published on the effect of VEGF antibodies in diabetic kidney disease. Treatment for 6 weeks in STZ-diabetic rats with an anti-VEGF monoclonal neutralizing antibody fully abolished the diabetes-associated hyperfiltration and partially abolished the increase in UAE.[196] VEGF-antibody treatment significantly decreased glomerular volume and tended to decrease kidney weight in diabetic rats.[196] No effect on metabolic control was seen in diabetic animals and no renal effects were seen in non-diabetic controls.[196] Further, VEGF-antibody administration in an obese mouse model of type 2 diabetes (i.e. *db/db* mice) showed amelioration of diabetic renal changes by attenuation of the diabetes-associated increases in kidney weight, glomerular volume and UAE, while the increase in basement membrane thickness and creatinine clearance was abolished. Finally, VEGF-antibody administration only tended to reduce total mesangial volume expansion.[197]

### AGE inhibition

In the study described above, in an experimental type 2 diabetic model,[179] it was shown that long-term treatment with OPB-9195 abolishes the enhanced renal VEGF immunoreactivity along with renoprotection, by restoring diabetes-induced renal collagen IV accumulation to normal and reducing the rise in UAE.[179]

## VASOACTIVE FACTORS

Several vasoactive hormones, such as kinin, prostaglandins, atrial natriuretic peptide, and nitric oxide, play a role in renal haemodynamic alterations that have been implicated in the initiation and progression of diabetic nephropathy.[198] The main focus in this review will be on angiotensin (Ang II), the renin-angiotensin system (RAS) and endothelin (ET), as Ang II and ET not only modulate vascular tone and glomerular filtration,[199] but also have mitogenic properties,[200,201] and because diabetes induces changes in several components of the RAS (Table 5.3).

## Angiotensin/renin-angiotensin-system

Apart from the well-known elements of the circulating RAS that regulate vascular tone, fluid and electrolyte balance,[202] many tissues appear to have a local, independently regulated RAS.[203] Ang II, the main mediator of the RAS, exerts both haemodynamic and non-haemodynamic effects,[204,205] and most

**Table 5.3 Vasoactive factors that have been implicated in the pathogenesis of diabetic kidney disease: list of different components of the angiotensin/renin-angiotensin system (RAS) and endothelin system, and known or potential inhibitors of these systems.**

| Vasoactive factors | Components | Inhibitors |
|---|---|---|
| Angiotensin/RAS | Renin, angiotensinogen, angiotensin II | *Angiotensin-converting enzyme inhibitors (ACEi)* |
| | *Enzyme:* angiotensin-converting enzyme | *Ang II AT$_1$-receptor antagonists:* losartan, eprosartan, candesartan |
| | *Receptors:* Ang II type 1, type 2, type 3, type 4 | |
| Endothelin | Endothelins ET-1, ET-2, ET-3 | *Endothelin antagonists:* selective (FR139317, LU 135252), non-selective (bosentan, PD 142893) |
| | *Receptors:* endothelin receptors A, B and C | *Others:* ACEi, PKC-inhibitor, vasodilators |

For further explanation and references, please see text.

of the intrarenal actions of Ang II are mediated by Ang II type 1 receptors ($AT_1$).[202,206,207] $AT_1$ receptors are coupled to traditional signal-transduction pathways, including activation of phospholipases $A_2$, C and D and PKC, $Ca^{2+}$ mobilization, inhibition of adenylate cyclase activity, and reduction of cAMP levels.[207] Growth stimulation by Ang II-mediated pathways involves tyrosine phosphorylation and activation of janus-activated kinase (JAK), signal transducer and activator of transcription pathway (STAT), and mitogen-activated protein (MAP) kinases.[207] The role of Ang II type 2 receptors ($AT_2$) in adult kidney has not yet been clearly defined, but $AT_2$ is involved in the production of cGMP,[208] nitric oxide[209] and prostaglandin $F_{2\alpha}$.[210] Various signal transduction pathways have been assigned to $AT_2$, including activation of guanylate cyclase, phosphatases and potassium channels.[202] $AT_2$ might also be involved in mediating proliferation and apoptosis,[211–213] differentiation,[214–216] and possibly vasodilatation,[217] and might counteract the effects of $AT_1$ receptors.[218] Recently, additional Ang II receptors, named $AT_3$ and $AT_4$, have been identified, but their functional role has not yet been elucidated.[219,220] All components of the RAS, renin, angiotensinogen, ACE, Ang II, $AT_1$, and $AT_2$, are expressed in the normal kidney.[221–223]

## Evidence for a role of RAS in diabetic kidney disease

*In vitro* blockade of the RAS in PTCs inhibits the stimulatory effects of hyperglycaemia on angiotensinogen expression, Ang II production, and cellular hypertrophy, supporting the notion that intrarenal Ang II formation may play a role in the development of renal hypertrophy in early diabetes.[224] It has previously been shown that ET and Ang II enhance protein tyrosine phosphorylation by PKC-dependent and -independent pathways in glomerular mesangial cells, and it was suggested that these vasoactive peptides share in the signalling pathways of growth factors.[225] Ang II-stimulated ET-1 production in glomerular mesangial cells is partially PKC-dependent[226] and plays a role in the mitogenic effect of Ang II.[227] Although the role of RAS in diabetic nephropathy is indisputable,[207] data concerning the influence of diabetes on systemic and intrarenal RAS have been conflicting. In experimental diabetes, plasma levels of RAS components have generally shown suppression of the system, and the local glomerular RAS seems to be activated, but data are variable,[207] a result which may be due to the

degree of hyperglycaemia or the time after onset of diabetes.[207] STZ-diabetic rats tend to have increased plasma and intrarenal levels of Ang II compared to control and insulin-treated rats.[221] Studies investigating mRNA for renin, angiotensinogen and ACE in the PT[221] and glomeruli[223] in rats with STZ diabetes for 2 weeks show only a significant increase in renin mRNA in the PT. Thus, a downregulation in Ang II receptor protein expression is reported, more specifically in cortical and PT $AT_1$,[221] and in $AT_2$ in all kidney regions,[223] suggesting that alterations in the balance of kidney $AT_1$ and $AT_2$ may contribute to Ang II-mediated diabetic glomerular injury. In transgenic rats overexpressing Ang II, diabetic renal pathology is associated with intense renin mRNA and protein in PTs and juxtaglomerular cells, along with overexpression of TGF-β1 and collagen IV mRNA in glomeruli and tubules, as well as a declining GFR and albuminuria.[222] In type 1 diabetic patients, hyperglycaemia is associated with increased plasma renin concentrations, while in patients with type 2 diabetes and nephropathy, plasma renin levels have been shown to be suppressed.[207] One study has found stronger signals for renin, angiotensinogen and ACE mRNA in mesangial and epithelial cells obtained by kidney biopsies in hypertensive patients and patients with renal pathology, including some with diabetes mellitus.[202] The prevention of glomerular growth in microalbuminuric type 1 diabetic patients treated with an ACEi is in agreement with experimental data and fits with the growth stimulatory effects of Ang II.[204,228] Microalbuminuric type 1 diabetic patients carrying the D-allele of the ACE gene have an increased progression of diabetic glomerulopathy[229] (see also Chapter 4). These clinical studies[228,229] provide indirect evidence for the role of the RAS in diabetic kidney disease, but due to the small number of patients, larger studies are needed to confirm the clinical significance of these findings.

## Treatment targeting AT

### Angiotensin-converting enzyme inhibitors (ACEi)

ACEis have been successfully used in the treatment of diabetic kidney disease, but are frequently associated with side effects due to accumulation of bradykinin and other peptides, since ACE inhibition interferes with their metabolism. Further, they do not provide a complete inhibition of Ang II activity, as Ang II can be formed through non-ACE pathways. Ang II $AT_1$-receptor antagonists have been developed, as they might exert a more specific and complete blockade of the RAS, through their inhibition of the actions of Ang II at the receptor site. Some of the beneficial effects of ACE inhibition and AT receptor blockade will be mentioned, but for a more extensive review, see Chapter 7. *In vitro*, the effects of high glucose on angiotensin gene expression and cellular hypertrophy are blocked by ACE inhibition and an $AT_1$ antagonist (losartan), but not by an $AT_2$ receptor blocker (PD123319).[224] In addition, losartan abolishes the Ang II-mediated increase of ET-1 production in rat glomerular mesangial cells.[226] ACEi and $AT_1$ antagonists consistently limit progressive renal injury in experimental models of renal disease progression, including STZ-induced diabetes.[230] The beneficial effect of ACE inhibition on proteinuria and renal function has also been confirmed in patients with diabetic and non-diabetic proteinuric glomerulopathies.[231–233] Recent studies have examined the effect of Ang II receptor blockers on renal functional parameters in healthy subjects. Eprosartan has a renal vasodilatory effect during hyperglycaemia, an effect which is consistent with activation of the intrarenal RAS.[234] Candesartan induces an increase in renal plasma flow and a remarkable rise in plasma renin activity, which is substantially larger than that in earlier studies with ACEi, providing additional evidence for non-ACE-dependent Ang II generation in the kidney.[235]

## Endothelin (ET)

Endothelins consist of a family of structurally and functionally related peptides, ET-1, the most potent vasoconstrictor known,[236] and ET-2 and ET-3.[237] Endothelins exert their effects through binding to specific receptors.[238] Endothelin receptors A ($ET_A$), relatively selective for ET-1,[239,240] are involved in vasoconstrictive and proliferative effects of ET, whereas endothelin receptors B ($ET_B$), non-specifically binding all three ETs,[241,242] mediate NO release among other effects.[243,244] More recently, a third type of ET receptor, $ET_C$, has been identified, with a higher affinity for ET-3 than ET-1.[245] ET-1 is found in all parts in the nephron.[226,246–253] ET-1 acts in both paracrine,[253] and autocrine[254] ways, and has a wide spectrum of biological activities in kidney.[246] ET-3 (mRNA and protein) has been detected in rat kidney and is distributed differently along the nephron than ET-1.[255] ET-3 mRNA is not detected in human tissues[237] nor in diabetic rat glomeruli,[256] suggesting that ET-3 does not play a pathophysiological role in diabetic glomerulopathy.[256] Both $ET_A$ and $ET_B$ receptor mRNAs are expressed in glomeruli.[256]

## Evidence for a role of endothelin in diabetic kidney disease

In cultured PTCs, the synthesis and release of ET-1 is increased by albumin and high-density lipoproteins, suggesting a link between proteinuria and tubular ET-1 metabolism.[230] Fibronectin, collagen type IV and laminin also induce ET-1 synthesis in cultured tubular cells.[230] Accumulation of ET-1, having vasoconstrictor and proliferating properties, might take part in interstitial ischaemia and fibrosis, and inflammation.[257] Other factors such as hyperglycaemia,[258] shear stress[259] due to glomerular hyperfiltration, and urine flow[260] have been shown to stimulate ET-1 synthesis or release. Studies examining systemic and intrarenal ET-1 in diabetes are rare and have yielded conflicting results. Plasma ET-1 levels have been described as either undetectable,[261] unchanged,[198] enhanced[260–263] or suppressed,[264] and renal ET-1 levels have been shown to be unchanged,[261] enhanced,[256] or reduced.[198] Accordingly, it is suggested that these changes are caused by the diabetic state, and differences may be due to the degree of hyperglycaemia, the renal localization, or varying duration of diabetes.[198] Glomerular ET-1 mRNA levels increase with progression of diabetic nephropathy in STZ-diabetic rats, whereas the mRNA levels for ET receptor A and B do not change in diabetes.[256] On the contrary, early after the induction of diabetes, renal ET-1 mRNA and protein expression have been reported to be reduced and plasma ET-1 levels unchanged, implying that the intrarenal ET-1 system may be affected independently of the systemic ET-1 system.[198] In early STZ-diabetic rats, no difference in glomerular $ET_A$ receptor characteristics has been found; however, a reduction in lower-affinity $ET_B$ density, as well as a reduction in glomerular Ang II receptor density, has been reported. Infusion of a specific PKC-inhibitor reverses the downregulation of ER-2 receptors.[265] Urinary ET-1 excretion is increased in STZ-diabetic rats, in parallel with enhanced proteinuria.[230] Upregulation of the renal ET system may favour the development of renal lesions, as suggested by *in vivo* studies in transgenic mice and rats.[230,266–268] In patients, the elevation of ET levels is associated with the onset of microalbuminuria.[262]

## Treatments targeting ET

### ET antagonists
The effects of ETs can be blocked by administration of selective $ET_A$ antagonists (FR 139317, BQ123, BMS193884, LU 135252) or non-selective ET receptor antagonists (bosentan, PD 142893). Some antagonists

have been reported to be renoprotective in various animal models of progressive renal disease, including experimental diabetes,[257] by normalizing blood pressure, reducing UAE, improving renal function and limiting glomerular injury.[230,245,269] PD 142893 reduces UAE in diabetic animals.[270] Selective $ET_A$ blockade has shown protective effects in experimental diabetic glomerulopathy.[263,271] LU 135252 prevents renal histological alterations in STZ-diabetic rats, and significantly decreases urinary ET-1 excretion, but has no effect on UAE.[272] The combination of LU 135252 and an ACEi has an additive renoprotective effect compared to single therapy.[273] In nondiabetic and diabetic (mRen-2)27 rats, a transgenic rat model overexpressing Ang II, oral administration of bosentan for 12 weeks normalizes systolic blood pressure and attenuates the diabetes-associated decline in GFR.[222] Despite producing normotension, severe diabetic renal pathology is not prevented by bosentan, suggesting dissociation of ET, albuminuria, and hypertension from the structural injury in this diabetic model.[222] It has been suggested that albuminuria per se may induce ET-1 secretion in the tubulointerstitium, an effect which may contribute to the interstitial lesions of diabetic nephropathy.[274] In diabetic rats, mRNA levels for various collagens, laminin, and growth factors are elevated[263] and glomerular PCNA, c-myc, c-fos, and c-jun mRNA levels increase with progression of diabetic nephropathy in STZ-diabetic rats.[275] These changes are reduced by $ET_A$ blockade with FR139317,[275] suggesting that ET may play a role in ECM production. Thus, ET inhibition may protect against diabetic glomerular injury, possibly by interference with growth factors and growth-related genes.[263]

*Others*

In rats with non-diabetic renal disease, ACEis not only normalize UAE, but also reduce ET-1-like immunoreactivity in urine, supporting a link between UAE and enhanced renal ET-1 synthesis.[230] In endothelial and mesangial cells, ET-1 production is inhibited by vasodilators such as atrial natriuretic peptide, ET-3, and prostaglandin $E_2$.[198] The PKC-inhibitor 1-(6-isoquinolinesulfonyl) piperazine normalizes the reduction in ET receptor density in association with normalization of PKC activity in STZ-diabetic rats.[265]

## MISCELLANEOUS FACTORS

Other factors with influence on diabetic kidney disease include blood pressure, dietary factors such as low-protein diet,[230] serum lipid abnormalities,[276] and

smoking.[277] Many of these factors and their related therapeutic measures will be discussed in the succeeding chapters on Treatment of Diabetic Nephropathy, Antihypertensive Treatment, Low-Protein Diet, and Control of Serum Lipids. Recently, the influence of smoking on the development and progression of diabetic kidney disease has been extensively reviewed.[278]

## CONCLUSIONS AND OUTLOOK

Despite intensified metabolic control and antihypertensive treatment of diabetic patients, the development of diabetic nephropathy remains a serious problem. There is increasing evidence for a multifactorial pathogenesis of diabetic kidney disease, including various metabolic factors, growth factors and cytokines, and vasoactive factors as active players. *In vitro* and *in vivo* studies have shown enhanced AGE levels in diabetic kidney that affect PKC activity, activation of transcription factors and subsequent gene expression. Further, beneficial effects have been reported with different AGE formation inhibitors, AGE-cross-link breakers, and more specifically with RAGE blockade. Activation of the AR/polyol pathway is believed to play a role in the pathogenesis of diabetic kidney disease, and seems to interact with non-enzymatic glycation. Various ARIs have been shown to be renoprotective in experimental diabetes. However, many failed to confirm their effects in clinical trials or proved to be toxic. Activation of the DAG–PKC pathway has been shown to be important in diabetes. Glucose-induced renal changes, such as increased prostaglandin production, and TGF-β, collagen and fibronectin expression, are PKC-dependent. Furthermore, PKC inhibitors, especially PKCβ inhibitors, have been shown to be effective in reducing the diabetes-associated changes in kidney structural and functional parameters. In addition, vitamin E is likely to have beneficial effects through its influence on the DAG–PKC system.

It is known today that growth factors and cytokines, through complex endocrine and paracrine systems, play an important role in the early and late renal changes in experimental and human diabetes. Treatment with specific antagonists of these systems, such as long-acting somatostatin analogues and GHR antagonists, is followed by renoprotection in diabetic animal models. Despite varying data in experimental diabetes, the RAS undoubtedly plays a role in diabetic kidney disease, and knowledge is still expanding with new receptors being identified. The effect of AT receptor antagonists compared to ACE inhibition has been investigated, as they may provide a more compete blockade of the RAS, and have yielded positive results so far. Recently, endothelin has been implicated in ECM production and development of proteinuria, and ET inhibition has been shown to protect against diabetic glomerular injury.

Various treatments targeting these specific pathways have shown their renoprotective effects *in vitro* and in experimental diabetic models, but need to be confirmed in future well-designed clinical trials to prove their usefulness in the treatment of human diabetic nephropathy. Furthermore, future research will elucidate how these pathways interact and influence each other. On the basis of this novel knowledge on mechanisms involved in diabetic kidney disease, new therapeutic strategies can be designed that may prove to be beneficial in preventing the development and progression of diabetic kidney disease. In addition, future experiments may show whether a combination of inhibitors with different points of action may be more effective than treatments that influence only one pathway.

## ACKNOWLEDGEMENTS

The work was supported by the Danish Medical Research Council (Grant no. 9700592), the Eva and Henry Frænkels Memorial Foundation, the Danish Kidney Foundation, the Ruth König Petersen Foundation, the Danish Diabetes Association, the Novo Foundation, the Nordic Insulin Foundation, the Johanne and Aage Louis Petersen Memorial Foundation, the Institute of Experimental Clinical Research, University of Aarhus, Denmark, and the Aarhus University-Novo Nordisk Centre for Research in Growth and Regeneration (Danish Medical Research Council Grant no. 9600822). B.F. Schrijvers is supported by a grant from the Institute for the Promotion of Innovation by Science and Technology in Flanders (IWT). A.S. De Vriese is supported by a grant from the Fund for Scientific Research, Flanders (N20/0).

## REFERENCES

1. The effect of intensive treatment of diabetes on the development and progression of long-term complications in insulin-dependent diabetes mellitus. The Diabetes Control and Complications Trial Research Group. *N Engl J Med* 1993; **329**: 977–86.
2. Ritz E, Keller C, Bergis K et al, Pathogenesis and course of renal disease in IDDM/NIDDM: differences and similarities. *Am J Hypertens* 1997; **10**: 202S–207S.
3. Schleicher E, Kolm V, Ceol M et al, Structural and functional changes in diabetic glomerulopathy. *Kidney Blood Press Res* 1996; **19**: 305–15.
4. Singh R, Barden A, Mori T et al, Advanced glycation end-products: a review. *Diabetologia* 2001; **44**: 129–46.
5. Fu MX, Wells-Knecht KJ, Blackledge JA et al, Glycation, glycoxidation, and cross-linking of collagen by glucose. Kinetics, mechanisms, and inhibition of late stages of the Maillard reaction. *Diabetes* 1994; **43**: 676–83.
6. Niwa T, Katsuzaki T, Miyazaki S et al, Immunohistochemical detection of imidazolone, a novel advanced glycation end product, in kidneys and aortas of diabetic patients. *J Clin Invest* 1997; **99**: 1272–80.
7. Schmidt AM, Yan SD, Yan SF et al, The biology of the receptor for advanced glycation end products and its ligands. *Biochim Biophys Acta* 2000; **1498**: 99–111.
8. Li YM, Mitsuhashi T, Wojciechowicz D et al, Molecular identity and cellular distribution of advanced glycation endproduct receptors: relationship of p60 to OST-48 and p90 to 80K-H membrane proteins. *Proc Natl Acad Sci USA* 1996; **93**: 11047–52.
9. Horiuchi S, Higashi T, Ikeda K et al, Advanced glycation end products and their recognition by macrophage and macrophage-derived cells. *Diabetes* 1996; **45** (Suppl 3): S73–6.
10. Cooper ME, Jerums G, Advanced glycation end-products and diabetic renal disease. In: *The Kidney and Hypertension in Diabetes Mellitus*, 4th edn (Mogensen CE, ed.). Kluwer: Boston, 1998; 257–62.
11. Vlassara H, Advanced glycation in diabetic renal and vascular disease. *Kidney Int Suppl* 1995; **51**: S43–4.
12. Di Mario U, Pugliese G, 15th Golgi lecture: from hyperglycaemia to the dysregulation of vascular remodelling in diabetes. *Diabetologia* 2001; **44**: 674–92.
13. Sakai H, Jinde K, Suzuki D et al, Localization of glycated proteins in the glomeruli of patients with diabetic nephropathy. *Nephrol Dial Transplant* 1996; **11** (Suppl 5): 66–71.
14. Soulis T, Cooper ME, Vranes D et al, Effects of aminoguanidine in preventing experimental diabetic nephropathy are related to the duration of treatment. *Kidney Int* 1996; **50**: 627–34.
15. Abel M, Ritthaler U, Zhang Y et al, Expression of receptors for advanced glycosylated end-products in renal disease. *Nephrol Dial Transplant* 1995; **10**: 1662–7.
16. Chen S, Cohen MP, Lautenslager GT et al, Glycated albumin stimulates TGF-beta 1 production and protein kinase C activity in glomerular endothelial cells. *Kidney Int* 2001; **59**: 673–81.
17. Scivittaro V, Ganz MB, Weiss MF, AGEs induce oxidative stress and activate protein kinase C-beta(II) in neonatal mesangial cells. *Am J Physiol Renal Physiol* 2000; **278**: F676–83.
18. Yeh CH, Sturgis L, Haidacher J et al, Requirement for p38 and p44/p42 mitogen-activated protein kinases in RAGE-mediated nuclear factor-kappaB transcriptional activation and cytokine secretion. *Diabetes* 2001; **50**: 1495–504.
19. Schmidt AM, Stern DM, RAGE: a new target for the prevention and treatment of the vascular and inflammatory complications of diabetes. *Trends Endocrinol Metab* 2000; **11**: 368–75.
20. Gugliucci A, Bendayan M, Reaction of advanced glycation end-products with renal tissue from normal and streptozotocin-induced diabetic rats: an ultrastructural study using colloidal gold cytochemistry. *J Histochem Cytochem* 1995; **43**: 591–600.
21. Soulis T, Thallas V, Youssef S et al, Advanced glycation end products and their receptors co-localise in rat organs susceptible to diabetic microvascular injury. *Diabetologia* 1997; **40**: 619–28.
22. Youssef S, Nguyen DT, Soulis T et al, Effect of diabetes and aminoguanidine therapy on renal advanced glycation end-product binding. *Kidney Int* 1999; **55**: 907–16.
23. Soulis T, Cooper ME, Sastra S et al, Relative contributions of advanced glycation and nitric oxide synthase inhibition to aminoguanidine-mediated renoprotection in diabetic rats. *Diabetologia* 1997; **40**: 1141–51.

24. Striker LJ, Striker GE, Administration of AGEs in vivo induces extracellular matrix gene expression. *Nephrol Dial Transplant* 1996; **11** (Suppl 5): 62–5.

25. Vlassara H, Fuh H, Makita Z et al, Exogenous advanced glycosylation end products induce complex vascular dysfunction in normal animals: a model for diabetic and aging complications. *Proc Natl Acad Sci USA* 1992; **89**: 12043–7.

26. Yamamoto Y, Kato I, Doi T et al, Development and prevention of advanced diabetic nephropathy in RAGE-overexpressing mice. *J Clin Invest* 2001; **108**: 261–8.

27. Berg TJ, Clausen JT, Torjesen PA et al, The advanced glycation end product Nepsilon-(carboxymethyl)lysine is increased in serum from children and adolescents with type 1 diabetes. *Diabetes Care* 1998; **21**: 1997–2002.

28. Berg TJ, Bangstad HJ, Torjesen PA et al, Advanced glycation end products in serum predict changes in the kidney morphology of patients with insulin-dependent diabetes mellitus. *Metabolism* 1997; **46**: 661–5.

29. Aoki S, Hasegawa G, Shigeta H et al, Crossline levels in serum and erythrocyte membrane proteins from patients with diabetic nephropathy. *Diabetes Res Clin Pract* 2000; **48**: 119–25.

30. Horie K, Miyata T, Maeda K et al, Immunohistochemical colocalization of glycoxidation products and lipid peroxidation products in diabetic renal glomerular lesions. Implication for glycoxidative stress in the pathogenesis of diabetic nephropathy. *J Clin Invest* 1997; **100**: 2995–3004.

31. Makino H, Shikata K, Kushiro M et al, Roles of advanced glycation end-products in the progression of diabetic nephropathy. *Nephrol Dial Transplant* 1996; **11** (Suppl 5): 76–80.

32. Suzuki D, Miyata T, Saotome N et al, Immunohistochemical evidence for an increased oxidative stress and carbonyl modification of proteins in diabetic glomerular lesions. *J Am Soc Nephrol* 1999; **10**: 822–32.

33. Slatter DA, Bolton CH, Bailey AJ, The importance of lipid-derived malondialdehyde in diabetes mellitus. *Diabetologia* 2000; **43**: 550–7.

34. Edelstein D, Brownlee M, Mechanistic studies of advanced glycosylation end product inhibition by aminoguanidine. *Diabetes* 1992; **41**: 26–9.

35. Takagi Y, Kashiwagi A, Tanaka Y et al, Significance of fructose-induced protein oxidation and formation of advanced glycation end product. *J Diabetes Complications* 1995; **9**: 87–91.

36. Soulis-Liparota T, Cooper M, Papazoglou D et al, Retardation by aminoguanidine of development of albuminuria, mesangial expansion, and tissue fluorescence in streptozocin-induced diabetic rat. *Diabetes* 1991; **40**: 1328–34.

37. Osicka TM, Yu Y, Lee V et al, Aminoguanidine and ramipril prevent diabetes-induced increases in protein kinase C activity in glomeruli, retina and mesenteric artery. *Clin Sci (Colch)* 2001; **100**: 249–57.

38. Soulis T, Sastra S, Thallas V et al, A novel inhibitor of advanced glycation end-product formation inhibits mesenteric vascular hypertrophy in experimental diabetes. *Diabetologia* 1999; **42**: 472–9.

39. Osicka TM, Kiriazis Z, Pratt LM et al, Ramipril and aminoguanidine restore renal lysosomal processing in streptozotocin diabetic rats. *Diabetologia* 2001; **44**: 230–6.

40. Osicka TM, Yu Y, Panagiotopoulos S et al, Prevention of albuminuria by aminoguanidine or ramipril in streptozotocin-induced diabetic rats is associated with the normalization of glomerular protein kinase C. *Diabetes* 2000; **49**: 87–93.

41. Appel G, Bolton K, Freedman B et al, Pimagedine (PG) lowers total urinary protein (TUP) and slows progression of overt diabetic nephropathy in patients with type 1 diabetes mellitus (DM). *J Am Soc Nephrol* 1999; **10**: 153A (abst).

42. Jain SK, Lim G, Pyridoxine and pyridoxamine inhibits superoxide radicals and prevents lipid peroxidation, protein glycosylation, and (Na$^+$ + K$^+$)-ATPase activity reduction in high glucose-treated human erythrocytes. *Free Radic Biol Med* 2001; **30**: 232–7.

43. Khalifah RG, Booth AA, Gattone VH et al, Effects of pyridoxamine, a novel post-Amadori AGE inhibitor, on nephropathy induced by glycated albumin. *J Am Soc Nephrol* 1997; **7**: 641A (abst).

44. Baynes JW, Degenhardt TP, Alderson NL et al, Pyridorin, a post-Amadori inhibitor of advanced glycation reactions, preserves renal function in diabetic rats. *J Am Soc Nephrol* 1998; **9**: 628A (abst).

45. Oturai PS, Christensen M, Rolin B et al, Effects of advanced glycation end-product inhibition and cross-link breakage in diabetic rats. *Metabolism* 2000; **49**: 996–1000.

46. Nakamura S, Makita Z, Ishikawa S et al, Progression of nephropathy in spontaneous diabetic rats is prevented by OPB-9195, a novel inhibitor of advanced glycation. *Diabetes* 1997; **46**: 895–9.

47. Oldfield MD, Bach LA, Forbes JM et al, Advanced glycation end products cause epithelial-myofibroblast transdifferentiation via the receptor for advanced glycation end products (RAGE). *J Clin Invest* 2001; **108**: 1853–63.

48. Forbes JM, Soulis T, Thallas V et al, Renoprotective effects of a novel inhibitor of advanced glycation. *Diabetologia* 2001; **44**: 108–14.

49. Cohen MP, Sharma K, Jin Y et al, Prevention of diabetic nephropathy in db/db mice with glycated albumin antagonists. A novel treatment strategy. *J Clin Invest* 1995; **95**: 2338–45.

50. Vasan S, Zhang X, Zhang X et al, An agent cleaving glucose-derived protein crosslinks in vitro and in vivo. *Nature* 1996; **382**: 275–8.

51. Cooper ME, Thallas V, Forbes J et al, The cross-link breaker, N-phenacylthiazolium bromide, prevents vascular advanced glycation end-product accumulation. *Diabetologia* 2000; **43**: 660–4.

52. Kass DA, Shapiro EP, Kawaguchi M et al, Improved arterial compliance by a novel advanced glycation end-product crosslink breaker. *Circulation* 2001; **104**: 1464–70.

53. Wolffenbuttel BH, Boulanger CM, Crijns FR et al, Breakers of advanced glycation end products restore large artery properties in experimental diabetes. *PNAS* 1998; **95**: 4630–4.

54. Bierhaus A, Illmer T, Kasper M et al, Advanced glycation end product (AGE)-mediated induction of tissue factor in cultured endothelial cells is dependent on RAGE. *Circulation* 1997; **96**: 2262–71.

55. Lander HM, Tauras JM, Ogiste JS et al, Activation of the receptor for advanced glycation end products triggers a p21(ras)-dependent mitogen-activated protein kinase pathway regulated by oxidant stress. *J Biol Chem* 1997; **272**: 17810–14.

56. Pugliese G, Pricci F, Romeo G et al, Upregulation of mesangial growth factor and extracellular matrix synthesis by advanced glycation end products via a receptor-mediated mechanism. *Diabetes* 1997; **46**: 1881–7.

57. Wautier JL, Zoukourian C, Chappey O et al, Receptor-mediated endothelial cell dysfunction in diabetic vasculopathy. Soluble receptor for advanced glycation end products blocks hyperpermeability in diabetic rats. *J Clin Invest* 1996; **97**: 238–43.

58. Hamada Y, Araki N, Horiuchi S et al, Role of polyol pathway in nonenzymatic glycation. *Nephrol Dial Transplant* 1996; **11** (Suppl 5): 95–8.

59. Soulis-Liparota T, Cooper ME, Dunlop M et al, The relative roles of advanced glycation, oxidation and aldose reductase inhibition in the development of experimental diabetic nephropathy in the Sprague-Dawley rat. *Diabetologia* 1995; **38**: 387–94.

60. Narayanan S, Aldose reductase and its inhibition in the control of diabetic complications. *Ann Clin Lab Sci* 1993; **23**: 148–58.

61. Burg MB, Kador PF, Sorbitol, osmoregulation, and the complications of diabetes. *J Clin Invest* 1988; **81**: 635–40.

62. McCormack AJ, Finn WF, The effects of aldose reductase inhibitors in diabetic nephropathy. *J Diabetes Complications* 1989; **3**: 18–26.

63. Sato S, Kador PF, Human kidney aldose and aldehyde reductases. *J Diabetes Complications* 1993; **7**: 179–87.

64. Sato S, Rat kidney aldose reductase and aldehyde reductase and polyol production in rat kidney. *Am J Physiol* 1992; **263**: F799–805.

65. Kicic E, Palmer TN, Is sorbitol dehydrogenase gene expression affected by streptozotocin-diabetes in the rat? *Biochim Biophys Acta* 1994; **1226**: 213–18.

66. Hamada Y, Odagaki Y, Sakakibara F et al, Effects of an aldose reductase inhibitor on erythrocyte fructose 3-phosphate and sorbitol 3-phosphate levels in diabetic patients. *Life Sci* 1995; **57**: 23–9.

67. Greene DA, Lattimer SA, Sima AA, Sorbitol, phosphoinositides, and sodium-potassium-ATPase in the pathogenesis of diabetic complications. *N Engl J Med* 1987; **316**: 599–606.

68. Williamson JR, Chang K, Frangos M et al, Hyperglycemic pseudohypoxia and diabetic complications. *Diabetes* 1993; **42**: 801–13.

69. Henry DN, Busik JV, Brosius FC III et al, Glucose transporters control gene expression of aldose reductase, PKCalpha, and GLUT1 in mesangial cells in vitro. *Am J Physiol* 1999; **277**: F97–104.

70. Raskin P, Rosenstock J, Aldose reductase inhibitors and diabetic complications. *Am J Med* 1987; **83**: 298–306.

71. Popp-Snijders C, Lomecky-Janousek MZ, Schouten JA et al, Myo-inositol and sorbitol in erythrocytes from diabetic patients before and after sorbinil treatment. *Diabetologia* 1984; **27**: 514–16.

72. Oates PJ, Mylari BL, Aldose reductase inhibitors: therapeutic implications for diabetic complications. *Expert Opin Investig Drugs* 1999; **8**: 2095–119.

73. Hotta N, Kakuta H, Ando F et al, Current progress in clinical trials of aldose reductase inhibitors in Japan. *Exp Eye Res* 1990; **50**: 625–8.

74. Keogh RJ, Dunlop ME, Larkins RG, Effect of inhibition of aldose reductase on glucose flux, diacylglycerol formation, protein kinase C, and phospholipase A$_2$ activation. *Metabolism* 1997; **46**: 41–7.

75. Averbuch M, Weintraub M, Liao JC et al, Red blood cell sorbitol lowering effects and tolerance of single doses of AL 1576 (HOE 843) in diabetic patients. *J Clin Pharmacol* 1988; **28**: 757–61.

76. Yabe-Nishimura C, Aldose reductase in glucose toxicity: a potential target for the prevention of diabetic complications. *Pharmacol Rev* 1998; **50**: 21–33.

77. Pedersen MM, Christiansen JS, Mogensen CE, Reduction of glomerular hyperfiltration in normoalbuminuric IDDM patients by 6 mo of aldose reductase inhibition. *Diabetes* 1991; **40**: 527–31.

78. Saxena AK, Srivastava P, Kale RK et al, Effect of vanadate administration on polyol pathway in diabetic rat kidney. *Biochem Int* 1992; **26**: 59–68.

79. Webb BLJ, Hirst SJ, Giembycz MA, Protein kinase C isoenzymes: a review of their structure, regulation and role in regulating airways smooth muscle tone and mitogenesis. *Br J Pharmacol* 2000; **130**: 1433–52.

80. Nishizuka Y, Intracellular signaling by hydrolysis of phospholipids and activation of protein kinase C. *Science* 1992; **258**: 607–14.

81. Idris I, Gray S, Donnelly R, Protein kinase C activation: isozyme-specific effects on metabolism and cardiovascular complications in diabetes. *Diabetologia* 2001; **44**: 659–73.

82. Mochly-Rosen D, Gordon AS, Anchoring proteins for protein kinase C: a means for isozyme selectivity. *FASEB J* 1998; **12**: 35–42.

83. Liscovitch M, Cantley LC, Lipid second messengers. *Cell* 1994; **77**: 329–34.

84. Nishizuka Y, Protein kinase C and lipid signaling for sustained cellular responses. *FASEB J* 1995; **9**: 484–96.

85. Koya D, King GL, Protein kinase C in diabetic renal involvement, the perspective of its inhibition. In: *The Kidney and Hypertension in Diabetes Mellitus*, 4th edn (Mogensen CE, ed.). Kluwer: Boston, 1998; 263–8.

86. Ganz MB, Saksa B, Saxena R, PDGF and IL-1 induce and activate specific protein kinase C isoforms in mesangial cells. *Am J Physiol* 1996; **271**: F108–13.

87. Yoshida Y, Huang FL, Nakabayashi H et al, Tissue distribution and developmental expression of protein kinase C isozymes. *J Biol Chem* 1988; **263**: 9868–73.

88. Igarashi M, Wakasaki H, Takahara N et al, Glucose or diabetes activates p38 mitogen-activated protein kinase via different pathways. *J Clin Invest* 1999; **103**: 185–95.

89. Koya D, Jirousek MR, Lin YW et al, Characterization of protein kinase C beta isoform activation on the gene expression of transforming growth factor-beta, extracellular matrix components, and prostanoids in the glomeruli of diabetic rats. *J Clin Invest* 1997; **100**: 115–26.

90. Craven PA, DeRubertis FR, Protein kinase C is activated in glomeruli from streptozotocin diabetic rats. Possible mediation by glucose. *J Clin Invest* 1989; **83**: 1667–75.

91. Williams B, Schrier RW, Glucose-induced protein kinase C activity regulates arachidonic acid release and eicosanoid production by cultured glomerular mesangial cells. *J Clin Invest* 1993; **92**: 2889–96.

92. Xia P, Kramer RM, King GL, Identification of the mechanism for the inhibition of Na+,K(+)-adenosine triphosphatase by hyperglycemia involving activation of protein kinase C and cytosolic phospholipase A$_2$. *J Clin Invest* 1995; **96**: 733–40.

93. Vasilets LA, Schwarz W, Structure-function relationships of cation binding in the Na+/K(+)-ATPase. *Biochim Biophys Acta* 1993; **1154**: 201–22.

94. Park CW, Kim JH, Lee JW et al, High glucose-induced intercellular adhesion molecule-1 (ICAM-1) expression through an osmotic effect in rat mesangial cells is PKC-NF-kappa B-dependent. *Diabetologia* 2000; **43**: 1544–53.

95. Ishii H, Jirousek MR, Koya D et al, Amelioration of vascular dysfunctions in diabetic rats by an oral PKC beta inhibitor. *Science* 1996; **272**: 728–31.

96. Koya D, Haneda M, Nakagawa H et al, Amelioration of accelerated diabetic mesangial expansion by treatment with a PKC beta inhibitor in diabetic db/db mice, a rodent model for type 2 diabetes. *FASEB J* 2000; **14**: 439–47.

97. Craven PA, Davidson CM, DeRubertis FR, Increase in diacylglycerol mass in isolated glomeruli by glucose from de novo synthesis of glycerolipids. *Diabetes* 1990; **39**: 667–74.

98. Way KJ, Chou E, King GL, Identification of PKC-isoform-specific biological actions using pharmacological approaches. *Trends Pharmacol Sci* 2000; **21**: 181–7.

99. Ishii H, Koya D, King GL, Protein kinase C activation and its role in the development of vascular complications in diabetes mellitus. *J Mol Med* 1998; **76**: 21–31.

100. Jirousek MR, Gillig JR, Gonzalez CM et al, (S)-13-[(dimethylamino)methyl]-10,11,14,15-tetrahydro-4,9:16, 21-dimetheno-1H,13H-dibenzo[e,k]pyrrolo[3,4-h][1,4,13]oxadiazacyclohexadecene-1,3(2H)-d ione (LY333531) and related analogues: isozyme selective inhibitors of protein kinase C beta. *J Med Chem* 1996; **39**: 2664–71.

101. Flyvbjerg A, Hill C, Nielsen B et al, Effect of protein kinase C

beta inhibition on renal morphology, urinary albumin excretion and renal transforming growth factor beta in experimental diabetes in rats. *J Am Soc Nephrol* 1999; **10**: A3445 (abst).

102. Wu HL, Albrightson C, Nambi P, Selective inhibition of rat mesangial cell proliferation by a synthetic peptide derived from the sequence of the C2 region of PKCbeta. *Peptides* 1999; **20**: 675–8.

103. Tran K, Proulx PR, Chan AC, Vitamin E suppresses diacylglycerol (DAG) level in thrombin-stimulated endothelial cells through an increase of DAG kinase activity. *Biochim Biophys Acta* 1994; **1212**: 193–202.

104. Lee IK, Koya D, Ishi H et al, d-Alpha-tocopherol prevents the hyperglycemia induced activation of diacylglycerol (DAG)-protein kinase C (PKC) pathway in vascular smooth muscle cell by an increase of DAG kinase activity. *Diabetes Res Clin Pract* 1999; **45**: 183–90.

105. Kunisaki M, Bursell SE, Clermont AC et al, Vitamin E prevents diabetes-induced abnormal retinal blood flow via the diacylglycerol-protein kinase C pathway. *Am J Physiol* 1995; **269**: E239–46.

106. Koya D, Lee IK, Ishii H, Prevention of glomerular dysfunction in diabetic rats by treatment with d-alpha-tocopherol. *J Am Soc Nephrol* 1997; **8**: 426–35.

107. Craven PA, DeRubertis FR, Kagan VE et al, Effects of supplementation with vitamin C or E on albuminuria, glomerular TGF-beta, and glomerular size in diabetes. *J Am Soc Nephrol* 1997; **8**: 1405–14.

108. Bursell SE, Clermont AC, Aiello LP et al, High-dose vitamin E supplementation normalizes retinal blood flow and creatinine clearance in patients with type 1 diabetes. *Diabetes Care* 1999; **22**: 1245–51.

109. Csukai M, Mochly-Rosen D, Pharmacologic modulation of protein kinase C isozymes: the role of RACKs and subcellular localisation. *Pharmacol Res* 1999; **39**: 253–9.

110. Ron D, Luo J, Mochly-Rosen D, C2 region-derived peptides inhibit translocation and function of beta protein kinase C in vivo. *J Biol Chem* 1995; **270**: 24180–7.

111. Flyvbjerg A, Putative pathophysiological role of growth factors and cytokines in experimental diabetic kidney disease. *Diabetologia* 2000; **43**: 1205–23.

112. Werner H, Shen-Orr Z, Stannard B et al, Experimental diabetes increases insulinlike growth factor I and II receptor concentration and gene expression in kidney. *Diabetes* 1990; **39**: 1490–7.

113. Flyvbjerg A, Nielsen S, Sheikh MI et al, Luminal and basolateral uptake and receptor binding of IGF-I in rabbit renal proximal tubules. *Am J Physiol* 1993; **265**: F624–33.

114. Shimasaki S, Shimonaka M, Zhang HP et al, Identification of five different insulin-like growth factor binding proteins (IGFBPs) from adult rat serum and molecular cloning of a novel IGFBP-5 in rat and human. *J Biol Chem* 1991; **266**: 10646–53.

115. Shimasaki S, Gao L, Shimonaka M et al, Isolation and molecular cloning of insulin-like growth factor-binding protein-6. *Mol Endocrinol* 1991; **5**: 938–48.

116. Hwa V, Oh Y, Rosenfeld RG, The insulin-like growth factor-binding protein (IGFBP) superfamily. *Endocr Rev* 1999; **20**: 761–87.

117. Carlsson B, Billig H, Rymo L et al, Expression of the growth hormone-binding protein messenger RNA in the liver and extrahepatic tissues in the rat: co-expression with the growth hormone receptor. *Mol Cell Endocrinol* 1990; **73**: R1–R6.

118. Landau D, Domene H, Flyvbjerg A et al, Differential expression of renal growth hormone receptor and its binding protein in experimental diabetes mellitus. *Growth Horm IGF Res* 1998; **8**: 39–45.

119. Bortz JD, Rotwein P, DeVol D et al, Focal expression of insulin-like growth factor I in rat kidney collecting duct. *J Cell Biol* 1988; **107**: 811–19.

120. Flyvbjerg A, Bornfeldt KE, Marshall SM et al, Kidney IGF-I mRNA in initial renal hypertrophy in experimental diabetes in rats. *Diabetologia* 1990; **33**: 334–8.

121. Murphy LJ, Bell GI, Friesen HG, Tissue distribution of insulin-like growth factor I and II messenger ribonucleic acid in the adult rat. *Endocrinology* 1987; **120**: 1279–82.

122. Pillion DJ, Haskell JF, Meezan E, Distinct receptors for insulin-like growth factor I in rat renal glomeruli and tubules. *Am J Physiol* 1988; **255**: E504–12.

123. Doi T, Striker LJ, Elliot SJ et al, Insulinlike growth factor-1 is a progression factor for human mesangial cells. *Am J Pathol* 1989; **134**: 395–404.

124. Moran A, Brown DM, Kim Y et al, Effects of IGF-I and glucose on protein and proteoglycan synthesis by human fetal mesangial cells in culture. *Diabetes* 1991; **40**: 1346–54.

125. Lupia E, Elliot SJ, Lenz O et al, IGF-1 decreases collagen degradation in diabetic NOD mesangial cells: implications for diabetic nephropathy. *Diabetes* 1999; **48**: 1638–44.

126. Tannenbaum GS, Growth hormone secretory dynamics in streptozotocin diabetes: evidence for a role for endogenous circulating somatostatin. *Endocrinology* 1981; **108**: 76–82.

127. Massa G, Verhaeghe J, Vanderschueren-Lodeweyckx M et al, Normalization of decreased plasma concentrations of growth hormone-binding protein by insulin treatment in spontaneously diabetic BB rats. *Horm Metab Res* 1993; **25**: 325–6.

128. Flyvbjerg A, Frystyk J, Osterby R et al, Kidney IGF-I and renal hypertrophy in GH-deficient diabetic dwarf rats. *Am J Physiol* 1992; **262**: E956–62.

129. Gronbaek H, Volmers P, Bjorn SF et al, Effect of GH/IGF-I deficiency on long-term renal changes and urinary albumin excretion in diabetic dwarf rats. *Am J Physiol* 1997; **272**: E918–24.

130. Flyvbjerg A, Bennett WF, Rasch R et al, Inhibitory effect of a growth hormone receptor antagonist (G120K-PEG) on renal enlargement, glomerular hypertrophy, and urinary albumin excretion in experimental diabetes in mice. *Diabetes* 1999; **48**: 377–82.

131. Flyvbjerg A, Orskov H, Kidney tissue insulin-like growth factor I and initial renal growth in diabetic rats: relation to severity of diabetes. *Acta Endocrinol (Copenh)* 1990; **122**: 374–8.

132. Segev Y, Landau D, Marbach M et al, Renal hypertrophy in hyperglycemic non-obese diabetic mice is associated with persistent renal accumulation of insulin-like growth factor I. *J Am Soc Nephrol* 1997; **8**: 436–44.

133. Landau D, Chin E, Bondy C et al, Expression of insulin-like growth factor binding proteins in the rat kidney: effects of long-term diabetes. *Endocrinology* 1995; **136**: 1835–42.

134. Flyvbjerg A, Kessler U, Dorka B et al, Transient increase in renal insulin-like growth factor binding proteins during initial kidney hypertrophy in experimental diabetes in rats. *Diabetologia* 1992; **35**: 589–93.

135. Flyvbjerg A, Kessler U, Kiess W, Increased kidney and liver insulin-like growth factor II/mannose-6-phosphate receptor concentration in experimental diabetes in rats. *Growth Regul* 1994; **4**: 188–93.

136. Flyvbjerg A, Role of growth hormone, insulin-like growth factors (IGFs) and IGF-binding proteins in the renal complications of diabetes. *Kidney Int Suppl* 1997; **60**: S12–19.

137. Cummings EA, Sochett EB, Dekker MG et al, Contribution of growth hormone and IGF-I to early diabetic nephropathy in type 1 diabetes. *Diabetes* 1998; **47**: 1341–6.

138. Sen A, Buyukgebiz A, Albumin excretion rate, serum insulin-like growth factor-I and glomerular filtration rate in type I diabetes mellitus at puberty. *J Pediatr Endocrinol Metab* 1997; **10**: 209–15.

139. Bacci S, De Cosmo S, Garruba M et al, Role of insulin-like growth factor (IGF)-1 in the modulation of renal haemodynamics in type I diabetic patients. *Diabetologia* 2000; **43**: 922–6.

140. Shinada M, Akdeniz A, Panagiotopoulos S et al, Proteolysis of insulin-like growth factor-binding protein-3 is increased in urine from patients with diabetic nephropathy. *J Clin Endocrinol Metab* 2000; **85**: 1163–9.

141. Flyvbjerg A, Frystyk J, Thorlacius-Ussing O et al, Somatostatin analogue administration prevents increase in kidney somatomedin C and initial renal growth in diabetic and uninephrectomized rats. *Diabetologia* 1989; **32**: 261–5.

142. Gronbaek H, Nielsen B, Frystyk J et al, Effect of lanreotide on local kidney IGF-I and renal growth in experimental diabetes in the rat. *Exp Nephrol* 1996; **4**: 295–303.

143. Gronbaek H, Nielsen B, Frystyk J et al, Effect of octreotide on experimental diabetic renal and glomerular growth: importance of early intervention. *J Endocrinol* 1995; **147**: 95–102.

144. Flyvbjerg A, Marshall SM, Frystyk J et al, Octreotide administration in diabetic rats: effects on renal hypertrophy and urinary albumin excretion. *Kidney Int* 1992; **41**: 805–12.

145. Gronbaek H, Vogel I, Osterby R et al, Effect of octreotide, captopril or insulin on renal changes and UAE in long-term experimental diabetes. *Kidney Int* 1998; **53**: 173–80.

146. Pedersen MM, Christensen SE, Christiansen JS et al, Acute effects of a somatostatin analogue on kidney function in type 1 diabetic patients. *Diabetic Med* 1990; **7**: 304–9.

147. Serri O, Beauregard H, Brazeau P et al, Somatostatin analogue, octreotide, reduces increased glomerular filtration rate and kidney size in insulin-dependent diabetes. *JAMA* 1991; **265**: 888–92.

148. Chen NY, Chen WY, Bellush L et al, Effects of streptozotocin treatment in growth hormone (GH) and GH antagonist transgenic mice. *Endocrinology* 1995; **136**: 660–7.

149. Liu ZH, Striker LJ, Phillips C et al, Growth hormone expression is required for the development of diabetic glomerulosclerosis in mice. *Kidney Int Suppl* 1995; **51**: S37–8.

150. Chen NY, Chen WY, Kopchick JJ, A growth hormone antagonist protects mice against streptozotocin induced glomerulosclerosis even in the presence of elevated levels of glucose and glycated hemoglobin. *Endocrinology* 1996; **137**: 5163–5.

151. Haylor J, Hickling H, El Eter E et al, JB3, an IGF-I receptor antagonist, inhibits early renal growth in diabetic and uninephrectomized rats. *J Am Soc Nephrol* 2000; **11**: 2027–35.

152. Bach LA, Dean R, Youssef S et al, Aminoguanidine ameliorates changes in the IGF system in experimental diabetic nephropathy. *Nephrol Dial Transplant* 2000; **15**: 347–54.

153. Nilsson AB, Nitescu N, Chen Y et al, IGF-I treatment attenuates renal abnormalities induced by neonatal ACE inhibition. *Am J Physiol Regul Integr Comp Physiol* 2000; **279**: R1050–60.

154. New JP, Canavan JP, Flyvbjerg A et al, Renal enlargement and insulin-like growth factor-1 accumulation in the Wistar rat model of experimental diabetes is not prevented by angiotensin converting enzyme inhibition. *Diabetologia* 1996; **39**: 166–71.

155. Lawrence DA, Transforming growth factor-beta: an overview. *Kidney Int Suppl* 1995; **49**: S19–23.

156. Wrana JL, Attisano L, Wieser R et al, Mechanism of activation of the TGF-beta receptor. *Nature* 1994; **370**: 341–7.

157. Nakamura T, Fukui M, Ebihara I et al, mRNA expression of growth factors in glomeruli from diabetic rats. *Diabetes* 1993; **42**: 450–6.

158. Hill C, Flyvbjerg A, Gronbaek H et al, The renal expression of transforming growth factor-beta isoforms and their receptors in acute and chronic experimental diabetes in rats. *Endocrinology* 2000; **141**: 1196–208.

159. Ziyadeh FN, Snipes ER, Watanabe M et al, High glucose induces cell hypertrophy and stimulates collagen gene transcription in proximal tubule. *Am J Physiol* 1990; **259**: F704–14.

160. Nakamura T, Miller D, Ruoslahti E et al, Production of extracellular matrix by glomerular epithelial cells is regulated by transforming growth factor-beta 1. *Kidney Int* 1992; **41**: 1213–21.

161. Roberts AB, McCune BK, Sporn MB, TGF-beta: regulation of extracellular matrix. *Kidney Int* 1992; **41**: 557–9.

162. Davies M, Thomas GJ, Martin J et al, The purification and characterization of a glomerular-basement-membrane- degrading neutral proteinase from rat mesangial cells. *Biochem J* 1988; **251**: 419–25.

163. Marti HP, Lee L, Kashgarian M et al, Transforming growth factor-beta 1 stimulates glomerular mesangial cell synthesis of the 72-kd type IV collagenase. *Am J Pathol* 1994; **144**: 82–94.

164. Shankland SJ, Scholey JW, Ly H et al, Expression of transforming growth factor-beta 1 during diabetic renal hypertrophy. *Kidney Int* 1994; **46**: 430–42.

165. Sharma K, Ziyadeh FN, Renal hypertrophy is associated with upregulation of TGF-beta 1 gene expression in diabetic BB rat and NOD mouse. *Am J Physiol* 1994; **267**: F1094–F1101.

166. Yamamoto T, Noble NA, Cohen AH et al, Expression of transforming growth factor-beta isoforms in human glomerular diseases. *Kidney Int* 1996; **49**: 461–9.

167. Yamamoto T, Nakamura T, Noble NA et al, Expression of transforming growth factor beta is elevated in human and experimental diabetic nephropathy. *Proc Natl Acad Sci USA* 1993; **90**: 1814–18.

168. Sharma K, Ziyadeh FN, Alzahabi B et al, Increased renal production of transforming growth factor-beta 1 in patients with type II diabetes. *Diabetes* 1997; **46**: 854–9.

169. Hellmich B, Schellner M, Schatz H et al, Activation of transforming growth factor-beta1 in diabetic kidney disease. *Metabolism* 2000; **49**: 353–9.

170. Ziyadeh FN, Sharma K, Ericksen M et al, Stimulation of collagen gene expression and protein synthesis in murine mesangial cells by high glucose is mediated by autocrine activation of transforming growth factor-beta. *J Clin Invest* 1994; **93**: 536–42.

171. Ziyadeh FN, Han DC, Cohen JA et al, Glycated albumin stimulates fibronectin gene expression in glomerular mesangial cells: involvement of the transforming growth factor-beta system. *Kidney Int* 1998; **53**: 631–8.

172. Sharma K, Jin Y, Guo J et al, Neutralization of TGF-beta by anti-TGF-beta antibody attenuates kidney hypertrophy and the enhanced extracellular matrix gene expression in STZ-induced diabetic mice. *Diabetes* 1996; **45**: 522–30.

173. Ziyadeh FN, Hoffman BB, Han DC et al, Long-term prevention of renal insufficiency, excess matrix gene expression, and glomerular mesangial matrix expansion by treatment with monoclonal antitransforming growth factor-beta antibody in db/db diabetic mice. *Proc Natl Acad Sci USA* 2000; **97**: 8015–20.

174. Kagami S, Border WA, Miller DE et al, Angiotensin II stimulates extracellular matrix protein synthesis through induction of transforming growth factor-beta expression in rat glomerular mesangial cells. *J Clin Invest* 1994; **93**: 2431–7.

175. Guh JY, Yang ML, Yang YL et al, Captopril reverses high-glucose-induced growth effects on LLC-PK1 cells partly by decreasing transforming growth factor-beta receptor protein expressions. *J Am Soc Nephrol* 1996; **7**: 1207–15.

176. Hill C, Logan A, Smith C et al, Angiotensin converting enzyme inhibitor suppresses glomerular transforming growth factor beta receptor expression in experimental diabetes in rats. *Diabetologia* 2001; **44**: 495–500.

177. Sharma K, Eltayeb BO, McGowan TA et al, Captopril-induced reduction of serum levels of transforming growth factor-beta 1 correlates with long-term renoprotection in insulin-dependent diabetic patients. *Am J Kidney Dis* 1999; **34**: 818–23.

178. Studer RK, Craven PA, DeRubertis FR, Antioxidant inhibition of protein kinase C-signaled increases in transforming growth factor-beta in mesangial cells. *Metabolism* 1997; **46**: 918–25.

179. Tsuchida K, Makita Z, Yamagishi S et al, Suppression of transforming growth factor beta and vascular endothelial growth factor in diabetic nephropathy in rats by a novel advanced glycation end product inhibitor, OPB-9195. *Diabetologia* 1999; **42**: 579–88.

180. Neufeld G, Cohen T, Gengrinovitch S et al, Vascular endothelial growth factor (VEGF) and its receptors. *FASEB J* 1999; **13**: 9–22.

181. Ferrara N, Houck KA, Jakeman LB et al, The vascular endothelial growth factor family of polypeptides. *J Cell Biochem* 1991; **47**: 211–18.

182. Senger DR, Connolly DT, Van de WL et al, Purification and NH2-terminal amino acid sequence of guinea pig tumor-secreted vascular permeability factor. *Cancer Res* 1990; **50**: 1774–8.

183. Kim KJ, Li B, Winer J et al, Inhibition of vascular endothelial growth factor-induced angiogenesis suppresses tumour growth in vivo. *Nature* 1993; **362**: 841–4.

184. Carmeliet P, Ferreira V, Breier G et al, Abnormal blood vessel development and lethality in embryos lacking a single VEGF allele. *Nature* 1996; **380**: 435–9.

185. Ferrara N, Carver-Moore K, Chen H et al, Heterozygous embryonic lethality induced by targeted inactivation of the VEGF gene. *Nature* 1996; **380**: 439–42.

186. Cooper ME, Vranes D, Youssef S et al, Increased renal expression of vascular endothelial growth factor (VEGF) and its receptor VEGFR-2 in experimental diabetes. *Diabetes* 1999; **48**: 2229–39.

187. Simon M, Rockl W, Hornig C et al, Receptors of vascular endothelial growth factor/vascular permeability factor (VEGF/VPF) in fetal and adult human kidney: localization and [125I]VEGF binding sites. *J Am Soc Nephrol* 1998; **9**: 1032–44.

188. Simon M, Grone HJ, Johren O et al, Expression of vascular endothelial growth factor and its receptors in human renal ontogenesis and in adult kidney. *Am J Physiol* 1995; **268**: F240–50.

189. Gruden G, Thomas S, Burt D et al, Interaction of angiotensin II and mechanical stretch on vascular endothelial growth factor production by human mesangial cells. *J Am Soc Nephrol* 1999; **10**: 730–7.

190. Pupilli C, Lasagni L, Romagnani P et al, Angiotensin II stimulates the synthesis and secretion of vascular permeability factor/vascular endothelial growth factor in human mesangial cells. *J Am Soc Nephrol* 1999; **10**: 245–55.

191. Williams B, A potential role for angiotensin II-induced vascular endothelial growth factor expression in the pathogenesis of diabetic nephropathy? *Miner Electrolyte Metab* 1998; **24**: 400–5.

192. Williams B, Gallacher B, Patel H et al, Glucose-induced protein kinase C activation regulates vascular permeability factor mRNA expression and peptide production by human vascular smooth muscle cells in vitro. *Diabetes* 1997; **46**: 1497–503.

193. Marumo T, Schini-Kerth VB, Busse R, Vascular endothelial growth factor activates nuclear factor-kappaB and induces monocyte chemoattractant protein-1 in bovine retinal endothelial cells. *Diabetes* 1999; **48**: 1131–7.

194. Malamitsi-Puchner A, Sarandakou A, Tziotis J et al, Serum levels of basic fibroblast growth factor and vascular endothelial growth factor in children and adolescents with type 1 diabetes mellitus. *Pediatr Res* 1998; **44**: 873–5.

195. Shulman K, Rosen S, Tognazzi K et al, Expression of vascular permeability factor (VPF/VEGF) is altered in many glomerular diseases. *J Am Soc Nephrol* 1996; **7**: 661–6.

196. Vriese AS, Tilton RG, Elger M et al, Antibodies against vascular

endothelial growth factor improve early renal dysfunction in experimental diabetes. *J Am Soc Nephrol* 2001; **12**: 993–1000.

197. Flyvbjerg A, Dagnaes-Hansen F, De Vriese AS et al, Amelioration of long-term renal changes by administration of a neutralizing VEGF-ab in obese type 2 diabetic mice. *Diabetes* 2002; **51**: 3090–4.

198. Shin SJ, Lee YJ, Lin SR et al, Decrease of renal endothelin 1 content and gene expression in diabetic rats with moderate hyperglycemia. *Nephron* 1995; **70**: 486–93.

199. Mene P, Simonson MS, Dunn MJ, Phospholipids in signal transduction of mesangial cells. *Am J Physiol* 1989; **256**: F375–86.

200. Taubman MB, Berk BC, Izumo S et al, Angiotensin II induces c-fos mRNA in aortic smooth muscle. Role of $Ca^{2+}$ mobilization and protein kinase C activation. *J Biol Chem* 1989; **264**: 526–30.

201. Simonson MS, Wann S, Mene P et al, Endothelin stimulates phospholipase C, $Na^+/H^+$ exchange, c-fos expression, and mitogenesis in rat mesangial cells. *J Clin Invest* 1989; **83**: 708–12.

202. Dinh DT, Frauman AG, Johnston CI et al, Angiotensin receptors: distribution, signalling and function. *Clin Sci (Colch)* 2001; **100**: 481–92.

203. Lai KN, Leung JC, Lai KB et al, Gene expression of the renin-angiotensin system in human kidney. *J Hypertens* 1998; **16**: 91–102.

204. Wolf G, Ziyadeh FN, The role of angiotensin II in diabetic nephropathy: emphasis on nonhemodynamic mechanisms. *Am J Kidney Dis* 1997; **29**: 153–63.

205. Leehey DJ, Singh AK, Alavi N et al, Role of angiotensin II in diabetic nephropathy. *Kidney Int* 2000; **58** (Suppl 77): S93–8.

206. Sasamura H, Hein L, Krieger JE et al, Cloning, characterization, and expression of two angiotensin receptor (AT-1) isoforms from the mouse genome. *Biochem Biophys Res Commun* 1992; **185**: 253–9.

207. Burns KD, Angiotensin II and its receptors in the diabetic kidney. *Am J Kidney Dis* 2000; **36**: 449–67.

208. Siragy HM, Carey RM, The subtype-2 (AT2) angiotensin receptor regulates renal cyclic guanosine 3', 5'-monophosphate and AT1 receptor-mediated prostaglandin $E_2$ production in conscious rats. *J Clin Invest* 1996; **97**: 1978–82.

209. Siragy HM, Carey RM, The subtype 2 (AT2) angiotensin receptor mediates renal production of nitric oxide in conscious rats. *J Clin Invest* 1997; **100**: 264–9.

210. Siragy HM, Carey RM, The subtype 2 angiotensin receptor regulates renal prostaglandin $F_2$ alpha formation in conscious rats. *Am J Physiol* 1997; **273**: R1103–7.

211. Meffert S, Stoll M, Steckelings UM et al, The angiotensin II AT2 receptor inhibits proliferation and promotes differentiation in PC12W cells. *Mol Cell Endocrinol* 1996; **122**: 59–67.

212. Cao Z, Kelly DJ, Cox A et al, Angiotensin type 2 receptor is expressed in the adult rat kidney and promotes cellular proliferation and apoptosis. *Kidney Int* 2000; **58**: 2437–51.

213. Yamada T, Akishita M, Pollman MJ et al, Angiotensin II type 2 receptor mediates vascular smooth muscle cell apoptosis and antagonizes angiotensin II type 1 receptor action: an in vitro gene transfer study. *Life Sci* 1998; **63**: L289–95.

214. Stroth U, Meffert S, Gallinat S et al, Angiotensin II and NGF differentially influence microtubule proteins in PC12W cells: role of the AT2 receptor. *Brain Res Mol Brain Res* 1998; **53**: 187–95.

215. Laflamme L, Gasparo M, Gallo JM et al, Angiotensin II induction of neurite outgrowth by AT2 receptors in NG108-15 cells. Effect counteracted by the AT1 receptors. *J Biol Chem* 1996; **271**: 22729–35.

216. Cote F, Laflamme L, Payet MD et al, Nitric oxide, a new second messenger involved in the action of angiotensin II on neuronal differentiation of NG108-15 cells. *Endocr Res* 1998; **24**: 403–7.

217. Csikos T, Chung O, Unger T, Receptors and their classification:

focus on angiotensin II and the AT2 receptor. *J Hum Hypertens* 1998; **12**: 311–18.

218. Siragy HM, AT(1) and AT(2) receptors in the kidney: role in disease and treatment. *Am J Kidney Dis* 2000; **36**: S4–S9.

219. Wright JW, Harding JW, Important role for angiotensin III and IV in the brain renin-angiotensin system. *Brain Res Brain Res Rev* 1997; **25**: 96–124.

220. Chaki S, Inagami T, Identification and characterization of a new binding site for angiotensin II in mouse neuroblastoma neuro-2A cells. *Biochem Biophys Res Commun* 1992; **182**: 388–94.

221. Zimpelmann J, Kumar D, Levine DZ et al, Early diabetes mellitus stimulates proximal tubule renin mRNA expression in the rat. *Kidney Int* 2000; **58**: 2320–30.

222. Kelly DJ, Skinner SL, Gilbert RE et al, Effects of endothelin or angiotensin II receptor blockade on diabetes in the transgenic (mRen-2)27 rat. *Kidney Int* 2000; **57**: 1882–94.

223. Wehbi GJ, Zimpelmann J, Carey RM et al, Early streptozotocin-diabetes mellitus downregulates rat kidney AT2 receptors. *Am J Physiol Renal Physiol* 2001; **280**: F254–65.

224. Zhang SL, To C, Chen X et al, Effect of renin-angiotensin system blockade on the expression of the angiotensinogen gene and induction of hypertrophy in rat kidney proximal tubular cells. *Exp Nephrol* 2001; **9**: 109–17.

225. Force T, Kyriakis JM, Avruch J et al, vasopressin, and angiotensin II enhance tyrosine phosphorylation by protein kinase C-dependent and -independent pathways in glomerular mesangial cells. *J Biol Chem* 1991; **266**: 6650–6.

226. Ikeda M, Kohno M, Takeda T, Endothelin production in cultured mesangial cells of spontaneously hypertensive rats. *Hypertension* 1995; **25**: 1196–201.

227. Bakris GL, Re RN, Endothelin modulates angiotensin II-induced mitogenesis of human mesangial cells. *Am J Physiol* 1993; **264**: F937–42.

228. Osterby R, Bangstad HJ, Rudberg S, Follow-up study of glomerular dimensions and cortical interstitium in microalbuminuric type 1 diabetic patients with or without antihypertensive treatment. *Nephrol Dial Transplant* 2000; **15**: 1609–16.

229. Rudberg S, Rasmussen LM, Bangstad HJ et al, Influence of insertion/deletion polymorphism in the ACE-I gene on the progression of diabetic glomerulopathy in type 1 diabetic patients with microalbuminuria. *Diabetes Care* 2000; **23**: 544–8.

230. Remuzzi G, Ruggenenti P, Benigni A, Understanding the nature of renal disease progression. *Kidney Int* 1997; **51**: 2–15.

231. Andersen S, Tarnow L, Rossing P et al, Renoprotective effects of angiotensin II receptor blockade in type 1 diabetic patients with diabetic nephropathy. *Kidney Int* 2000; **57**: 601–6.

232. Lacourciere Y, Belanger A, Godin C et al, Long-term comparison of losartan and enalapril on kidney function in hypertensive type 2 diabetics with early nephropathy. *Kidney Int* 2000; **58**: 762–9.

233. Ruggenenti P, Remuzzi G, Angiotensin-converting enzyme inhibitor therapy for non-diabetic progressive renal disease. *Curr Opin Nephrol Hypertens* 1997; **6**: 489–95.

234. Osei SY, Price DA, Laffel LM et al, Effect of angiotensin II antagonist eprosartan on hyperglycemia-induced activation of intrarenal renin-angiotensin system in healthy humans. *Hypertension* 2000; **36**: 122–6.

235. Lansang MC, Osei SY, Price DA et al, Renal hemodynamic and hormonal responses to the angiotensin II antagonist candesartan. *Hypertension* 2000; **36**: 834–8.

236. Yanagisawa M, Kurihara H, Kimura S et al, A novel potent vasoconstrictor peptide produced by vascular endothelial cells. *Nature* 1988; **332**: 411–15.

237. Inoue A, Yanagisawa M, Kimura S et al, The human endothelin family: three structurally and pharmacologically distinct isopeptides predicted by three separate genes. *Proc Natl Acad Sci USA* 1989; **86**: 2863–7.

238. Sakurai T, Yanagisawa M, Masaki T, Molecular characterization of endothelin receptors. *Trends Pharmacol Sci* 1992; **13**: 103–8.

239. Adachi M, Yang YY, Furuichi Y et al, Cloning and characterization of cDNA encoding human A-type endothelin receptor. *Biochem Biophys Res Commun* 1991; **180**: 1265–72.

240. Arai H, Hori S, Aramori I et al, Cloning and expression of a cDNA encoding an endothelin receptor. *Nature* 1990; **348**: 730–2.

241. Lin HY, Kaji EH, Winkel GK et al, Cloning and functional expression of a vascular smooth muscle endothelin 1 receptor. *Proc Natl Acad Sci USA* 1991; **88**: 3185–9.

242. Sakurai T, Yanagisawa M, Takuwa Y et al, Cloning of a cDNA encoding a non-isopeptide-selective subtype of the endothelin receptor. *Nature* 1990; **348**: 732–5.

243. Ohlstein EH, Arleth A, Bryan H et al, The selective endothelin ETA receptor antagonist BQ123 antagonizes endothelin-1-mediated mitogenesis. *Eur J Pharmacol* 1992; **225**: 347–50.

244. Simonson MS, Endothelin peptides and compensatory growth of renal cells. *Curr Opin Nephrol Hypertens* 1994; **3**: 73–85.

245. Benigni A, Remuzzi G, Endothelin receptor antagonists: which are the therapeutic perspectives in renal diseases? *Nephrol Dial Transplant* 1998; **13**: 5–7.

246. Kedzierski RM, Yanagisawa M, Endothelin system: the double-edged sword in health and disease. *Annu Rev Pharmacol Toxicol* 2001; **41**: 851–76.

247. Zoja C, Orisio S, Perico N et al, Constitutive expression of endothelin gene in cultured human mesangial cells and its modulation by transforming growth factor-beta, thrombin, and a thromboxane A2 analogue. *Lab Invest* 1991; **64**: 16–20.

248. Kohan DE, Production of endothelin-1 by rat mesangial cells: regulation by tumor necrosis factor. *J Lab Clin Med* 1992; **119**: 477–84.

249. Kasinath BS, Fried TA, Davalath S et al, Glomerular epithelial cells synthesize endothelin peptides. *Am J Pathol* 1992; **141**: 279–83.

250. Kitamura K, Tanaka T, Kato J et al, Regional distribution of immunoreactive endothelin in porcine tissue: abundance in inner medulla of kidney. *Biochem Biophys Res Commun* 1989; **161**: 348–52.

251. Uchida S, Takemoto F, Ogata E et al, Detection of endothelin-1 mRNA by RT-PCR in isolated rat renal tubules. *Biochem Biophys Res Commun* 1992; **188**: 108–13.

252. Sakamoto H, Sasaki S, Nakamura Y et al, Regulation of endothelin-1 production in cultured rat mesangial cells. *Kidney Int* 1992; **41**: 350–5.

253. Marsden PA, Dorfman DM, Collins T et al, Regulated expression of endothelin 1 in glomerular capillary endothelial cells. *Am J Physiol* 1991; **261**: F117–25.

254. Simonson MS, Wang Y, Dunn MJ, Cellular signaling by endothelin peptides: pathways to the nucleus. *J Am Soc Nephrol* 1992; **2**: S116–25.

255. Terada Y, Tomita K, Nonoguchi H et al, Expression of endothelin-3 mRNA along rat nephron segments using polymerase chain reaction. *Kidney Int* 1993; **44**: 1273–80.

256. Fukui M, Nakamura T, Ebihara I et al, Gene expression for endothelins and their receptors in glomeruli of diabetic rats. *J Lab Clin Med* 1993; **122**: 149–56.

257. Benigni A, Perico N, Remuzzi G, Endothelin antagonists and renal protection. *J Cardiovasc Pharmacol* 2000; **35**: S75–8.

258. Yamauchi T, Ohnaka K, Takayanagi R et al, Enhanced secretion of endothelin-1 by elevated glucose levels from cultured bovine aortic endothelial cells. *FEBS Lett* 1990; **267**: 16–18.

259. Hocher B, Thone-Reineke C, Bauer C et al, The paracrine endothelin system: pathophysiology and implications in clinical medicine. *Eur J Clin Chem Clin Biochem* 1997; **35**: 175–89.

260. Hocher B, Lun A, Priem F et al, Renal endothelin system in diabetes: comparison of angiotensin- converting enzyme inhibition and endothelin-A antagonism. *J Cardiovasc Pharmacol* 1998; **31** (Suppl 1): S492–5.

261. Takahashi K, Suda K, Lam HC et al, Endothelin-like immunoreactivity in rat models of diabetes mellitus. *J Endocrinol* 1991; **130:** 123–7.

262. Neri S, Bruno CM, Leotta C et al, Early endothelial alterations in non-insulin-dependent diabetes mellitus. *Int J Clin Lab Res* 1998; **28:** 100–3.

263. Nakamura T, Ebihara I, Fukui M et al, Effect of a specific endothelin receptor A antagonist on mRNA levels for extracellular matrix components and growth factors in diabetic glomeruli. *Diabetes* 1995; **44:** 895–9.

264. Hu RM, Levin ER, Pedram A et al, Insulin stimulates production and secretion of endothelin from bovine endothelial cells. *Diabetes* 1993; **42:** 351–8.

265. Awazu M, Parker RE, Harvie BR et al, Down-regulation of endothelin-1 receptors by protein kinase C in streptozotocin diabetic rats. *J Cardiovasc Pharmacol* 1991; **17** (Suppl 7): S500–2.

266. Liefeldt L, Bocker W, Schonfelder G et al, Regulation of the endothelin system in transgenic rats expressing the human endothelin-2 gene. *J Cardiovasc Pharmacol* 1995; **26** (Suppl 3): S32–3.

267. Hocher B, Thone-Reineke C, Rohmeiss P et al, Endothelin-1 transgenic mice develop glomerulosclerosis, interstitial fibrosis, and renal cysts but not hypertension. *J Clin Invest* 1997; **99:** 1380–9.

268. Hocher B, Liefeldt L, Thone-Reineke C et al, Characterization of the renal phenotype of transgenic rats expressing the human endothelin-2 gene. *Hypertension* 1996; **28:** 196–201.

269. Benigni A, Zoja C, Corna D et al, A specific endothelin subtype A receptor antagonist protects against injury in renal disease progression. *Kidney Int* 1993; **44:** 440–4.

270. Benigni A, Colosio V, Brena C et al, Unselective inhibition of endothelin receptors reduces renal dysfunction in experimental diabetes. *Diabetes* 1998; **47:** 450–6.

271. Cameron NE, Dines KC, Cotter MA, The potential contribution of endothelin-1 to neurovascular abnormalities in streptozotocin-diabetic rats. *Diabetologia* 1994; **37:** 1209–15.

272. Dhein S, Hochreuther S, Aus Dem SC et al, Long-term effects of the endothelin(A) receptor antagonist LU 135252 and the angiotensin-converting enzyme inhibitor trandolapril on diabetic angiopathy and nephropathy in a chronic type I diabetes mellitus rat model. *J Pharmacol Exp Ther* 2000; **293:** 351–9.

273. Benigni A, Corna D, Maffi R et al, Renoprotective effect of contemporary blocking of angiotensin II and endothelin-1 in rats with membranous nephropathy. *Kidney Int* 1998; **54:** 353–9.

274. Benigni A, Remuzzi G, How renal cytokines and growth factors contribute to renal disease progression. *Am J Kidney Dis* 2001; **37:** S21–4.

275. Nakamura T, Ebihara I, Tomino Y et al, Alteration of growth-related proto-oncogene expression in diabetic glomeruli by a specific endothelin receptor A antagonist. *Nephrol Dial Transplant* 1996; **11:** 1528–31.

276. Groop P, Lipidaemia and diabetic renal disease. In: *The Kidney and Hypertension in Diabetes Mellitus* (Mogensen CE, ed.). Boston: Kluwer, 1998; 357–69.

277. Sawicki PT, Smoking and diabetic nephropathy. In: *The Kidney and Hypertension in Diabetes Mellitus* (Mogensen CE, ed.). Boston: Kluwer, 1998; 209–16.

278. Orth SR, Smoking—a renal risk factor. *Nephron* 2000; **86:** 12–26.

# II

## Therapeutic measures in patients with diabetic nephropathy

# 6

# Treatment of diabetic nephropathy: the role of strict glucose control

Stephen Thomas, Mike Krimholtz and GianCarlo Viberti

## INTRODUCTION

Epidemiologically, the development of all stages of diabetic nephropathy is related to the degree of glycaemic control (Figure 6.1).[1,2] The importance of strict glycaemic control in preventing diabetic nephropathy has been confirmed by large clinical trials in both type 1 and type 2 diabetes.[3,4] In the Diabetes Control and Complications Trial (DCCT) in type 1 diabetes, a reduction in HbA1c to a mean of 7.2% reduced the risk of developing microalbuminuria by 34%, as compared to conventional therapy with a mean HbA1c of 9%.[3] This benefit was maintained for up to 4 years even once the difference in glycaemic control between the groups had waned.[5]

Similarly, the UK Prospective Diabetes Study of type 2 diabetes reported a 34% reduction in the risk of developing proteinuria in the intensively treated group (mean HbA1c of 7%), as compared with the conventionally treated group (mean HbA1c of 7.9%).[4]

The benefits of strict glycaemic control in the management of patients who already have nephropathy are less clear. There is considerable evidence that other factors, such as rising blood pressure, may then drive the progression. This has led to the concept of a 'metabolic point of no return'. It is true, however, that diabetic nephropathy progresses towards end-stage renal failure in the majority of patients despite good blood-pressure control, albeit at a much slower rate, suggesting that many factors may operate in driving the kidney damage. In this review, we will confine ourselves to whether we can affect the course of the kidney complication by attention to glycaemic control.

We will examine the role of glycaemic control from the early functional changes of hyperfiltration and renal enlargement, the effect on urinary albumin excretion (UAE) and the decline in the glomerular filtration rate (GFR), and renal structural damage.

## EFFECT OF IMPROVED GLYCAEMIC CONTROL ON HYPERFILTRATION AND RENAL ENLARGEMENT

Patients with type 1 diabetes have a GFR on average 20–40% above that of age-matched normal subjects,[6] and many have a GFR above the limit of the age- and sex-adjusted normal range.[7] A phase of hyperfiltration also occurs in type 2 diabetes.[8]

Hyperfiltration is related to blood-glucose control, and an acute rise in GFR occurs as blood glucose rises to around 14 mmol/l (240 mg/dl).[9] At higher blood-glucose values, the GFR tends to be normal or low. This hyperfiltration is reversible with intensified insulin treatment and good metabolic control within weeks to months in both type 1 and type 2 diabetes.[10,11]

The relationship of kidney size to glycaemic control is less clear than that of the GFR, and some conflicting results are seen. Overall, there is evidence that increased kidney size may be reversible in newly diagnosed patients with both type 1 and type 2 diabetes by intensive insulin therapy for up to 3 months.[12,13] The situation may be less reversible in patients with longer-term diabetes. In one study of patients with type 1 diabetes, intensified insulin treatment for 1 year had no effect on kidney size despite a reduction in GFR.[10] However, other studies differ from this conclusion.[14] This phenomenon is also seen in animal models of diabetes where kidney enlargement is reversed only if insulin treatment is started soon after induction of diabetes.[15] After a month of hyperglycaemia, renal enlargement seems to be irreversible in the diabetic animal.[16] This suggests that there may be differing mechanisms which underlie the initial renal enlargement, possibly significant renal hyperplasia and an increase in kidney fluid, and that these mechanisms may be more sensitive to normalization of the metabolic environment. The significance of the later stages of renal hypertrophy that are not responsive to glycaemic control remains unclear.

## EFFECT OF IMPROVED GLYCAEMIC CONTROL ON UAE

Overall, studies in the phase of microalbuminuria (UAE of 20–200 μg/min) suggest a benefit in terms of retardation rather than absolute prevention of progression to overt diabetic nephropathy.

### Can improved glycaemic control reverse increased UAE?

Early increases in UAE are promptly reversible by improved glycaemic control and are likely to be functional.[17,18] In longer-term studies, there are somewhat conflicting results, although the majority suggest that improved glycaemic control is associated with a reduction in UAE.

In the prospective, controlled Kroc collaborative study of continuous subcutaneous insulin infusion (CSII) treatment, 20 of the patients had microalbuminuria (mean UAE of 193 μg/min) at baseline and 39 had normal UAE (mean of 13 μg/min). CSII improved glycaemic control, with mean HbA1 levels of 8.1% compared to a mean of 10% in a conventionally treated group. Mean UAE fell significantly in the CSII group by 4 months, persisting for at least 8 months in those patients with microalbuminuria, although there was no change in those with normal UAE.[19] Similarly, in another study of 45 patients with type 1 diabetes, UAE was significantly reduced in patients using CSII, as compared to conventional control, an effect, which was sustained for up to 8 years. Similarly, in the DCCT, where the majority had normal UAE, intensive treatment decreased UAE by 15% after the first year of therapy (6.5 vs 7.7 μg/min).[3]

In contrast, in a 12-month Steno study of CSII in 36 patients with type 1 diabetes and microalbuminuria, there was no significant change in UAE despite a fall in the HbA1c from 9.5% to 7.3%.[20] One possible confounding issue in this study was a rise in the mean arterial pressure (MAP) from 98 to 101 mmHg in the CSII group.

## Can improved glycaemic control retard progression from microalbuminuria to overt diabetic nephropathy?

Several studies have investigated whether tight glycaemic control affects the progression to overt diabetic nephropathy (UAE >200 μg/min, the phase at which the GFR starts to fall below the normal range.

In the Steno study described, although no fall in UAE was seen, delayed progression was demonstrated in the group treated with CSII, overt diabetic nephropathy developing in five patients in the conventional-treatment group, but none in the CSII group.[21]

However, neither of the largest studies done to date with a combined total of 143 patients has demonstrated any benefit of tight glycaemic control in the prevention of progression to overt diabetic nephropathy.[3,22] One study randomized 70 patients to intensive or conventional glycaemic control for around 5 years[22] with a 1.4% fall in HbA1c in the intensive therapy group. Six patients progressed to 'overt' nephropathy in each group. Interestingly, even in this study of glycaemic control, a MAP above 93.6 mmHg predicted progression to clinical albuminuria, whereas HbA1c did not. By modern standards, MAP was rather high in this study, a feature which may have confounded the results.

Similarly, in 73 subjects in the DCCT secondary

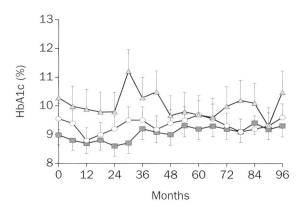

**Figure 6.1** Seven year prospective study of patients with type 1 diabetes and normal AER at baseline. Those who develop microalbuminuria have higher HbA1c prior to the development of microalbuminuria than those who remain normoalbuminuric (2) (modified).
▲, Those who develop persistent microalbuminuria;
○, Those who develop intermittent microalbuminuria;
■, Those who remain normoalbuminuric.

cohort, with UAE between 28 and 139 µg/min at baseline, intensive treatment did not reduce progression to overt nephropathy as occurred in eight intensively treated and eight conventionally treated patients.[3]

Conversely, a meta-analysis of 16 randomized trials analysed the effects of intensive blood-glucose control on either nephropathy or retinopathy, or both in type 1 diabetes. The risk of progression of UAE was significantly reduced by intensive therapy compared to conventional treatment (odds ratio 0.34 CI 0.25–0.58). Interestingly, the benefits of intensive treatment appeared to be clearer in terms of nephropathy progression than retinopathy progression, although this may relate to the accuracy of the definition.[23]

There are even fewer data in type 2 diabetes, although one study based in Japan randomized 110 patients with type 2 diabetes, and 55 with retinopathy and microalbuminuria to receive either multiple injection therapy (MIT) or conventional insulin (CIT) over a 6-year period. The cumulative percentage of the progression of nephropathy in the MIT group was 11.5%, as compared with 32.0% in the CIT group.[24]

The main drawback to all these studies is the sample size. It has been calculated that for 80% power to demonstrate a 50% reduction in the progression from microalbuminuria to albuminuria, 206 subjects would be required in each group.[25] Furthermore, many of these studies were conducted in the face of suboptimal and changing blood-pressure control by modern

standards. Nevertheless, it may be permissible to conclude that there is an effect of intensified glycaemic control on the risk of progression to overt nephropathy, but it is likely to be modest when compared to other factors such as blood-pressure treatment.

## CAN IMPROVED GLYCAEMIC CONTROL AFFECT THE DECLINE IN GFR?

The effect of glycaemic control on the rate of decline of renal function is also controversial. Observational data show that worse glycaemic control is associated with a faster rate of GFR decline, but interventional data demonstrating that improvement of glycaemic control reduces the rate of kidney function loss are relatively lacking. In the phase of microalbuminuria when the GFR tends to be in the normal range but may still be declining, there is evidence that good glycaemic control may arrest the fall in GFR. In a combined analysis of the two Steno studies of CSII treatment in type 1 diabetes, data on 69 of the 70 patients were analysed after 5–8 years of follow-up. CSII treatment resulted in around a 2% improvement in HbA1c. The annual change in GFR was −0.1 ml/min per 1.73 m² in the CSII group and −3.7 ml/min per 1.73 m² in the conventionally treated group.[26]

At the later stage of overt diabetic nephropathy, there is much conflicting evidence. In the late 1980s, Nyberg et al prospectively followed 18 patients with type 1 diabetes and diabetic nephropathy for 21 months.[27] There was a direct relationship between the fall in GFR and the HbA1c, with the greatest fall in GFR occurring in those with highest HbA1c. The mean supine blood pressure was 154/88 mmHg, and differences in HbA1c explained one-third of the loss of GFR. In contrast, in a prospective study of 115 patients with diabetes and renal impairment—50 with type 1 diabetes and 65 with type 2 diabetes—no relationship between HbA1c and fall in creatinine clearance was seen over a 7-year period.[28] Similarly, a London cohort also failed to demonstrate any relationship between HbA1 and fall in GFR. Twenty-four patients were followed for an average of 43 months, blood pressure being the main determinant of the rate of decline of GFR.[29] However, in a later analysis of the same but enlarged London cohort of 54 patients, there was a linear relationship between higher HbA1c and faster rate of fall of GFR over a mean follow-up of 7 years[30] (Figure 6.2). Similarly, in a retrospective analysis of 158 patients with type 1 diabetes and overt nephropathy, the rate of fall of GFR over a median of 8 years was related to both blood pressure and HbA1c.[31] The cohort had a mean

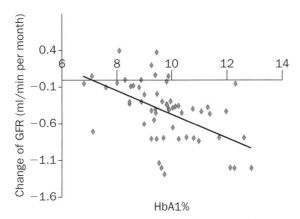

**Figure 6.2** Relationship between glycaemic control (HbA1) and rate of fall of GFR over 7 years in 54 patients with type 1 diabetes and renal failure. Adapted from *Nephrology, Dialysis, Transplantation* with permission.[30]

blood pressure of 143/82 and a mean rate of fall of GFR of 3.8 ml/min per year. In contrast, the rate of fall of GFR in patients with HbA1c of <8% and diastolic blood pressure of <85 mmHg was around 1.7 ml min per year.

One likely explanation for the contradictory findings in the different cohorts is differences in blood-pressure control. In the London cohort, there were significantly lower blood pressures in the late 1990s, a mean MAP of 96 mmHg, as compared to 106 mmHg in the 1980s, reflecting better understanding of appropriate blood-pressure treatment targets and maybe better therapeutic strategies.

Thus, the association between worse glycaemic control and faster loss of GFR is more discernible on a background of improved blood-pressure control, as the powerful association between raised blood pressure and the rate of GFR decline may mask the less powerful association with blood-glucose control.

There are relatively few studies examining the effects of glycaemic control in patients with type 2 diabetes, although two prospective studies have found that poor glycaemic control was associated with a faster fall of GFR.[32,33] Other studies, however, did not find any relationship between the two.[34,35]

Overall, the epidemiological data seem to support an association between worse glycaemic control and faster rate of fall of GFR, albeit a weaker relationship than exists between arterial pressure and fall of GFR.

To date, there is a paucity of randomized controlled intervention studies (category 1 data) to determine conclusively the benefits of improved glycaemic control.

In small self-controlled or parallel-group studies of CSII treatment in overt nephropathy, there was no discernible effect on the rate of fall of GFR. In type 1 diabetes, the longest study to date studied six patients with clinical proteinuria and established retinopathy on CSII, as compared with six patients on conventional treatment for up to 24 months.[36] Despite a significant improvement of glycaemic control, there was no change in either the rise in serum creatinine or the fall of GFR, although in one individual a considerable slowing of the rate of loss of kidney function was noted.

It is remarkable that no large trial of intensive therapy has ever been carried out in overt nephropathy, whether in type 1 or type 2 diabetes. Two possible reasons for this are the highly significant retarding effect and relative 'ease' of antihypertensive therapy and the complexity of delivering tight glycaemic control, and the increased risk of hypoglycaemia even with CSII regimens.[37]

## EFFECT OF GLYCAEMIC CONTROL ON STRUCTURAL KIDNEY DAMAGE

A number of small renal biopsy studies have provided information on the benefits of glycaemic control on renal structure. In a 2–3-year study of patients with type 1 diabetes and microalbuminuria, patients were randomized either to intensive treatment by CSII or to conventional therapy, with a resultant fall in HbA1c and overall lower HbA1c in the CSII group. Although basement membrane thickness increased in both groups, it increased most in those on conventional therapy. Similarly, mesangial matrix volume fraction and matrix star volume increased only in those on conventional therapy.[38] This suggests that stabilization of the structural lesion is possible at the stage of microalbuminuria by intensification of glycaemic control.

With the normalization of glycaemic control seen in solitary pancreas transplantation, regression of disease may be seen, at least in those patients with microalbuminuria or normal AER. Structural regression is not seen after 5 years,[39] but by 10 years there is regression of glomerular and tubular basement membrane thickening and reduction of mesangial fractional volume, mostly because of a reduction in mesangial matrix (Figure 6.3).[40] These changes were associated with a fall in the median UAE from 103 mg/day at baseline to 30 mg/day after 5 years and 20 mg/day after 10 years. There was also a fall in the mean creatinine clearance from 108 ml/min

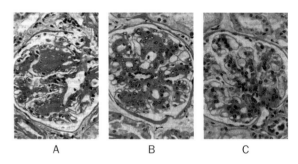

A       B       C

**Figure 6.3** Reversal of diabetic nephropathy after pancreas transplantation. Sequential renal biopsies (periodic acid-Schiff, ×120) from a patient who received a solitary pancreas transplant section are shown. A: Before the transplant, biopsy shows marked mesangial matrix expansion, B: 5 years after transplant, biopsy shows still considerable mesangial expansion; C: 10 years after transplant, biopsy shows marked regression of mesangial matrix. Adapted from *New England Journal of Medicine* with permission.[40]

per 1.73 m² at baseline to 74 ml/min per 1.73 m² at 5 years, and this value was stable thereafter. However, some of these changes may be multifactorial and related to other factors in the transplant regimen such as immunosuppression.

## EFFECT OF IMPROVED GLYCAEMIC CONTROL IN PATIENTS WITH END-STAGE RENAL FAILURE

Clearly, at this stage of disease, the benefits or not of good glycaemic control must be assessed in the context of the non-renal complications. In a retrospective analysis, good glycaemic control in the 6 months prior to starting dialysis was associated with significantly increased 1-year, 3-year and 5-year survival rates. There have also been at least two prospective studies, one in continuous ambulatory peritoneal dialysis (CAPD) and one in haemodialysis (HD), suggesting that better predialysis glycaemic control was associated with less hospitalization and longer survival on dialysis.[41,42]

In one prospective observational study of 150 patients with diabetes on HD in Japan, cumulative survival was lower in those whose HbA1c was over 7.5% before starting HD as compared to those with HbA1c under 7.5%.[43]

However, one of the complications of intensification of glycaemic control in this group of patients is difficulty in the assessment of glycaemic control and increased dangers of hypoglycaemia;[44] again, interventional studies to assess the benefits of intensified control are required.

## SUMMARY

There is no doubt that intensification of glycaemic control is an effective primary prevention strategy that reduces the risk of diabetic nephropathy in both type 1 and type 2 diabetes by around one-third.

Robust interventional data are lacking at all stages of established diabetic nephropathy, and what studies there are lack power to detect a modest but significant clinical effect.

In particular, older studies may be hampered by the overpowering effect of higher blood pressures, muting the benefits of better glycaemic control. Whether a properly powered randomized trial will ever be performed to determine the effect of intensification of control in diabetic nephropathy remains to be seen. Presently, it seems reasonable to conclude that there is likely to be added renal benefit from improved gly-

caemic control as part of a multifactorial approach of blood-pressure reduction and lipid-lowering therapy, as is now being advocated in several studies.[45,46]

## REFERENCES

1. Mattock MB, Barnes DJ, Viberti G et al, Microalbuminuria and coronary heart disease in NIDDM: an incidence study, *Diabetes* (1998) **47:** 1786–92.
2. Predictors of the development of microalbuminuria in patients with Type 1 diabetes mellitus: a seven-year prospective study. The Microalbuminuria Collaborative Study Group. *Diabet Med* (1999) **16:** 918–25.
3. Effect of intensive therapy on the development and progression of diabetic nephropathy in the Diabetes Control and Complications Trial. The Diabetes Control and Complications (DCCT) Research Group, *Kidney Int* (1995) **47:** 1703–20.
4. UK Prospective Diabetes Study (UKPDS) Group. Intensive blood-glucose control with sulphonylureas or insulin compared with conventional treatment and risk of complications in patients with type 2 diabetes (UKPDS 33). UK Prospective Diabetes Study (UKPDS) Group, *Lancet* (1998) **352:** 837–53.
5. Retinopathy and nephropathy in patients with type 1 diabetes four years after a trial of intensive therapy. Diabetes Control and Complications Trial/Epidemiology of Diabetes Interventions and Complications Research Group. *N Engl J Med* (2000) **342:** 381–9.
6. Mogensen CE, Glomerular filtration rate and renal plasma flow in short-term and long-term juvenile diabetes mellitus, *Scand J Clin Lab Invest* (1971) **28:** 91–100.
7. Cotroneo P, Manto A, Todaro L et al, Hyperfiltration in patients with type I diabetes mellitus: a prevalence study, *Clin Nephrol* (1998) **50:** 214–17.
8. Marre M, Hallab M, Roy J, Glomerular hyperfiltration in type I, type II, and secondary diabetes, *J Diabetes Complications* (1992) **6:** 19–24.
9. Wiseman MJ, Viberti GC, Keen H, Threshold effect of plasma glucose in the glomerular hyperfiltration of diabetes, *Nephron* (1984) **38:** 257–60.
10. Wiseman MJ, Saunders AJ, Keen H et al, Effect of blood glucose control on increased glomerular filtration rate and kidney size in insulin-dependent diabetes, *N Engl J Med* (1985) **312:** 617–621.
11. Vora JP, Dolben J, Williams JD et al, Impact of initial treatment on renal function in newly-diagnosed type 2 (non-insulin-dependent) diabetes mellitus. *Diabetologia* (1993) **36:** 734–40.
12. Tuttle KR, Bruton JL, Perusek MC et al, Effect of strict glycemic control on renal hemodynamic response to amino acids and renal enlargement in insulin-dependent diabetes mellitus, *N Engl J Med* (1991) **324:** 1626–32.
13. Mogensen CE, Andersen MJ, Increased kidney size and glomerular filtration rate in untreated juvenile diabetes: normalization by insulin-treatment, *Diabetologia* (1975) **11:** 221–4.
14. Feldt-Rasmussen B, Hegedus L, Mathiesen ER et al, Kidney volume in type 1 (insulin-dependent) diabetic patients with normal or increased urinary albumin excretion: effect of long-term improved metabolic control, *Scand J Clin Lab Invest* (1991) **51:** 31–6.
15. Rasch R, Prevention of diabetic glomerulopathy in streptozotocin diabetic rats by insulin treatment. Kidney size and glomerular volume, *Diabetologia* (1979) **16:** 125–8.
16. Seyer-Hansen K, Renal hypertrophy in streptozotocin-diabetic rats, *Clin Sci Mol Med Suppl* (1976) **51:** 551–5.

17. Viberti G, Pickup JC, Bilous RW et al, Correction of exercise-induced microalbuminuria in insulin-dependent diabetics after 3 weeks of subcutaneous insulin infusion, *Diabetes* (1981) **30:** 818–23.

18. Viberti GC, Pickup JC, Jarrett RJ et al, Effect of control of blood glucose on urinary excretion of albumin and beta2 microglobulin in insulin-dependent diabetes, *N Engl J Med* (1979) **300:** 638–41.

19. Bending JJ, Viberti GC, Bilous RW et al, Eight-month correction of hyperglycemia in insulin-dependent diabetes mellitus is associated with a significant and sustained reduction of urinary albumin excretion rates in patients with microalbuminuria, *Diabetes* (1985) **34** (Suppl 3): 69–73.

20. Feldt-Rasmussen B, Mathiesen ER, Hegedus L et al, Kidney function during 12 months of strict metabolic control in insulin-dependent diabetic patients with incipient nephropathy, *N Engl J Med* (1986) **314:** 665–70.

21. Feldt-Rasmussen B, Mathiesen ER, Deckert T, Effect of two years of strict metabolic control on progression of incipient nephropathy in insulin-dependent diabetes, *Lancet* (1986) **2:** 1300–4.

22. Intensive therapy and progression to clinical albuminuria in patients with insulin dependent diabetes mellitus and microalbuminuria. Microalbuminuria Collaborative Study Group, United Kingdom, *BMJ* (1995) **311:** 973–7.

23. Wang PH, Lau J, Chalmers TC, Meta-analysis of effects of intensive blood-glucose control on late complications of type I diabetes, *Lancet* (1993) **341:** 1306–9.

24. Ohkubo Y, Kishikawa H, Araki E et al, Intensive insulin therapy prevents the progression of diabetic microvascular complications in Japanese patients with non-insulin-dependent diabetes mellitus: a randomized prospective 6-year study, *Diabetes Res Clin Pract* (1995) **28:** 103–17.

25. Chaturvedi N, Fuller JH, Effect of intensive treatment in insulin dependent diabetes mellitus with microalbuminuria. Sample size was too small, *BMJ* (1996) **312:** 253.

26. Feldt-Rasmussen B, Mathiesen ER, Jensen T et al, Effect of improved metabolic control on loss of kidney function in type 1 (insulin-dependent) diabetic patients: an update of the Steno studies, *Diabetologia* (1991) **34:** 164–70.

27. Nyberg G, Blohme G, Norden G, Impact of metabolic control in progression of clinical diabetic nephropathy, *Diabetologia* (1987) **30:** 82–6.

28. Jerums G, Cooper ME, Seeman E et al, Comparison of early renal dysfunction in type I and type II diabetes: differing associations with blood pressure and glycaemic control, *Diabetes Res Clin Pract* (1988) **4:** 133–41.

29. Viberti G, Keen H, Dodds R et al, Metabolic control and progression of diabetic nephropathy, *Diabetologia* (1987) **30:** 481–2.

30. Alaveras AE, Thomas SM, Sagriotis A et al, Promoters of progression of diabetic nephropathy: the relative roles of blood glucose and blood pressure control, *Nephrol Dial Transplant* (1997) **12** (Suppl 2): 71–4.

31. Mulec H, Blohme G, Grande B et al, The effect of metabolic control on rate of decline in renal function in insulin-dependent diabetes mellitus with overt diabetic nephropathy, *Nephrol Dial Transplant* (1998) **13:** 651–5.

32. Nielsen S, Schmitz A, Rehling M et al, The clinical course of renal function in NIDDM patients with normo- and micro-albuminuria, *J Intern Med* (1997) **241:** 133–41.

33. Hasslacher C, Stech W, Wahl P et al, Blood pressure and metabolic control as risk factors for nephropathy in type 1 (insulin-dependent) diabetes, *Diabetologia* (1985) **28:** 6–11.

34. Gall MA, Nielsen FS, Smidt UM et al, The course of kidney function in type 2 (non-insulin-dependent) diabetic patients with diabetic nephropathy, *Diabetologia* (1993) **36:** 1071–8.

35. Nelson RG, Bennett PH, Beck GJ et al, Development and progression of renal disease in Pima Indians with non-insulin-dependent diabetes mellitus. Diabetic Renal Disease Study Group, *N Engl J Med* (1996) **335:** 1636–42.

36. Viberti GC, Bilous RW, Mackintosh D et al, Long term correction of hyperglycaemia and progression of renal failure in insulin dependent diabetes, *BMJ* (1983) **286:** 598–602.

37. Bending JJ, Pickup JC, Viberti GC et al, Glycaemic control in diabetic nephropathy, *BMJ (Clin Res Edn)* (1984) **288:** 1187–91.

38. Bangstad HJ, Osterby R, Dahl-Jorgensen K et al, Improvement of blood glucose control in IDDM patients retards the progression of morphological changes in early diabetic nephropathy, *Diabetologia* (1994) **37:** 483–90.

39. Fioretto P, Mauer SM, Bilous RW et al, Effects of pancreas transplantation on glomerular structure in insulin-dependent diabetic patients with their own kidneys, *Lancet* (1993) **342:** 1193–6.

40. Fioretto P, Steffes MW, Sutherland DE et al, Reversal of lesions of diabetic nephropathy after pancreas transplantation, *N Engl J Med* (1998) **339:** 69–75.

41. Tzamaloukas AH, The relationship between glycaemic control and morbidity and mortality for diabetics on dialysis, *ASAIO J* (1993) **39:** 880–5.

42. Tzamaloukas AH, Yuan ZY, Murata GH et al, Clinical associations of glycemic control in diabetics on CAPD, *Adv Perit Dial* (1993) **9:** 291–4.

43. Morioka T, Emoto M, Tabata T et al, Glycemic control is a predictor of survival for diabetic patients on hemodialysis, *Diabetes Care* (2001) **24:** 909–13.

44. Mehmet S, Quan G, Thomas S et al, Important causes of hypoglycaemia in patients with diabetes on peritoneal dialysis, *Diabet Med* (2001) **18:** 679–82.

45. Gaede P, Vedel P, Parving HH et al, Intensified multifactorial intervention in patients with type 2 diabetes mellitus and microalbuminuria: the Steno type 2 randomised study, *Lancet* (1999) **353:** 617–22.

46. Manto A, Cotroneo P, Marra G et al, Effect of intensive treatment on diabetic nephropathy in patients with type I diabetes, *Kidney Int* (1995) **47:** 231–5.

# 7

# Treatment of diabetic nephropathy: antihypertensive treatment

Mordechai Ravid and Rita Rachmani

## INTRODUCTION

Diabetic nephropathy and hypertension are closely linked; they are found together in about 40–50% of the diabetic population on cross-sectional surveys, the prevalence depending on the definition of hypertension.[1] This prevalence increases, however, both with age and with the duration of diabetes. After 10 years of diabetes, elevated blood-pressure levels will be present in 60% of the patients.[2] This rate will increase to 80% after 20 years. Eventually, therefore, if they live long enough, most, if not all, diabetic patients will become hypertensive.

Hypertension may precede diabetic nephropathy, since diabetic patients are obviously not immune to essential hypertension and all other secondary forms of hypertension. In particular, the accelerated atherosclerosis that accompanies the course of diabetes may result in renovascular hypertension, which may either cause an elevation of initially normal blood-pressure levels or worsen the course of previously existing hypertension and turn it into a resistant disease that is difficult to control.

In type 1 diabetes, microalbuminuria usually precedes the gradual rise in blood-pressure readings by 3–5 years. Any increase in urinary albumin excretion, even within the normal range (e.g., an increase from 10 to 20 mg/24 hr), indicates renal as well as general vascular damage, and predicts subsequent acceleration in the rate of progression of renal damage. It also predicts an increase in blood pressure and a rise in the combined cardiovascular event rate.[3]

One of the issues in the current debate about the therapeutic strategies for diabetes in general is therefore related to the appropriate stage for the introduction of vasodilatory interventions with angiotensin-converting enzyme (ACE) inhibitors and similar agents.

In type 2 diabetes, there is no consistent pattern of the course of elevation of blood-pressure levels as related to renal disease. The elevation in blood-pressure levels precedes the rise in albumin excretion rate in about 40% of the patients. In most of these patients, however, the signs of renal damage will soon follow, and the rate of progression will be two to six times greater than the decline in renal function over time in normoalbuminuric, normotensive patients. It is noteworthy, however, that observational follow-up studies show that in initially normotensive subjects the progression to microalbuminuria is predicted by the initial albumin excretion rate, by body-mass index (BMI) or waist:hip ratio, and by plasma lipid levels, but not by initial blood-pressure levels.[4] The type 2 diabetic subjects, in whom microalbuminuria precedes the rise in blood pressure, run a more predictable course, which is similar in principle to the course observed in type 1 patients. The type 2 patients are 15–20 years older, are usually overweight, have more associated diseases and are often much more difficult to manage. One must also keep in mind that hypertension is already present in 25–30% of patients with type 2 diabetes at the time of diagnosis of diabetes. In type 2 diabetes, however, hyperglycemia usually exists 2–5 years prior to its diagnosis, and insulin resistance may have been present for many years, together with the alterations in the lipoprotein composition: increases in small dense low-density lipoprotein (LDL), oxidized LDL, and triglycerides and, especially, low high-density lipoprotein (HDL) cholesterol.[5] Type 2 diabetic patients, therefore, may already have fairly advanced vascular disease at the time of diagnosis. In many patients, in fact, diabetes is first diagnosed during an acute myocardial infarction or a cerebrovascular event.

The overall risk of the combination of diabetes

and hypertension is best deduced from the data of the MRFIT study.[6] This study summarized 10 years' follow-up data in over 300 000 men aged 35–55 years on initial examination. The total 10-year mortality rate in initially nondiabetic, normotensive (<140/90 mmHg) men was 6:1000. In nondiabetic, hypertensive men the 10-year mortality was 14:1000. In diabetic, initially normotensive men, it was 15:1000, while in men with both diabetes and hypertension initially the 10-year mortality rate was 48:1000, eight times the mortality rate of the healthy population. The second half of the 20th century witnessed a gradual and steady decline in cardiovascular mortality. The age-adjusted mortality rates for both cerebrovascular and coronary events declined by 60% from the early 1970s to the mid-1990s. This trend flattened somewhat during the last decade of the 20th century.[7] The diabetic population, however, did not benefit from this generally favorable trend. The coronary and cerebrovascular morbidity remain very high, and the mortality rate is more than double that of nondiabetic subjects.[8] Looking specifically at the progression of renal disease reveals the profound impact of blood-pressure levels on the annual decline in glomerular filtration rate (GFR). As compared to a rate of decline in GFR of 1–2 ml·min$^{-1}$ year$^{-1}$ in normotensive, normoalbuminuric patients, an elevation in blood pressure is accompanied by a decline in GFR of 7–20 ml·min$^{-1}$ year$^{-1}$.[4] Therefore, for successful management of patients with diabetes mellitus, it is imperative both to identify the first stages in the development of hypertension and to institute treatment without delay.

The opinions of various investigators vary as to the role of intervention in normotensive patients, the practical ways to implement nonpharmacological therapeutic modalities, and the choice of initial therapy as well as the order of preference in the use of additional agents. The two most important issues in the treatment of hypertension, particularly in the diabetic patient, are how to increase the percentage of patients that are being treated, and how to make sure that the blood pressure is reduced to target levels. Primary-care physicians, rather than experts in diabetes, ought to be the target professional group towards whom efforts should be directed to increase the early identification of microalbuminuria and hypertension in diabetic subjects. These physicians should promptly institute measures to control blood pressure with or without professional consultation.

In this context, the responsibility of public-health authorities also needs to be discussed. The investment in health-care interventions such as the treatment of hypertension is long term. It is often difficult to convince the political and public-service ranks of the importance of prevention-orientated policies, as these put a continuous demand on the budget without producing demonstrable results in the short term. It is the duty of leading researchers in this field to lobby for the appropriate allocation of funds and effort in the various health-care systems to improve the prognosis and quality of life of diabetic patients by early and aggressive treatment of hypertension. There is now sufficient evidence that such a policy is not only clinically sound but also cost-effective.[8] These efforts directed toward policy decision makers are at least as important as, or no less important than, further data generation and development of new therapeutic modalities.

## Target values of blood pressure

The positive relationships between systolic and diastolic blood pressure and cardiovascular risk and progression of renal disease have long been recognized. This relationship is unequivocal, continuous and independent of other confounding factors in the general population, and especially, with a much stronger correlation, in patients with diabetes mellitus. The correlation between blood-pressure values and prognosis is not linear but exponential. The search for a threshold value beyond which there is a sharp rise in the risk of cardiovascular and microvascular (retinal and renal) endpoints has not yielded any mathematically verifiable turning points. The choice of blood-pressure values for commencement of treatment, as well as the treatment target values, remain arbitrary. Long-term observational studies and some early randomized, placebo-controlled studies provide information which establishes the significantly greater blood-pressure-dependent progression of vascular changes at all levels in diabetic than nondiabetic subjects. It was only logical therefore to set the target values of blood pressure in diabetic patients lower than in nondiabetic patients. Furthermore, long-term follow-up studies of initially normotensive diabetic subjects without renal disease showed a blood-pressure-dependent decline in GFR with blood-pressure levels within the normal range.[9] Thus, diabetic patients with low normal mean arterial blood-pressure (MAP) levels (MAP is defined as diastolic blood pressure (DBP) + 1/3 pulse pressure) below 97 mmHg rarely developed microalbuminuria and showed an annual decline in GFR close to the 'normal' rate of 1–1.5 ml·min$^{-1}$ year$^{-1}$. Patients with MAP values of 97–107 mmHg (corresponding to 130/80 to 140/90 mmHg) showed a greater decline in GFR

(2–10 ml·min$^{-1}$ year$^{-1}$), and about 30% of these patients developed micro- or macroalbuminuria over an observation period of 12–15 years. The accelerated, blood-pressure-dependent decline in GFR seen in patients with albuminuria prompted nephrologists to suggest that in these patients the levels of blood pressure should be kept even lower than in normoalbuminuric patients. In patients with significant proteinuria, in excess of 1 gm/24 hr, it has been suggested that one keep blood-pressure levels below 125/75.[10,15]

These overall graded clinical recommendations suggest, therefore, that one should intensify the control of blood pressure alongside the progression of vascular and renal disease. While this approach helps to define high-risk groups and may be cost-effective in the short term, its basic philosophy may be questioned. In principle, this policy is based on the assumption that a more rigorous control of blood pressure will retard the progress towards cardiovascular and renal complications. Why, then, should we wait for the clinical manifestations of the vascular derangement in order to intensify therapy when we have ample evidence of its presence in asymptomatic diabetic subjects? Why not strive to maintain optimal levels of blood pressure (≤125/75 mmHg) in all patients with diabetes? However, the ratio of adequately controlled patients according to the presently recommended criteria is alarmingly low, at 10–35% in different surveys.[2,12] There is, therefore, a long way to go before tightening the recommendations for target values of blood pressure.

The official recommendations about the target levels of blood pressure in diabetes were first published in the sixth report of the Joint National Committee on Prevention, Detection, Evaluation and Treatment of High Blood Pressure in 1997.[1] They were to maintain blood pressure levels at or below 130/85 mmHg. These recommendations were adopted by the American Diabetes Association in 1999.[10] However, the consensus report of the National Kidney Foundation (NKF) suggests that the goal should be a blood pressure of less than 130/80 mmHg.[11] In fact, in a recently published study, Schrier et al[13] found that intensive treatment of normotensive, type 2 diabetic patients to a blood pressure of approximately 125/75 mmHg, with nisoldipine or enalapril, resulted in a slowing of progression to incipient and overt diabetic nephropathy, decreased the progression of retinopathy and diminished the incidence of stroke. It should be noted that only 30% of the patients in the intensive therapy group and 35% in the moderate therapy group had microalbuminuria or overt proteinuria at entry to the study.

In patients with isolated systolic hypertension, who are mainly elderly patients (≥65 years of age), a two-stage approach is currently recommended. In patients with systolic blood pressure (SBP) ≥180 mmHg, the target value should be ≤160 mmHg. In patients with 160–179 mmHg, the SBP should be lowered by 20 mmHg. When these levels are stabilized and well tolerated, further lowering may be indicated to SBP levels of 120 or 130 mmHg. This is particularly true for patients with comorbid conditions, mainly albuminuria and congestive heart failure. It has been suggested, since publication of the HOT study, that the universally accepted target value of 130/85 mmHg be further reduced to 130/80 mmHg.[14]

The main objectives of the HOT study were as follows:

1) to define the optimal target blood pressure for reducing the incidence of major cardiovascular events, such as fatal and nonfatal myocardial infarction and stroke
2) to assess the effect of low-dose acetylsalicylic acid (75 mg/day of aspirin) as compared with placebo on the incidence of cardiovascular events.

The study comprised close to 19 000 subjects, 1501 of whom had diabetes. Subjects were randomly assigned to one of three groups, with target DBP values of <90, <85 or <80 mmHg. Felodipine was used as initial treatment and other drugs, mainly angiotensin-converting enzyme (ACE) inhibitors and beta-blockers, were added according to a five-step predetermined regimen. The event rate of all major cardiovascular events declined, although without significant differences between the DBP target values of 85 and 80 mmHg. Among the patients with diabetes, however, the difference in the incidence of stroke and fatal myocardial infarction was significantly lower in the group assigned to a DBP target value of <80 mmHg than in the groups with target DBP of <90 and <85 mmHg. The further decline in cardiovascular event rate for the lowest target DBP group was, thus, observed only in subjects with diabetes, a finding that highlighted the higher risk of cardiovascular disease among diabetic patients. The validity of the conclusions of the HOT study has been questioned because the total event rate in that study was low, but mainly because the actual differences in mean DBP values between the two groups with the lowest target DBP were very small, no more than 2 mmHg (the actual mean DBP values were 82.3 and 81.3 mmHg in the <85 and <80 mmHg groups, respectively).

It is, therefore, unclear how far the blood pressure should be lowered. The rule that the lower the better comes from epidemiological studies in essential hypertension, in which mortality was positively associated with blood-pressure levels also within the normotensive range. However, the issue of further lowering of blood-pressure levels in normotensive patients was never addressed in interventional studies. Elderly patients and patients with coronary heart disease may be adversely affected by excessive lowering of blood pressure. Some evidence suggests an increase of ischemic cardiac events in patients with DBP levels below 85 mmHg.[12] The exact mechanism by which blood-pressure values below a critical level might increase the risk of cardiovascular events is not known. It has been suggested that at low diastolic filling pressure the coronary blood flow may be compromised. This may prove critical in patients with occlusive coronary disease, especially when oxygen demand is increased in the presence of left ventricular hypertrophy. It has also been reported in a few studies that excessive lowering of blood pressure is associated with increased viscosity and platelet adhesiveness predisposing to thrombus formation near atherosclerotic plaques.[12] The progression of nephropathy was found to be retarded in type 1 and, in one study, also in type 2 diabetic subjects with further lowering of initially normal blood-pressure levels.[15] In these studies, the number of patients was not large enough and the follow-up periods were not long enough to permit valid conclusions as to the influence of the therapeutic interventions on cardiovascular events or on mortality.

A careful analysis of some studies documenting cardiovascular outcomes in hypertensive patients shows that when the initial or the mean values of systolic, diastolic or pulse pressure over the period of the study are considered, the best cardiovascular risk-predictive parameter is the pulse pressure.[16] Thus, in subjects with equal SBP values, the risk ratio for cardiovascular morbidity and mortality is inversely correlated with DBP values. There is, however, no conclusive evidence from interventional studies to suggest that lowering of initially elevated or initially normal DBP values by antihypertensive treatment is associated with increased cardiovascular or cerebrovascular event rates. Pharmacological preparations which lower blood pressure via central as well as peripheral vasodilatory mechanisms lower SBP substantially more than DBP.

In conclusion, it is now generally agreed that in subjects with diabetes the SBP should be kept at 130 mmHg or lower, except in patients with albuminuria or concomitant congestive heart failure, in whom the SBP should best be lowered to 125 mmHg (the figure stated in most consensus reports).[11] There is a general agreement that DBP values of 85 mmHg or lower are associated with reduced cardiovascular mortality in diabetes. In spite of the fact that the latest guidelines suggest that the target should be to reduce DBP to below 80 mmHg, this has not been substantiated adequately in clinical studies.

## General therapeutic considerations

In 1984, two leading diabetologists, Viberti and Keen, published a review discussing proteinuria in diabetes mellitus.[17] The only therapeutic intervention to slow the progression of nephropathy that was discussed in that article published nearly 20 years ago was improved glycemic control. Blood pressure was not even mentioned. We have come a long way since that concise review. It is now generally accepted that all three major interventions—control of hyperglycemia, dyslipidemia and hypertension—are important to retard micro- and macrovascular disease in diabetes. Since all three aspects are unequivocally crucial both to the quality of life and to the life expectancy of patients with diabetes mellitus, it is perhaps redundant to discuss priorities in the choice and commencement of therapeutic interventions.

### Cost-effectiveness
Clinical considerations are rarely exclusive, however. The financial aspects of the various therapeutic regimens must also be considered. Therapies are therefore chosen on the basis of cost-effectiveness, and preferably on the prospect of cost saving as much as on the basis of clinical effectiveness. The overall effect of finance on the outcome of disease in affluent societies is exemplified by the UK national data, which show a strong inverse association between social class and the risk of death from diabetes.[18]

In the USA, the prevalence of the main complications of diabetes is higher in ethnic minorities than in the general population. The prevalence of obesity and diabetes is also highest among the poor. Analysis of cost-effectiveness assumes that there are clinically effective treatments, with a range of different treatment options and limited budgets. Cost-effectiveness is generally greatest among those with highest risk, and is closely related to the concept of number-needed-to-treat. Various risk charts and risk engines have therefore been proposed in order to help decision makers draw up appropriate therapeutic guidelines. In an analysis of cost-effectiveness, the direct added-cost of therapy is compared to the potential saving by prevention of complications. The theoretical saving by adding a year of life, or by having a complication-free year, is thus estimated. Various societies deem acceptable different sums for these potential savings. There is, however, no official policy in any country that helps clinicians and economists decide on the acceptability of different treatments by criteria of effectiveness and cost. In the USA, the figure of $100 000 for a life-year saved is often quoted as acceptable. In the UK, the figure of £20 000 was unofficially quoted by the National Health Service authorities as acceptable for a treatment or a drug to be included in the national arsenal. The most appropriate use of cost-effectiveness analysis, which may also yield the most reliable results, is by comparing two or more alternative treatments or medications on a disease condition in a given population. These head-to-head trials are rarely done, however, since manufacturers prefer salesmanship to comparative cost-effectiveness analysis. Public health-care authorities, which should be the most interested in the results of such studies, do not often find their funding to be of high enough priority.

## Clinical considerations

Since effective treatment of patients with diabetes must take into consideration the control of hyperglycemia, lipids and blood pressure, the antihypertensive medications must be evaluated not only for their direct antihypertensive effect and untoward side-effect profile but also for their influence on carbohydrate and lipid metabolism. Diabetic patients always end up being treated with multiple drugs; thus, possible interactions play a major role in choosing the therapeutic regimen. About 75% of diabetic patients with hypertension require at least two drugs to control their blood pressure.[14,19] There is, therefore, an increasing trend among pharmaceutical manufacturers to market fixed combination preparations. This approach does not really reduce the troublesome polypharmacy of treating of diabetes, but, at least, the patient has to consume fewer tablets, thus possibly helping to increase compliance. Some, if not all, of the combined preparations are comparatively cost-effective because their cost is lower than that of the two components when purchased separately. Untoward side effects in patients treated with combination drugs may pose some management problems. Both patients and physicians tend to forget the particular components of the combination drugs, leading to late identification of side effects and drug interactions. The most commonly available combina-

tions of medications include an antihypertensive agent together with a low-dose diuretic, and two antihypertensive agents (e.g., a beta-blocker and a calcium-channel blocker). The rate of appearance of new combination therapies renders any discussion about individual preparations irrelevant. By the time this book appears, many new combinations will already be available.

The antihypertensive efficacy of most of the currently used preparations is very similar. Short-term studies have shown that in the early phase of treatment most drugs, after dose titration, lower both SBP and DBP to the same degree, with the maximal effect obtained after 4–8 weeks. About 50% of nondiabetic patients are controlled initially with monotherapy.[20] Thus, the choice of the initial treatment depends by and large on the individual's preferences. The factors that should be taken into consideration include the patient's age, gender, renal function and metabolic status; the presence of cardiac, vascular or other diseases; and the other medications that the patient may be receiving. Reduction of blood pressure to the target values is relatively infrequent following the use of monotherapy in diabetic patients with mild to moderate hypertension. In fact, a suitable response may be expected in no more than 20% of the cases.[19] This proportion may be even lower in patients with diabetic nephropathy.

A question which becomes more and more relevant is whether treatment should be started with a single preparation, with two drugs or with a combination drug. The combination drugs are rapidly gaining popularity. There are few data available in the literature which compare combination drugs with single agents. One study examined the added antihypertensive effect of 12.5 mg of hydrochlorothiazide (HCTZ) in patients with diabetic nephropathy and GFR values within the normal range.[21] The patients were initially treated with an ACE inhibitor (cilazapril) or an alpha-blocker (doxazosin). A mean decline of 15 mm in SBP and 8 mm in DBP was obtained. The addition of HCTZ resulted in a further decline in SBP of 8 mmHg and in DBP of 5 mmHg. There was also a further reduction in urinary albumin excretion rate. Several short-term studies examined the additional antihypertensive effect of various doses of HCTZ in patients treated with angiotensin receptor blockers.[22] Daily doses of 6.25, 12.5 and 25 mg of HCTZ were compared, and it was shown that the 12.5- and 5-mg doses were equally effective and significantly superior to the 6.25-mg dose. It has thus become accepted to add 12.5 mg of HCTZ to most antihypertensive regimens, either in combination or as an additional drug. Experienced clinicians, when confronted with patients with diabetic nephropathy or even with microalbuminuria, will consider the use of combination drugs right from the start, thus aiming at more rigorous control of blood pressure within a shorter time frame.

Patients with diabetic nephropathy at any stage are already at high risk of developing further renal, as well as other micro- and macrovascular, complications.[4] The degree of concordance of nephropathy with diabetic retinopathy is high, 50–70% at diagnosis of microalbuminuria in different studies.[23] Effective antihypertensive treatment has been repeatedly demonstrated to slow the progression of retinopathy.[24] The presence of diabetic retinopathy may, therefore, encourage a more aggressive antihypertensive regimen, thus potentially justifying the initial use of a combination preparation or two or more agents. In the UKPDS study,[24] intensive antihypertensive therapy was associated with a 21% reduction in the incidence of new cases of retinopathy. Since the SBP and DBP values in those 'intensive' patients were higher by 12 and 2 mmHg, respectively, than currently accepted target values for patients with diabetes, effective antihypertensive treatment may be expected to reduce further the incidence and to retard the progression of diabetic retinopathy. It should be remembered, in this context, that normotensive patients with type 1 diabetes, as well as type 2 patients with nephropathy who were treated with ACE inhibitors, showed a 25–40% reduced incidence of retinopathy and also a retardation in the progression of existing retinopathy (EUCLID study).[25] The presence of retinopathy may therefore influence the selection of initial therapy.

### Twenty-four-hour ambulatory blood-pressure monitoring (ABPM)

With the development of user-friendly digital monitoring devices, this method became very popular among physicians involved in the care of hypertensive patients in general and in susceptible populations, such as patients with diabetic nephropathy.[26] ABPM may be useful in detecting patients in whom the mean nocturnal blood pressure does not decline as compared to the mean daytime values (nondippers). These patients have been reported to be at greater cardiovascular risk than those who show a decline in mean nocturnal blood pressure (dippers), even when the mean 24-hr pressures were equal.[27] Furthermore, some reports have highlighted the role of ABPM in revealing patients with normal mean 24-hr blood pressure levels among those with elevated clinic blood-pressure ('white-coat' hypertension).[28] Since it has been shown that patients with white-coat

hypertension share a higher risk of developing cardiovascular endpoints, this distinction may now be less relevant.[29] Patients with diabetic nephropathy, who are at increased risk of cardiovascular events, should receive antihypertensive treatment early, even at the stage of white-coat hypertension. ABPM is thus indicated in patients with diabetic nephropathy in order to decide whether treatment is indicated in a patient with borderline hypertension; to ascertain the correct blood pressure in patients in whom there is a big difference between self-measured home values and office recordings; to decide whether a patient is really controlled, for research purposes; and to determine the circadian effects of different drugs. Home self-measurement of blood pressure should be considered an appropriate method for assessing response to therapy. Home blood-pressure determinations are, no doubt, cost-effective when compared to ABPM. Moreover, the patients' active participation in the therapeutic process may help to improve compliance. ABPM should be reserved for the conditions mentioned above.

Another general question for consideration is the therapeutic policy for patients with diabetic nephropathy and severe hypertension. There are no controlled studies which address this question. A patient with nephropathy and severe hypertension should best be regarded as a medical emergency, perhaps comparable to a patient with malignant hypertension. It is the authors' experience that, if not aggressively managed, these patients deteriorate very rapidly to end-stage renal disease. Thus, patients with nephropathy who present with DBP values higher than 110 mmHg or SBP values higher than 210 mmHg (these are, needless to say, arbitrary values) should be treated in hospital with rapidly acting vasodilators. Patients with diabetic nephropathy in whom an unexplained rise in blood pressure is detected should be thoroughly investigated. These patients often have a significant degree of arteriosclerosis, with possibly associated renal artery stenosis.

## Non-pharmacological treatment

Two main approaches need to be considered under this heading: physical activity, and weight control via dietary measures.

### Physical activity

Patients with diabetic nephropathy represent a very high-risk group among hypertensive patients similar to those who have survived a major coronary event. In these patients, therefore, any additional management approach which has proven beneficial effects is of the utmost importance since the magnitude of the effects of any given intervention is directly proportional to the initial risk. The effect of methodical physical activity on the risk ratio of coronary events has not been specifically examined in patients with diabetic nephropathy. It is now well established, however, that in the middle-aged population at large, when divided into four categories of physical fitness (estimated by interpreting answers to mailed questionnaires), the cardiovascular mortality in the fittest group approximated 50% that of the least fit group with a sedentary lifestyle.[30] It is also well known that regular physical activity results in lower blood-pressure values, and in reduced insulin resistance.[31] These effects last as long as the patients remain active and return to baseline values within less than 2 weeks of inactivity. Encouraging patients to maintain accepted regimens of regular physical activity (e.g., walking 30–45 minutes four to five times a week) may have a profound impact on their well-being, as well as facilitate the effect of antihypertensive therapy and improve survival.

## Weight maintenance

The average body-mass index (BMI) (weight/ height$^2$) of patients with type 2 diabetes in most reported series is 29–30 kg/m$^2$.[32] About 35% of the patients are grossly obese with BMI values above 35 kg/m$^2$. Antihypertensive therapy in obese patients is often problematic. Firstly, the measurement of blood pressure may not reflect the true values of arterial pressure when the examination is performed with a standard-size cuff in obese patients. Secondly, gross obesity may be associated with albuminuria and peripheral edema, resulting in an inability to estimate the severity of the renal derangement. Finally, grossly obese patients require larger doses of medications and have an increased ratio of untoward effects. Encouraging loss of weight is therefore an essential component of doctor–patient encounters with diabetic or hypertensive patients in general, and especially so in patients with nephropathy. It is much easier to achieve weight loss when a low-calorie diet is combined with physical activity.

A weight loss of 3–4 kg is usually accompanied by a decrease of 5–10 mmHg in SBP and 2–4 mmHg in DBP.[33] This new balance is maintained for a period of up to 1–3 years. In the vast majority of patients, blood-pressure values will gradually rise to prediet values, even in those patients who maintain their weight and do not regain the lost kilograms. Most patients, however, return to the original weight and often gain more weight over time. The UKPDS and other studies showed that weight gain was steady and more pronounced in those patients who were randomized to the intensive hypoglycemic treatment.[34] The only documented hypoglycemic agent which is not associated with a gain in weight is metformin.[32] Patients with nephropathy tolerate this drug well. However, metformin should not be taken when serum creatinine exceeds 1.5 mg/dl (133 μmol/l) in males and 1.3 mg/dl (115 μmol/l) in females. Thus, metformin is only of transient benefit in patients with diabetic nephropathy.

The relationship between weight loss and hypertension is complex. A decline in SBP has been observed as early as 24 hr after starting a hypocaloric diet, before any weight loss could have taken place.[35] The rapid changes in basal metabolic rate which accompany early caloric deficit and the reduced heat production associated with a low-calorie diet result in decreased sympathetic activity and a fall in blood pressure. When the negative caloric balance transforms into a new equilibrium, the sympathetic activity is restored, followed by the return of original levels of blood pressure. Whatever the theoretical explanation, the reality is that while loss of weight is very desirable in patients with diabetic nephropathy, it seldom occurs. A detailed discussion of the low-salt diet is beyond the scope of this chapter. There are, nevertheless, some data worthy of examination. Carefully controlled studies have recently shown that in hypertensive diabetic patients reducing salt consumption from 10 to 6 g per day results in sustained decline of 6–10 and 2–5 mmHg in SBP and DBP, respectively.[36] It is also well known that a diet rich in salt (in excess of 14 g/day) abrogates the effects of antihypertensive therapy.[37] A recommendation to limit the consumption of salt is therefore reasonable, especially in high-risk patients. The prospective benefits must be weighed against quality-of-life issues. Salt intake must be properly monitored, especially in patients who use diuretics.

## Low-protein diet

The unresolved issue of the long-term kidney-function-sparing effect of a moderate low-protein diet, especially in view of the controversial results of the MDRD study,[38] is beyond the scope of the present discussion and is discussed in Chapter 19. A moderately low-protein diet is, however, associated with increased effectiveness of antihypertensive therapy.

## Potassium supplements

The decline in blood-pressure values that follows sodium restriction may be, at least, partially attributed to added potassium since many of the salt substitutes are potassium salts. The addition of oral potassium supplements to normokalemic hypertensive patients results in a fall in blood-pressure values equivalent to the degree of decline obtained with a moderate low-salt diet.[20] This effect of potassium is lost in patients on low sodium intake. This observation led to the hypothesis that the effect of potassium supplementation is partially mediated through natriuresis at the level of the distal renal tubule. Furthermore, a diet rich in potassium results in a decrease in renin-induced release of angiotensin and norepinephrine.[39] In patients with diabetic nephropathy, potassium supplements should be restricted to those who develop diuretic-induced hypokalemia. The development of clinically significant hyperkalemia may be rapid and unexpected, even in patients with normal GFR.

### Vegetarian diet

Vegetarian and fiber-rich diets have been repeatedly reported to possess a mild blood-pressure-lowering effect.[39] There has been no clinical trial, however, in which the hypotensive effect of a vegetarian diet was tested when the subjects consumed 90–100 mmol of sodium per day. Vegetarian diets tend to be rich in potassium, and patients with diabetic nephropathy should be cautioned accordingly. It is noteworthy in this context that about 20% of patients with renal diseases also consult naturopaths or other alternative-medicine therapists. Some of the alternative healers use fruit juice, especially grape juice. We have observed several patients with extreme, life-threatening hyperkalemia induced by fruit juice.

### Alcohol

The 'one drink a day' rule has never been tested specifically in patients with diabetic nephropathy. However, reduced cardiovascular mortality has been documented in mild alcohol drinkers (including diabetics) as compared to nonusers.[40] However, excessive intake of alcohol has been associated with increased blood pressure, and reducing alcohol intake results in a reduction in blood pressure.

### Coffee

It has been accepted for over a decade that habitual coffee drinkers do not have higher blood pressure than those who abstain from coffee. A recent, long-term, large study in Finland, documented a marginal (but significant) survival benefit for coffee drinkers.[28] There is, at present, no evidence to support any restriction on consumption of coffee in diabetic subjects with or without nephropathy.

## DRUG THERAPY

Antihypertensive medications now form the largest group of prescription drugs in western countries. However, their widespread use does not reflect adequate control of blood pressure.

Traditional recommendations highlight the role of the nonpharmacological interventions, mainly changes in lifestyle. It is often advocated that one withhold pharmacotherapy in patients with mild to moderate hypertension in order to encourage them to adopt physical activity and dietary modifications. Antihypertensive medications are then offered when these measures have failed or have produced suboptimal results. Patients with diabetic nephropathy are at the highest risk of developing cardio- and cerebrovascular events, as well as worsening retinopathy, and they manifest a rapid rate of decline of GFR, progressing to ESRD. In these patients, therefore, all lifestyle modifications should be recommended and encouraged alongside drug therapy, which should be initiated as soon as blood-pressure values exceed the accepted target values. There should be a very strong message from the physician to the patient that maintenance of normal blood-pressure levels is critical and indispensable to the preservation of health. Strict compliance with therapeutic recommendations, adequate monitoring and recording of blood pressure, and timely response to changes in monitored parameters and untoward effects will facilitate control of blood pressure.

Achieving satisfactory blood-pressure levels is often a prolonged, time-dependent process. The maximal antihypertensive effect of all drugs is obtained only after 4–8 weeks. This requires the patience of both the patient and the physician, frequent visits or telephone (Internet) contact, and careful individual adjustment of the antihypertensive drugs. Postural hypotension, with a prevalence among diabetic subjects double that of an age-matched general population, also constitutes a limiting factor, especially when therapy aims to achieve normotension. The various preparations differ in their effect on baroreceptor regulation. Clinically significant large-vessel disease exists in a large proportion of patients with diabetic nephropathy. Lowering blood pressure may decrease perfusion pressure to various organs, resulting in a clinically important decline in organ perfusion. Drug-induced effects on peripheral resistance and flow across atherosclerotic arteries should also be considered when selecting antihypertensive agents especially for elderly or clinically atherosclerotic patients.

## Comparative efficacy of different agents

All presently available antihypertensive agents are approved by health authorities (e.g., the US Federal Drug Administration [FDA]) only after clinical testing in a large number of patients, usually 2000 or more. The doses of the drugs are adjusted to produce a 10% decline in SBP and DBP. Furthermore, the doses of individual tablets are so designed as to avoid excessive or too rapid lowering of blood pressure. Contrary to the belief of many doctors, the mean antihypertensive potency of an agent is not an important factor in the choice of the initial preparation to be used. A direct head-to-head comparison between most of the commonly used classes of antihypertensive medications was performed in the TOHMS study (Treatment of Mild Hypertension), the final results of which were published in 1993.[41] Diuretics, CCBs, beta-blockers, alpha-blockers and ACE inhibitors were compared. The blood-pressure-lowering effect of the different classes was similar, as was the ratio of patients who needed a second drug. Individual patients may react differently, however. It was repeatedly shown that, in patients of African descent, CCBs were the most effective whereas ACE inhibitors were more effective in males of Caucasian origin. Beta-blockers were found to be more effective in women and in older men. Other studies claim that CCBs are more effective in an elderly population, especially with isolated systolic hypertension.[42-44] It was postulated in the early 1990s that short-term testing or the response to a single dose may predict individual response to a given agent. These methods have gained little popularity. Long-term response is rarely predictable; furthermore, it is frequently inconsistent. The main issues in tailoring individual drug therapy are the patient's sense of well-being, the side-effect profile and associated compliance issues. In patients with diabetic nephropathy, a single-agent therapy is often inadequate, and second and third drugs must be added. The subtle differences in individual agent potency are therefore of limited clinical relevance.

### Dose-response regulation

Newly introduced antihypertensive agents were often used initially in excessively high doses in order to promote efficacy. The most prominent examples, summarized in the excellent book on clinical hypertension by Norman Kaplan,[45] are hydrochlorothiazide (HCTZ) and captopril. Doses of 50–100 mg of HCTZ were used in the early 1980s. A myriad of side effects was observed, including severe hypokalemia, reduced glucose tolerance, elevation of LDL cholesterol, and elevation of uric acid. The dose

was gradually reduced and, at present, the standard recommended daily dose is 12.5 mg. Likewise, captopril was first used in doses of up to 600 mg/day. It is now often used in doses of 75 mg or less per day. The doses of beta-blockers were also reduced substantially. The aim of the dose adjustment should be to identify the dose range with the best efficacy and lowest risk of side effects.

The biological response curves of most agents follow the pattern of an S-shaped curve where the hemodynamic response is log-linear with the dose only within a narrow dose-range, while the risk of side effects rises continuously (Figure 7.1). The manufacturers of antihypertensive agents have been slow to respond to the dose adjustments borne out by clinical experience. Thus, atenolol, for example, is still marketed in 100- and 50-mg tablets, and only recently was a 25-mg tablet introduced, while the optimal dose range in most patients is probably 12.5–25 mg. The newer drugs are now manufactured as tablets of appropriate dosages in order to reduce the need to split tablets.

In patients with diabetic nephropathy, a degree of arteriosclerosis must always be assumed, even when there are no overt indications of vasculopathy. The autoregulatory mechanisms which maintain relatively constant perfusion of the brain, the heart and the kidney may have shifted to adjust to the elevated perfusion pressure. Pharmacological reduction of blood pressure must, therefore, be gradual in order to allow enough time for readjustment of the autoregulatory mechanisms in the perfusion of vital organs.

In isolated systolic hypertension in elderly patients, the recommendations are first to lower SBP to a level of 160 mmHg or by 20 mmHg pressure and only after stabilization to consider further attempts to lower SBP to target values. In patients with diabetic nephropathy, the gradual approach should always be adopted. The process of lowering blood pressure should be guided by cerebral and renal parameters which are readily detected and also by careful assessment of cardiac performance. Lightheadedness, dizziness and impairment of cognitive performance may follow the initial, drug-induced, fall in blood pressure. Such phenomena should promote readjustment of dosage until equilibrium is obtained, and then further reduction of blood pressure should be attempted until target values are reached or symptoms return and prohibit further reduction in blood pressure. Likewise, an initial drop in GFR or a rise in serum creatinine should not deter further attempts to approach target values. This is particularly true for treatment with ACE

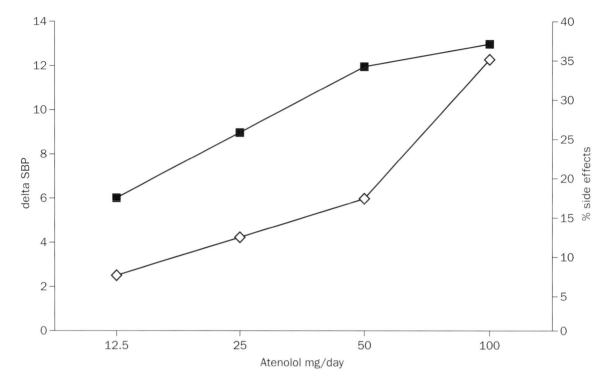

**Figure 7.1** The added blood-pressure-lowering effect of atenolol decreases with each increase in the daily dose while the proportion of patients reporting side effects increases exponentially. Data are based on the authors' registry, comprising 1100 patients with diabetes mellitus and hypertension treated with atenolol. delta SBP: percentage of initial value; % side effects: percentage of patients reporting side effects via a standard questionnaire; ■ delta: systolic blood pressure; ◇ percentage of patients with side effects.

inhibitors. Serum levels of creatinine should be followed monthly for the first few months. An initial rise in serum creatinine of up to 20% above the initial value should be expected. Treatment should be altered only if there is a continuous rise on consecutive examinations or a rapid doubling in serum creatinine levels suggestive of hemodynamically significant bilateral renal artery stenosis.

*Impotence*
In males with diabetic nephropathy, some degree of erectile dysfunction is present in about 50% of patients under 60 years of age. The effect of antihypertensive drugs on erectile function must, therefore, be carefully considered. A detailed explanation to the patient of the expected effects of individual agents is mandatory in order to avoid the discontinuation of drugs by the patients in the belief that they are responsible for the appearance or worsening of erectile dysfunction.

Both diabetic neuropathy and vascular changes are the underlying causes of erectile failure.

Therefore, the lowering of blood pressure is at times associated with erectile problems. Drugs which are associated with reduced blood flow, especially beta-blockers, may aggravate impotence. The introduction of sildenafil has led to an alleviation of this problem in some patients.[46,47] The use of vasodilating agents, especially alpha-blockers and ACE inhibitors, may bring some relief by restoring a positive response to sildenafil.[48] Young patients with moderate to severe impotence may often be persuaded to inject vasodilatory agents (e.g., alprostadil or preparations containing papaverine) into the corpus cavernosum. Older patients are rarely prepared to use this method.

## Antihypertensive agents

*Diuretics*
Two classes of diuretics will be discussed, thiazides and loop diuretics. There is no question that thiazide diuretics should be preferred as antihypertensive

agents, while loop diuretics should be used only in patients who do not respond to thiazides either because of renal failure or in the presence of congestive heart failure.

## Thiazide diuretics

The three most frequently used agents in this class are HCTZ, indapamide and chlorthalidone. These agents, especially HCTZ, have been tested in prospective clinical studies; thus the data on their efficacy and long-term effects and side effects are reliable.[49]

Historically, thiazide diuretics were the most frequently prescribed therapy in patients with hypertension. Since the mid-1980s their use has been declining. Reports about their adverse metabolic effects, both on glucose and on lipids, deterred many physicians from using these agents, especially in patients with diabetes. The realization that lower doses maintain an adequate antihypertensive effect with only a fraction of the side effects described with high doses has led to a reversal in this trend and to a rise in the use of low-dose thiazides. HCTZ is the agent most frequently included in combination preparations, with ACE inhibitors, ARBs, CCBs or beta-blockers.

## Mechanism of action

Thiazide diuretics inhibit sodium and chloride transport across the membrane of the first segment of the distal convoluted tubule in the kidney. The increase in sodium, chloride and water excretion is followed by intravascular and extracellular volume depletion, resulting in compensatory renin and aldosterone secretion. Plasma volume returns to near normal or normal values within 7–10 days, and the increase in diuresis is only transient. Thus, the long-term effect of thiazides is dependent on a reduction in peripheral resistance. There have been numerous attempts to correlate the endocrine response to the individual antihypertensive effect. No consistent correlation has ever been shown between either the pretreatment renin-angiotensin status or the initial response to treatment and the sustained blood-pressure-lowering effect of thiazides. It should be noted that patients whose initial response to thiazides, when given as a single agent, is marginal, will still benefit significantly from the thiazide drug when used in conjunction with another agent, especially a vasodilator.

## Indapamide

Indapamide has diuretic and antihypertensive potencies similar to HCTZ. This agent is lipid neutral, and it has been experimentally shown to possess antioxi-

dant activity. It can probably be used as a safe substitute for HCTZ. The clinical experience with this agent in patients with diabetic nephropathy is limited.

## Chlorthalidone

A daily dose of 12.5 mg chlorthalidone resulted in a decline of 17 mmHg in SBP in patients with mild to moderate hypertension.[22,50] The side-effect profile is similar to that of HCTZ. Chlorthalidone was used in several studies in elderly diabetic patients with micro- and macroalbuminuria and with isolated systolic hypertension, and it was as effective as CCBs and beta-blockers.[51] The overall experience with this agent is limited. There is no reason, however, to avoid its use.

## Metabolic effects

Continuous use of chlorothiazide, the first thiazide agent, and later also of HCTZ, was associated with reduced glucose tolerance in nondiabetic subjects and with increased hyperglycemia in diabetic subjects. This effect was found in early studies when large doses (50–100 mg/day of HCTZ) were used. The hyperglycemic effect was reversible upon cessation of the drug and was also abrogated by the addition of potassium. No adverse effect on glucose metabolism was ever demonstrated with HCTZ doses lower than 25 mg/day. Early, short-term studies have shown a rise in total serum cholesterol, LDL cholesterol and triglyceride levels. Large doses were used in those studies. Long-term studies failed to demonstrate any effect of thiazide diuretics on plasma lipid composition.[52] Nevertheless, the failure to reduce the ratio of coronary events in early controlled studies of treatment of hypertension with thiazides was attributed to the adverse metabolic effects of these agents, which were thought to counteract the benefits conferred by their antihypertensive action. The impact on clinicians of these studies, most of which were performed in the early 1980s, is so strong that even at the beginning of the 21st century, when low-dose thiazides are universally recognized as effective antihypertensive agents, these agents are included in the therapeutic regimen in only 20% of diabetic hypertensive patients.

## Efficacy and dosage

As already stated, the dose of HCTZ should be kept low, preferably at 12.5 mg/day. This dose should produce about 80–85% of the maximal effect with a major reduction in side effects and without any detectable metabolic abnormalities. Hypokalemia may occur but is rarely severe. Furthermore, the prevalence of impotence, which was reported in over 6% of patients on large doses of thiazides, does not exceed that reported with placebo. Further reduction of the dose of HCTZ to 6.25 mg results in reduced, but not absent, antihypertensive efficacy.

HCTZ or chlorthalidone, when used as a single drug, was shown to reduce SBP by 11–17 mmHg.[53] In long-term studies, there was a mean reduction of 20–24% in left ventricular mass, comparable to the decline observed with CCBs or ACE inhibitors when used as single agents. However, these studies must be considered in the context that the doses of both CCBs and ACE inhibitors were low in those studies. When low-dose thiazides were added to monotherapy with a CCB, an ACE inhibitor, an alpha-blocker or an ARB, there was always a further reduction in UAE, without a change in GFR. These effects were maintained for at least 1 year.[21,54]

### Side effects

Low-dose thiazide treatment results, in the long term, in a slight depletion in total body potassium, with serum $K^+$ levels declining by less than 0.4 mmol/l. Significant hypokalemia is rarely encountered. Hyperuricemia and hypercalcemia are infrequent.

Since there are no long-term studies specifically performed in patients with diabetic nephropathy, no side-effect profile has been reported in this group of patients. The addition of low-dose thiazides to other agents had a negligible effect on the incidence of side effects.

### Furosemide

This is the most widely used loop diuretic. It is included in the antihypertensive arsenal in patients with diabetic nephropathy when they cease to respond to thiazides, usually when serum creatinine levels rise beyond 2.5 mg/dl (220 μmol/l). There are no data on the antihypertensive efficacy of furosemide under these circumstances nor on the side-effect profile because this agent has never been used as monotherapy. It was first reported in an antihypertensive regimen, together with enalapril and metoprolol, by Bjorck et al in 1992.[55] In nondiabetic patients, the antihypertensive efficacy of furosemide is equal to or less than that of HCTZ, with an increased prevalence of side effects. Furosemide should therefore be used only in patients with advanced renal impairment (GFR <30 ml/min) or in patients with congestive heart failure. In patients with hyporeninemic hypoaldosteronism, where hyperkalemia may pose a problem, especially if ACE inhibitors are also used, the addition of furosemide

may help to maintain normal serum potassium levels, whereas a thiazide may not be as effective. The main side effects of furosemide include hypokalemia, hyperuricemia with provocation of attacks of gouty arthritis, hypocalcemia and hypomagnesemia, hearing impairment, rare occasions of pancreatitis and allergic reactions, including Henoch–Schönlein purpura.

## Angiotensin-converting enzyme inhibitors (ACE inhibitors)

The synthesis of this class of antihypertensive agents followed the isolation of the first ACE inhibitor from the venom of a Brazilian viper. During the late 1970s and early 1980s, several effective ACE inhibitors became available and rapidly gained acceptance as effective antihypertensive agents. Their specific effects in diabetic nephropathy, reduction in urinary albumin excretion (UAE) and preservation of renal function, in addition to and beyond their blood-pressure-lowering effect, became clear in the late 1980s through the pioneering work of Mogensen, Parving, Bjorck and others.[55–57] Numerous studies in diabetic patients with and without nephropathy have since provided additional evidence of this beneficial effect.[9,15,58–61]

ACE inhibitors are now considered to be the drugs of choice for the treatment of hypertension in diabetes and for retarding the decline in renal function in nephropathy in type 1 and most probably also in type 2 diabetes. These agents were also shown to reverse left ventricular hypertrophy in hypertensive patients and to reduce the total cardiovascular event rate in patients with diabetes with hypertension, and also in diabetic patients with microalbuminuria who initially had normal or normalized blood pressure levels (MICRO-HOPE study).[60]

### Chemical composition

ACE inhibitors can be classified into three chemical classes according to the ligand to the zinc ion of the ACE molecule. The first ACE inhibitor in clinical use, captopril, has a sulfhydryl group; one agent, fosinopril, has a phosphinyl group; and all other agents (e.g., enalapril, cilazapril, lisinopril and ramipril) contain a carboxyl group. Furthermore, ramipril has a pentane ring attached to the pyrol group, which renders the molecule more lipophilic than the other carboxyl drugs. Some ACE inhibitors (e.g., enalapril, ramipril) are absorbed as prodrugs and metabolized to the active form.

## Mode of action

ACE is widely expressed on the endothelium of blood vessels and is thus accessible to inhibitors which cause a significant reduction in blood angiotensin II levels. All the components of the renin-angiotensin system (RAS) are found in various tissues, thus allowing both autocrine and paracrine effects (heart, brain, kidney). The penetration of the various ACE inhibitors may theoretically be important in reducing local angiotensin II availability. This may be especially important in patients with diabetic nephropathy, in whom there may be a reduction in tissue perfusion in both the myocardium and the kidney. Some ACE inhibitors also show higher affinity to ACE than others. Blocking the ACE enzyme also leads to increased concentration of the vasodilator, bradykinin, which activates the arachidonic acid cascade, resulting in the synthesis of vasodilating prostaglandins as well as stimulation of nitric oxide (NO) release, probably through induction of the expression of endothelial NO synthase (eNOS). The potentiation of the bradykinin action through the blockade of its degradation is thought to augment the vasodilatory and antihypertensive potential of ACE inhibitors. ACE inhibition also decreases plasma concentration of the plasminogen activator inhibitor (PAI-1), while there is no decrease in tissue plasminogen activator (tPA).[62] Beyond the direct antihypertensive effect due to lowered blood levels of angiotensin II, several other effects which indirectly influence blood pressure and tissue perfusion also occur. For example, a decrease in aldosterone secretion may have more significance than just reducing sodium reabsorption. Blocking aldosterone secretion improves endothelial dysfunction. The addition of low-dose spironolactone to ACE inhibitor-treated patients with albuminuria results in a further significant decline in UAE, without a further reduction in blood pressure.[63]

ACE inhibitor-induced vasodilation and the fall in blood pressure take place without an increase in heart rate. Unlike with other vasodilators (e.g., hydralazine, isosorbide dinitrate), the sympathetic activity does not increase and cardiac output does not rise. However, the sympathetic surge on changing body position from supine to erect is not blunted by ACE inhibitors. It was repeatedly shown in diabetic and in elderly patients that postural hypotension, usually aggravated by antihypertensive treatment, is often alleviated by ACE inhibitors.[64] A major postulated effect of ACE inhibitors in diabetic nephropathy is the reduction of glomerular capillary pressure through vasodilation of the efferent arterioles.[65] Lowering of the glomerular perfusion pressure not only reduces shear stress and direct vascular damage but may also reduce growth-factor expression with resultant retardation of mesangial proliferation and glomerular expansion, thus slowing further renal damage. These agents also act directly on the endothelium, enhancing vasodilation, and partially improving endothelial function as manifested by improved charge-selectivity and reduced albumin excretion. Since, in diabetic nephropathy, albuminuria evokes a self-propagating process of further renal damage, reducing albumin excretion is a very important adjuvant to the lowering of blood pressure.[65]

ACE inhibitors vary in their absorption from 25% (lisinopril) to 75% (captopril) and also in the elimination half-life from 2 hr (captopril) to 40 hr (cilazapril).[45] All agents are eliminated by the kidneys both unchanged and as metabolites. The lipophilic agent ramipril is also eliminated via the liver. Most agents therefore require dose reduction when the GFR falls below 25 ml/min. In patients with severe liver disease, some increase in the dose should be expected due to reduced transformation from the prodrug to the active form. It may be safely stated, however, that most of these differences in chemical composition, absorption, elimination and degradation, as well as differential tissue penetration, are of only marginal clinical relevance. The clinically important points are as follows: captopril has to be administered twice or, preferably, three times a day in order to maintain a sustained hypotensive and vasodilatory effect; enalapril, should, in most patients, be administered twice daily especially if the early morning rise in blood pressure is to be prevented, and the same is probably true also for fosinopril. All other currently available ACE inhibitors maintain adequate 24-hr blood-pressure control when appropriate doses are used. Adjustment of dosage may be anticipated in such unstable patients as those with diabetic nephropathy due to a large variety of changing circumstances such as renal function, cardiac output, glucose control, changes in weight, concomitant diseases and other medications. It is therefore unnecessary, in most cases, to study the metabolism of a given agent in detail, but rather to respond promptly to alterations in clinical parameters, especially blood-pressure readings, postural hypotension, and serum potassium levels.

## Metabolic effects

ACE inhibitors are, most probably, metabolically neutral. Some early papers quoted reduction of HbA1c in the order of 0.2–0.4%, mainly in type 2 diabetic patients. Well-controlled trials have failed to confirm this observation. The CAPPP study, which compared a beta-blocker to an ACE inhibitor, found fewer newly diagnosed diabetic subjects among the ACE inhibitor-treated patients.[59] Further analysis of this and another study (HOPE) has been interpreted as representing a diabetes-enhancing effect of beta-blockers rather than a diabetes-sparing effect of ACE inhibitors.[60] A reduction in insulin resistance has been suggested in some studies,[66] but the effects observed appear to be of minimal clinical significance.

### Control of blood pressure

When appropriate dose adjustment is made over a period of 4–6 weeks, a reduction of 15–25% in SBP will take place in about one-half to two-thirds of the patients. The addition of low-dose HCTZ will increase this proportion of responding patients by an additional 10–15%. Several short-term studies in which various ACE inhibitors were compared to each other in a random design failed to demonstrate significant differences between the agents. When fixed doses were used, however, the results sometimes favored one agent over another. When enalapril was compared to ramipril, the trough-to-peak blood-pressure ratio was better for ramipril (50% and 64% DBP and SBP, respectively) than for enalapril (40% and 46%, respectively).[67] Since enalapril has a known shorter half-life, these results may not imply true differences in antihypertensive efficacy. Comparisons involving randomized clinical trials with appropriate dose adjustments have seldom been performed. All the cumulative clinical data indicate that when used judiciously all ACE inhibitors will produce similar results in terms of lowering blood pressure.

### Renoprotection

In most studies of patients with diabetes, in general or with nephropathy, the blood-pressure values in those receiving ACE inhibitors fell short of the recommended target values. This was due to the fact that these studies were planned prior to the present consensus on target values or because the treatment consisted of a fixed-dose regimen. Early studies in small numbers of patients with overt diabetic nephropathy showed a marked attenuation of the annual decline in GFR and a decrease in albuminuria with ACE inhibitors, both captopril and enalapril.[55] Retardation of the decline in GFR was also shown with other antihypertensive medications, but the effect on albuminuria was most prominent with ACE inhibitors.

The evidence that ACE inhibitors were indeed renoprotective in patients with type 1 diabetes and nephropathy came from the study by Lewis et al published in 1993. That study demonstrated a significant decline in the primary endpoints (doubling of serum creatinine and the development of ESRD) in the group treated with captopril.[61] Seven years later, the EUCLID study,[25] which was performed in 18 European centers, randomized type 1 patients with normo- or microalbuminuria to treatment with an ACE inhibitor (lisinopril) or placebo.[25] After 24 months, there was a significant difference in favor of the lisinopril patients both in terms of mean UAE and in the ratio of transition from normo- to microalbuminuria. However, SBP values were 3 mmHg less in the lisinopril-treated patients. In type 2 diabetes, there have been several studies which demonstrated a significant retardation of the progression of UAE and the decline in GFR in enalapril-treated patients with microalbuminuria and also in initially normoalbuminuric patients.[9,15] These studies were done in diabetic patients who were usually normotensive. Several studies on hypertensive patients with nephropathy showed a clear decline in UAE in the order of 30–40% and a slower rate of decline in GFR or parallel endpoints.[68,69] These studies comprised a small number of patients and did not extend beyond 3 years. Therefore, although in type 1 diabetes ACE inhibitors were clearly demonstrated to be renoprotective, the issue in type 2 diabetic patients was not as clearly defined. The difficulty in obtaining unequivocal results in type 2 diabetic subjects may partly relate to the diversity in the clinical and pathological disease processes which occur in these patients. The MICRO-HOPE study comprised 1140 patients with type 2 diabetes and microalbuminuria randomized to ramipril 10 mg/day or placebo.[60] The blood pressure of all patients was to be kept at normal (target) values and could include the addition of other medications. The aim of the study was to determine whether ACE inhibition has organ-protective effects independent of its antihypertensive action. Indeed, the ramipril-treated patients had, at 4.5 years, a combined primary outcome risk reduction of 25%, myocardial infarction being reduced by 22%, stroke by 33%, cardiovascular death by 37% and total mortality by 24%. The renal outcome was less dramatic but, nevertheless, significant. There was a slower rise in UAE in the ramipril-treated patients, and fewer patients on ramipril progressed from normo- to micro- and from micro- to macroalbuminuria. The proportion of patients who required laser photocoagulation tended to be less in those treated with ramipril.

## Side effects

The side-effect profile of ACE inhibitors is not different in patients with diabetic nephropathy than in the general population. During the first weeks of treatment, in association with the decline in blood pressure, a 10% reduction in GFR is to be anticipated. The GFR rises to pretreatment values upon discontinuation of treatment. However, in the long term, the cumulative decline in GFR will be less than observed with antihypertensive agents. However, not all investigators agree that ACE inhibitors are superior to other agents. Several studies in both type 1 and type 2 diabetes of 2–3 years' duration have reported that the decline in GFR is similar between ACE inhibition and other antihypertensive agents.[57]

The typical dry cough is the most common untoward effect, reported in about 10% of the patients. This side effect leads to discontinuation of ACE inhibitor in one-half to two-thirds of those patients. Most if not all patients in whom ACE inhibitors have to be discontinued due to side effects are now transferred to treatment with ARBs. Rare cases of angioneurotic edema and bone-marrow dyscrasia have also been reported. Renal artery stenosis is probably more common in patients with diabetic nephropathy than in nondiabetic patients.[70] Treating physicians must thus be aware of the possibility of bilateral or bilateral renal artery stenosis, which may need to be excluded before starting therapy. In addition, serum creatinine should be measured repeatedly in the first months of treatment in high-risk patients. Case reports of ACE inhibitor-induced acute renal failure in patients with bilateral renal artery stenosis has dissuaded many physicians from prescribing ACE inhibitors in diabetic patients with impaired renal function. However, these patients may benefit most from these agents. A systematic screening for the presence of bilateral renal artery stenosis in patients treated by ACE inhibitors and subsequent follow-up showed that in 75% of these patients there was no worsening of renal function.[71] Thus, patients with diabetic nephropathy who have clinical signs of vascular disease, such as carotid stenosis, intermittent claudication or vascular bruits, on physical examination should be investigated for the presence of renal artery stenosis prior to administration of ACE inhibitors. Ultrasound-Doppler examination of the abdominal arterial tree should be used as a screening test in patients who are thought to have vascular involvement. Nevertheless, even with normal findings on ultrasound-Doppler examination, it is imperative to monitor serum creatinine levels.

## Angiotensin II receptor blockers (ARBs)

ARBs are a relatively new class of antihypertensive agents that inhibit the renin-angiotensin system by selectively blocking the $AT_1$ subtype of $A_{II}$ receptors. Furthermore, blockade of the $AT_1$ may possibly divert more angiotensin II molecules to the AT2 receptor subtype. The beneficial effects of the ARBs are thought to be as a result of blocking the vasoconstriction, smooth-muscle proliferation, procoagulation and other effects mediated through the $AT_1$ receptor. In addition, augmenting vasodilation by nitric oxide production mediated by the AT2 receptor subtype may provide additional antihypertensive efficacy of these agents.[72]

The first oral ARB was the nonpeptide, imidazole derivative, losartan, which became available in 1993. It has moderate antihypertensive efficacy at a dose of 50 mg, comparable to 10 mg of enalapril. It soon became clear that this agent and the others which followed had a major advantage over ACE inhibitors in terms of the side-effect profile. ARBs do not block bradykinin degradation, and therefore, do not reduce the threshold for cough.[73] The excellent side-effect profile was the main reason that ARBs became the obvious substitutes for ACE inhibitors in patients who develop cough.

### Metabolic effects

Some observations have suggested a decrease in insulin resistance with ARBs, but these effects have not been reported to be of significant clinical relevance.

### Potency and dose

ARBs were found to be effective antihypertensive agents. Compared to ACE inhibitors, a similar reduction in blood pressure was obtained when the dose was adjusted appropriately. Losartan, the first ARB in clinical use, is the least potent of the currently available agents of this class. Furthermore, an increase in daily dose from 50 to 100 mg results in only a marginal increase in antihypertensive potency. This may be due to the small proportion, about 15%, of the drug which is converted to the active metabolite. The newer ARBs irbesartan and candesartan have a clearer dose-dependent profile and are at least as effective as ACE inhibitors, albeit with a side-effect profile equal to placebo. Candesartan 8 and 16 mg and irbesartan 150 and 300 mg are equipotent to enalapril 15 and 30 mg or lisinopril 10 and 20 mg.

Were it not for the comparatively high cost of these agents, ARBs would be considered the drugs of choice for the treatment of hypertension and possibly, congestive heart failure and diabetic nephropathy.

The cardioprotective effects of ARBs were at first thought to be superior to those of ACE inhibitors (ELITE 1 study).[74] However, when tested in a larger and better-controlled study which comprised over 3000 subjects, losartan had no advantage over enalapril (ELITE 2 study).[75] Several small studies had demonstrated a decrease in albuminuria in patients with diabetic nephropathy similar to the effect obtained with ACE inhibitors.[76,77] A renoprotective effect was not proven, however, until the results of three large international prospective controlled studies (3818 patients in total) were published in one issue of the *New England Journal of Medicine*.[78–80] These three studies enrolled patients with microalbuminuria[79] or with overt proteinuria and renal impairment,[78,80] and established the renoprotective effect of irbesartan and losartan by showing that these agents not only reduced albuminuria but also, over periods of 2–4 years, significantly retarded the decline in GFR and the proportion of patients developing end-stage renal failure. The RENAAL study[78] enrolled 1519 patients with type 2 diabetes, proteinuria and hypertension. The patients were randomized to treatment with losartan or placebo, while the blood pressure was controlled, in both groups, with other drugs. Treatment with losartan was associated with a risk reduction of 28% of developing ESRD, and a decline of 32% of developing any of the combined cardiovascular endpoints. Losartan treatment also reduced UAE by 35%. In the RENAAL study, losartan was noted to be effective in all subjects with nephropathy independent of baseline serum creatinine levels. In the three-arm IDNT study,[80] the effect of irbesartan was also compared to that of amlodipine. The risk of renal deterioration or death was 20–23% lower in the patients receiving irbersartan than that of those receiving placebo or amlodipine. In the RENAAL and IDNT studies, blood-pressure values were controlled by additional medications. Further analysis indicated that the effect of angiotensin II receptor blockade was greater than predicted just from the blood-pressure-lowering effect. In the IRMA-2 study, 590 patients with type 2 diabetes, hypertension and microalbuminuria were randomized to receive irbesartan (150 or 300 mg/day) or placebo. Both doses of irbesartan were found to be renoprotective when compared to placebo. The higher dose had a superior effect.[79]

Although the authors of all three studies phrased their conclusions as relevant to the specific agent and the dose (irbesartan 300 mg/day or losartan 100 mg/day), the conclusions can, most probably, be extrapolated to other, equally potent ARBs and also to ACE inhibitors. These studies, together with the ELITE and MICRO-HOPE studies, provide the rationale to use ACE inhibitors and ARBs in diabetic patients with nephropathy.[60,75,81]

Given the high price of ARBs, ACE inhibitors are often preferred and ARBs are considered only in those patients who cannot tolerate ACE inhibitors. The question whether ACE inhibitors and ARBs, if administered together, would have a more pronounced clinical effect was tested in the CALM study.[82] This study comprised 199 patients with type 2 diabetes, hypertension and microalbuminuria. The patients were randomized to 16 mg candersartan, 20 mg lisinopril, or both. The short-term, 24-week outcome showed candesartan and lisinopril to be equipotent in lowering blood pressure and in reducing albuminuria. As expected, the combination treatment was more effective than either drug alone in reducing blood pressure. Rossing et al[83] added an ARB to a group of type 2 diabetic patients, who were receiving ACE-I in addition to other medications and who had a blood pressure ≥135/85 mmHg or albuminuria >1000 mg/24 hr. The dual blockade of the RAS resulted in a reduction in albuminuria and in blood pressure. Both the CALM study and the study of Rossing used fixed doses of the tested medications. Thus, one cannot compare the efficacy of the combination to the maximal dose of each drug. If future studies do indeed demonstrate a superior effect of the combination of an ACE inhibitor with an angiotensin-receptor antagonist over maximal doses of each drug alone, then the standard antihypertensive medication may be an ARB-ACE inhibitor combination.

## Calcium-channel blockers (CCBs)

CCBs have been widely used for the treatment of cardiovascular disease, particularly angina pectoris, arrhythmias and hypertension. Their beneficial effects are related to systemic vasodilation, caused by inhibition of the inward-flow of calcium ions through the L-type calcium channels in the cell membrane. CCBs were introduced first as antianginal agents in the early 1970s and approved as antihypertensive drugs in the early 1980s.

### Composition

Three main classes of CCBs, classified according to their chemical structure, are in current use: benzothiazepines (diltiazem), phenylalkylamines (verapamil) and dihydropyridines (nifedipine, felodipine, amlodipine, lercanidipine, lacidipine, etc.). Verapamil and diltiazem show a significant affinity to cardiac muscle fibers as well as to vascular smooth muscle. They slow heart rate and have a negative inotropic effect. The dihydropyridine derivatives, as their generation advances, have become more vascular-selective with less detectable direct cardiac effects.

## Efficacy

CCBs are universally recognized as effective antihypertensive agents. They have been used in mild, moderate and severe hypertension, in young and old patients, male and female, and white and black subjects. In the Afro-American population, CCBs are more effective than ACE inhibitors. CCBs have been examined in isolated systolic hypertension in elderly patients and were found to be effective in reducing cardiovascular endpoints (the HOT study), particularly in the diabetic cohort.[84]

The early preparations of CCBs were short-acting formulations of nifedipine. These agents have been reported to be associated with an increase in the rate of sudden death in cardiac patients.[85] All currently used dihydropyridine CCBs are long-acting with a 24-hr antihypertensive effect and a trough-to-peak ratio of 0.6–0.8, which is favorable when compared to other antihypertensive classes. In contrast to ACE inhibitors, a low-sodium diet does not potentiate the antihypertensive effect of CCBs (some studies have even demonstrated a reduced activity). However, most studies have shown a potentiation of the antihypertensive effect by the addition of thiazide diuretics to CCBs.[86] This added potentiation is comparable to the effect of adding a diuretic to a beta-blocker but weaker than the combined effect of a diuretic with an ACE inhibitor.

## Renal effects

CCBs induce systemic vasodilation. In the kidney, the dilation of the afferent arterioles increases renal plasma flow and GFR. It has been postulated that this increase in glomerular perfusion may be harmful to the kidney, especially in the presence of hypertension-promoting nephrosclerosis and progressive loss of renal function. Experimental and clinical studies on the renal effect of CCBs have yielded conflicting results. This may relate to the balance between the beneficial antihypertensive effect and the damage induced by hyperperfusion.

The effect of CCBs on the diabetic kidney has been examined in many studies, both placebo-controlled and in comparison with other agents including ACE inhibitors, diuretics and beta-blockers. A reduction in UAE has been demonstrated, parallel to the lowering of blood pressure in patients with incipient as well as established diabetic nephropathy in some of these studies.[76,87] Most of these studies were small, comprising only 20–40 patients in each group, and seldom extended beyond a duration of 1 year. The role of CCBs in the treatment of diabetic nephropathy, therefore, remains undetermined. Nondihydropyridines have been shown to lead to a reduction in UAE, while the dihydropyridines have in general cases not been associated with a decrease in UAE. However, these agents may preserve renal function without reducing proteinuria, as was suggested in a study by Parving's group comparing nisoldipine to lisinopril.[88] However, the recent findings from the IDNT study provide evidence that dihydropyridines do not confer a similar degree of renoprotection to agents which interrupt the renin-angiotensin system.[80]

## Metabolic effects

Both glucose-induced insulin secretion and liver glucose release are calcium-mediated. α-Adrenergic receptor glycogenolysis is also calcium-mediated. These experimental findings of the effects of calcium on glucose metabolism alerted clinical researchers to determine whether calcium blockers could influence glucose control. Despite early reports to the contrary, long-term studies have failed to show any significant effect of CCBs on glucose homeostasis. CCBs are now the sole class of antihypertensive for which a consensus has been established that these agents are neutral in terms of glucose metabolism. These drugs also do not interact significantly with insulin or with any of the oral hypoglycemic agents.

## Side effects

The newer slow-release CCBs show an improved side-effect profile. Most of the side effects are related to vasodilation. They include leg edema, facial flushes, headache and palpitations. CCBs also worsen postural hypotension, especially in patients with diabetic neuropathy.[89]

## Clinical considerations

The decision to add a calcium-blocking agent to the treatment of a patient with diabetic nephropathy is complex. CCBs have been shown to reduce the incidence of cardiovascular complications in patients with hypertension. The risk reduction of cerebrovascular events is more pronounced with CCBs than with any other antihypertensive treatment.[90] In patients with coexistent angina pectoris, CCBs are also often used. The new dihydropyridine agents may also be safely administered in patients with congestive heart failure. Though few authorities would, at present, choose CCBs as first-line treatment in hypertensive patients with diabetic nephropathy, these drugs may be safely included in a multiagent antihypertensive regimen in patients with resistant hypertension unresponsive to other agents, or when other conditions, especially angina pectoris, provide an indication for their use. Furthermore, CCBs, especially the nondihydropyridines, may have a synergistic effect with ACE inhibitors or with ARBs in the treatment of diabetic nephropathy.

## Beta-blockers

Developed in the late 1950s by chemical modification of beta-agonists, the β-adrenergic receptor blocking agents rapidly became the most popular antihypertensive agents and maintained this position for more than two decades until the CCBs and ACE inhibitors began to dominate this arena. The antihypertensive potency of beta-blockers is equivalent to that of diuretics, and, contrary to early beliefs, the cardiovascular protection in treated patients matched that seen with diuretic treatment.

Following the introduction of beta-blockers in the early 1960s, about 20 different agents of this class were developed, each claiming an advantage over the other drugs, due to either pharmacodynamic or pharmacokinetic differences. Over the subsequent 30 years, clinicians and pharmaceutical companies were engaged in numerous studies examining the efficacy of the various beta-blockers in different populations and in different clinical settings. In retrospect, re-evaluating this large body of data, one can safely summarize that, though there are some differences between specific agents, the overall antihypertensive and cardioprotective effects of the various beta-blockers are similar if proper dose-adjustments are made. The early hypothesis, for example, that selective beta-blockers would be superior to nonselective agents was not validated, nor was the assumption that intrinsic sympathomimetic activity (ISA) would be clinically significant. The commercial success of one or other of these agents in relation to the others may be attributed mainly to the promotion by the manufacturers and sometimes as the result of a successful controlled study which had used a specific beta-blocker. Head-to-head comparisons between various beta-blockers were seldom done. In one such study, the antihypertensive potency and side effects of a nonselective agent (propranolol) were compared to selective agents without ISA (atenolol, metoprolol) and to an agent with ISA (oxprenolol).[91] The study was double-blinded with a crossover design. Atenolol, metoprolol and propranolol were equipotent (100, 200 and 160 mg/day, respectively) while oxprenolol was a weaker antihypertensive agent. There were no significant differences in side effects.

Carvedilol, a nonselective beta-blocker with alpha-blocking activity, has been widely used to treat patients with congestive heart failure. A significant decline in mortality largely due to a reduced incidence of sudden death was observed.[92] Similar results were obtained with metoprolol, a selective agent without alpha-blocking activity.[93] Numerous studies have also demonstrated a reduced short-term and 1-year mortality after acute myocardial infarction as well as after acute coronary events.[94] Both lipophilic and hydrophilic agents were used in these trials, and no difference could be found between the various agents. Beta-blockers are effective antianginal drugs, and they reduce intraocular pressure in glaucoma. Certain patients with migraine and with essential tremor benefit from beta-blockade, as do patients with tachyarrhythmia due to hyperthyroidism and patients with atrial fibrillation.

### Mode of action

The inhibition of β-adrenergic activity results in a reduction in cardiac output, a decrease in renin release, some decrease in central sympathetic activity with a decline in catecholamine release, and a variable influence on peripheral vascular resistance. The dual cardiac effect of beta-blockers, reduction in contractility and slowing the heart rate, is somewhat dose-dependent. With lower doses, the effect on the conduction system prevails while the effect on contractility diminishes. Thus, the use of relatively low doses of beta-blockers has become a mainstay in the therapy of patients with congestive heart failure and postcoronary events. Most of the beta-blockers in current use increase peripheral vascular resistance, resulting in a decline in the perfusion of partially occluded vessels. This effect is transient, however, and with continued use peripheral resistance returns to pretreatment values. When high doses of beta-blockers were in use, peripheral vascular disease was considered a major contraindication to their use. Since peripheral vascular disease (PVD) is so common among patients with diabetic nephropathy, and it usually coexists with coronary disease, this effect of beta-blocking agents can be of clinical relevance. However, the currently used smaller doses (e.g., atenolol 25 mg, metoprolol 95 mg, carvedilol ≤25 mg) have not been shown clinically to worsen perfusion in patients with PVD.

## Metabolic effects

β-Adrenergic blockers have been under scrutiny for more than three decades. Under experimental conditions, nonselective beta-blockers such as propranolol decrease insulin sensitivity by more than 30%. The selective preparations such as atenolol and metoprolol have a marginally weaker effect in the order of 20–25%, and those agents with intrinsic sympathetic activity (e.g., pindolol) are associated with a decline in muscle glucose uptake in the order of 15%. Controlled clinical studies, however, have failed to show a constant effect of these agents on $HbA_{1c}$. In type 1 diabetes, there is probably a diminished awareness of the development of hypoglycemia. This concept is very difficult to test and remains anecdotal. Therefore, this issue should not deter the use of beta-blockers when otherwise indicated. An interesting but as yet not fully explained observation in two recent large studies in nondiabetic hypertensive subjects (CAPPP and HOPE studies) was that those on beta-blockers have been at significantly greater risk of developing type 2 diabetes than those treated by other drugs, including thiazide diuretics (risk ratio of 1.4 on beta-blockers as compared to all other drugs).[59,60,95]

## Side effects

The most common side effects are those related to the central nervous system, including insomnia, nightmares, depression and some worsening of cognitive function, especially in elderly patients. Another relevant side effect in diabetic males is impotence.

## Beta-blockers in diabetic nephropathy

The direct effect of beta-blockers on the diabetic kidney has not been adequately examined. The only large controlled study in diabetic patients in which beta-blockers (atenolol) were used to treat hypertension was the UKPDS.[96] In this widely quoted study, there was no difference in the combined renal outcome between patients treated with atenolol and captopril as the initial antihypertensive agent. The results of this study, however, are difficult to interpret. The incidence of renal disease was low; thus, the differences between the two agents may not have become apparent. Furthermore, the blood-pressure levels of the patients in the intensive treatment arm (144/82 mmHg) were significantly higher than currently accepted target values. Finally, in the majority of subjects, at least two and often three drugs were used. Therefore, this study cannot be considered a true comparison of beta-blockade and ACE inhibition. The use of beta-blockers in hypertension has

been on the decline for over two decades. The very conservative, noncommittal report of the Joint National Committee (JNCVI) does not recommend beta-blockers for initial treatment of hypertension in diabetes.[1] However, many patients with diabetic nephropathy are treated with beta-blockers for other indications, such as angina pectoris, congestive heart failure or atrial fibrillation, or sinus tachycardia induced by ACE inhibitors or CCBs. One has, therefore, to be familiar with both the beneficial and the untoward effects of this class of agents.

## α- and β-receptor blockers

Two agents of this class are currently in use, carvedilol and labetalol. Carvedilol has become a very popular agent in congestive heart failure. Its use was associated with reduced mortality in patients with all degrees of heart failure (New York Heart Association classes II–IV).[92] The effect of carvedilol has been attributed partially to the vasodilation induced by the alpha-blockade. Similar results were, however, obtained with metoprolol, a beta-blocker without alpha-blocking activity.[93] Moreover, the alpha-blocking effect of carvedilol fades away with continuous use while the cardioprotective effect remains.

The other agent in this category is labetalol, a lipid-soluble, nonselective beta-blocker with selective alpha$_1$-blocking activity similar to prazosin. Unlike other beta-blockers, labetalol is a vasodilating agent which reduces peripheral resistance. It is a potent antihypertensive agent, especially when administered intravenously, and it is eliminated mainly by the liver. It can therefore be safely used in patients with ESRD. Labetalol is popular among nephrologists and is also used in diabetic patients with renal impairment or ESRD and resistant hypertension. In these patients, the potentially adverse metabolic effects of labetalol are less relevant. The main side effect of labetalol is postural hypotension, limiting its use to patients with resistant hypertension. Labetalol should be administered twice daily, and the dose range is 200–1000 mg/day. There are no data as to the specific effects of this class of medications in diabetic patients.

## α-Receptor blockers

Selective alpha-blockers were never used to a large extent in the treatment of hypertension, possibly because the first generation of these agents (e.g., prazosin) were short-acting and induced postural hypotension. At present, a long-acting representative of this class, doxazosin, has gained a significant share of the market due to its effect in alleviating the obstructive symptoms of benign prostatic hypertrophy, apparently by relaxing the tone of the prostatic muscle. This agent is, therefore, often considered in elderly hypertensive males. In addition, its mild lipid-lowering effect and its reduction of insulin-resistance by alpha-blockers have earned some popularity for doxazosin among diabetologists. Well-controlled patients may develop hypoglycemic episodes when an alpha-blocker is added to their therapeutic regimen. Minor adjustments in insulin regimens may be necessary.

Doxazosin is less lipid-soluble than prazosin and has a lower affinity to α-receptors in the vascular smooth muscle. Therefore, the onset of the blood-pressure-lowering effect is more gradual. The gradual vasodilation allows adjustment of cardiac output, thus preventing the postural fall in blood pressure. Doxazosin is therefore used in patients with congestive heart failure, especially those who require additional therapy to ACE inhibitors.

### Use in diabetic nephropathy
The use of doxazosin and other agents of this group in patients with diabetic nephropathy is associated with a decline in UAE parallel to the decline in blood-pressure levels.[21] When used in moderate doses (e.g., doxazosin 2–6 mg/day) and in combination with other agents, there is an added antihypertensive effect with a minimal increase in untoward effects. When used alone, alpha-blockers induce a continuous vasodilation, a reactive surge in aldosterone secretion with resultant increase in plasma volume sometimes manifested by peripheral edema, and thus a time-dependent decrease in the antihypertensive effect. It has, therefore, been common knowledge among internists who used alpha-blockers that these agents should be accompanied by a thiazide, or other diuretics. This clinical experience was neglected by the designers of the ALLHAT study. This NIH-sponsored study was designed to compare various antihypertensive agents and included over 15000 diabetic patients.[97] The arm initially randomized to doxazosin was prematurely interrupted due to a large number of cases of congestive heart failure. Had the study-organizing committee taken into account previous clinical experience with alpha-blockers this adverse outcome may have been anticipated and prevented. The editorials which later cautioned against the use of doxazosin in hypertensive diabetic subjects also disregarded an important lesson from the ALLHAT results—this is that rather than avoiding doxazosin, this agent should always be used in conjunction with low-dose HCTZ.

## Effects of the main antihypertensive agents on lipid metabolism

It should be stated at the outset that no antihypertensive medication has been proven to have clinically significant, beneficial or negative effects on plasma lipids. There are, however, some effects which, though minor quantitatively, may have a long-term influence on diabetic patients with nephropathy at high risk of vascular disease.

### CCBs
Analysis of lipoprotein profiles in long-term studies failed to demonstrate changes of any clinical significance. Antioxidant properties were repeatedly ascribed to several agents in this group, implying a possible antiatherogenic effect of such drugs.[98] An improvement in carotid atheromatous lesions, manifested by reduction in the intima/media index, was found in amlodipine-treated patients after 12 months.[99] Whether this is a direct effect on atherogenesis or a by-product of the lowering of blood pressure remains an open question. The CCB lercanidipine has been reported to retard atherosclerosis in several animal models.[100] The investigator proposed that this effect was related to its antioxidant property. In a clinical study, lercanidipine was found to reduce significantly the propensity of the serum of diabetic patients with nephropathy to oxidize LDL.[101]

### Beta-blockers
Subtle changes in lipoprotein composition, a decline in HDL cholesterol and an increase in LDL cholesterol and in triglyceride concentrations were reported with the use of both selective and nonselective beta-blockers. There are no long-term controlled studies in which the effect of beta-blockers on plasma lipids was the primary endpoint. Lipid levels were, nevertheless reported in many studies with neither a significant nor a consistent pattern.[102] The known cardioprotective effects of beta-blockers in patients after myocardial infarction and in those with congestive heart failure largely outweigh any untoward effect on lipoprotein metabolism. These agents are therefore freely administered in patients with dyslipidemia.

### ACE inhibitors
ACE inhibitors are generally considered to be lipid-neutral. In patients with albuminuria, a small but consistent decline in total cholesterol levels in plasma was observed in long-term clinical studies in type 2 diabetes.[103] In one study, this decline was found to be

proportional to the decrease in urinary albumin excretion rate.[87] Some early studies found an increase in HDL/total cholesterol ratio in hypertensive patients treated with captopril.

### ARBs

No significant alterations in lipoprotein metabolism have been reported with the use of this class of agent.

### Alpha-blockers

A significant decrease in plasma levels of triglycerides was observed in clinical studies and was associated with the decrease in insulin resistance, and an improvement of the removal of triglyceride-rich lipoproteins through an increase in lipoprotein lipase activity. The effect on lipoprotein lipase is probably not direct but rather secondary to the increased sensitivity to insulin action or to the dilatation of muscular arterioles and resultant increase in capillary blood flow. This effect was sustained also after 12 months of treatment.[103,104]

### The debate: CCBs in comparison with ACE inhibitors

The effect of both CCBs and ACE inhibitors on the renal outcome in patients with diabetes has been examined in many clinical studies, with conflicting results. Several reasons for the disparity of results have been advanced. These include differences in the study population, duration of the studies, fixed doses of the different drugs, and lack of specific endpoints with the study design. The first meta-analysis of 100 clinical trials on diabetic patients was published in 1993.[105] ACE inhibitors were found to decrease proteinuria and preserve GFR beyond their effect on blood pressure, while the effects of CCBs and other agents on proteinuria could be entirely accounted for by their blood-pressure-lowering effect.

This opinion was not universally accepted, however, and a series of controlled trials was launched in which CCBs and ACE inhibitors were compared directly. In most of these studies, if adequate blood-pressure control was maintained, the differences in renal outcome between the newer dihydropyridine CCBs and ACE inhibitors were marginal. Some of these studies (CAPPP, FACET, ABCD, and HOPE) demonstrated that ACE inhibitor-based regimens were significantly superior in reducing cardiovascular risk.[59,60,106,107] An extensive meta-analysis[58] published in 2001 showed that when well-designed,

double-blinded studies were analyzed, CCB-based antihypertensive treatment was associated, in diabetic patients, with a higher cardiovascular event rate and higher cardiovascular mortality than ACE inhibitor-based treatment. In fact, this analysis also demonstrated that, in terms of cardiovascular outcome, CCBs were also inferior to the conventional beta-blocker–diuretic-based regimens. Moreover, the recently published IDNT showed that in the patients receiving amlodipine the progression of the renal disease was no better than in those receiving placebo and significantly worse than in those receiving irbesartan. It should be noted that blood-pressure control was similar in all three groups.[80] The present consensus reflects these conclusions. The guidelines of the American Diabetes Association[10] and of other official bodies include ACE inhibitors as the drugs of choice for the treatment of hypertension in patients with diabetes, and especially so for those with diabetic nephropathy. CCBs are recommended for use whenever a specific indication exists, mainly angina pectoris, and also when additional drugs are required to control resistant hypertension. It is also the authors' strong belief that presently available data do not support the use of CCBs as first-choice antihypertensive agents in patients with diabetic nephropathy.

### Experimental agents

### Vasopeptidase inhibitors

A new class of antihypertensive agents currently being evaluated in clinical studies are the vasopeptidase inhibitors. These agents cause simultaneous inhibition of the neutral endopeptidases (NEP) and ACE.[108] These agents, in addition to inhibiting ACE, block the degradation of the vasodilatory peptides (mainly atrial, brain and c-type natriuretic peptides), via inhibition of NEP, thus augmenting their endothelial vasodilatory and antiproliferative activity. Though theoretically very promising, the results of limited clinical trials have hitherto been modest.[109] The first available agent of this class, omapatrilat, was found to be equipotent to an ACE inhibitor in terms of its antihypertensive effect. In patients with congestive heart failure, short-term results indicate a trend towards reduced mortality in comparison with ACE inhibitor treatment. The side-effect profile is similar to that of ACE inhibitors,[110] although the preliminary findings from the OCTAVE study suggest at least a twofold increase in angioedema when compared to enalapril.[111] However, this side effect was still rare in this hypertensive population. The documented experience with this class of agents in diabetic nephropathy is limited. Short-term results show a decrease in UAE similar to that of ACE inhibitors.

## Endothelin receptor blockers

Since endothelin-1 is the major endothelium derived, several nonselective and selective endothelin inhibitors have been synthesized. Animal experiments indicate that these agents may have potential as vasodilatory, antiproliferative and antiatherogenic agents. Human studies have so far been partly limited by an unacceptably high side-effect rate and possibly less antihypertensive potency than currently available agents.[112]

## REFERENCES

1. Joint National Committee. The Sixth Report of the Joint National Committee on Prevention, Detection, Evaluation, and Treatment of High Blood Pressure. *Arch Intern Med* 1997; **157:** 2413–46.

2. Geiss LS, Rolka DB, Engelgau MM, Elevated blood pressure among U.S. adults with diabetes, 1988–1994. *Am J Prev Med* 2002; **1:** 42–8.

3. Viberti G, Prognostic significance of microalbuminuria. *Am J Hypertens* 1994; **7:** S69–72.

4. Mogensen CE, Microalbuminuria, blood pressure and diabetic renal disease: origin and development of ideas. *Diabetologia* 1999; **42:** 263–85.

5. Fujimoto WY, The importance of insulin resistance in the pathogenesis of type 2 diabetes mellitus. *Am J Med* 2000; **108:** S9–14.

6. Stamler J, Vaccaro O, Neaton JD et al, Diabetes, other risk factors, and 12-yr cardiovascular mortality for men screened in the Multiple Risk Factor Intervention Trial. *Diabetes Care* 1993; **16:** 434–44.

7. Centers for Disease Control and Prevention. Decline in deaths from heart disease and stroke—United States, 1900–1999. *JAMA* 1999; **282:** 724–6.

8. Zimmet P, Alberti KG, Shaw J, Global and societal implications of the diabetes epidemic. *Nature* 2001; **414:** 782–7.

9. Ravid M, Savin H, Jutrin I et al, Long-term stabilizing effect of angiotensin-converting enzyme inhibition on plasma creatinine and on proteinuria in normotensive type II diabetic patients. *Ann Intern Med* 1993; **118:** 577–81.

10. American Diabetes Association. Diabetic nephropathy. *Diabetes Care* 1999; **22:** S66–9.

11. Bakris GL, Williams M, Dworkin L, Preserving renal function in adults with hypertension and diabetes: a consensus approach. National Kidney Foundation Hypertension and Diabetes Executive Committees Working Group. *Am J Kidney Dis* 2000; **36:** 646–61.

12. Sawicki PT, Heise T, Berger M, Antihypertensive treatment and mortality in diabetic patients. What is the evidence? *Diabetologia* 1997; **40** (Suppl 2): S134–7.

13. Schrier RW, Estacio RO, Esler A et al, Effects of aggressive blood pressure control in normotensive type 2 diabetic patients on albuminuria, retinopathy and strokes. *Kidney Int* 2002; **61:** 1086–97.

14. Hansson L, Zanchetti A, Carruthes SG et al, Effects of intensive blood-pressure lowering and low-dose aspirin in patients with hypertension: principal results of the Hypertension Optimal

15. Treatment (HOT) randomised trial. *Lancet* 1998; **351:** 1755–62.

15. Ravid M, Brosh D, Levi Z et al, Use of enalapril to attenuate decline in renal function in normotensive, normoalbuminuric patients with type 2 diabetes mellitus: a randomized, controlled trial. *Ann Intern Med* 1998; **128:** 982–8.

16. Millar JA, Lever AF, Burke V, Pulse pressure as a risk factor for cardiovascular events in the MRC Mild Hypertension Trial. *J Hypertens* 1999; **8:** 1065–72.

17. Viberti G, Keen H, The patterns of proteinuria in diabetes mellitus. Relevance to pathogenesis and prevention of diabetic nephropathy. *Diabetes* 1984; **33:** 686–92.

18. Robinson N, Lloyd CE, Stevens LK, Social deprivation and mortality in adults with diabetes mellitus. *Diabetic Med* 1998; **3:** 205–12.

19. Bakris GL, A practical approach to achieving recommended blood pressure goals in diabetic patients. *Arch Intern Med* 2001; **161:** 2661–7.

20. Siani A, Strazzullo P, Giacco A et al, Increasing the dietary potassium intake reduces the need for antihypertensive medications. *Ann Intern Med* 1991; **115:** 753–9.

21. Rachmani R, Levi Z, Slavachevsky I et al, Effect of an α-adrenergic blocker, and ACE inhibitor and hydrochlorothiazide on blood pressure and on renal function in type 2 diabetic patients with hypertension and albuminuria. *Nephron* 1998; **80:** 175–82.

22. Black HR, The evolution of low-dose diuretic therapy. *Am J Med* 1996; **101:** S47–52.

23. Sessa A, Battini G, Meroni M et al, Renal-retinal diabetic syndrome. *Nephron* 1999; **83:** 285–6.

24. Stratton IM, Kohner EM, Aldington SJ et al, UKPDS 50: risk factors for incidence and progression of retinopathy in type II diabetes over 6 years from diagnosis. *Diabetologia* 2001; **44:** 156–63.

25. Chaturvedi N, Sjolie AK, Stephenson JM et al, Effect of lisinopril on progression of retinopathy in normotensive people with type 1 diabetes. The EUCLID Study Group. *Lancet* 1998; **351:** 28–31.

26. Pinkney H, Foyle WJ, Denver AE et al, The relationship of urinary albumin excretion rate to ambulatory blood pressure and erythrocyte sodium-lithium countertransport in NIDDM. *Diabetologia* 1995; **38:** 356–62.

27. Ohkubo T, Imai Y, Tsuji I et al, Relation between nocturnal decline in blood pressure and mortality. The Ohasama Study. *Am J Hypertens* 1997; **11:** 1201–7.

28. Kleemola P, Jousilahti P, Pietinen P et al, Coffee consumption and the risk of coronary heart disease and death. *Arch Intern Med* 2000; **160:** 3393–400.

29. Strandberg TE, Saloma V, White coat effect, blood pressure and mortality in men: prospective cohort study. *Eur Heart J* 2000; **20:** 1714–18.

30. Rosengren A, Wilhilmsen L, Physical activity protects against coronary death and deaths from all causes in middle-aged men. Evidence from a 20-year follow-up of the Primary Prevention Study in Göteborg. *Ann Epidemiol* 1997; **7:** 69–75.

31. Mayer-Davis EF, D'Agostino R Jr, Karter AJ, Intensity and amount of physical activity in relation to insulin sensitivity. The Insulin Resistance Atherosclerosis Study. *JAMA* 1998; **279:** 669–74.

32. Clarke P, Gray A, Adler A et al, Cost-effectiveness analysis of intensive blood-glucose control with metformin in overweight patients with type II diabetes (UKPDS No. 51). *Diabetologia* 2001; **44:** 298–304.

33. Corry DB, Tuck ML, The effects of weight loss and other non-pharmacologic interventions on blood pressure. *Curr Hypertens Rep* 1999; **1:** 118.

34. UK Prospective Diabetes Study (UKPDS) Group. Intensive blood-glucose control with sulphonylureas or insulin compared with conventional treatment and risk of complications in patients with type 2 diabetes (UKPDS 33). UK Prospective

Diabetes Study (UKPDS) Group. *Lancet* 1998; **352**: 837–53.

35. UK Prospective Diabetes Study Group. Efficacy of atenolol and captopril in reducing risk of macrovascular and microvascular complications in type 2 diabetes: UKPDS 39. *BMJ* 1998; **317**: 713–20.

36. Alderman MH, Salt, blood pressure, and human health. *Hypertension* 2000; **36**: 890–3 (review).

37. Weir MR, Chrysant SG, McCarron DA, Influence of race and dietary salt on the antihypertensive efficacy of an angiotensin-converting enzyme inhibitor or a calcium channel antagonist in salt-sensitive hypertensives. *Hypertension* 1998; **31**: 1088–96.

38. Levey AS, Greene T, Beck GJ et al, Dietary protein restriction and the progression of chronic renal disease: what have all of the results of the MDRD study shown? Modification of Diet in Renal Disease Study Group. *J Am Soc Nephrol* 1999; **10**: 2426–39 (review).

39. Hermansen K, Diet, blood pressure and hypertension. *Br J Nutr* 2000; **83**: S113–19 (review).

40. Murray RP, Connett JE, Tyas SL et al, Alcohol volume, drinking pattern, and cardiovascular disease morbidity and mortality: is there a U-shaped function? *Am J Epidemiol* 2002; **155**: 242–8.

41. Neaton JD, Grimm RH Jr, Prineas RJ et al, Treatment of Mild Hypertension Study. Final results. Treatment of Mild Hypertension Study Research Group. *JAMA* 1993; **270**: 713–24.

42. Richardson AD, Piepho RW, Effect of race on hypertension and antihypertensive therapy. *Int J Clin Pharmacol Ther* 2000; **38**: 75–9.

43. Ferdinand KC, Update in pharmacologic treatment of hypertension. *Cardiol Clin* 2001; **19**: 279–94.

44. Reckelhoff JF, Gender differences in the regulation of blood pressure. *Hypertension* 2001; **37**: 1199–208.

45. Kaplan NM, *Clinical Hypertension*, 6th edn. Williams & Wilkins: Baltimore, 1994.

46. Boulton AJ, Selam JL, Sweeney M et al, Sildenafil citrate for the treatment of erectile dysfunction in men with type II diabetes mellitus. *Diabetologia* 2001; **44**: 1296–301.

47. Fedele D, Lamonica M, Bax G, Experience with sildenafil in diabetes. *Diabetes Nutr Metab* 2002; **15**: 49–52.

48. Olsson AM, Persson CA, Efficacy and safety of sildenafil citrate for the treatment of erectile dysfunction in men with cardiovascular disease. *Int J Clin Pract* 2001; **55**: 171–6.

49. EUCLID Study Group. Randomised placebo-controlled trial of lisinopril in normotensive patients with insulin-dependent diabetes and normoalbuminuria or microalbuminuria. *Lancet* 1997; **349**: 1787–92.

50. Savage PJ, Pressel SL, Curb JD et al, Influence of long-term, low-dose, diuretic-based, antihypertensive therapy on glucose, lipid, uric acid, and potassium levels in older men and women with isolated systolic hypertension: the Systolic Hypertension in the Elderly Program. SHEP Cooperative Research Group. *Arch Intern Med* 1998; **158**: 741–51.

51. Lindholm LH, Hansson L, Ekbom T et al, Comparison of antihypertensive treatments in preventing cardiovascular events in elderly diabetic patients: results from the Swedish Trial in Old Patients with Hypertension—2. STOP Hypertension—2 Study Group. *J Hypertens* 2000; **18**: 1671–5.

52. Lakshman MR, Reda DJ, Materson BJ et al, Diuretics and beta-blockers do not have adverse effects at 1 year on plasma lipid and lipoprotein profiles in men with hypertension. Department of Veterans Affairs Cooperative Study Group on Antihypertensive Agents. *Arch Intern Med* 1999; **159**: 551–8.

53. Reyes AJ, Diuretics in the therapy of hypertension. *J Hum Hypertens* 2002; **16**: S78–83.

54. Pedersen MM, Christensen CK, Hansen KW et al, ACE-inhibition and renoprotection in early diabetic nephropathy. Response to enalapril acutely and in long-term combination

with conventional antihypertensive treatment. *Clin Invest Med* 1991; **14**: 642–51.

55. Bjorck S, Mulec H, Johnsen SA et al, Renal protective effect of enalapril in diabetic nephropathy. *BMJ* 1992; **304**: 339–43.

56. Mogensen CE, Angiotensin converting enzyme inhibitors and diabetic nephropathy. *BMJ* 1992; **304**: 327–8.

57. Parving HH, Rossing P, Hommel E et al, Angiotensin-converting enzyme inhibition in diabetic nephropathy: ten years experience. *Am J Kidney Dis* 1995; **26**: 99–107.

58. ACE Inhibitors in Diabetic Nephropathy Trialist Group. Should all patients with type I diabetes mellitus and microalbuminuria receive angiotensin-converting enzyme inhibitors? A meta-analysis of individual patients data. *Ann Intern Med* 2001; **134**: 370–9.

59. Hansson L, Lindholm LH, Niskanen L et al, Effect of angiotensin-converting-enzyme inhibition compared with conventional therapy on cardiovascular morbidity and mortality in hypertension: Captopril Prevention Project (CAPPP) randomised trial. *Lancet* 1999; **353**: 611–16.

60. Heart Outcomes Prevention Evaluation (HOPE) Study Investigators. Effects of ramipril on cardiovascular and microvascular outcomes in people with diabetes mellitus: results of the HOPE study and MICRO-HOPE substudy. *Lancet* 2000; **355**: 253–9.

61. Lewis EJ, Huniscker LG, Bain RP et al, The effect of angiotensin-converting-enzyme inhibition on diabetic nephropathy. *N Engl J Med* 1993; **329**: 1456–62.

62. Vaughan DE, Angiotensin and vascular fibrinolytic balance. *Am J Hypertens* 2002; **15**: 3S-8S.

63. Chrysostomou A, Becker G, Spironolactone in addition to ACE inhibition to reduce proteinuria in patients with chronic renal disease. *N Engl J Med* 2001; **345**: 925–6.

64. Slavachevsky I, Rachmani R, Levi Z et al, Effect of enalapril and nifedipine on orthostatic hypotension in older hypertensive patients. *J Am Geriatr Soc* 2000; **48**: 807–10.

65. Remuzzi G, Ruggeneti P, Perico N, Chronic renal disease: renoprotective benefits of rennin-angiotensin system inhibition. *Ann Intern Med* 2002; **136**: 604–15.

66. Feldman RD, Schmidt ND, Quinapril treatment enhances vascular sensitivity to insulin. *J Hypertens* 2001; **19**: 113–18.

67. Yasky J, Verho M, Erasmus TP et al, Efficacy of ramipril versus enalapril in patients with mild to moderate essential hypertension. *Br J Clin Pract* 1996; **50**: 302–10.

68. Bakris G, Barnhill BW, Sadler R, Treatment of arterial hypertension in diabetic humans: importance of therapeutic selection. *Kidney Int* 1992; **41**: 912–19.

69. Kasiske BL, Kalil RSN, Ma JZ et al, Effect of antihypertensive therapy on the kidneys in patients with diabetes: a metaregression analysis. *Ann Intern Med* 1993; **118**: 129–38.

70. Courreges JP, Bacha J, Aboud E et al, Prevalence of renal artery stenosis in type 2 diabetes. *Diabetes Metab* 2000; **4**: S90–6.

71. Gilbert RE, Cooper ME, Krum H, Drug administration in patients with diabetes mellitus. Safety considerations. *Drug Saf* 1998; **18**: 441–55.

72. Li D, Chen H, Mehta JL, Angiotensin II via activation of type 1 receptor upregulates expression of endoglin in human coronary artery endothelial cells. *Hypertension* 2001; **38**: 1062–7.

73. Pylypchuk GB, ACE inhibitor- versus angiotensin II blocker-induced cough and angioedema. *Ann Pharmacother* 1998; **32**: 1060–6 (review).

74. Houghton AR, Harrison M, Cowley AJ, Haemodynamic, neurohumoral and exercise effects of losartan vs. captopril in chronic heart failure: results of an ELITE trial substudy. Evaluation of Losartan in the elderly. *Eur J Heart Fail* 1999; **4**: 385–93.

75. Pitt B, Poole-Wilson PA, Segal R et al, Effect of losartan compared with captopril on mortality in patients with symptomatic

heart failure: randomised trial— the Losartan Heart Failure Survival Study ELITE II. *Lancet* 2000; **355**: 1582–7.

76. Chan JC, Critchley JA, Tomlinson B et al, Antihypertensive and anti-albuminuric effects of losartan potassium and felodipine in Chinese elderly hypertensive patients with or without non-insulin-dependent diabetes mellitus. *Am J Nephrol* 1997; **17**: 72–80.

77. Andersen S, Tarnow L, Rossing P et al, Renoprotective effects of angiotensin II receptor blockade in type 1 diabetic patients with diabetic nephropathy. *Kidney Int* 2000; **57**: 601–6.

78. Brenner BM, Cooper ME, de Zeeuw D et al, Effects of losartan on renal and cardiovascular outcomes in patients with type 2 diabetes and nephropathy. *N Engl J Med* 2001; **345**: 861–9.

79. Parving HH, Lehnert H, Brochner-Mortensen J et al, The effect of irbesartan on the development of diabetic nephropathy in patients with type 2 diabetes. *N Engl J Med* 2001; **345**: 870–8.

80. Lewis EJ, Unsicker LG, Clarke WR et al, Renoprotective effect of the angiotensin-receptor antagonist irbesartan in patients with nephropathy due to type 2 diabetes. *N Engl J Med* 2001; **345**: 851–60.

81. Sica DA, Bakris GL, Current concepts of pharmacotherapy in hypertension: type 2 diabetes: RENAAL and IDNT—the emergence of new treatment options. *J Clin Hypertens* 2002; **4**: 52–7.

82. Mogensen CE, Neldam S, Tikkanen I et al, Randomised controlled trial of dual blockade of renin-angiotensin system in patients with hypertension, microalbuminuria, and non-insulin dependent diabetes: the candesartan and lisinopril microalbuminuria (CALM) study. *BMJ* 2000; **321**: 1440–4.

83. Rossing K, Christensen PK, Jensen BR et al, Dual blockade of the rennin-angiotensin system in diabetic nephropathy. *Diabetes Care* 2002; **25**: 95–100.

84. Ruilope LM, Cardiovascular and renal risks of calcium-channel blockers— news from the HOT study. *Nephrol Dial Transplant* 1999; **14**: 286–7.

85. Friedmann J, Behar S, Reicher H, Two cases of sudden death documented by Holter monitor during Secondary Prevention Reinfarction Nifedipine Trial (SPRINT). *Am Heart J* 1986; **111**: 1011–13.

86. Morgan TO, Anderson AI, MacInnis RJ, ACE inhibitors, beta-blockers, calcium blockers, and diuretics for the control of systolic hypertension. *Am J Hypertens* 2001; **14**: 241–7.

87. Bakris GL, Smith AC, Richardson DJ et al, Impact of an ACE inhibitor and calcium antagonist on microalbuminuria and lipid subfractions in type 2 diabetes: a randomized, multi-centre pilot study. *J Hum Hypertens* 2002; **16**: 185–91.

88. Tarnow L, Rossing P, Jensen C et al, Long-term renoprotective effect of nisoldipine and lisinopril in type 1 diabetic patients with diabetic nephropathy. *Diabetes Care* 2000; **23**: 1725–30.

89. Lichtlen PR, Risks and benefits of calcium antagonists. *Lancet* 1995; **346**: 962–3.

90. Doyle AE, A review of the short-term benefits of antihypertensive treatment with emphasis on stroke. *Am J Hypertens* 1993; **6**: S6–S8.

91. Ravid M, Lang R, Jutrin I, The relative antihypertensive potency of propranolol, oxprenolol, atenolol, and metoprolol given once daily. *Arch Intern Med* 1985; **145**: 1321–5.

92. Joglar JA, Acusta AP, Shusterman NH et al, Effect of carvedilol on survival and hemodynamics in patients with atrial fibrillation and left ventricular dysfunction: retrospective analysis of the US Carvedilol Heart Failure Trials Program. *Am Heart J* 2001; **142**: 498–501.

93. Sabio JM, Jimenez-Alonso J, Effects of beta-blocker therapy in severe chronic heart failure. *N Engl J Med* 2001; **345**: 998–9.

94. Wikstrand J, Berglund G, Tuomilehto J, Beta-blockade in the primary prevention of coronary heart disease in hypertensive patients. Review of present evidence. *Circulation* 1991; **84**: VI93–100 (review).

95. Gress TW, Nieto FJ, Shahar E et al, Hypertension and antihypertensive therapy as risk factors for type 2 diabetes mellitus. Atherosclerosis Risk in Communities Study. *N Engl J Med* 2000; **342**: 905–12.

96. Diabetes Study Group. Efficacy of atenolol and captopril in reducing risk of macrovascular and microvascular complications in type 2 diabetes: UKPDS 39. *BMJ* 1998; **317**: 713–20.

97. Antihypertensive and Lipid-Lowering Treatment to Prevent Heart Attack Trial (ALLHAT). Major cardiovascular events in hypertensive patients randomized to doxazosin vs chlorthalidone. *JAMA* 2000; **283**: 1967–75.

98. Kramsch DM, Sharma RC, Limits of lipid-lowering therapy: the benefits of amlodipine as an anti-atherosclerotic agent. *J Hum Hypertens* 1995; **9**: S3–S9 (review).

99. Koshiyama H, Tanaka S, Minamikawa J, Effect of calcium channel blocker amlodipine on the intimal-medial thickness of carotid arterial wall in type 2 diabetes. *J Cardiovasc Pharmacol* 1999; **33**: 894–6.

100. Bellosta S, Bernini F, Lipophilic calcium antagonists in antiatherosclerotic therapy. *Curr Atheroscler Rep* 2000; **2**: 76–81.

101. Digiesi V, Fiorillo C, Cosmi L et al, Reactive oxygen species and antioxidant status in essential arterial hypertension during therapy with dihydropyridine calcium channel antagonists. *Clin Ter* 2000; **151**: 15–18.

102. Maitland-van der Zee AH, Klungel OH, Kloosterman JM et al, The association between antihypertensive drug therapies and plasma lipid levels in the general population. *J Hum Hypertens* 2001; **15**: 701–5.

103. Kasiske BL, Ma JZ, Kalil RS et al, Effects of antihypertensive therapy on serum lipids. *Ann Intern Med* 1995; **122**: 133–41.

104. Waite MA, Alpha I blockers: antihypertensives whose positive metabolic profile with regard to hyperinsulinaemia and lipid metabolism cannot be ignored. *J Intern Med* 1991; **735**: S113–17.

105. Kasiske BL, Kalil RS, Ma JZ et al, Effect of antihypertensive therapy on the kidney in patients with diabetes: a meta-regression analysis. *Ann Intern Med* 1993; **118**: 129–38.

106. Estacio RO, Schrier RE, Antihypertensive therapy in type 2 diabetes: implications of the Appropriate Blood Pressure Control in Diabetes (ABCD) trial. *Am J Cardiol* 1998; **82**: 9R–14R.

107. Tatti P, Pahor M, Byington RP, Outcome results of the Fosinopril versus Amlodipine Cardiovascular Events Randomized Trial (FACET) in patients with hypertension and NIDDM. *Diabetes Care* 1998; **21**: 597–603.

108. Nawarskas J, Rajan V, Frishman WH, Vasopeptidase inhibitors, and dual inhibitors of angiotensin-converting enzyme and neutral endopeptidase. *Heart Dis* 2001; **3**: 378–85.

109. Nathisuwan S, Talbert RL, A review of vasopeptidase inhibitors: a new modality in the treatment of hypertension and chronic heart failure. *Pharmacotherapy* 2002; **22**: 27–42.

110. Rouleau JL, Pfeffer MA, Stewart DJ et al, Comparison of vasopeptidase inhibitor, omapatrilat, and lisinopril on exercise tolerance and morbidity in patients with heart failure: IMPRESS randomised trial. *Lancet* 2000; **356**: 615–20.

111. Messerli FH, Nussberger J, Vasopeptidase inhibition and angio-oedema. *Lancet* 2000; **356**: 608–9.

112. Drum H, Viskoper RJ, Lacourciere Y et al, The effect of an endothelin-receptor antagonist, bosentan, on blood pressure in patients with essential hypertension. Bosentan Hypertension Investigator. *N Engl J Med* 1998; **338**: 784–90.

# 8

# Treatment of diabetic nephropathy: low-protein diet

Norman R Waugh and Aileen Robertson

## BACKGROUND

The story of protein restriction in renal disease goes back to at least the work of Addis in 1948, and is summarized by Simini.[1] Addis hypothesized that protein restriction would not only relieve the symptoms of uraemia, but would also prevent further damage by reducing the load on the remaining nephrons. Brenner et al[2] took the story forward by documenting the rise in glomerular capillary pressure and hyperfiltration due to high dietary protein intake, and then Remuzzi and Bertani[3] showed that increased protein traffic across the glomerulus could cause progression of renal disease. Attention then focused on the effect of antihypertensive therapies such as ACE inhibitors (for review, see Kasiske et al,[4] or Chapter 7), both in hypertensive and non-hypertensive diabetic subjects. These so-called non-hypertensive subjects may not actually be normotensive, and the effect of these agents may be via lowering of blood pressure rather than an intrarenal mechanism.[5] There was perhaps a loss of interest in low-protein diets (LPD), especially following the largest ever trial of protein restriction, the Modification of Diet in Renal Disease (MDRD) study,[6] which reported that protein restriction did not appear to affect the decline in renal function. However, there were only 25 patients with type 2 diabetes in the MDRD (those with type 1 were excluded from the trial); glomerulonephritis and polycystic disease made up about half, and there was some evidence of variation in response according to the aetiology of the renal impairment. Furthermore, compliance with the LPD was shown to be possible, and when a secondary analysis was performed, taking into account compliance and not intention to treat, the results were more promising.[7]

Given previous trials showing some benefit in diabetes, albeit with small numbers,[8] and the publication of some new studies, another review is indicated.

## NORMAL DIETARY PROTEIN INTAKE

Current dietary protein intake in people with type 1 diabetes was reported to be 1.5 g/kg per day in the EuroDiab Complications Study;[9] about 70% was from animal protein. This was similar to that in the USA.[10] Other studies have reported lower intakes. Gall et al[11] found an average intake of 0.88 g/kg per day in a small group of patients with type 2 diabetes and nephropathy. A survey from the UK[12] noted that Asian people with diabetes had a lower protein intake than Europeans (47 versus 76 g per day), though the difference declined with increasing length of residence in the UK.

The method of estimating protein intake affects the reported level. Snetselaar et al[13] found that healthy clinical staff tended to underestimate protein consumption in food diaries when the actual intake of protein was estimated with biological markers. The protein content of the diabetic diet has been reviewed by Henry.[14]

It has long been known that protein restriction is effective in alleviating the symptoms of uraemia[15] and that it can delay the onset of dialysis.[16] The key question to be addressed in this chapter is whether protein restriction is useful not just for symptomatic relief in patients with ESRF, but whether its use in early diabetic nephropathy (characterized by either microalbuminuria or frank proteinuria) can prevent or delay the onset of ESRF.

## GRADES OF EVIDENCE

It is generally agreed that the highest quality of evidence comes from properly conducted randomized, controlled trials (RCTs), since, by the avoidance of conscious or unconscious bias, these provide more reliable results. However, in situations such as diabetic nephropathy, where the natural history of a disease process shows invariable progression[17–20] even though individuals progress at different rates, it can be argued that an RCT is not necessary since other forms of comparison such as before and after, or crossover, trials, are sufficiently reliable.[21] Indeed Mogensen[17] argues this in his paper: 'Such measurements of rate of progression would also allow for control studies of possible therapeutical trials.'

However, patients who take part in RCTs may be a selected group in whom compliance with treatment may be better than average, and so even if the results are internally valid, caution is required when generalizing them to all patients.

The progression rate without treatment has been reported to be a decline in GFR of 9–14 ml/min per year in type 1 DM with proteinuria[17,22,23] but to be slower in patients with type 2 diabetes with nephropathy—a decline of about 6 ml/min per year in a Danish study.[11] The latter finding is in line with earlier work by Fabre et al,[24] who reported that patients with type 2 diabetes developed proteinuria earlier in the known duration of diabetes but progressed more slowly. These rates yield a baseline which should be sufficient to detect a clinically useful effect of protein restriction.

There have been many studies of protein restriction but many have been very short term—some only a few days, or even after a single meal. These may be able to show efficacy, but trials of much longer duration are needed to demonstrate convincingly real-life effectiveness, which will depend on efficacy, practicality and tolerability. Another problem is that almost all studies have been in type 1 diabetes. Although the risk of nephropathy is less in type 2 diabetes, the absolute numbers of patients mean that in Europe and the USA as many as or more patients with type 2 than type 1 are starting ESRF treatment.[25–27]

Other problems with evidence include the following:

- what is meant by protein restriction, in terms of gram per day or g/kg per day, and whether body weight is actual or ideal
- whether studies assess the extent of compliance
- what other dietary changes occur, such as a shift from animal to vegetable protein, or alterations in phosphate intake
- what non-dietary therapeutic changes occur, such as antihypertensive treatment
- the outcome used and how it is measured
- the definition and stage of nephropathy (microalbuminuria, raised creatinine, etc.)
- study design—numbers, representativeness, etc.

The ideal study might be a randomized trial of different levels and types of restriction, done with large numbers of patients, both type 1 and type 2, already optimally treated with an ACE inhibitor, over a period of perhaps 10 years, with time to ESRF as the outcome measure. We have found no such studies.

The best outcome measure available at present is the glomerular filtration rate (GFR). Most studies have used creatinine clearance, although there is some tubular secretion of creatinine, which leads to an overestimation of GFR. There are thus theoretical reasons for preferring more accurate methods such as the clearance of iothalamate, EDTA or some other suitable marker.[28,29] Another problem is that protein restriction eventually results in the reduction of serum creatinine.[30] However, what matters for present purposes is the rate of decline, and although creatinine clearance may somewhat overestimate renal function when compared to other methods, there is a high correlation between the rates of decline.[31] Some studies used cimetidine to block tubular transport of creatinine, resulting in a clearance value, which approximates that of GFR. More recent studies such as the MDRD[6] tend to use the more accurate measurements of GFR or a mathematical estimation of the GFR using serum creatinine.

## METHODS

We have reviewed studies which have examined the effects of dietary protein restriction in diabetic patients. Full details of methods such as search strategies will be given in the updated Cochrane review.[8] In brief, we have included both RCTs and before and after studies. Since creatinine clearance takes several months to reach equilibrium,[32] we have excluded studies with duration less than 4 months, and those in which changes in other treatment, particularly antihypertensives, confounded the results. We have used GFR (using best method if it was estimated by more than one in the study) as the main outcome measure; have included both type 1 and type 2; have excluded studies if details of the diet were not given; have searched English language (searches 1997 and 2000) and Italian (1999) (because many of the best studies come from Italy); and have looked for details of measurement of compliance, preferably by a biological method rather than self-reporting. Assessment of compliance is important for two reasons: firstly, as a guide to what patients can tolerate over long periods; secondly, as a guide to actual, rather than prescribed intake, since if a trial shows benefit, we need to know what level of restriction was efficacious. There was no restriction on size of study, since even small studies, if otherwise sound, can contribute to a meta-analysis.

## RESULTS

Most of the trials in the literature are very short term. Table 8.1 lists those which met our criteria.[33–41] It is pleasing to see a trial[38] in subjects with type 2 diabetes, though it should be noted that this study included mainly patients without microalbuminuria.

Nearly all the trials showed that protein restriction slows the decline in renal function. The average decline with LPD in the type 1 studies was 11 ml/min a year less than that on usual diets, or 8 ml/min less if the Ciavarella et al study[36] is excluded. (It is a bit of an outlier, showing a dramatic difference, and was a small study with mean follow-up of only 4.5 months, a fact which meant it only just met our criteria.) Since the usual decline in GRF is around 10 ml/min per year, this implies that patients who comply with the LPD can delay dialysis by, on average, 10 months, using the 8 ml/min figure. However, that average conceals marked variation among patients.

The number of patients with type 1 diabetes who were on LPD was only 100 (93 if the Ciavarella et al study is excluded). The study in type 2 diabetes by Pijls and colleagues[38] gave disappointing results, because the patients did not comply with the diet. However, the Walker et al[40] and Zeller et al[41] studies show that compliance is possible for most patients over a 3-year period, though both of those studies had less protein restriction than some of the shorter-term ones. The largest benefits were seen in the short-term studies, and the longer-term ones,[34,40,41] with follow-up for 2 years or more, are probably more representative of what would be seen in routine care, with an average reduction in decline of about 8 ml/min per year

## DISCUSSION

The questions usually asked in a health technology assessment are as follows:

- does it work?
- at what cost?
- is it worth it?

The answer to the first is that trials of protein restriction in type 1 diabetes are consistent in showing that there is benefit, in terms of slowing of progression. The only exception is the Dullaart et al study,[37] in which those on the LPD did worse. We have no good evidence of efficacy in type 2, because of lack of compliance with diet in the Pijls et al study.[38]

The question of cost refers not just to health-care costs, which would be minimal—mainly dietetic time, since patients would be having regular follow-up at diabetic clinics anyway. But there would be monetary and non-monetary costs to patients. People with diabetes already have various dietary restrictions, and we know that adherence to diet is already imperfect, with most people in two studies exceeding the recommended level of protein.[42,43] Adding protein restriction to the existing restrictions makes life more difficult. With very low levels such as 0.3 g/kg per day, special foods and supplements are needed. Intake of dairy produce has to be restricted to reduce phosphate intake. With the 40-g protein diet, calorie intake has to be maintained with low-protein, high-calorie foods. A 40-g protein diet allows only 200 ml of milk, 100 g meat, and 100 g bread, a day. We sent a questionnaire to renal dieticians in Scotland in 1997, asking about actual policies. Most used only modest restriction, to 0.8–1.0 g/kg per day.

The third question – is it worth it – depends on the balance between delaying the onset of renal replacement therapy, usually dialysis, and the costs to patients. The mean delay in decline towards ESRF was about 8 months. However, there might now be less to gain because of treatment with ACE inhibitors (ACEIs), which, in patients with proteinuria, slow progression[5] (see Chapter 7). One cannot be sure that the effects of protein restriction and ACEIs are independent. If protein restriction works by reducing the load on the kidney and hence reducing hyperfiltration, would it provide additional benefits in patients already on an ACEI?

A fourth and important question is whether we could achieve almost as much by changing the type of protein in the diet, rather than the amount. Jibani et al[44] found that albumin excretion rates fell when patients with microalbuminuria were given a predominantly vegetarian diet, although the results

**Table 8.1 Included studies.**

| Study | No. of patients | Design | UPD g/kg/day | LPD g/kg/day | Duration | GFR change on UPD | GFR change on LPD | Difference | Reduction in decline per year |
|---|---|---|---|---|---|---|---|---|---|
| Barsotti et al 1988[33] | 8, type 1 | Before and after | >1.2 | 0.3 vegetarian | 11 months | −1.48 ml/min/ month | −0.13 ml/min/ month | 1.33 | 16 ml/min |
| Barsotti et al 1998[34] | 32 and 22 type 1; 10 type 2 | Before and after | Not stated | 0.3 or 0.7 | 2–8 years | −0.9 | −0.22 | 0.68 | 8.2 ml/min |
| Brouhard and LaGrone 1990[35] | 15 type 1 | RCT | 1.0 | 0.6 | 12 months | −0.68 | 0.28 | 0.4 | 4.8 |
| Ciavarella et al 1987[36] | 16 type 1 | RCT | 1.5 | 0.7 | 4.5 months | −0.9 | +3.3 | 4.1 | 49 |
| Dullaart et al 1993[37] | 30 type 1 | RCT | 1.1 | 0.7 | 2 years | −0.42 | −0.75 | −0.33 | Increased decline by 4 ml/min |
| Pijls et al 1999[38] | 160 type 2 (40 dropped out) | RCT | 1.2 | 0.8 (see note 2) | 12 months | −0.1 | −0.2 | −0.1 | Insignificant increase in decline |
| Raal et al 1994[39] | 32 type 1 | RCT | 1.6 or over | 0.8 | 6 months | −1.3 | +0.5 | 1.8 | 22 |
| Walker et al 1989[40] | 15 type 1 (see note 1) | Before and after | 1.13 | 0.67 | 33 months | −0.54 | −0.17 | 0.37 | 4.4 |
| Zeller et al 1991[41] | 35 type 1 | RCT | 1 or more | 0.6 | 35 months | 1.0 | 0.26 | 0.74 | 8.9 |

UPD: usual protein diet; LPD: low-protein diet.
1. In the study by Walker et al,[40] 19 patients were included, but four were started on antihypertensive treatment while on the low-protein diet; these patients have been excluded in the table above.
2. The diets given were as prescribed. In the Pijls et al study,[38] compliance was poor and the true difference in intake was only 0.03 g/kg per day at 12 months.
3. Where GFR was measured by more than one method, we have used the more reliable one, rather than creatinine clearance.

were confounded by a sizeable drop in total protein intake, from 1.4 to 1.0 g/kg per day. Pecis et al[45] compared three diets—usual diet with 1.4 g/kg per day, an LPD with 0.5 g/kg per day, and a test diet in which chicken and fish replaced red meat. They found that the chicken and fish diet had similar effects on GFR to the LPD, but was much more acceptable. However, this was a short-term study with only 3 weeks on each diet. They hypothesize that this is due to the much lower levels of glycine, alanine and arginine in chicken and fish compared to red meat, these being the amino acids with greatest effect on GFR. If such diets are as effective as low-protein ones, then compliance becomes less of an issue.

## Research needs

We agree with Cooper[46] that a large prospective study is needed, and that compliance is important. Compliance may be much better with changes in type of protein (chicken, fish, vegetarian) and future studies should have three arms—usual diet, LPD, and usual level but different types. Trials need to be longer-term, and we need more in type 2 diabetes. We also need to find out whether the benefits are still seen in those treated with ACE or ACII inhibitors.

## CONCLUSION

The present body of evidence suggests that protein restriction can slow progression in early nephropathy, although the effect is fairly modest, and that it has a place in treatment.

## ACKNOWLEDGEMENTS

We thank Karla Bergerhoff of the Cochrane Metabolic and Endocrine Disorders Group for doing the main searches for this review, and Elizabeth Hodges for assistance in obtaining the studies.

## REFERENCES

1. Simini B, Proteins and pathogenesis of renal disease progression. *Lancet* 1998; **352:** 1315.
2. Brenner BM, Meyer TW, Hostetter TH, Dietary protein intake and the progressive nature of kidney disease. *N Engl J Med* 1982; **307:** 652–9.
3. Remuzzi G, Bertani T, Is glomerulosclerosis a consequence of altered glomerular permeability to macromolecules? *Kidney Int* 1990; **38:** 384–94.
4. Kasiske BL, Kalil RS, Ma JZ et al, Effect of antihypertensive therapy on the kidney in patients with diabetes: a meta-regression analysis. *Ann Intern Med* 1993; **118:** 129–38.
5. Lovell H, Are angiotensin converting enzyme inhibitors useful for normotensive diabetic patients with microalbuminuria? Cochrane Database of Systematic Reviews, 1999.
6. Klahr S, Levey AS, Beck GJ et al, The effects of dietary protein restriction and blood pressure control on the progression of chronic renal disease. *N Engl J Med* 1994; **330:** 877–84.
7. Levey AS, Adler S, Caggiula AW, for the Modification of Diet in Renal Disease Study Group. Effects of dietary protein restriction on the progression of advanced renal disease. *Am J Kidney Dis* 1996; **27:** 652–63.
8. Waugh NR, Robertson A, Protein restriction for diabetic renal disease. Cochrane Database of Systematic Reviews, 1997.
9. Toeller M, Buyken A, Heitkamp G et al for the EURODIAB IDDM Complications Study Group. Protein intake and urinary albumin excretion rates in the EURODIAB IDDM Complications Study. *Diabetologia* 1997; **40:** 1219–26.
10. Breyer JA, Medical management of nephropathy in type 1 diabetes mellitus: current recommendations. *J Am Soc Nephrol* 1995; **6:** 1523–9.
11. Gall M-A, Nielsen FS, Smidt UM et al, The course of kidney function in type 2 diabetic patients with diabetic nephropathy. *Diabetologia* 1993; **36:** 1071–8.
12. Tindall H, Martin P, Nagi D et al, Higher levels of microproteinuria in Asian compared with European patients with diabetes mellitus and their relationship to dietary protein intake and diabetic complications. *Diabetic Med* 1993; **11:** 37–41.
13. Snetselaar LG, Chenard CA, Hunsicker LG et al, Protein calculation from food diaries of adult humans underestimates values determined using a biological marker. *J Nutr* 1995; **125:** 2333–40.
14. Henry RR, Protein content of the diabetic diet. *Diabetes Care* 1994; **17:** 1502–13.
15. Attman P-O, Bucht H, Larsson O et al, Protein-reduced diet in diabetic renal failure. *Clin Nephrol* 1983; **19:** 217–20.
16. Walser M, Hill S, Can renal replacement therapy be deferred by a supplemented very low protein diet? *J Am Soc Nephrol* 1999; **10:** 110–16.
17. Mogensen C, Progression of nephropathy in long-term diabetics with proteinuria and effect of initial anti-hypertensive treatment. *Scand J Clin Lab Invest* 1976; **36:** 383–8.
18. Parving H-H, Smidt UM, Friisberg B et al, A prospective study of glomerular filtration rate and arterial blood pressure in insulin-dependent diabetics with diabetic nephropathy. *Diabetologia* 1981; **20:** 457–61.
19. Jones RH, Hayakawa H, Mackay JD et al, Progression of diabetic nephropathy. *Lancet* 1979; **i:** 1105–6.
20. Berglund J, Lins L-E, Lins P-E, Predictability in diabetic nephropathy. *Acta Med Scand* 1984; **215:** 263–70.
21. Waugh NR, Grades of evidence. *Health Bull (Edin)* 1999; **57:** 53–63.
22. Viberti GC, Bilous RW, Mackintosh D et al, Monitoring glomerular function in diabetic nephropathy. *Am J Med* 1983; **74:** 256–64.
23. Sampson MJ, Griffith VS, Drury PL, Blood pressure, diet and the progression of nephropathy in patients with type 1 diabetes and hypertension. *Diabetic Med* 1993; **11:** 150–4.
24. Fabre J, Balant LP, Dayer PG et al, The kidney in maturity onset diabetes mellitus: a clinical study of 510 patients. *Kidney Int* 1982; **21:** 730–8.
25. Raine AEG, The rising tide of diabetic nephropathy— the warning before the flood? *Nephrol Dial Transplant* 1995; **10:** 460–1.
26. Rettig B, Teutsch SM, The incidence of end-stage renal disease

in type 1 and type 2 diabetes mellitus. *Diabet Nephrop* 1984; **3:** 26–7.

27. Catalano C, Postorino M, Kelly PJ et al, Diabetes mellitus and renal replacement therapy in Italy: prevalence, main characteristics and complications. *Nephrol Dial Transplant* 1990; **5:** 788–96.

28. Shemesh O, Golbetz H, Kriss JP et al, Limitations of creatinine as a filtration marker in glomerulopathetic patients. *Kidney Int* 1985; **28:** 830–88.

29. Walser M, Drew HH, La France ND, Creatinine measurements often yielded false estimates of progression in chronic renal failure. *Kidney Int* 1988; **34:** 412–18.

30. Westberg G, Protein restriction in chronic renal failure. *Lancet* 1985; **i:** 102.

31. Norden G, Diabetic nephropathy: a clinical study of risk factors in type 1 diabetes mellitus. *Scand J Urol Nephrol* 1988 (Suppl 116).

32. Zeller KR, Low protein diets in renal disease. *Diabetes Care* 1991; **14:** 856–66.

33. Barsotti G, Navalesi R, Giampietro O et al, Effects of a vegetarian, supplemented diet on renal function, proteinuria, and glucose metabolism in patients with overt diabetic nephropathy and renal insufficiency. *Contr Nephrol* 1988; **65:** 87–94.

34. Barsotti G, Cupisti A, Barsotti M et al, Dietary treatment of diabetic nephropathy with chronic renal failure. *Nephrol Dial Transplant* 1998; **13:** 49–52.

35. Brouhard BH, LaGrone L, Effect of dietary protein restriction on functional renal reserve in diabetic nephropathy. *Am J Med* 1990; **89:** 427–31.

36. Ciavarella A, Di Mizio G, Stefoni S et al, Reduced albuminuria after dietary protein restriction in insulin-dependent diabetic patients with clinical nephropathy. *Diabetes Care* 1987; **10:** 407–13.

37. Dullaart RBF, Beusekamp BJ, Miejer S et al, Long-term effects of protein-restricted diet on albuminuria and renal function in IDDM patients without clinical nephropathy and hypertension. *Diabetes Care* 1993; **16:** 483–92.

38. Pijls LKT, de Vries H, Donker AJM et al, The effect of protein restriction on albuminuria in patients with type 2 diabetes mellitus: a randomised trial. *Nephrol Dial Transplant* 1999; **14:** 1445–53.

39. Raal FJ, Kalk WJ, Lawson M et al, Effect of moderate dietary restriction on the progression of overt diabetic nephropathy: a 6 month prospective study. *Am J Clin Nutr* 1994; **60:** 579–85.

40. Walker JD, Dodds RA, Murrells TJ et al, Restriction of dietary protein and progression of renal failure in diabetic nephropathy. *Lancet* 1989; **ii:** 1411–14.

41. Zeller K, Whittaker E, Sullivans L et al, Effect of restricting dietary protein on the progression of renal failure in patients with insulin-dependent diabetes mellitus. *N Engl J Med* 1991; **324:** 78–84.

42. Close EJ, Wiles PG, Lockton JA et al, Diabetic diets and nutritional recommendations: what happens in real life? *Diabetic Med* 1992; **9:** 181–8.

43. Pearson G, Rowley J, Walker L et al, Are we achieving the dietary recommendations for diabetic patients? *J Hum Nutr Diet* 1996; **9:** 181–7.

44. Jibani MM, Bloodworth E, Foden E et al, Predominantly vegetarian diet in patients with incipient and early clinical diabetic nephropathy: effects on albumin excretion rate and nutritional status. *Diabetic Med* 1991; **8:** 949–53.

45. Pecis M, de Azevedo MJ, Gross JL, Chicken and fish diet reduces glomerular hyperfiltration in IDDM patients. *Diabetes Care* 1994; **17:** 665–72.

46. Cooper ME, Pathogenesis, prevention and treatment of diabetic nephropathy. *Lancet* 1998; **352:** 213–18.

# 9

# Treatment of diabetic nephropathy: control of serum lipids

Karin Jandeleit-Dahm and Fabrice Bonnet

It has been suggested that hyperlipidaemia may contribute to renal disease in diabetes. A number of experimental studies have described the presence of renal lesions associated with abnormal lipid metabolism and suggested the potential influence of dyslipidaemia on the formation of renal injury.[1-4] Over the past decade, some clinical studies have attempted to assess the role of lipids in the progression of diabetic nephropathy, in both type 1 and type 2 diabetes.[5-7] This chapter reviews the available evidence for a possible role of hyperlipidaemia in the progression of diabetic nephropathy and cardiovascular disease, and addresses the effects of lipid-lowering treatment on the clinical course of diabetic micro- and macrovascular complications.

## ROLE OF LIPIDS IN THE PATHOGENESIS OF DIABETIC RENAL LESIONS

A number of experimental studies have suggested a link between hyperlipidaemia and the development of glomerulosclerosis. Hypercholesterolaemia induced by diet has been associated with a premature development of focal glomerulosclerosis in several animal models.[1-4] In the obese Zucker rat, hyperlipidaemia induced glomerular injury independently of glomerular haemodynamics.[8] Recently, it has been shown that progressive podocyte damage and macrophage infiltration are early events in the development of diabetic nephropathy in the obese hyperlipidaemic Zucker rat.[9] Lipid-lowering treatment has been shown to attenuate renal lesions in Zucker rats and in the subtotal nephrectomy model, emphasizing a possible pivotal role for lipids in the pathogenesis of progressive renal disease.[10,11] The mechanisms by which lipids cause or exacerbate glomerular injury remain poorly understood.

## PROPOSED MECHANISMS OF LIPID-ENHANCED RENAL INJURY

Mesangial and epithelial cells express scavenger receptors,[12,13] which are involved in the uptake of modified, glycosylated and oxidized low-density lipoprotein (LDL) and in the formation of mesangial foam cells.[14,15] This effect has also been observed in diabetes.[14,15] Exposure to oxidized lipoproteins has been reported to stimulate mesangial cell secretion of various chemotactic factors and adhesion molecules (M-CSF, ICAM-1 and VCAM-1), stimulating the renal recruitment of macrophages.[16] These intramesangial macrophages may, in turn, further oxidize LDL, creating a self-perpetuating cycle resulting in progressive renal injury. Renal activated macrophages have been shown to stimulate the release of reactive oxygen species and the expression of prosclerotic and proliferative cytokines such as transforming growth factor β1 (TGF-β1) and platelet-derived growth factor-AB (PDGF-AB). The deleterious role of these cytokines in the pathogenesis of diabetic nephropathy has been well characterized.[17] In vitro studies have demonstrated that LDL and oxidized LDL stimulate TGF-β1 gene expression in both human glomerular mesangial and epithelial cells.[18,19]

Finally, dietary cholesterol supplementation in animals has been associated with haemodynamic effects such as an increase in efferent arteriole resistance and a subsequent elevation in intraglomerular pressure, an effect considered deleterious in diabetic nephropathy.[20]

It has been demonstrated that hyperlipidaemia causes tubulointerstitial injury in animal models.[21] Tubulointerstitial injury is also pivotal for the development of diabetic nephropathy and is an independent risk factor for the progressive decline of renal function.[22] It has been reported that lipid-associated tubulointerstitial injuries in Zucker rats parallel the development of glomerulosclerosis,[4] precede glomerular changes or even occur independently of the glomerular lesions.[21] In these experimental studies, hyperlipidaemia-induced chronic tubulointerstitial damage was associated with significant interstitial macrophage infiltration and a parallel increase in TGF-β1 gene expression in interstitial cells, suggesting a cytokine-mediated role for lipids in the development or aggravation of tubulointerstitial lesions.[16,21] In conditions associated with proteinuria, including overt diabetic nephropathy, experimental *in vivo* studies have suggested that the tubular uptake and metabolism of the lipid component of filtered lipoproteins leads to tubulointerstitial injury via increased expression of inflammatory chemokines and cytokines.[23]

## ROLE OF LIPIDS IN THE PROGRESSION OF CLINICAL DIABETIC NEPHROPATHY

In both type 1 and type 2 diabetes, only a few prospective and case-control studies have attempted to establish a correlation between hyperlipidaemia and the decline of renal function in diabetic nephropathy.

### Type 1 diabetes

Mulec et al reported the effect of serum lipids on the subsequent decline in glomerular filtration rate (GFR) in a prospective study involving 30 type 1 diabetic patients with advanced renal disease and proteinuria over a 2.5-year period.[8] All patients were on antihypertensive treatment with either enalapril or metoprolol. In this study, the decline in GFR was negatively correlated to initial values of plasma total cholesterol, triglycerides and apolipoprotein B, and it was positively correlated to Apo AI.[8] There was no correlation between Lp(a) level and the decline in renal function. In a stepwise regression analysis taking into account multiple covariates, including glycosylated haemoglobin, arterial blood pressure and albuminuria, the strongest factors linked to decline in GFR were serum cholesterol and the type of antihypertensive treatment.

Parving et al found a significant positive correlation in univariate analysis between serum cholesterol level and the rate of decline in GFR in a 10-year prospective study of ACE inhibitors in diabetic nephropathy.[24] These patients were all hypertensive with persistent albuminuria without evidence of

chronic renal failure. However, this association with serum cholesterol levels did not remain significant after a stepwise multiple regression analysis which included other variables such as mean arterial blood pressure, albuminuria and glycaemic control.

Krolewski et al examined the determinants of progression to chronic renal failure in 439 patients with diabetic nephropathy in a post hoc analysis of the prospective Diabetic Retinopathy Study. All these patients had intermittent or persistent proteinuria in addition to severe diabetic retinopathy.[10] Only one-third of the patients experienced a rapid loss of renal function. Only serum cholesterol level and diastolic blood pressure at entry were significantly associated with a rapid loss of renal function. These correlations remained significant in a multiple logistic regression analysis. A recent randomized, double-blind, placebo-controlled study by Fried et al compared the effect of simvastatin and diet versus placebo and diet on albuminuria in 39 type 1 diabetic patients without overt nephropathy.[25] Simvastatin treatment slowed the rise in albuminuria over a 2-year observation period compared to placebo, but this change was not significant. Furthermore, simvastatin treatment was associated with a slower progression of other diabetes-associated microvascular complications such as diabetic neuropathy and retinopathy.

### Type 2 diabetes

Ravid et al have followed prospectively 94 normotensive patients with microalbuminuria and normal renal function. These patients were randomized to receive either enalapril or placebo and were followed for 5 years.[11] A significant correlation between baseline and mean study values of serum total cholesterol and the subsequent evolution of renal function (expressed as the ratio of initial to final reciprocal serum creatinine values) was observed. This association persisted after stratification for blood pressure in both the enalapril and placebo-treated groups. Initial and mean plasma total cholesterol and mean blood pressure were also significant predictors of the subsequent increase in albuminuria.[11,26] No correlation was found in that study between serum HDL cholesterol or triglyceride levels and either the renal outcome or the increase in albuminuria. Although some investigators have reported a significant independent influence of serum triglyceride levels on progression of microalbuminuria in type 2 diabetes and progressive loss of renal function in diabetic nephropathy,[27] a number of other observational studies have failed to demonstrate an independent effect of any serum lipid parameter on either evolution of albuminuria or the decline in renal function.[28–30]

# INTERVENTION STUDIES WITH LIPID-LOWERING THERAPY IN DIABETIC NEPHROPATHY

## Experimental models

Lipid-lowering agents have been shown to exert a certain degree of renoprotection in animal models of renal disease,[7,31] but their role in experimental diabetes remains unclear. Indeed, most of the studies which have assessed the renal effects of lipid-lowering agents in experimental diabetic models have evaluated HMG CoA reductase inhibitors. With this class of agent, it remains difficult to determine whether the potential renal effect of these agents was directly related to lipid lowering or to other specific biological properties of this class of drugs.

Lovastatin treatment has been shown to be associated with a significant preservation of GFR in streptozotocin-induced diabetic rats compared to placebo-treated control rats.[31] This renoprotective effect of the HMG CoA reductase inhibitor was similar to that conferred by an ACE inhibitor and was associated with a significant reduction in mesangial histological lesions. However, the renoprotective effects of lovastatin appeared to be independent of plasma lipid-level changes.[31] Similarly, Kim et al have recently reported in this same diabetic rat model that 12 months' treatment with lovastatin suppressed the increase in albuminuria, kidney weight and glomerular volume despite chronic hyperglycaemia.[32] The investigators demonstrated that lovastatin directly blunted the increase in glomerular TGFβ1 gene expression observed in untreated diabetic rats. These results are consistent with those reported in experimental models of non-diabetic renal disease in which HMG CoA reductase inhibitors have been reported to reduce urine albumin excretion and to attenuate the development of glomerulosclerosis.[33–35] A number of mechanisms for these beneficial effects of HMG CoA reductase inhibitors have been proposed, including antiproliferative effects on mesangial cells[36] and a reduction in the expression of chemokines and cytokines.[33,35] Although these results may be relevant to a possible beneficial action of HMG CoA reductase inhibitors in diabetic nephropathy, these findings cannot be considered as definitive evidence for a renoprotective effect of lipid-lowering intervention *per se*.

## Clinical studies

The potential renoprotective properties of lipid-lowering treatments in diabetic nephropathy remain controversial. Initial uncontrolled studies suggested a beneficial effect of the HMG CoA reductase inhibitor pravastatin on progression of albuminuria.[37,38] But, as shown in Table 9.1, most of the placebo-controlled and crossover studies with HMG CoA reductase inhibitors have reported no or only a minimal effect on proteinuria over weeks to months in both type 1 and type 2 diabetes.[39–47] A majority of these studies had a short follow-up, limiting the relevance of their conclusions.

In a prospective, single-blind, placebo-controlled study, Lam et al showed in type 2 diabetic patients that the decline in renal function (assessed by GFR) was significantly attenuated by lovastatin treatment, in comparison to placebo after 2 years of treatment.[41] However, the 24-hr albumin excretion rate and serum creatinine levels increased in both groups, and the statistical analysis applied in that study has been disputed.[48] Furthermore, that study included a relatively heterogeneous group of 34 patients with either microalbuminuria or overt proteinuria. In a crossover study with 1-year simvastatin treatment, Tonolo et al have shown, in moderately hypercholesterolaemic, microalbuminuric type 2 diabetic patients with normal renal function, that simvastatin significantly decreased plasma total and LDL cholesterol levels. This lipid-lowering effect was associated with no changes in renal function, but a concomitant 25% decrease in albuminuria and a rebound in albuminuria after cessation of simvastatin.[42] These results must be interpreted with caution since only 19 patients were included. By contrast, no similar benefit of HMG CoA reductase inhibition has been observed in several studies in type 1[43–45] and type 2 diabetes.[46]

One randomized, controlled trial has specifically evaluated the triglyceride-lowering effects of a fibrate on progression of microalbuminuria in diabetic nephropathy.[47] Fifteen normotensive type 2 diabetic patients with both hypertriglyceridaemia and microalbuminuria received either placebo or gemfibrozil treatment over 12 months. Lipid-lowering treatment was associated with an improvement in hypertriglyceridaemia, and progression of albuminuria was reduced, albeit not statistically significantly, in the gemfibrozil-treated subjects when compared to the placebo group. In comparison to patients with stable or increasing triglyceride levels, the subgroup with a marked reduction in triglyceride concentrations had a significantly lower rate of progression of

**Table 9.1 Effects of lipid-lowering treatment on progression of albuminuria in diabetic patients with micro- and macroalbuminuria**

| Type of diabetes | Agent used | n | Duration | Effect on albuminuria | Reference |
|---|---|---|---|---|---|
| *Patients with microalbuminuria* | | | | | |
| Type 1 | simvastatin | 39 | 2 years | → | Fried et al[50] |
| Type 1 | pravastatin | 20 | 12 weeks | → | Zhang et al[44] |
| Type 1 | simvastatin | 22 | 18–30 weeks | → | Barnes et al[45] |
| Type 2 | simvastatin | 18 | 36 weeks | → | Nielsen et al[46] |
| Type 2 | simvastatin | 19 | 1 year | ↓ | Tonolo et al[42] |
| Type 2 | gemfibrozil | 15 | 1 year | ↓ | Smulders et al[47] |
| Type 2 | bezafibrate/ pravastatin | 71 | 4 years | → | Nagai et al[49] |
| *Patients with proteinuria* | | | | | |
| Type 1 | simvastatin | 26 | 12 weeks | → | Hommel et al[43] |
| Type 2 | pravastatin | 19 | 12 weeks | ↓ | Sasaki et al[39] |
| Type 2 | pravastatin | 12 | 12 weeks | ↓ | Shoji et al[40] |
| Type 2 | lovastatin | 34 | 2 years | ↓ | Lam et al[41] |

albuminuria.[47] This small study supports a potential specific benefit of triglyceride-lowering therapy on the progression of albuminuria in diabetic nephropathy but requires confirmation by a larger randomized trial of longer duration. Most of these studies were of short duration, were restricted to the effects of lipid-lowering treatment on progression of albuminuria and did not address decline in renal function. Recently, Nagai et al showed in a longer study period over 4 years that there was no increase in albuminuria in 71 type 2 diabetic patients with hypercholesteraemia treated with either bezafibrate or pravastatin, a result which could be interpreted as indicating a renoprotective effect of both lipid-lowering drugs in diabetes. However, there was no placebo control group in that study.[49]

Recently, a meta-analysis of lipid-lowering therapy on the progression of renal disease has been reported. Thirteen prospective controlled trials, including seven of the above-mentioned studies exclusively performed in diabetic patients (Table 9.1), which examined the effects of antilipaemic agents on renal function, proteinuria or albuminuria were analysed.[50]

This meta-analysis showed that lipid lowering was associated with a lower rate of the decline in renal function compared to controls (p=0.008) which was comparable to the beneficial effect of an ACE inhibitor on preservation of renal function. The studies were statistically homogeneous, and in a regression analysis, the effect of treatment on GFR did not correlate with the type of lipid-lowering agent or the cause of renal disease. The effects of lipid-lowering treatment on proteinuria were less clear in this meta-analysis, as the studies were statistically heterogeneous. However, there was a tendency for a favourable effect of anti-lipidaemic treatment to be observed with respect to proteinuria and albuminuria.[50]

## DIABETES, HYPERLIPIDAEMIA AND MACROVASCULAR DISEASE

Numerous studies in non-diabetic patients have demonstrated that lipid abnormalities greatly increase the risk of atherosclerosis and that the correction of dyslipoproteinaemia reduces the risk of coronary artery disease in primary as well as in secondary prevention studies.[51–54] Diabetes is associated with a high cardiovascular risk profile. This is partly due to a pro-atherosclerotic dyslipidaemia consisting of a low high-density lipoprotein (HDL) level, increased triglyceride levels in association with normal or increased LDL levels, a preponderance of small, dense LDL and compositional changes in very low-density lipoprotein (VLDL) and HDL. The diabetes-associated dyslipidaemia further accelerates macrovascular complications in the diabetic patient.

Some of the large clinical trials in hyperlipidaemia including the Scandinavian Simvastatin Survival Study (4S)[54] and the CARE study,[53] had diabetic subgroups, clearly showing the evidence of lipid-lowering benefits with statins on cardiovascular morbidity and mortality in the diabetic population. Studies specifically evaluating the effect of lipid-lowering treatment in diabetic patients are limited. The recent Diabetes Atherosclerosis Intervention Study (DAIS) was designed to assess the effects of fenofibrate on progression of coronary atherosclerosis in type 2 diabetic patients with mild lipoprotein abnormalities. In this placebo-controlled study, the fenofibrate-treated group had significantly reduced angiographic progression of coronary artery disease compared to the placebo group.[51] These benefits were associated with a parallel correction of lipoprotein abnormalities in patients treated with the fibrate.

Some studies are currently investigating multifactorial interventions including antihypertensive and lipid-lowering treatments. In the ALLHAT study,[55] the effect of the HMG CoA reductase inhibitor pravastatin on all-cause and cardiovascular mortality in mildly hypercholesteraemic patients will be evaluated. The study includes a significant proportion of diabetic patients.

The classic mixed dyslipidaemia in type 2 diabetes is part of the metabolic syndrome which includes insulin resistance, hyperinsulinaemia, glucose intolerance and hypertension. Although optimization of glycaemic control and aggressive blood-pressure reduction can reduce macrovascular complications in diabetic patients,[56,57] the cardiovascular risk of the diabetic patient is still significantly increased. Similar to the international guidelines for the treatment of hypertension in diabetes, lower target levels of LDL and total cholesterol are required in the diabetic population than in non-diabetic patients, aiming at a total cholesterol of less than 5 mmol/l and an LDL of less than 3 mmol/l.[58,59]

For the treatment of hypercholesteraemia in the diabetic context, preference should be given to an HMG CoA reductase inhibitor because of the clinical evidence of the large studies. Alternative treatment choices include bile acid sequestrants, nicotinic acid derivatives, fibric acid derivatives or probucol. If hypertriglyceridaemia with a low HDL level is pre-dominant, a fibrate can be used, although the clinical evidence on cardiovascular outcomes is more limited. As cited earlier, the DAIS trial demonstrated an angiographic benefit of fenofibrate in type 2 diabetic patients, yet it was not powered to examine clinical endpoints. The placebo-controlled Veterans Affairs Cooperative Studies Program High-Density Lipoprotein Cholesterol Intervention Trial (VA-HIT) showed that treatment with the fibrate gemfibrozil in men with coronary heart disease and a low HDL level significantly reduced the incidence of non-fatal myocardial infarction and stroke compared to the placebo group.[52] These benefits conferred by the fibrate were observed in the subgroup of patients with diabetes as well, yet with a less significant p value (p = 0.05). Similar results were previously reported for primary intervention with gemfibrozil in the Helsinki Heart Study, showing a 34% reduction in the incidence of coronary heart disease over 5 years in the gemfibrozil group compared to placebo.[60]

Enhanced lipid lowering is achieved with combinations of lipid-modifying drugs which differ in their mode of action. However, potential side effects are more likely if both agents are used in combination and/or in the context of impaired renal function. Statins and fibrates both may elevate liver enzymes and can cause myopathy associated with increased creatine phosphokinase levels. It remains in dispute whether combination therapy with a statin and a fibrate requires routine monitoring of liver function tests and creatine phosphokinase. It has been suggested that the combination of an HMG CoA reductase inhibitor and nicotinic acid should be avoided because of increased risk of myopathy, although studies aiming at such combinations, including these in diabetic subjects, have been previously described.[61] Fibrates may cause acute deterioration of renal function in patients with initially increased serum creatinine levels; therefore, they should not be used in patients with overt diabetic nephropathy and impaired renal function.[62] Furthermore, caution has to be exercised regarding potential drug interactions which have been reported for HMG CoA reductase inhibitors with cyclosporin A, erythromycin, itraconazole, protease inhibitors and warfarin.

## CONCLUSION

Dyslipidaemia in diabetic patients has been clearly demonstrated to be an important risk factor for the development of vascular disease. The potential influence of hyperlipidaemia on the subsequent decline in renal function and/or the progression of albuminuria in diabetic nephropathy remains controversial and needs to be further assessed in larger clinical studies of longer duration. The results of those studies will determine whether HMG CoA reductase inhibitors should be considered as additional renoprotective agents in diabetic nephropathy. Furthermore, clinical studies specifically designed for the diabetic population are now required to assess whether lipid-lowering therapy is particularly beneficial in this group of patients at high risk of cardiovascular disease.

## REFERENCES

1. French SW, Yamanaka W, Ostwald R, Dietary induced glomerulosclerosis in the guinea pig. *Arch Pathol* 1967; **83**: 204–10.
2. Wellmann KF, Volk BW, Renal changes in experimental hypercholesterolemia in normal and in subdiabetic rabbits. II. Long term studies. *Lab Invest* 1971; **24**: 144–55.
3. Peric-Golia L, Peric-Golia M, Aortic and renal lesions in hypercholesterolemic adult, male, virgin Sprague-Dawley rats. *Atherosclerosis* 1983; **46**: 57–65.
4. Kasiske BL, O'Donnell MP, Schmitz PG et al, Renal injury of diet-induced hypercholesterolemia in rats. *Kidney Int* 1990; **37**: 880–91.
5. Kasiske BL, Cleary MP, Keane WF, Effects of genetic obesity on renal structure and function in the Zucker rat. *J Lab Clin Med* 1995; **106**: 598–604.
6. Kasiske BL, O'Donnell MP, Cleary MP et al, Treatment of hyperlipidemia reduces glomerular injury in obese Zucker rats. *Kidney Int* 1988; **33**: 667–72.
7. Kasiske BL, O'Donnell MP, Garvis WJ et al, Pharmacologic treatment of hyperlipidemia reduces glomerular injury in rat 5/6 nephrectomy model of chronic renal failure. *Circ Res* 1988; **62**: 367–74.
8. Mulec H, Johnsen SA, Wiklund O et al, Cholesterol: a renal risk factor in diabetic nephropathy? *Am J Kidney Dis* 1993; **22**: 196–201.
9. Coimbra TM, Janssen U, Grone HJ et al, Early events leading to renal injury in obese Zucker (fatty) rats with type II diabetes. *Kidney Int* 2000; **57**: 167–82.
10. Krolewski AS, Warram JH, Christlieb AR, Hypercholesterolemia—a determinant of renal function loss and deaths in IDDM patients with nephropathy. *Kidney Int Suppl* 1994; **45**: S125–31.
11. Ravid M, Neumann L, Lishner M, Plasma lipids and the progression of nephropathy in diabetes mellitus type II: effect of ACE inhibitors. *Kidney Int* 1995; **47**: 907–10.
12. Wheeler DC, Fernando RL, Gillett MP et al, Characterisation of the binding of low-density lipoproteins to cultured rat mesangial cells. *Nephrol Dial Transplant* 1991; **6**: 701–8.
13. Grone HJ, Walli AK, Grone E et al, Receptor mediated uptake of apo B and apo E rich lipoproteins by human glomerular epithelial cells. *Kidney Int* 1990; **37**: 1449–59.
14. Takemura T, Yoshioka K, Aya N et al, Apolipoproteins and lipoprotein receptors in glomeruli in human kidney diseases. *Kidney Int* 1993; **43**: 918–27.
15. Schlondorff D, Cellular mechanisms of lipid injury in the glomerulus. *Am J Kidney Dis* 1993; **22**: 72–82.
16. Grone HJ, Walli AK, Grone EF, The role of oxidatively modified lipoproteins in lipid nephropathy. *Contrib Nephrol* 1997; **120**: 160–75.
17. Cooper ME, Pathogenesis, prevention, and treatment of diabetic nephropathy. *Lancet* 1998; **352**: 213–19.
18. Studer RK, Craven PA, DeRubertis FR, Low-density lipoprotein stimulation of mesangial cell fibronectin synthesis: role of protein kinase C and transforming growth factor-beta. *J Lab Clin Med* 1995; **125**: 86–95.
19. Ding G, van Goor H, Ricardo SD et al, Oxidized LDL stimulates the expression of TGF-beta and fibronectin in human glomerular epithelial cells. *Kidney Int* 1997; **51**: 147–54.
20. Bank N, Aynedjian HS, Role of thromboxane in impaired renal vasodilatation response to acetylcholine in hypercholesterolemic rats. *J Clin Invest* 1992; **89**: 1636–42.
21. Grone HJ, Hohbach J, Grone EF, Modulation of glomerular sclerosis and interstitial fibrosis by native and modified lipoproteins. *Kidney Int Suppl* 1996; **54**: S18–22.
22. Gilbert RE, Cooper ME, The tubulointerstitium in progressive diabetic kidney disease: more than an aftermath of glomerular injury? *Kidney Int* 1999; **56**: 1627–37.
23. Remuzzi G, Ruggenenti P, Benigni A, Understanding the nature of renal disease progression. *Kidney Int* 1997; **51**: 2–15.
24. Parving HH, Rossing P, Hommel E et al, Angiotensin-converting enzyme inhibition in diabetic nephropathy: ten years' experience. *Am J Kidney Dis* 1995; **26**: 99–107.
25. Fried LF, Forrest KY, Ellis D et al, Lipid modulation in insulin-dependent diabetes mellitus: effect on microvascular outcomes. *J Diabetes Complications* 2001; **15**: 113–19.
26. Smulders YM, Rakic M, Stehouwer CD et al, Determinants of progression of microalbuminuria in patients with NIDDM. A prospective study. *Diabetes Care* 1997; **20**: 999–1005.
27. Hasslacher C, Bostedt-Kiesel A, Kempe HP et al, Effect of metabolic factors and blood pressure on kidney function in proteinuric type 2 (non-insulin-dependent) diabetic patients. *Diabetologia* 1993; **36**: 1051–6.
28. Viswanathan VV, Snehalatha C, Ramachandran A et al, Proteinuria in NIDDM in south India: analysis of predictive factors. *Diabetes Res Clin Pract* 1995; **28**: 41–6.
29. Wirta OR, Pasternack AI, Mustonen JT et al, Urinary albumin excretion rate and its determinants after 6 years in non-insulin-dependent diabetic patients. *Nephrol Dial Transplant* 1996; **11**: 449–56.
30. Oue T, Namba M, Nakajima H et al, Risk factors for the progression of microalbuminuria in Japanese type 2 diabetic patients— a 10 year follow-up study. *Diabetes Res Clin Pract* 1999; **46**: 47–55.
31. Inman SR, Stowe NT, Cressman MD et al, Lovastatin preserves renal function in experimental diabetes. *Am J Med Sci* 1999; **317**: 215–21.
32. Kim SI, Han DC, Lee HB, Lovastatin inhibits transforming growth factor-beta1 expression in diabetic rat glomeruli and cultured rat mesangial cells. *J Am Soc Nephrol* 2000; **11**: 80–7.
33. Jandeleit-Dahm K, Cao Z, Cox AJ et al, Role of hyperlipidemia in progressive renal disease: focus on diabetic nephropathy. *Kidney Int Suppl* 1999; **71**: S31–6.
34. Lee SK, Jin SY, Han DC et al, Effects of delayed treatment with enalapril and/or lovastatin on the progression of glomerulosclerosis in 5/6 nephrectomized rats. *Nephrol Dial Transplant* 1993; **8**: 1338–43.
35. Park YS, Guijarro C, Kim Y et al, Lovastatin reduces glomerular macrophage influx and expression of monocyte chemoattractant Protein-1 mRNA in nephrotic rats. *Am J Kidney Dis* 1998; **31**: 190–4.
36. O'Donnell MP, Kasiske BL, Kim Y et al, Lovastatin inhibits proliferation of rat mesangial cells. *J Clin Invest* 1993; **91**: 83–8.
37. Rabelink AJ, Hene RJ, Erkelens DW et al, Partial remission of

nephrotic syndrome in patient on long-term simvastatin. *Lancet* 1990; **335:** 1045–6.

38. Rayner BL, Byrne MJ, Smit RV, A prospective clinical trial comparing the treatment of idiopathic membranous nephropathy and nephrotic syndrome with simvastatin and diet, versus diet alone. *Clin Nephrol* 1996; **46:** 219–24.

39. Sasaki T, Kurata H, Nomura K et al, Amelioration of proteinuria with pravastatin in hypercholesterolemic patients with diabetes mellitus. *Jpn J Med* 1990; **29:** 156–63.

40. Shoji T, Nishizawa Y, Toyokawa A et al, Decreased albuminuria by pravastatin in hyperlipidemic diabetics [letter]. *Nephron* 1991; **59:** 664–5.

41. Lam KS, Cheng IK, Janus ED et al, Cholesterol-lowering therapy may retard the progression of diabetic nephropathy. *Diabetologia* 1995; **38:** 604–9.

42. Tonolo G, Ciccarese M, Brizzi P et al, Reduction of albumin excretion rate in normotensive microalbuminuric type 2 diabetic patients during long-term simvastatin treatment. *Diabetes Care* 1997; **20:** 1891–5.

43. Hommel E, Andersen P, Gall MA et al, Plasma lipoproteins and renal function during simvastatin treatment in diabetic nephropathy. *Diabetologia* 1992; **35:** 447–51.

44. Zhang A, Vertommen J, Van Gaal L et al, Effects of pravastatin on lipid levels, in vitro oxidizability of non-HDL lipoproteins and microalbuminuria in IDDM patients. *Diabetes Res Clin Pract* 1995; **29:** 189–94.

45. Barnes DJ, Stephens EG, Mattock MB et al, The effect of simvastatin on the progression of renal disease in IDDM patients with elevated urinary albumin excretion. *Proceedings European Diabetic Nephropathy Study Group*, 11th meeting, 1998.

46. Nielsen S, Schmitz O, Moller N et al, Renal function and insulin sensitivity during simvastatin treatment in type 2 (non-insulin-dependent) diabetic patients with microalbuminuria. *Diabetologia* 1993; **36:** 1079–86.

47. Smulders YM, van Eeden AE, Stehouwer CD et al, Can reduction in hypertriglyceridaemia slow progression of microalbuminuria in patients with non-insulin-dependent diabetes mellitus? *Eur J Clin Invest* 1997; **27:** 997–1002.

48. Parving HH, Cholesterol-lowering therapy may retard the progression of diabetic nephropathy [letter]. *Diabetologia* 1996; **39:** 367–8.

49. Nagai T, Tomizawa T, Nakajima K et al, Effect of bezafibrate or pravastatin on serum lipid levels and albuminuria in NIDDM patients. *J Atheroscler Thromb* 2000; **7:** 91–6.

50. Fried LF, Orchard TJ, Kasiske BL, Effect of lipid reduction on the progression of renal disease: a meta-analysis. *Kidney Int* 2001; **59:** 260–9.

51. Effect of fenofibrate on progression of coronary-artery disease in type 2 diabetes: the Diabetes Atherosclerosis Intervention Study, a randomised study. *Lancet* 2001; **357:** 905–10.

52. Rubins HB, Robins SJ, Collins D et al, Gemfibrozil for the secondary prevention of coronary heart disease in men with low levels of high-density lipoprotein cholesterol. Veterans Affairs High-Density Lipoprotein Cholesterol Intervention Trial Study Group. *N Engl J Med* 1999; **341:** 410–18.

53. Sacks FM, Pfeffer MA, Moye LA et al, The effect of pravastatin on coronary events after myocardial infarction in patients with average cholesterol levels. Cholesterol and Recurrent Events Trial investigators. *N Engl J Med* 1996; **335:** 1001–9.

54. Randomised trial of cholesterol lowering in 4444 patients with coronary heart disease: the Scandinavian Simvastatin Survival Study (4S). *Lancet* 1994; **344:** 1383–9.

55. Davis BR, Cutler JA, Gordon DJ et al, Rationale and design for the Antihypertensive and Lipid Lowering Treatment to Prevent Heart Attack Trial (ALLHAT). ALLHAT Research Group. *Am J Hypertens* 1996; **9:** 342–60.

56. Gerstein HC, Yusuf S, Mann JFE et al, Effects of ramipril on cardiovascular and microvascular outcomes in people with diabetes mellitus: results of the HOPE study and MICRO-HOPE substudy. *Lancet* 2000; **355:** 253–9.

57. Hansson L, Zanchetti A, Carruthers SG et al, for the HOT Study Group. Effects of intensive blood-pressure lowering and low-dose aspirin in patients with hypertension: principal results of the Hypertension Optimal Treatment (HOT) randomised trial. *Lancet* 1998; **351:** 1755–62.

58. Wood D, De Backer G, Faergeman O et al, Prevention of coronary heart disease in clinical practice: recommendations of the Second Joint Task Force of European and other Societies on Coronary Prevention. *Atherosclerosis* 1998; 140: 199–270.

59. Joint British recommendations on prevention of coronary heart disease in clinical practice. British Cardiac Society, British Hyperlipidaemia Association, British Hypertension Society, endorsed by the British Diabetic Association. *Heart* 1998; **80** (Suppl 2): S1–29.

60. Frick MH, Elo O, Haapa K et al, Helsinki Heart Study: primary-prevention trial with gemfibrozil in middle-aged men with dyslipidemia. Safety of treatment, changes in risk factors, and incidence of coronary heart disease. *N Engl J Med* 1987; **317:** 1237–45.

61. Tsalamandris C, Panagiotopoulos S, Sinha A et al, Complementary effects of pravastatin and nicotinic acid in the treatment of combined hyperlipidaemia in diabetic and non-diabetic patients. *J Cardiovasc Risk* 1994; **1:** 231–9.

62. Lipscombe J, Lewis GF, Cattran D et al, Deterioration in renal function associated with fibrate therapy. *Clin Nephrol* 2001; **55:** 39–44.

# 10

# Diabetic nephropathy: treatment of cardiac complications

Riccardo Candido and Piyush Srivastava

## INTRODUCTION

Patients with diabetes mellitus (DM) have a high prevalence of cardiac morbidity and mortality, with up to 75% of mortality being from cardiovascular disease (CVD).[1,2]

Specific vascular, myopathic and neuropathic alterations have been suggested as being responsible for the excessive cardiovascular (CV) morbidity and mortality in diabetes.[3–5] These alterations manifest themselves clinically as coronary heart disease (CHD), congestive heart failure (CHF) and/or sudden cardiac death (SCD). Previous studies have shown that age-adjusted relative risk of death due to CV events in persons with diabetes is threefold higher than in the general population.[1,6] Furthermore, diabetic patients without any history of CHD have the same risk of CHD death as a nondiabetic patient with a previous acute myocardial infarction (AMI).[1] Diabetes acts as an independent risk factor for several forms of CVD. To make matters worse, when patients with diabetes develop clinical CVD, they sustain a worse prognosis for survival than do CVD patients without diabetes.[1,7,8] Moreover, prospective studies[9,10] show that not only diabetes, but also impaired glucose tolerance, is a risk factor for CVD. Diabetes is associated with a relatively greater risk of CVD in women than in men.[11] Furthermore, women with diabetes seem to lose most of their inherent protection against developing CVD. When adjusted for other risk factors, the risk rate for increased mortality is 2.4 times greater for diabetic men and 3.5 times greater for diabetic women.[2,11] Diabetes, notably type 2 diabetes, is on the rise in children and adolescents, thereby increasing the likelihood that they will develop premature CVD.

The major cardiovascular risk factors—elevated low-density lipoprotein (LDL) cholesterol, hypertension, smoking, and sex—remain important determinants of CVD in patients with diabetes. Nevertheless, within the Multiple Risk Factor Intervention Trial (MRFIT),[12] the occurrence of CV death at the 12-year follow-up was about three times more in diabetic men than in their nondiabetic controls, regardless of systolic blood pressure, age, cholesterol, ethnic group or smoking status. This study also confirmed that systolic hypertension, elevated cholesterol, and cigarette smoking were independent predictors of mortality, and the presence of at least one of these risk factors had a greater impact on increasing CV mortality in persons with diabetes than in those without diabetes, suggesting a key role for the management of CV risk factors in these patients.

In addition, emerging risk factors, such as fibrinogen, degree of glycemia, extent of insulin resistance, and presence of subclinical atherosclerosis, appear further to affect risk in individuals with diabetes. Among the emerging risk factors, an independent risk factor for the development of CVD morbidity and mortality in the diabetic population is microalbuminuria, which links cardiac damage to the renal injury. Albuminuria has been shown to be a marker for increased CV mortality in both diabetic and nondiabetic subjects,[13–17] recent studies showing that the degree and rate of progression of albuminuria correlate with increased CV event rates in diabetic patients.[18,19] Hence albuminuria may be used as a marker to identify diabetic subjects at high risk of CVD events manifesting as CHD, CHF, SCD and/or stroke. Moreover, every study of mortality in dialysis patients has shown that diabetic patients have a worse survival rate than their nondiabetic counterparts with end-stage renal disease, and that about half of this excess mortality can be attributed to CV causes.[20,21] When diabetes is present, CVD is the leading cause of death among patients with end-stage renal disease, suggesting that CV complications are particularly important in patients with diabetic nephropathy.[22–24] The recent results of large multi-center, multinational, randomized, controlled trials in patients with diabetes and albuminuria (IRMA2, IDNT and RENAAL) have shown a renoprotective effect of blockade of the angiotensin receptor.[25–27] However, none of these trials were able to show a significant improvement in CV mortality and morbidity, apart from heart failure admissions in the RENAAL study. In contrast, blockade of angiotensin-converting enzyme (ACE) has a proven cardioprotective effect in diabetic and nondiabetic patients. In the Heart Outcomes Prevention Evaluation (HOPE) trial, in which 9297 high-risk patients were enrolled, a subgroup of 3577 subjects had diabetes. There was an overall 30% reduction in CVD mortality in non-diabetics, and a 37% reduction in diabetic patients, including a 22% risk reduction in myocardial infarction. In the MICRO-HOPE substudy (microalbuminuria, CV and renal outcomes), there was a 22% risk reduction for the development of overt nephropathy, and a 15% reduction in microvascular complications.[28,29] Hence, albuminuria is likely to identify a subset of diabetic patients at an increased risk of CV morbidity and mortality. To date, there have been limited trials focusing upon the cardiac management of diabetic patients with albuminuria. The remaining sections will cover current management approaches to primary and secondary prevention of CHD events in diabetic patients as well as the pathophysiology and current treatment options for acute coronary syndrome, CHF and/or risk of SCD.

## CORONARY HEART DISEASE (CHD)

Both type 1 and type 2 diabetes are independent risk factors for the development of CHD.[30] CHD in diabetic subjects arises from known cardiac risk factors, which include hypertension, smoking, dyslipidemia, hyperglycemia and genetic factors (family history of CHD). However autopsy, coronary angiographic and, more recently, electron-beam computed tomography (EBCT) studies have shown that the coronary arteries of diabetic patients exhibit a diffuse accelerated atherosclerotic process with increased atherosclerotic disease burden and severity of lesions.[30–34] Furthermore, CHD in diabetic patients has an increased incidence, as well as earlier onset, with clinical presentation in younger age groups and among female patients.[35,36]

Atherosclerotic lesions are almost invariably present in patients who have had diabetes for 5–10 years or longer, and increase with age and duration of the diabetes. Moreover, atherosclerotic lesions tend to develop 10–12 years earlier in diabetic than in nondiabetic patients.[35,37] In a recent coronary angiographic study in diabetic subjects with symptomatic CHD, the degree of albuminuria (none, microalbuminuria, overt nephropathy) correlated with the atherosclerotic disease burden and restenosis rates of angioplastied segments,[38] suggesting that albuminuric diabetic patients have an even more accelerated underlying atherosclerotic process. The risk of CHD is also substantially increased in patients with asymptomatic hyperglycemia.[39] Furthermore, there is an unusually high incidence of subclinical diabetes among patients with premature CHD.[40] These observations provide further evidence for the close interactions among hyperglycemia, atherosclerosis and CHD. Moreover, myocardial ischemia due to CHD commonly occurs without symptoms in patients with diabetes.[41] As a result, multivessel atherosclerosis often is present before ischemic symptoms occur and before treatment is instituted. Delayed recognition of various forms of coronary heart disease undoubtedly worsens the prognosis of survival for many diabetic patients.[42] Hence the need for primary prevention of CHD events in albuminuric diabetics is paramount to their survival.

## Pathophysiology of CHD

Not much is known about plaque differences in subjects with and without diabetes. Indeed, it is yet to be clarified whether the atherosclerotic lesion in the diabetic patient has the same pathologic features as in nondiabetic subjects. In atherectomy specimens, the cell-rich and necrotic areas are increased in de novo lesions in persons with diabetes.[43] In restenotic areas, an increased content of collagen has been found in vessels from subjects with diabetes.[44] In a series of coronary arteries examined after sudden death, the extent of the necrotic core of plaques, calcification, and healed ruptures were increased in patients with type 2 diabetes.[45] However, in type 1 diabetes, an increased content of fibrous tissue and reduced number of foam cells in plaques may provide relative stability to atherosclerotic lesions.[46] Recently, evidence has been obtained of an increased content of macrophages in the atherosclerotic lesions of diabetic subjects.[47] This is probably the consequence of an increase in recruitment of macrophages into the vessel wall due to the higher levels of cytokines present in diabetes. In an experimental model of type 1 diabetes, our group has recently demonstrated that in long-term diabetes there is not only an acceleration in the development of atherosclerosis but also an increase in the complexity of the atherosclerotic plaques, characterized by increased macrophage infiltration, cellular proliferation, smooth-muscle cell migration and collagen content.[48] It is still controversial as to whether there is a difference in plaque pathology between type 1 and 2 diabetic subjects, type 1 diabetic patients having more fibrous and calcified atherosclerotic lesions and type 2 diabetic patients having more cellular and lipid-containing lesions.

The pathogenesis of the accelerated atherosclerosis observed in the diabetic context is still incompletely understood. As mentioned previously, there is an increased prevalence of other cardiac risk factors, such as hypertension, dyslipidemia and obesity, among diabetic patients.[49] Nevertheless, epidemiologic studies suggest that these risk factors, although more prevalent in diabetes, do not fully account for the increased risk of CHD.[49,50] Furthermore, although hyperglycemia, the primary clinical manifestation of diabetes, is considered to contribute to the accelerated development of atherosclerosis, the Diabetes Control and Complications Trial Research studies and, more recently, the UK Prospective Diabetes Study (UKPDS) did not detect statistically significant effects of intensified glycemic control on macrovascular disease.[51,52] Therefore, the increased atherosclerotic disease burden in diabetic patients raises the likelihood that factors specific to diabetes other than hyperglycemia contribute to the increased CHD mortality and morbidity. Several clinical and experimental observations suggest that the pathogenesis of atherosclerosis in diabetes is complex and multifactorial.[47] Five general areas of pathogenetic mechanisms have been recently identified by the American Heart Association.[53]

The first area, *metabolic factors,* is based on the principle that hyperglycemia results from both insulin deficiency and insulin resistance. The insulin-resistance syndrome is a composite of numerous biochemical and clinical abnormalities, which include increased flux of free fatty acids, dyslipidemia (increased very low-density lipoprotein (VLDL), and decreased high-density lipoprotein (HDL) and small dense lipoproteins), hyperinsulinemia, and hypertension. Importantly, hyperglycemia results in increased rates of glycation and oxidation.

The second area, excessive *oxidation/glucoxidation,* is a consequence of abundant protein glycation in the setting of increased oxygen radicals, with subsequent accumulation of advanced glycation end-products

(AGEs). The presence of AGEs is closely related to hyperglycemia, and their pathobiochemistry could explain many of the changes observed in diabetes-related complications. These AGEs have effects on lipids, lipid metabolism and the development of atherosclerosis, effects which could influence diabetes-related CHD. AGEs have been observed in fatty streaks, atherosclerotic lesions, lipid-containing smooth-muscle cells and macrophages from diabetic subjects.[54,55] A correlation between tissue AGE concentrations and the severity of atherosclerotic lesions has also been shown.[55] AGE accumulation in the extracellular matrix of atheromatous arteries might result in enhanced subintimal protein and lipoprotein deposition, with covalent trapping of LDL as well as nitric oxide depletion.[55,56] Moreover, through AGE receptor-dependent mechanisms, AGE induction of cytokines and growth factors has been implicated in contributing to the pathogenesis of diabetes-associated atherosclerosis.[57] Animal studies using soluble receptor for AGEs (RAGE) to block the RAGE receptor resulted in suppression of vascular lesion formation and reduced vascular permeability, independently of lipid and glycemic control, confirming that other mechanisms are important for vascular lesion formation.[57] Susceptibility to atherosclerotic lesion formation by AGE has been shown in in vitro studies demonstrating endothelial dysfunction manifesting as changes in vascular permeability, coagulation and increased adherence or migration of macrophages and T lymphocytes into the intima, with the initiation of a prolonged subinflammatory response.[55,58] Endothelial migration of monocytes, considered to be one of the first steps in atherogenesis, is dependent on the upregulation of vascular cell adhesion molecule-1 (VCAM-1).[59] AGEs have been shown to increase VCAM-1 expression, confirming an important role for AGEs in inducing diabetes-associated atherosclerosis.[60]

LDL can exist as oxidized LDL, glycated LDL and glycoxidated LDL. AGE linked to lipids has been shown to initiate oxidative modification with the formation of oxidized LDL and VLDL.[56,61] In diabetes, a greater portion of LDL is glycated and oxidized.[62,63] The LDL receptor does not recognise modified LDL, which is taken up by macrophage scavenger receptors or AGE receptors, resulting in lipid-laden foam cells in the arterial intima and the promotion of atherosclerosis.[64] Furthermore, a positive correlation has been shown between arterial wall AGE and AGE-modified LDL in the blood of diabetic subjects.[55] Furthermore, recent human clinical studies have shown a link between AGEs and diastolic dysfunction (via increased myocardial stiffness) in type 1

DM[65] and CHD in type 2 diabetic subjects.[66] Recently, it has been observed that Lp(a), an independent risk factor for CVD, undergoes glycation in diabetic subjects.[67] Moreover, in vitro studies demonstrated that glycation of Lp(a) attenuates fibrinolysis by inducing expression of plasminogen activator inhibitor (PAI-1) and reducing generation of tissue-plasminogen activator.

The third pathogenetic mechanism, *endothelial dysfunction*, is known to occur with hyperglycemia, dyslipidemia and hypertension. It is an important initiator of the atherosclerotic process. Diabetic vasculopathy appears to be partly due to the altered expression of adhesion molecules and growth factors, resulting in increased vascular permeability.[68] Furthermore, insulin resistance and hyperinsulinemia have been shown to cause endothelial dysfunction and hence contribute to ischemic cardiac events.[69]

Fourthly, a diabetes-induced increase in the process of *inflammation* is also involved in the pathogenesis of atherosclerosis. This, in part, relates to the excessive amount of adipose tissue, an important source of interleukin-6, a precursor of C-reactive protein generation. Recently, an important role in inducing an activation of the inflammatory process in the diabetic vessels has been demonstrated for the renin-angiotensin system (RAS) by our group. Several clinical trials have shown that ACE inhibitors prevent or retard the development of diabetic macrovascular complications, suggesting the role of the RAS in the pathogenesis of CHD.[29,70–72] Our group has demonstrated an activation of the local RAS within the aorta in diabetic apolipoprotein E knockout mice, predominantly within the plaques and the medial layer.[48] This activation of the local RAS within the plaques was associated with a significant increase in the development and progression of diabetes-induced atherosclerosis. In our study, blockade of the RAS with an ACE inhibitor, despite a modest effect on blood pressure and no significant influence on the lipid profile or glycemic control, was demonstrated to prevent the development of this accelerated atherosclerosis by mechanisms involving inhibition of proinflammatory adhesion molecules such as VCAM-1 and the prosclerotic cytokine connective-tissue growth factor.[48] These findings suggest that the local RAS is implicated in the development and progression of diabetes-associated atherosclerosis.

Finally, diabetes is also considered to be a *prothrombotic state*. Diabetic serum has been studied and shown to have increased platelet turnover and glycoprotein IIb/IIIa receptors, with raised levels of procoagulant factors such as thromboxane, von Willebrand factor (vWf), fibrinogen and PAI 1, and diminished levels of anticoagulants such as antithrombin III.[73] This imbalance in prothrombotic, anticoagulant and antifibrinolytic processes results in hyperaggregable serum with increased sensitivity to agonists such as thromboxane. Moreover, abnormalities in platelet function, coagulation, and fibrinolysis may favor intraluminal thrombosis at the site of plaque fissuring or rupture.[74] These are some of the pathophysiological factors important to the development of CHD, CHF and SCD in diabetic patients. The management of these factors, which may be divided into chronic or preventative strategies and acute management strategies, is discussed below.

## PRIMARY PREVENTION OF CVD

The increasing prevalence and cost of diabetes-related cardiac mortality and morbidity have led to an increased focus on CVD risk assessment and prevention of diabetic complications in patients.[75–77] Furthermore, recent studies have shown that the risk of silent myocardial ischemia is increased in patients with microalbuminuria compared with normoalbuminuric diabetic subjects,[78] providing further evidence that albuminuria may identify a subset of diabetic patients who are at further increased risk of CVD events. Hence, greater emphasis should be placed upon the primary prevention of CVD, potentially achievable via lifestyle change and medical management of cardiac risk factors.

### Lifestyle modification

Diabetic patients should be encouraged to make lifestyle modifications that have proven efficacy in reducing CVD mortality and morbidity, such as cessation of smoking,[79] regular physical exercise, and weight reduction with a low-salt and lipid-lowering diet.[80] The American Diabetes Association (ADA) has published guidelines for patients considering an exercise regimen, giving specific recommendations according to the type and presence or absence of diabetic complications. It is also recommended that treadmill exercise testing for the detection of myocardial ischemia and arrhythmia be performed in patients about to undertake a moderate to vigorous exercise regimen if they satisfy one or more of the following criteria:[81]

- age greater than 35 years
- type 2 diabetes of 10 years' duration or type 1

diabetes of 15 years' duration
- presence of any additional risk factor for coronary artery disease
- presence of microvascular disease (proliferative retinopathy or nephropathy, including microalbuminuria)
- presence of peripheral vascular disease
- presence of autonomic neuropathy
- presence of typical or atypical cardiac symptoms
- resting ECG suggestive of ischemia or infarction.

Smoking in diabetic patients has been linked to microvascular complications and the development of type 2 diabetes.[82] Furthermore, given the strong link between CVD and smoking, cessation of smoking should be strongly encouraged in all patients, and this can be implemented via assessment of smoking status, with counseling on smoking prevention and cessation by the treating physician at clinic reviews. To increase the likelihood of achieving cessation, an effective system for the delivery of education on the cessation of smoking should be available to the patient and treating doctor.[79]

## Medical management of cardiac risk factors

The medical management of cardiac risk factors revolves around reinforcement of lifestyle modifications as well as achieving and maintaining adequate control of lipid, blood pressure and glucose profiles, as detailed in earlier chapters.[53,83–85] Given the increasing recognition of raised CV risk in diabetic subjects, there has been a lowering of targets for blood pressure control (130/85, JNC VI)[86,87] and lipid-lowering therapy (National Cholesterol Education Program [NCEP] and Adult Treatment Panel [ATP] III guidelines).[83,85,88] In particular, the recent ATP III guidelines recommend that diabetic patients be treated as a 'CHD risk equivalent' due to the greater than 20% per 10-year risk of CHD events in diabetic subjects; that is, it should be assumed that all diabetic patients require secondary prevention.[88,89]

The recent Heart Protection Study (HPS) of 20 536 high-risk patients with total cholesterol (TC) of >3.5 mmol/l included 5963 patients with diabetes, 1981 with prior CHD and 3982 without prior CHD. Participants were randomized to 40 mg simvastatin or placebo and followed for an average of 5 years. The overall findings were a significant reduction in all-cause mortality, driven mainly by a 24% reduction in CV events. A similar effect was found in the diabetic subgroup.[90] Furthermore, there is some evidence that therapy to lower LDL may reduce the rate of progression of diabetic nephropathy.[91,92] These recent trial findings suggest that a further refinement in lipid-therapy guidelines for diabetic patients may be necessary. Specifically, in addition to treating to targets, one may also treat to achieve a specific reduction in lipid parameters; that is, reducing total or LDL cholesterol by 1 mmol/l.

The use of aspirin for primary prevention was studied in the US Physicians' Health Study, and compared aspirin (325 mg every other day) to placebo in male physicians. There was a 44% risk reduction in the treated group, and subgroup analyses in the diabetic physicians revealed a reduction in myocardial infarction from 10.1% to 4.0% in the aspirin-treated arm.[93,94] For secondary prevention, a recent meta-analysis of antiplatelet trials with a diabetic substudy revealed a 25% reduction in events with an estimated prevention of $38 \pm 12$ vascular events per 1000 diabetic patients treated.[95] The use of antiplatelet therapy in diabetic subjects alone for primary and secondary prevention has been studied only in those with retinopathy and hypertension, and is recommended for use in these high-risk subgroups.[96–98] Hence, aspirin therapy should be initiated in patients requiring secondary prevention of CV events. In addition, diabetic patients at high risk of CVD events should consider aspirin therapy. Such subjects include those with:[31]

- a family history of CHD
- cigarette smoking
- hypertension
- obesity (>120% desirable weight); BMI of >27.3 kg/m$^2$ in women, >27.8 kg/m$^2$ in men
- albuminuria (micro- or macro-)
- dyslipidemia
  — cholesterol of >200 mg/dl
  — LDL cholesterol of ≥100 mg/dl
  — HDL cholesterol of <45 mg/dl in men and <55 mg/dl in women
  — triglycerides of >200 mg/dl
- age over 30 years.

Diabetic subjects with contraindications to aspirin therapy should be considered for alternative antiplatelet therapy such as clopidogrel. Despite the available evidence, the use of antiplatelet therapy in diabetic subjects has been shown to be suboptimal.[99–101]

Recent studies have shown that despite education and regular monitoring the percentage of diabetic patients achieving optimal control of CVD risk factors with use of antiplatelet therapy is low, less than 3.2%.[102,103] This situation requires further improvement, and this will involve education, counselling and motivational approaches by health-care professionals and diabetic patients. In summary, the benefits of primary prevention to be obtained in diabetic subjects with albuminuria are likely to lead to larger absolute benefits, given the higher baseline risk of CV events in this group.

## SECONDARY PREVENTION OF CVD

Patients with prior acute coronary syndromes (ACS) represent some of those with the highest risk of recurrence and subsequent mortality and morbidity. These patients require aggressive cardiac risk-factor modification, as outlined above for primary prevention. In addition, the targets for risk-factor control are more aggressive, with targets for lipid control including a TC of <4.0 mmol/l, a HDL of >1.0 mmol/l and a LDL of <2.5 mmol/l in Australia. However, in the USA, lipid targets remain unchanged as per NCEP guidelines (LDL of <2.6 mmol/l, HDL of >1.15 mmol/l and non-HDL cholesterol [total cholesterol-HDL cholesterol] of <3.4 mmol/l).[85,88,89]

After a CV event, all patients should be prescribed antiplatelet therapy, β-blockers and ACE inhibitors.[104] These agents have a proven role in reducing cardiac mortality and morbidity, and are likely to provide even greater benefits in those at most risk, that is, albuminuric diabetic patients. The role of angiotensin-receptor blockers (ARBs) in diabetic patients in the setting of prior myocardial infarction and/or CHF has not been extensively studied to date. It is anticipated that one recently reported and another pending trial in diabetic and nondiabetic subjects will provide further information on ARBs in diabetic patients in the context of myocardial infarction. OPTIMAAL, a superiority trial comparing losartan to captopril, found a non-significant difference in total mortality in favor of captopril, the investigators recommending that ACE inhibitors remain the first-line choice in the treatment of patients after complicated acute myocardial infarction.[105] VALIANT is an ongoing superiority and non-inferiority trial assessing valsartan, captopril or the combination after myocardial infarction.[106]

In subjects with CHF, the CHARM trial is currently comparing candesartan with or without ACE inhibition versus placebo and an ACE inhibitor arm.[107] Other ACE-ARB comparison studies to date have included ELITE I and the more definitive ELITE II, which have shown that losartan is not superior to captopril in CHF. In the setting of CHF and ACE-ARB combination therapy, the Val-HeFT study has shown a positive reduction in the composite mortality/morbidity endpoint, driven mainly by a 27% reduction in hospitalization for CHF.[108–110] An observation from Val-HeFT was that much of the benefit from ARB therapy was observed in those patients who were not on either an ACE inhibitor or a β-blocker. Only 7% of the patients enrolled in Val-HeFT were not on ACE inhibitors, but these patients showed significant improvement with the addition of valsartan (45% versus 12% reduction). Only 35% of enrolled patients were on β-blockers, and patients who were not on β-blockers also had significant improvement when treated with valsartan. However, there was an important finding in patients who were taking all three neurohumoral blockers (ACE, ARB, and β-blocker), these patients tending to have a negative outcome.[111,112] Hence, until the results of the trials currently underway are available, the role of ARB in secondary prevention should be only in patients who are intolerant of ACE inhibitors, and combination therapy should be considered only in those intolerant of β-blockers.

## ACUTE MANAGEMENT OF CHD

In patients with DM, CHD can manifest acutely as an ACS. This is subclassified into ST segment elevation infarction (STEMI), non-STEMI (NSTEMI) or unstable angina (UA) in these patients. Treatment options vary according to the type of coronary syndrome, the major aim being stabilization and cardiac risk stratification for secondary prevention.

### ST segment elevation infarction (STEMI)

Patients with DM have an increased frequency and prevalence of STEMI with increased complication rates and subsequent raised morbidity and mortality.[1,113] The management of a diabetic patient presenting with a STEMI follows guidelines similar to that of a nondiabetic patient. The primary aim is urgent restoration of flow to the occluded coronary artery (revascularization) to limit the amount of myocardial necrosis. This may be achieved by thrombolytic therapy or, if facilities are available, percutaneous coronary intervention (PCI).[104] A recent report on the diabetic substudy of the CAPTIM study (Comparison of Primary Angioplasty and Prehospital Thrombolysis in Patients with Acute Myocardial Infarction) found that the incidence of the primary composite endpoint (death, recurrent AMI and stroke at 30 days) was 14.6% in diabetic and 5.6% in nondiabetic subjects, with a tripling in mortality in the diabetic subgroup (8.7% versus 3.2%). At 30 days, the composite end-point occurred in 5.8% of those randomized to PCI as compared to 21.7% in those randomized to thrombolysis, suggesting that primary angioplasty would be preferable if facilities were available.[114]

Proliferative diabetic retinopathy is no longer considered an absolute contraindication to thrombolytic therapy in diabetic subjects. In conjunction with thrombolysis and/or PCI, antiplatelet therapy in the form of aspirin, clopidogrel and/or heparin should be commenced immediately.

The role of glucose-insulin therapy in the acute management of STEMI has been reported in the DIGAMI study. In this study, 620 diabetic patients with an acute STEMI and plasma glucose of >11 mmol/l on admission were randomized to the usual glycemic therapy or an intensified regimen. The intensified regimen comprised an intravenous glucose-insulin infusion, acutely for at least 24 hr followed by long-term multidose insulin treatment. There was no difference detected for in-hospital mortality, but there was a significant 30% (11% absolute) reduction in 12-month mortality in the intensive regimen group with no difference in revascularization or readmission. Furthermore, the greatest benefit was seen in those patients not taking insulin previously and with a lower risk profile.[115–118] This study has raised many further issues. What is the mechanism for the derived benefit? Why did low-risk patients benefit the most? Why was the effect not present until 12 months? What effect was attributable to glucose-insulin therapy, to multidose insulin therapy and to removal of oral hypoglycemic agents? These questions regarding the role of glucose-insulin therapy in the management of coronary syndromes should be further delineated once the results of trials currently underway, including DIGAMI2, are available.

Diabetic patients recovering from myocardial infarction attend cardiac rehabilitation classes where they are counseled and educated on therapies for secondary prevention of CVD. Their medical therapy should include medications with proven efficacy in reducing cardiac morbidity and mortality, including ACE inhibition, β-blockade and lipid-lowering therapy. In patients with diabetic nephropathy, the introduction of an ACE inhibitor should include monitoring for hyperkalemia.

## Unstable angina (UA) or non-ST segment elevation infarction (NSTEMI)

The management of a diabetic patient presenting with UA or NSTEMI follows guidelines for that of a nondiabetic patient.[119] The major goal is stabilization and risk stratification of the patient, with identification of those at high risk. In patients without serious comorbidities, the markers of increased risk that would warrant an early invasive strategy with PCI include:

1. recurrent angina/ischemia at rest or with low-level activities despite intensive anti-ischemic therapy
2. elevated troponin levels
3. new ST-segment depression
4. recurrent angina/ischemia with CHF symptoms
5. high-risk findings on noninvasive stress testing
6. depressed left-ventricular systolic function (for example, ejection fraction (EF) less than 0.40 on noninvasive study)
7. hemodynamic instability
8. sustained ventricular tachycardia
9. PCI within 6 months.
10. prior coronary artery bypass grafting (CABG).

In conjunction with PCI, these patients should have antiplatelet therapy initiated with aspirin administered at presentation and continued indefinitely. Clopidogrel should be administered to patients who are unable to take aspirin because of hypersensitivity or major gastrointestinal intolerance. Anticoagulation with heparin should be added to antiplatelet therapy with aspirin and/or clopidogrel. Consideration should be given to the addition of a platelet glycoprotein (GP) IIb/IIIa antagonist in patients already receiving heparin, aspirin, and clopidogrel in whom PCI is planned.

In patients for whom a conservative, noninterventional approach is planned due to low risk or multiple comorbidities, aspirin and heparin should be administered. Consideration should also be given to the administration of clopidogrel in addition to aspirin soon after admission. If commenced, clopidogrel should be continued for at least 1 month and up to 9–12 months, as the CURE and CREDO study results have shown benefits with treatment for this length of time.[120,121]

## Revascularization of a diabetic patient

The choice of method for revascularization in a diabetic patient is dependent upon a variety of factors including extent of disease (diffuse or localized), severity of disease (one-vessel versus three-vessel) and presence of ventricular dysfunction.

Recently, data for the 18-year follow-up of the diabetic cohort from the CASS (Coronary Artery Surgery Study) study have been reported. In this study 24 958 patients were stratified to a surgical versus medical therapy with 2613 having diabetes. Diabetic patients fared worse in both arms than nondiabetics. However, diabetic subjects with three-vessel disease that underwent CABG did significantly better, with no advantage for surgery demonstrated for one- or two-vessel disease.[122] PCI in diabetic subjects was initially reported in the BARI study.[123,124] That study noted better outcome in subjects randomized to surgery than PCI. However, this study was performed at a time when current methodologies and equipment were not in use (stents and GP IIb/IIIA inhibitors), making the results difficult to apply to current practice. Nevertheless, the implication of this and other studies is that complete revascularization is paramount to obtaining survival benefit in patients with multivessel disease. Diabetic patients undergoing coronary artery bypass surgery have increased rates of morbidity (wound infection), but not mortality, in the immediate perioperative period. In the longer term, the patency and benefits of arterial conduits have been proven in diabetic patients.[125–128] These data serve to reinforce the fact that, regardless of choice of revascularization therapy, diabetic patients fare worse than nondiabetic patients with increased CV event rates. In addition, in patients with three-vessel involvement and poor ventricular function, coronary artery bypass surgery with use of arterial conduits should be recommended.[129]

Inhibition of the platelet GP IIb/IIIa receptor prevents platelet aggregation and ultimately limits the formation of thrombus. The use of stents and GP IIb/IIIa agents has been shown to reduce target-vessel revascularization and major cardiac events in diabetic patients.[130,131] In addition, the development of newer techniques with promising results to minimize restenosis, such as intracoronary irradiation and drug-coated or eluting stents, is likely to reduce further the major cardiac adverse event rate. However, given that albuminuric diabetics have a higher incidence of restenosis,[38] careful consideration should be given to the choice of method of revascularization in diabetic patients with one- or two-vessel CHD. The BARI 2D study, which is comparing immediate aggressive revascularization with conservative therapy and glycemic control with insulin sensitizers in diabetic subjects, should provide further insight into this issue.

## CONGESTIVE HEART FAILURE (CHF)

CHF, which is more prevalent in patients with diabetes,[132–134] presents with diastolic and/or systolic dysfunction. Diabetic patients with albuminuria are more likely to develop symptomatic heart failure.[19] The etiology and mechanisms of this CHF are multifactorial in nature, incorporating ischemic, dilated, hypertensive, autonomic and/or 'diabetic cardiomyopathic' etiologies. The concept of a 'diabetic cardiomyopathy' in which DM, independently of hypertension or CHD, affects cardiac structure and function was first documented by Rubler et al in 1972.[135] Subsequent human and animal data have led to increasing evidence for this condition.[5,136–144] The exact mechanism is still under intense investigation, with evidence accumulating that DM leads to a worsening cascade of myocardial fibrosis/hypertrophy, left-ventricular diastolic dysfunction and finally systolic dysfunction.[145–149] In this section, we shall review the pathophysiology of diabetic cardiomyopathy and the current management of CHF in diabetes.

## Pathophysiology of diabetic cardiomyopathy

While it was once thought that ischemic heart disease was mainly responsible for the increased incidence of CHF in diabetic patients, recent data suggest that one of the major adverse complications of diabetes is the development of specific cardiomyopathy, characterized by both diastolic and systolic left-ventricular dysfunction. Indeed, epidemiologic, anatomic, experimental and human studies are consistent with the existence of a specific diabetic myocardial disease,[136] independent of coronary atherosclerosis.

Several studies have been dedicated to the evaluation of morphologic changes in the diabetic heart.[150] Anatomic studies have shown that diabetic cardiomyopathy is mainly characterized by alterations in the microvasculature and myocardial interstitium.[143,151] In the initial stages of the disease, interstitial changes with preserved myocytes and microvascular structure and function may predominate and lead to the observed reduction in myocardial compliance.[152,153] With disease progression, salient findings include left-ventricular hypertrophy with perivascular, interstitial and replacement fibrosis, and accumulation of periodic acid-Schiff (PAS)-positive material. Arteriolar or capillary involvement typical of diabetic microangiopathy, including increased thickening of the myocardial capillary-basement membrane and microaneurysms, occurs later in association with more severe myocardial dysfunction.[154] These lesions are not characteristic of diabetes only and appear to be synergistic with the structural changes usually observed in arterial hypertension. This fact might be particularly relevant in the light of the positive effects of antihypertensive therapy in diabetic patients observed in the UKPDS[155] and HOT[156] studies.

The pathophysiology of diabetic cardiomyopathy remains largely unknown, but several hypotheses have been investigated. Contributing to its development is the depressed calcium-ATPase activity of myosin and actomyosin, thus accounting for the decreased shortening velocity of cardiac muscle, which is associated with a myosin isoenzyme shift from the more active V1 to the less active V3 form.[157] Calcium homeostasis also appears to be defective in the diabetic heart. While calcium transport by the sarcolemmal and sarcoplasmatic reticular calcium pumps is minimally affected by diabetes, significant impairment occurs in $Na^+$–$Ca^{2+}$ exchanger activity. This defect limits the ability of the diabetic heart to extrude calcium, contributing to an elevation in intracellular calcium. A decrease in $Na^+$, $K^+$-ATPase activity, which is known to increase intracellular calcium secondary to a rise in intracellular sodium, may also promote the accumulation of calcium by the diabetic cell.[157] It is very likely that these defects are related to aberrations of glucose and/or lipid metabolism that involve membrane changes, such as phosphatidylethanolamine N-methylation and protein phosphorylation, which, in turn, determine myocyte metabolic dysfunction.

The adverse cardiac effects of diabetes could also be due to other factors. Carbohydrate and lipid metabolism alterations consequent to diabetes are closely linked to the intracellular accumulation of potentially toxic intermediates such as various acyl-carnitine and coenzyme derivatives.[158,159] Abnormally high amounts of metabolic intermediates could cause disturbances in calcium homeostasis, which, as previously mentioned, in the long term, can eventually lead to cardiac dysfunction.[159] In this context, lowering raised plasma triglycerides and free fatty acid levels could therefore decrease the heart's reliance on fatty acids and overcome the fatty-acid inhibition of myocardial glucose utilization. In fact, increased levels of citrate, produced by free fatty-acid oxidation, inhibit phosphofructokinase, leading to decreased glycolysis and promotion of glycogen synthesis. Impaired glucose oxidation also leads to lactic acid accumulation that further promotes the degradation of free fatty acids.

Nonenzymatic glycosylation of proteins is another explanation for the interstitial accumulation of PAS-positive material and increased content of collagen resistant to proteolysis in diabetic hearts.[160]

Reduced myocardial blood flow has been clearly shown in diabetes,[161] independently of frank epicardial coronary disease, and is linked to impaired endothelial function.[162–164] Acute hyperglycemia may further impair endothelial-derived vasodilation.[165] Indeed, the inability to increase myocardial blood flow appears to be independently related to long-term blood-glucose control,[166] suggesting that hyperglycemia per se is of considerable importance for impaired vascular function. Hyperinsulinemia, by increasing the production of endothelial factors such as endothelins,[167] will also adversely affect the evolution of CVD. In the long term, impaired coronary flow reserve, in the presence of the already described metabolic alterations, might well determine and aggravate a cardiomyopathic process.

Cardiac autonomic dysfunction (see below) has also been proposed as a possible pathogenetic mechanism for the development of diabetic cardiomyopathy.[137] Finally, recent observations suggest that local cardiac increases in angiotensin II in the context of diabetes may enhance oxidative damage, activating cardiac cell apoptosis and necrosis that lead to myocardial dysfunction.[168]

In summary, the pathophysiological mechanisms responsible for a specific diabetic cardiomyopathy are likely to be multifactorial, including both metabolic and vascular components.

## Management of CHF

### Left-ventricular systolic dysfunction and systolic heart failure

Patients with systolic left-ventricular dysfunction should be investigated to exclude the presence of reversible myocardial ischemia amenable to revascularization by functional testing or coronary angiography. In addition, significant valvular heart disease should be excluded by an echocardiographic examination in all patients. Furthermore, primary and secondary CV preventive strategies should be employed as described above. Education and counseling should be provided. This will include low-salt and fluid intake, cessation of alcohol intake, and regular weighing to assess fluid status. Patients should be encouraged to exercise to minimize fluid retention. Pharmacologic therapy should revolve around drugs shown to improve mortality titrated to maximal dose (ACE inhibitors, β-blockers and spironolactone, hydralazine and monosodium nitrate—in those intolerant of ACE inhibitors) as well as agents for symptom relief (diuretics and nitrates). The use of ARBs has been discussed above. Medications to avoid in these patients include most antiarrhythmics (except β-blockers and amiodarone), centrally acting-calcium-channel blockers (negatively inotropic), tricyclic antidepressants (proarrhythmic), and non-steroidal anti-inflammatory agents and cyclo-oxygenase inhibitors (fluid retention). Other issues that may require a specific cardiologic opinion include the use of positive inotropic therapy, thromboembolic prophylaxis and arrhythmia management with consideration of pharmacologic antiarrhythmic therapy, implantable cardiac defibrillators and/or cardiac resynchronization therapy. Finally, surgical options may also need to be considered, such as cardiomyoplasty, volume reduction, mitral regurgitation and heart transplantation surgery.[132,169–173]

### Left-ventricular diastolic dysfunction and diastolic heart failure

Diastolic heart failure defined as symptomatic heart failure with preserved systolic function is reported in 20–40% of patients with CHF. The etiology is related to abnormal diastolic ventricular function arising from impaired relaxation and compliance properties of the ventricle. Predisposing conditions include hypertension and diabetes, as discussed previously. The prevalence of left-ventricular diastolic dysfunction in diabetic patients was reported as about 30% in early studies.[147,174] However, with the recent development of new echocardiographic techniques such as tissue Doppler imaging and color M mode Doppler, the prevalence appears to be much higher.[175–177] Indeed, our group has found a prevalence of cardiac abnormalities, as defined by specific echocardiographic parameters, in an unselected diabetic population of greater than 60%, with diastolic dysfunction present in over 50% of subjects. This higher prevalence is almost entirely due to improved differentiation of patients with pseudonormal diastolic dysfunction from normal diastolic function.[178] To date, there have been few studies on the natural history and no randomized clinical trials on the treatment of diastolic heart failure in diabetes. Numerous studies are currently underway to treat diastolic dysfunction in both nondiabetic and diabetic patients (I-PRESERVE, CHARM and ADEPT). Currently, the management of a patient with diastolic heart failure is based on adequate blood pressure control with use of an ACE inhibitor, β-blocker and/or calcium antagonist with symptomatic treatment with diuretics. Finally, in patients with atrial fibrillation, an attempt should be made for reversion to sinus rhythm.

## SUDDEN CARDIAC DEATH (SCD)

Patients with diabetes are at an increased risk of SCD, due to the increased prevalence of silent myocardial ischemia and cardiac autonomic neuropathy predisposing patients to ventricular tachyarrhythmias.[179]

### Silent myocardial ischemia

'Silent myocardial ischemia' is a term usually used to describe myocardial ischemia in the absence of pain but in the presence of other evidence of ischemia.[180] Patients with silent ischemia have been classified by Cohn:[181] patients with only painless ischemia, asymptomatic with no history of myocardial infarction or angina; patients presenting with a 'silent myocardial infarction', with evidence of a new myocardial infarction on the electrocardiogram or with abnormalities of ventricular function and no antecedent history of ischemia; and patients with both symptomatic ischemia (angina) and episodes of painless ischemia. All diabetic patients are at an increased risk of silent myocardial ischemia with a further rise in risk of this condition in those with albuminuria.[182]

The perception of pain during ischemia in diabetic subjects may be reduced by several factors. Langer et al[183] have demonstrated that silent myocardial ischemia in asymptomatic diabetic men occurred frequently and in association with autonomic dysfunction, suggesting that diabetic autonomic neuropathy might be implicated in the mechanism of silent ischemia. Furthermore, the same authors observed that diabetic subjects with silent myocardial ischemia had evidence of a diffuse abnormality in metaiodobenzylguanidine (MIBG) uptake, suggesting that abnormalities in pain perception might be linked to sympathetic denervation.[184] Studying the anginal perceptual threshold, Ambepityia et al[185] observed that altered perception of myocardial ischemia in diabetic patients might result from damage to the sensory innervation of the heart. Another possible factor responsible for silent myocardial ischemia in diabetes is a disorder of central pain perception. Rosen et al[186] demonstrated that abnormal central processing of afferent pain messages plays an important role in silent myocardial ischemia. Moreover, Hikita et al[187] demonstrated that β-endorphin level and pain thresholds were significantly higher in nondiabetic patients with silent ischemia than in diabetic patients.

In summary, there could be several explanations for different patterns of symptoms in patients with diabetes, including central mechanisms, such as different thresholds of pain sensitivity and β-endorphin levels, and peripheral mechanisms, such as the presence of autonomic neuropathy leading to sensory denervation.

There are limited prognostic data in diabetic patients with silent myocardial ischemia. Weiner et al[188] demonstrated that when myocardial ischemia (whether silent or symptomatic) was present during exercise testing, the long-term survival among diabetic patients was worse than in nondiabetic subjects. In contrast, when ischemia was absent, there was no higher mortality risk for diabetic patients. Importantly, survival rates among patients with silent ischemia were similar to those of symptomatic patients regardless of diabetic status. These findings are consistent with another survival analysis by Pancholy et al,[189] which demonstrated no significant difference in the event-free survival in patients with symptomatic or silent ischemia over a time period of 2 years. The extent of perfusion abnormality and history of diabetes were the most important predictors of events. Thus, the limited prognostic data in the literature point to a worse outcome among patients with diabetes and silent ischemia than patients without ischemia.

Treadmill exercise testing is recommended for symptomatic patients as well as for asymptomatic diabetic patients older than 35 years with albuminuria and wishing to commence an exercise regimen.[81] However, this testing is not recommended for routine screening of diabetic patients. Newer modalities of screening, such as EBCT and nuclear, echocardiographic and magnetic resonance techniques, have been used to identify the prevalence of silent myocardial ischemia and/or atherosclerotic disease burden, but are not recommended for routine screening purposes.[190] This is due to the mixed outcome data in diabetic patients with silent myocardial ischemia, ranging from poor to good. Furthermore, revascularization outcome data are available only in symptomatic, and not asymptomatic, patients. Hence, this group of asymptomatic diabetic patients requires further evaluation.

## Cardiac autonomic neuropathy (CAN)

Peripheral somatic neuropathy is a commonly recognized complication of DM. Autonomic neuropathy also occurs in diabetes, leading to diarrhea, vomiting, sexual dysfunction and other disturbances. A form of autonomic dysfunction involves the heart and is generally termed 'cardiac autonomic neuropathy' (CAN).[191] Autonomic dysfunction due to true CAN should be distinguished from the autonomic dysfunction related to coronary artery disease, myocardial infarction or CHF because all these conditions can cause similar abnormalities in autonomic function tests.[192–195] Data from the Honolulu Heart Program indicate that diabetes is a predictor of sudden death and that this predisposition is related to an increased risk of SCD from arrhythmias.[196] Imbalance of the autonomic nervous system of the heart, with decreased vagal activity or increased sympathetic activity, contributes to the genesis of ventricular arrhythmia and sudden death[197] and constitutes an independent risk factor for death among survivors of acute myocardial infarction.[198,199] Absent heart rate variability secondary to diabetic autonomic neuropathy is predictive of both left-ventricular failure and increased mortality.[200] Moreover, left-ventricular function has been reported to be depressed in 59% of diabetic subjects with diabetic CAN compared with only 8% of those without CAN.[201] Thus, CAN secondary to diabetes is a predictor of the development of CHF and SCD.[200]

CAN may be divided into two categories: clinically based with objective signs or subjective symptoms, and subclinical, as detected in asymptomatic patients by autonomic testing.[202] Although clinical features of autonomic neuropathy generally occur only in patients with diabetes of long duration, it has become increasingly evident that subclinical diabetic autonomic neuropathy, mainly in the form of CAN, may evolve early in the course of diabetes,[202–204] and in the absence of other microvascular complications.[204–206] The balance of activity between the cardiac sympathetic and parasympathetic nervous systems has a key role in the functional and structural performance of the diabetic heart.[207] CAN may involve the sympathetic nervous system and/or the parasympathetic nervous system. Clinical studies have shown that cardiac denervation in diabetes closely resembles the pattern of denervation that is thought to predispose to malignant arrhythmias:[208–210] protective parasympathetic tone is decreased and sympathetic myocardial innervation is most preserved in regions incapable of vasodilating during adenosine stimulation.[211] Recent observations suggest that diabetes may result in left-ventricular sympathetic denervation with proximal hyperinnervation complicating distal denervation.[212] This exaggerated sympathetic imbalance may contribute to the accelerated rate of SCD in diabetes.[212] Moreover, using positron-emission tomography (PET), Stevens et al[211] recently demonstrated that regional sympathetic myocardial denervation in diabetes is associated with abnormal patterns of myocardial blood flow. In type 2 diabetes, although less studied, the pattern of cardiac sympathetic denervation is similar to that observed in type 1 diabetic patients.[184] There is, however, evidence that the extent of denervation is less pronounced in type 2 than in type 1 diabetes.[207,213]

Several studies suggest a multifactorial pathogenesis of CAN with a complex interaction between metabolic,[160,214–216] vascular,[215,217] rheological[215] and immunologic[218–220] abnormalities. The 'sorbitol pathway' by which glucose is converted to sorbitol and fructose under hyperglycemic conditions has been shown to lead to reduction of myoinositol, which in turn may reduce the activity of $Na^+,K^+$-ATPase, an enzyme known to be important for nerve conduction velocity.[221,222] Deficiencies of dihomo-γ-linolenic acid, as well as N-acetyl-L-carnitine, have also been suggested as a possible pathogenetic mechanism. In addition, oxidative stress has been implicated in the pathogenesis of diabetic autonomic neuropathy. In particular, free radicals may impair the endothelium-dependent vasodilation, either by changes in the generation and bioactivity of nitric oxide or by a reduced synthesis of vasodilating prostaglandins.[215,223] The diminished generation of vasodilating mediators may lead to a reduced endoneurial blood flow, which, in turn, causes the endoneurial hypoxia and/or ischemia that are responsible for the neuronal damage.[215,223,224] Another important aspect in the progression of diabetic neuropathy is the impaired ability of damaged nerve fibers to regenerate.[225] Indeed, the levels of several neurotrophic factors, including nerve growth factor (NGF), ciliary neurotrophic factor, brain-derived neurotrophic factor and insulin growth factor, which are assumed to be essential for nerve regeneration, have been shown to be reduced in diabetic neuropathy.[226,227] In particular, in subjects with diabetic autonomic neuropathy, serum NGF levels are reduced,[227] and it has been suggested that NGF autoantibodies may play a role in the development of autonomic dysfunction.[228] Schmid et al[229] have recently demonstrated that diabetic-induced distal left-ventricular denervation is associated with a proximal-to-distal gradient of myocardial NGF protein depression, providing evidence of a key role for the regional fluctuations of left-ventricular NGF protein in determining the heterogeneous cardiac sympathetic denervation complicating diabetes. In type 1 diabetes, immunologic

factors, as evidenced by autoantibodies against sympathetic ganglia, have been reported to be associated with cardiac sympathetic dysfunction.[218–220,230] These antibodies seem to be rather specific for cardioneuropathy of type 1 diabetic patients and occur independently of those against islet cells, GAD or protein tyrosine phosphatase-like molecules, such as ICA512.[230] Autoantibodies against autonomic nervous tissues are not detected significantly in type 2 diabetes, either with or without cardiac sympathetic dysfunction.[230,231] The specificity of autoantibodies against sympathetic ganglia in type 1 diabetes supports the view that autoantibodies against sympathetic postganglionic neurons cause local damage and subsequently promote deterioration of neuronal function in these patients.

Cardiac autonomic dysfunction may be diagnosed by direct and indirect means. The recent development of scintiscanning techniques has allowed cardiac nerves to be visualized directly with radionuclide tracer materials. Advanced single-photon-emission computed tomography (SPECT) and PET with the radiopharmaceuticals I123 MIBG and 11C-hydroxyephedrine (HED) enable the characterization of the pattern and extent of cardiac sympathetic denervation.[232–234] These techniques have demonstrated that sympathetic neuronal damage occurs early in the development of diabetic autonomic neuropathy and often before CV reflex abnormalities are apparent.[235] Until recently, the diagnosis of CAN was indirect and based on CV responses and rhythms, including:

1. resting heart rate (after 15-min rest) of 100 beats/min or more
2. lack of heart rate variability on electrocardiographic recording of ≤10 beats/min
3. a ratio of the longest R-R interval to the shortest of 1.10 or less during the Valsalva maneuver
4. a ratio of the R-R interval of the 30th beat to 15th beat after standing of 1 or less
5. QT interval length that has been demonstrated to be significantly longer in patients with diabetic autonomic neuropathy
6. a fall in systolic blood pressure of 30 mmHg or more after 1 min of standing
7. left-ventricular dysfunction.[191,236–239]

Treatment strategies to minimize the effects of silent myocardial ischemia and CAN should be employed, and they include primary prevention strategies as previously outlined. Furthermore, in diabetic patients considered to be at high risk (survivors of sudden cardiac arrest, impaired systolic ventricular function—that is, ejection fraction under

30%—and ventricular tachycardia on HOLTER monitoring), electrophysiological studies with a view to implantable cardiac defibrillators should be considered.[240]

# REFERENCES

1. Haffner S, Mortality from coronary heart disease in subjects with type 2 diabetes and in nondiabetic subjects with and without prior myocardial infarction, *N Engl J Med* (1998) **339:** 229–34.

2. Garcia MJ, McNamara PM, Gordon T et al, Morbidity and mortality in diabetics in the Framingham population. Sixteen year follow-up study, *Diabetes* (1974) **23:** 105–11.

3. Bell DS. Diabetic cardiomyopathy. A unique entity or a complication of coronary artery disease?, *Diabetes Care* (1995) **18:** 708–14.

4. Raman M, Nesto RW, Heart disease in diabetes mellitus, *Endocrinol Metab Clin North Am* (1996) **25:** 425–38.

5. Mahgoub MA, Abd-Elfattah AS, Diabetes mellitus and cardiac function, *Mol Cell Biochem* (1998) **180:** 59–64.

6. Sowers JR, Epstein M, Risk factors for arterial disease in diabetes: hypertension. In: Tooke JE, ed., *Diabetic Angiopathy.* (Arnold: London, 1999) 45–63.

7. Singer DE, Moulton AW, Nathan DM, Diabetic myocardial infarction. Interaction of diabetes with other preinfarction risk factors, *Diabetes* (1989) **38:** 350–7.

8. Stone PH, Muller JE, Hartwell T et al, The effect of diabetes mellitus on prognosis and serial left ventricular function after acute myocardial infarction: contribution of both coronary disease and diastolic left ventricular dysfunction to the adverse prognosis. The MILIS Study Group, *J Am Coll Cardiol* (1989) **14:** 49–57.

9. Haffner SM, Impaired glucose tolerance, insulin resistance and cardiovascular disease, *Diabet Med* (1997) **14** (Suppl 3): S12–S18.

10. Laakso M, Lehto S, Epidemiology of risk factors for cardiovascular disease in diabetes and impaired glucose tolerance, *Atherosclerosis* (1998) **137** (Suppl): S65–73.

11. Sowers JR, Diabetes mellitus and cardiovascular disease in women, *Arch Intern Med* (1998) **158:** 617–21.

12. Stamler J, Vaccaro O, Neaton JD et al, Diabetes, other risk factors, and 12-yr cardiovascular mortality for men screened in the Multiple Risk Factor Intervention Trial, *Diabetes Care* (1993) **16:** 434–44.

13. Borch-Johnsen K, Feldt-Rasmussen B, Strandgaard S et al, Urinary albumin excretion. An independent predictor of ischemic heart disease, *Arterioscler Thromb Vasc Biol* (1999) **19:** 1992–7.

14. Gerstein HC, Mann JF, Pogue J et al, Prevalence and determinants of microalbuminuria in high-risk diabetic and nondiabetic patients in the Heart Outcomes Prevention Evaluation Study. The HOPE Study Investigators, *Diabetes Care* (2000) **3** (Suppl 2): B35–B39.

15. Hanninen J, Takala J, Keinanen-Kiukaanniemi S, Albuminuria and other risk factors for mortality in patients with non-insulin-dependent diabetes mellitus aged under 65 years: a population-based prospective 5-year study, *Diabetes Res Clin Pract* (1999) **43:** 121–6.

16. Wachtell K, Olsen MH, Dahlof B et al, Microalbuminuria in hypertensive patients with electrocardiographic left ventricular hypertrophy: the LIFE study, *J Hypertens* (2002) **20:** 405–12.

17. Hillege HL, Fidler V, Diercks GF et al, Urinary albumin excretion predicts cardiovascular and noncardiovascular mortality in general population, *Circulation* (2002) **106:** 1777–82.

18. Spoelstra-de Man AM, Brouwer CB, Stehouwer CD et al, Rapid progression of albumin excretion is an independent predictor of cardiovascular mortality in patients with type 2 diabetes and microalbuminuria, *Diabetes Care* (2001) **24:** 2097–101.

19. Gerstein HC, Mann JF, Yi Q et al, Albuminuria and risk of cardiovascular events, death, and heart failure in diabetic and nondiabetic individuals, *JAMA* (2001) **286:** 421–6.

20. Perneger TV, Brancati FL, Whelton PK et al, End-stage renal disease attributable to diabetes mellitus, *Ann Intern Med* (1994) **121:** 912–18.

21. Foley RN, Culleton BF, Parfrey PS et al, Cardiac disease in diabetic end-stage renal disease, *Diabetologia* (1997) **40:** 1307–12.

22. McMillan MA, Briggs JD, Junor BJ, Outcome of renal replacement treatment in patients with diabetes mellitus, *BMJ* (1990) **301:** 540–4.

23. Hirschl MM, Heinz G, Sunder-Plassmann G et al, Renal replacement therapy in type 2 diabetic patients: 10 years' experience, *Am J Kidney Dis* (1992) **20:** 564–8.

24. Rischen-Vos J, van der Woude FJ, Tegzess AM et al, Increased morbidity and mortality in patients with diabetes mellitus after kidney transplantation as compared with non-diabetic patients, *Nephrol Dial Transplant* (1992) **7:** 433–7.

25. Rodby RA, Rohde RD, Clarke WR et al, The Irbesartan Type II Diabetic Nephropathy Trial: study design and baseline patient characteristics. For the Collaborative Study Group, *Nephrol Dial Transplant* (2000) **15:** 487–97.

26. Lewis EJ, Hunsicker LG, Clarke WR et al, Renoprotective effect of the angiotensin-receptor antagonist irbesartan in patients with nephropathy due to type 2 diabetes, *N Engl J Med* (2001) **345:** 851–60.

27. Brenner BM, Cooper ME, de Zeeuw D et al, Effects of losartan on renal and cardiovascular outcomes in patients with type 2 diabetes and nephropathy, *N Engl J Med* (2001) **345:** 861–9.

28. Gerstein HC, Reduction of cardiovascular events and microvascular complications in diabetes with ACE inhibitor treatment: HOPE and MICRO-HOPE, *Diabetes Metab Res Rev* (2002) **18** (Suppl 3): S82–5.

29. Heart Outcomes Prevention Evaluation Study Investigators, Effects of ramipril on cardiovascular and microvascular outcomes in people with diabetes mellitus: results of the HOPE study and MICRO-HOPE substudy, *Lancet* (2000) **355:** 253–9.

30. Burchfiel CM, Reed DM, Marcus EB et al, Association of diabetes mellitus with coronary atherosclerosis and myocardial lesions. An autopsy study from the Honolulu Heart Program. *Am J Epidemiol* (1993) **137:** 1328–40.

31. Meigs JB, Larson MG, D'Agostino RB et al, Coronary artery calcification in type 2 diabetes and insulin resistance: the Framingham offspring study, *Diabetes Care* (2002) **25:** 1313–19.

32. Waller BF, Palumbo PJ, Lie JT et al, Status of the coronary arteries at necropsy in diabetes mellitus with onset after age 30 years. Analysis of 229 diabetic patients with and without clinical evidence of coronary heart disease and comparison to 183 control subjects, *Am J Med* (1980) **69:** 498–506.

33. Vigorita VJ, Moore GW, Hutchins GM, Absence of correlation between coronary arterial atherosclerosis and severity or duration of diabetes mellitus of adult onset, *Am J Cardiol* (1980) **46:** 535–42.

34. Goldschmid MG, Barrett-Connor E, Edelstein SL et al, Dyslipidemia and ischemic heart disease mortality among men and women with diabetes, *Circulation* (1994) **89:** 991–7.

35. Dash H, Johnson RA, Dinsmore RE et al, Cardiomyopathic syndrome due to coronary artery disease. II. Increased prevalence in patients with diabetes mellitus: a matched pair analysis, *Br Heart J* (1977) **39:** 740–7.

36. Jarrett RJ, Risk factors for coronary heart disease in diabetes mellitus, *Diabetes* (1992) **41** (Suppl 2): 1–3.

37. Manson JE, Colditz GA, Stampfer MJ et al, A prospective study of maturity-onset diabetes mellitus and risk of coronary heart disease and stroke in women, *Arch Intern Med* (1991) **151:** 1141–7.

38. Heper G, Durmaz T, Murat SN et al, Clinical and angiographic outcomes of diabetic patients after coronary stenting: a comparison of native vessel stent restenosis rates in different diabetic subgroups, *Angiology* (2002) **53:** 287–95.

39. Stamler R, Stamler J, Dyer A et al, Asymptomatic hyperglycemia and cardiovascular diseases in three Chicago epidemiologic studies, *Diabetes Care* (1979) **2:** 142–3.

40. West KM, Epidemiology of diabetes and its macrovascular complications, *Diabetes Care* (1979) **2:** 63–4.

41. Wingard DL, Barrett-Connor EL, Scheidt-Nave C et al, Prevalence of cardiovascular and renal complications in older adults with normal or impaired glucose tolerance or NIDDM. A population-based study, *Diabetes Care* (1993) **16:** 1022–5.

42. Grundy SM, Benjamin IJ, Burke GL et al, Diabetes and cardiovascular disease: a statement for healthcare professionals from the American Heart Association, *Circulation* (1999) **100:** 1134–46.

43. Moreno PR, Murcia AM, Palacios IF et al, Coronary composition and macrophage infiltration in atherectomy specimens from patients with diabetes mellitus, *Circulation* (2000) **102:** 2180–4.

44. Moreno PR, Fallon JT, Murcia AM et al, Tissue characteristics of restenosis after percutaneous transluminal coronary angioplasty in diabetic patients, *J Am Coll Cardiol* (1999) **34:** 1045–9.

45. Burke AP, Varghese PJ, Peterson E et al, Large lipid core and extensive plaque burden are features of coronary atherosclerosis in patients with non-insulin dependent diabetes mellitus, *J Am Coll Cardiol* (2001) **37:** 257A (abst).

46. Mautner SL, Lin F, Roberts WC, Composition of atherosclerotic plaques in the epicardial coronary arteries in juvenile (type I) diabetes mellitus, *Am J Cardiol* (1992) **70:** 1264–8.

47. Eckel RH, Wassef M, Chait A et al, Prevention Conference VI: diabetes and cardiovascular disease: Writing Group II: pathogenesis of atherosclerosis in diabetes, *Circulation* (2002) **105:** e138–43.

48. Candido R, Jandeleit-Dahm KA, Cao Z et al, Prevention of accelerated atherosclerosis by angiotensin-converting enzyme inhibition in diabetic apolipoprotein E-deficient mice, *Circulation* (2002) **106:** 246–53.

49. Uusitupa MI, Niskanen LK, Siitonen O et al, 5-Year incidence of atherosclerotic vascular disease in relation to general risk factors, insulin level, and abnormalities in lipoprotein composition in non-insulin-dependent diabetic and nondiabetic subjects, *Circulation* (1990) **82:** 27–36.

50. Laakso M, Hyperglycemia and cardiovascular disease in type 2 diabetes, *Diabetes* (1999) **48:** 937–42.

51. Diabetes Control and Complications Trial Research Group, The effect of intensive treatment of diabetes on the development and progression of long-term complications in insulin-dependent diabetes mellitus, *N Engl J Med* (1993) **329:** 977–86.

52. UK Prospective Diabetes Study (UKPDS) Group, Intensive blood-glucose control with sulphonylureas or insulin compared with conventional treatment and risk of complications in patients with type 2 diabetes (UKPDS 33), *Lancet* (1998) **352:** 837–53.

53. Grundy SM, Howard B, Smith S Jr et al, Prevention Conference VI: diabetes and cardiovascular disease: executive summary: conference proceeding for healthcare professionals from a special writing group of the American Heart Association, *Circulation* (2002) **105:** 2231–9.

54. Friedman EA, Advanced glycosylated end products and hyperglycemia in the pathogenesis of diabetic complications, *Diabetes Care* (1999) **22** (Suppl 2): B65–71.

55. Stitt AW, He C, Friedman S et al, Elevated AGE-modified ApoB in sera of euglycemic, normolipidemic patients with atherosclerosis: relationship to tissue AGEs, *Mol Med* (1997) **3:** 617–27.

56. Hoff HF, Whitaker TE, O'Neil J, Oxidation of low density lipoprotein leads to particle aggregation and altered macrophage recognition, *J Biol Chem* (1992) **267:** 602–9.

57. Schmidt AM, Yan SD, Wautier JL et al, Activation of receptor for advanced glycation end products: a mechanism for chronic vascular dysfunction in diabetic vasculopathy and atherosclerosis, *Circ Res* (1999) **84:** 489–97.

58. Stitt AW, Bucala R, Vlassara H, Atherogenesis and advanced glycation: promotion, progression, and prevention, *Ann N Y Acad Sci* (1997) **811:** 115–29.

59. Libby P, Ridker PM, Maseri A, Inflammation and atherosclerosis, *Circulation* (2002) **105:** 1135–43.

60. Kunt T, Forst T, Wilhelm A et al, Alpha-lipoic acid reduces expression of vascular cell adhesion molecule-1 and endothelial adhesion of human monocytes after stimulation with advanced glycation end products, *Clin Sci (Lond)* (1999) **96:** 75–82.

61. Mamo JC, Szeto L, Steiner G, Glycation of very low density lipoprotein from rat plasma impairs its catabolism, *Diabetologia* (1990) **33:** 339–45.

62. Bucala R, Lipid and lipoprotein modification by advanced glycosylation end-products: role in atherosclerosis, *Exp Physiol* (1997) **82:** 327–37.

63. Makita Z, Yanagisawa K, Kuwajima S et al, The role of advanced glycosylation end-products in the pathogenesis of atherosclerosis, *Nephrol Dial Transplant* (1996) **11:** 31–3.

64. Sobal G, Sinzinger H, Menzel EJ, Binding of long-term glycated low density lipoprotein and AGE-albumin by peripheral monocytes and endothelial cells, *J Recept Signal Transduct Res* (1999) **19:** 267–81.

65. Berg T, Serum levels of advanced glycation end products are associated with left ventricular diastolic function in patients with type 1 diabetes, *Diabetes Care* (1999) **22:** 1186–90.

66. Kiuchi K, Nejima J, Takono T et al, Increased serum concentrations of advanced glycation end products: a marker of coronary artery disease activity in type 2 diabetic patients, *Heart* (2001) **85:** 87–91.

67. Zhang J, Ren S, Shen GX, Glycation amplifies lipoprotein(a)-induced alterations in the generation of fibrinolytic regulators from human vascular endothelial cells, *Atherosclerosis* (2000) **150:** 299–308.

68. Esposito C, Gerlach H, Brett J et al, Endothelial receptor-mediated binding of glucose-modified albumin is associated with increased monolayer permeability and modulation of cell surface coagulant properties, *J Exp Med* (1989) **170:** 1387–407.

69. Nitenberg A, Valensi P, Sachs R et al, Impairment of coronary vascular reserve and ACh-induced coronary vasodilation in diabetic patients with angiographically normal coronary arteries and normal left ventricular systolic function, *Diabetes* (1993) **42:** 1017–25.

70. Zuanetti G, Latini R, Maggioni AP et al, Effect of the ACE inhibitor lisinopril on mortality in diabetic patients with acute myocardial infarction: data from the GISSI-3 study, *Circulation* (1997) **96:** 4239–45.

71. UK Prospective Diabetes Study Group, Efficacy of atenolol and captopril in reducing risk of macrovascular and microvascular complications in type 2 diabetes: UKPDS 39, *BMJ* (1998) **317:** 713–20.

72. Hansson L, Lindholm LH, Niskanen L et al, Effect of

angiotensin-converting-enzyme inhibition compared with conventional therapy on cardiovascular morbidity and mortality in hypertension: the Captopril Prevention Project (CAPPP) randomised trial, *Lancet* (1999) **353:** 611–16.

73. Sobol A, The role of platelets in diabetes related vascular complication, *Diabetes Res Clin Practice* (2000) **50:** 1–16.

74. MacRury SM, Lowe GD, Blood rheology in diabetes mellitus, *Diabet Med* (1990) **7:** 285–91.

75. Caro JJ, Ward AJ, O'Brien JA, Lifetime costs of complications resulting from type 2 diabetes in the US, *Diabetes Care* (2002) **25:** 476–81.

76. Nichols GA, Glauber HS, Brown JB, Type 2 diabetes: incremental medical care costs during the 8 years preceding diagnosis, *Diabetes Care* (2000) **23:** 1654–9.

77. Nichols GA, Brown JB, The impact of cardiovascular disease on medical care costs in subjects with and without type 2 diabetes, *Diabetes Care* (2002) **25:** 482–6.

78. Rutter MK, McComb JM, Brady S et al, Silent myocardial ischemia and microalbuminuria in asymptomatic subjects with non-insulin-dependent diabetes mellitus, *Am J Cardiol* (1999) **83:** 27–31.

79. American Diabetes Association, Smoking and diabetes, *Diabetes Care* (2002) **25** (Suppl 1): 80–1.

80. Grundy SM, Garber A, Goldberg R et al, Prevention Conference VI: diabetes and cardiovascular disease: Writing Group IV: lifestyle and medical management of risk factors, *Circulation* (2002) **105:** e153–8.

81. American Diabetes Association, Diabetes mellitus and exercise, *Diabetes Care* (2002) **25** (Suppl 1): 64.

82. Haire-Joshu D, Glasgow RE, Tibbs TL, Smoking and diabetes, *Diabetes Care* (1999) **22:** 1887–98.

83. American Diabetes Association, Treatment of hypertension in adults with diabetes, *Diabetes Care* (2002) **25** (Suppl 1): 71–3.

84. American Diabetes Association, Standards of medical care for patients with diabetes mellitus, *Diabetes Care* (2002) **25** (Suppl 1): 33–49.

85. American Diabetes Association, Management of dyslipidemia in adults with diabetes, *Diabetes Care* (2002) **25** (Suppl 1): 74–7.

86. Sheps SG, Overview of JNC VI: new directions in the management of hypertension and cardiovascular risk, *Am J Hypertens* (1999) **12:** 65S-72S.

87. Elliott WJ, Weir DR, Black HR, Cost-effectiveness of the lower treatment goal (of JNC VI) for diabetic hypertensive patients. Joint National Committee on Prevention, Detection, Evaluation, and Treatment of High Blood Pressure, *Arch Intern Med* (2000) **160:** 1277–83.

88. Expert Panel on Detection and Treatment of High Blood Cholesterol in Adults, Executive summary of the third report of the National Cholesterol Education Program (NCEP) Expert Panel on detection, evaluation, and treatment of high blood cholesterol in adults (Adult Treatment Panel III), *JAMA* (2001) **285:** 2486–97.

89. Gotto AM, Lipid management in diabetic patients: lessons from prevention trials, *Am J Med* (2002) **112** (Suppl 8A): 19S-26S.

90. Heart Protection Study Collaborative Group, MRC/BHF heart protection study of antioxidant vitamin supplementation in 20,536 high-risk individuals: a randomised placebo-controlled trial, *Lancet* (2002) **360:** 23–33.

91. Lam KS, Cheng IK, Janus ED et al, Cholesterol-lowering therapy may retard the progression of diabetic nephropathy, *Diabetologia* (1995) **38:** 604–9.

92. Parving HH, Cholesterol-lowering therapy may retard the progression of diabetic nephropathy, *Diabetologia* (1996) **39:** 367–8.

93. Cook NR, Cole SR, Hennekens CH, Use of a marginal structural model to determine the effect of aspirin on cardiovascular mortality in the Physicians' Health Study, *Am J Epidemiol* (2002) **155:** 1045–53.

94. Group SCotPHSR, Final report on the aspirin component of the ongoing Physicians' Health Study, *N Engl J Med* (1989) **321:** 129–35.

95. Collaborative overview of randomised trials of antiplatelet therapy. I: Prevention of death, myocardial infarction, and stroke by prolonged antiplatelet therapy in various categories of patients. Antiplatelet Trialists' Collaboration, *BMJ* (1994) **308:** 81–106.

96. Rolka DB, Fagot-Campagna A, Narayan KM, Aspirin use among adults with diabetes: estimates from the Third National Health and Nutrition Examination Survey, *Diabetes Care* (2001) **24:** 197–201.

97. American Diabetes Association, Aspirin therapy in diabetes, *Diabetes Care* (1997) **20:** 1772–3.

98. Mehta JL, Aspirin for the primary prevention of coronary events, *N Engl J Med* (2002) **347:** 948.

99. Krein SL, Vijan S, Pogach LM et al, Aspirin use and counseling about aspirin among patients with diabetes, *Diabetes Care* (2002) **25:** 965–70.

100. Akbar DH, Ahmed MM, Siddique AM, Low aspirin use in diabetics, *Saudi Med J* (2002) **23:** 457–60.

101. Colwell JA, Aspirin therapy in diabetes is underutilized, *Diabetes Care* (2001) **24:** 195–6.

102. McFarlane SI, Jacober SJ, Winer N et al, Control of cardiovascular risk factors in patients with diabetes and hypertension at urban academic medical centers, *Diabetes Care* (2002) **25:** 718–23.

103. Grant RW, Cagliero E, Murphy-Sheehy P et al, Comparison of hyperglycemia, hypertension, and hypercholesterolemia management in patients with type 2 diabetes, *Am J Med* (2002) **112:** 603–9.

104. Bonow RO, Mitch WE, Nesto RW et al, Prevention Conference VI: diabetes and cardiovascular disease: Writing Group V: management of cardiovascular-renal complications, *Circulation* (2002) **105:** e159–64.

105. Dickstein K, Kjekshus J, Effects of losartan and captopril on mortality and morbidity in high-risk patients after acute myocardial infarction: the OPTIMAAL randomised trial. Optimal Trial in Myocardial Infarction with Angiotensin II Antagonist Losartan, *Lancet* (2002) **360:** 752–60.

106. Pfeffer MA, McMurray J, Leizorovicz A et al, Valsartan in acute myocardial infarction trial (VALIANT): rationale and design, *Am Heart J* (2000) **140:** 727–50.

107. Swedberg K, Pfeffer M, Granger C et al, Candesartan in heart failure – assessment of reduction in mortality and morbidity (CHARM): rationale and design. Charm-Programme Investigators, *J Card Fail* (1999) **5:** 276–82.

108. McMurray JJ, Angiotensin II receptor antagonists for the treatment of heart failure: what is their place after ELITE-II and Val-HeFT?, *J Renin Angiotensin Aldosterone Syst* (2001) **2:** 89–92.

109. Dickstein K, ELITE II and Val-HeFT are different trials: together what do they tell us?, *Curr Control Trials Cardiovasc Med* (2001) **2:** 240–3.

110. Willenheimer R, Angiotensin receptor blockers in heart failure after the ELITE II trial, *Curr Control Trials Cardiovasc Med* (2000) **1:** 79–82.

111. Maggioni AP, Anand I, Gottlieb SO et al, Effects of valsartan on morbidity and mortality in patients with heart failure not receiving angiotensin-converting enzyme inhibitors, *J Am Coll Cardiol* (2002) **40:** 1414.

112. Cohn JN, Tognoni G, A randomized trial of the angiotensin-receptor blocker valsartan in chronic heart failure, *N Engl J Med* (2001) **345:** 1667–75.

113. Miettinen H, Lehto S, Salomaa V et al, Impact of diabetes on mortality after the first myocardial infarction. The FINMONICA Myocardial Infarction Register Study Group, *Diabetes Care* (1998) **21:** 69–75.

114. Bonnefoy E, Leborgne L, Dupouy P et al, Evidence that primary angioplasty is more effective than prehospital fibrinolysis in diabetics with acute myocardial infarction. A captim substudy, *Circulation* (2002) **106:** 698.

115. Almbrand B, Johannesson M, Sjostrand B et al, Cost-effectiveness of intense insulin treatment after acute myocardial infarction in patients with diabetes mellitus; results from the DIGAMI study, *Eur Heart J* (2000) **21:** 733–9.

116. Malmberg K, McGuire DK, Diabetes and acute myocardial infarction: the role of insulin therapy, *Am Heart J* (1999) **138:** S381–6.

117. Malmberg K, Prospective randomised study of intensive insulin treatment on long term survival after acute myocardial infarction in patients with diabetes mellitus. DIGAMI (Diabetes Mellitus, Insulin Glucose Infusion in Acute Myocardial Infarction) Study Group, *BMJ* (1997) **314:** 1512–15.

118. Malmberg K, Ryden L, Hamsten A et al, Effects of insulin treatment on cause-specific one-year mortality and morbidity in diabetic patients with acute myocardial infarction. DIGAMI Study Group. Diabetes Insulin-Glucose in Acute Myocardial Infarction, *Eur Heart J* (1996) **17:** 1337–44.

119. Braunwald E, Antman EM, Beasley JW et al, ACC/AHA guideline update for the management of patients with unstable angina and non-ST-segment elevation myocardial infarction 2002. Summary article: A report of the American College of Cardiology/American Heart Association Task Force on Practice Guidelines (Committee on the Management of Patients with Unstable Angina), *Circulation* (2002) **106:** 1893–1900.

120. Budaj A, Yusuf S, Mehta SR et al, Benefit of clopidogrel in patients with acute coronary syndromes without ST-segment elevation in various risk groups, *Circulation* (2002) **106:** 1622–6.

121. Steinhubl SR, Berger PB, Mann JT, 3rd et al, Early and sustained dual oral antiplatelet therapy following percutaneous coronary intervention: a randomized controlled trial, *JAMA* (2002) **288:** 2411–20.

122. Singh M, Fry RL, Ballman KV et al, Influence of diabetes mellitus on long-term survival in patients with coronary artery disease: eighteen years' follow-up data from Coronary Artery Surgery Study (CASS) group, *Circulation* (2002) **106:** 508.

123. Feit F, Brooks MM, Sopko G et al, Long-term clinical outcome in the Bypass Angioplasty Revascularization Investigation Registry: comparison with the randomized trial. BARI Investigators, *Circulation* (2000) **101:** 2795–2802.

124. Berger PB, Velianou JL, Aslanidou Vlachos H et al, Survival following coronary angioplasty versus coronary artery bypass surgery in anatomic subsets in which coronary artery bypass surgery improves survival compared with medical therapy. Results from the Bypass Angioplasty Revascularization Investigation (BARI), *J Am Coll Cardiol* (2001) **38:** 1440–9.

125. Schwartz L, Kip KE, Frye RL et al, Coronary bypass graft patency in patients with diabetes in the Bypass Angioplasty Revascularization Investigation (BARI), *Circulation* (2002) **106:** 2652–8.

126. Hirotani T, Kameda T, Kumamoto T et al, Effects of coronary artery bypass grafting using internal mammary arteries for diabetic patients, *J Am Coll Cardiol* (1999) **34:** 532–8.

127. Yamamoto T, Hosoda Y, Takazawa K et al, Is diabetes mellitus a major risk factor in coronary artery bypass grafting? The influence of internal thoracic artery grafting on late survival in diabetic patients, *Jpn J Thorac Cardiovasc Surg* (2000) **48:** 344–52.

128. Taggart DP, D'Amico R, Altman DG, Effect of arterial revascularisation on survival: a systematic review of studies comparing bilateral and single internal mammary arteries, *Lancet* (2001) **358:** 870–5.

129. Abizaid A, Costa MA, Centemero M et al. Clinical and economic impact of diabetes mellitus on percutaneous and surgical treatment of multivessel coronary disease patients: insights from the Arterial Revascularization Therapy Study (ARTS) trial, *Circulation* (2001) **104:** 533–8.

130. Roffi M, Chew DP, Mukherjee D et al. Platelet glycoprotein IIb/IIIa inhibitors reduce mortality in diabetic patients with non-ST-segment-elevation acute coronary syndromes, *Circulation* (2001) **104:** 2767–71.

131. Smith SC, Jr, Faxon D, Cascio W et al, Prevention Conference VI: diabetes and cardiovascular disease: Writing Group VI: revascularization in diabetic patients, *Circulation* (2002) **105:** e165–9.

132. Lavine SJ, Gellman SD, Treatment of heart failure in patients with diabetes mellitus, *Drugs* (2002) **62:** 285–307.

133. Nichols GA, Hillier TA, Erbey JR et al, Congestive heart failure in type 2 diabetes: prevalence, incidence, and risk factors, *Diabetes Care* (2001) **24:** 1614–19.

134. Dries DL, Sweitzer NK, Drazner MH et al, Prognostic impact of diabetes mellitus in patients with heart failure according to the etiology of left ventricular systolic dysfunction, *J Am Coll Cardiol* (2001) **38:** 421–8.

135. Rubler S, Dlugash J, Yuceoglu YZ et al, New type of cardiomyopathy associated with diabetic glomerulosclerosis, *Am J Cardiol* (1972) **30:** 595–602.

136. Galderisi M, Anderson KM, Wilson PW et al, Echocardiographic evidence for the existence of a distinct diabetic cardiomyopathy (the Framingham Heart Study), *Am J Cardiol* (1991) **68:** 85–98.

137. Spector KS, Diabetic cardiomyopathy, *Clin Cardiol* (1998) **21:** 885–7.

138. Malone JI, Schocken DD, Morrison AD et al, Diabetic cardiomyopathy and carnitine deficiency, *J Diabetes Complications* (1999) **13:** 86–90.

139. Francis GS, Diabetic cardiomyopathy: fact or fiction?, *Heart* (2001) **85:** 247–8.

140. Joffe II, Travers KE, Perreault-Micale CL et al, Abnormal cardiac function in the streptozotocin-induced non-insulin-dependent diabetic rat: noninvasive assessment with doppler echocardiography and contribution of the nitric oxide pathway, *J Am Coll Cardiol* (1999) **34:** 2111–19.

141. Robillon JF, Sadoul JL, Jullien D et al, Abnormalities suggestive of cardiomyopathy in patients with type 2 diabetes of relatively short duration, *Diabete Metab* (1994) **20:** 473–80.

142. Uusitupa MI, Mustonen JN, Airaksinen KE, Diabetic heart muscle disease, *Ann Med* (1990) **22:** 377–86.

143. Zarich SW, Nesto RW, Diabetic cardiomyopathy, *Am Heart J* (1989) **118:** 1000–12.

144. Kawaguchi M, Techigawara M, Ishihata T et al, A comparison of ultrastructural changes on endomyocardial biopsy specimens obtained from patients with diabetes mellitus with and without hypertension, *Heart Vessels* (1997) **12:** 267–74.

145. Lee SL, Ostadalova I, Kolar F et al, Alterations in Ca(2+)-channels during the development of diabetic cardiomyopathy, *Mol Cell Biochem* (1992) **109:** 173–9.

146. Liu X, Takeda N, Dhalla NS, Myosin light-chain phosphorylation in diabetic cardiomyopathy in rats, *Metabolism* (1997) **46:** 71–5.

147. Astorri E, Fiorina P, Contini GA et al, Isolated and preclinical impairment of left ventricular filling in insulin-dependent and non-insulin-dependent diabetic patients, *Clin Cardiol* (1997) **20:** 536–40.

148. Devereux RB, Roman MJ, Liu JE et al, Congestive heart failure

despite normal left ventricular systolic function in a population-based sample: the Strong Heart Study, *Am J Cardiol* (2000) **86:** 1090–6.

149. Grossman E, Messerli FH, Diabetic and hypertensive heart disease, *Ann Intern Med* (1996) **125:** 304–10.

150. Hardin NJ, The myocardial and vascular pathology of diabetic cardiomyopathy, *Coron Artery Dis* (1996) **7:** 99–108.

151. Regan TJ, Lyons MM, Ahmed SS et al, Evidence for cardiomyopathy in familial diabetes mellitus, *J Clin Invest* (1977) **60:** 884–99.

152. Fein FS, Sonnenblick EH, Diabetic cardiomyopathy, *Prog Cardiovasc Dis* (1985) **27:** 255–70.

153. Shimizu M, Umeda K, Sugihara N et al, Collagen remodelling in myocardia of patients with diabetes, *J Clin Pathol* (1993) **46:** 32–6.

154. Factor SM, Okun EM, Minase T, Capillary microaneurysms in the human diabetic heart, *N Engl J Med* (1980) **302:** 384–8.

155. UK Prospective Diabetes Study Group, Tight blood pressure control and risk of macrovascular and microvascular complications in type 2 diabetes: UKPDS 38, *BMJ* (1998) **317:** 703–13.

156. Hansson L, Zanchetti A, Carruthers SG et al, Effects of intensive blood-pressure lowering and low-dose aspirin in patients with hypertension: principal results of the Hypertension Optimal Treatment (HOT) randomised trial. HOT Study Group, *Lancet* (1998) **351:** 1755–62.

157. Schaffer SW, Cardiomyopathy associated with noninsulin-dependent diabetes, *Mol Cell Biochem* (1991) **107:** 1–20.

158. Fragasso G, Margonato A, Recent advances in the diagnosis and treatment of diabetic cardiomyopathy, *Ital Heart J* (2001) **2** (Suppl 3): 7S–11.

159. Rodrigues B, Cam MC, McNeill JH, Myocardial substrate metabolism: implications for diabetic cardiomyopathy, *J Mol Cell Cardiol* (1995) **27:** 169–79.

160. Brownlee M, Cerami A, Vlassara H, Advanced glycosylation end products in tissue and the biochemical basis of diabetic complications, *N Engl J Med* (1988) **318:** 1315–21.

161. Pitkanen OP, Nuutila P, Raitakari OT et al, Coronary flow reserve is reduced in young men with IDDM, *Diabetes* (1998) **47:** 248–54.

162. Johnstone MT, Creager SJ, Scales KM et al, Impaired endothelium-dependent vasodilation in patients with insulin- dependent diabetes mellitus, *Circulation* (1993) **88:** 2510–16.

163. Calver A, Collier J, Vallance P, Inhibition and stimulation of nitric oxide synthesis in the human forearm arterial bed of patients with insulin-dependent diabetes, *J Clin Invest* (1992) **90:** 2548–54.

164. Williams SB, Cusco JA, Roddy MA et al, Impaired nitric oxide-mediated vasodilation in patients with non-insulin-dependent diabetes mellitus, *J Am Coll Cardiol* (1996) **27:** 567–74.

165. Williams SB, Goldfine AB, Timimi FK et al, Acute hyperglycemia attenuates endothelium-dependent vasodilation in humans in vivo, *Circulation* (1998) **97:** 1695–1701.

166. Yokoyama I, Momomura S, Ohtake T et al, Reduced myocardial flow reserve in non-insulin-dependent diabetes mellitus, *J Am Coll Cardiol* (1997) **30:** 1472–7.

167. Piatti PM, Monti LD, Galli L et al, Relationship between endothelin-1 concentration and metabolic alterations typical of the insulin resistance syndrome, *Metabolism* (2000) **49:** 748–52.

168. Frustaci A, Kajstura J, Chimenti C et al, Myocardial cell death in human diabetes, *Circ Res* (2000) **87:** 1123–32.

169. Norhammar A, Malmberg K, Heart failure and glucose abnormalities: an increasing combination with poor functional capacity and outcome, *Eur Heart J* (2000) **21:** 1293–4.

170. Iribarren C, Karter AJ, Go AS et al, Glycemic control and heart failure among adult patients with diabetes, *Circulation* (2001) **103:** 2668–73.

171. Bell DS, Treatment of heart failure in patients with diabetes: clinical update, *Ethn Dis* (2002) **12:** S1–12–8.

172. Hunt SA, Baker DW, Chin MH et al, ACC/AHA guidelines for the evaluation and management of chronic heart failure in the adult: executive summary. A report of the American College of Cardiology/American Heart Association Task Force on Practice Guidelines (Committee To Revise the 1995 Guidelines for the Evaluation and Management of Heart Failure), *J Am Coll Cardiol* (2001) **38:** 2101–13.

173. Krum H, New and emerging pharmacological strategies in the management of chronic heart failure, *Curr Opin Pharmacol* (2001) **1:** 126–33.

174. Di Bonito P, Cuomo S, Moio N et al, Diastolic dysfunction in patients with non-insulin-dependent diabetes mellitus of short duration, *Diabet Med* (1996) **13:** 321–4.

175. Zabalgoitia M, Ismaeil MF, Anderson L et al, Prevalence of diastolic dysfunction in normotensive, asymptomatic patients with well-controlled type 2 diabetes mellitus, *Am J Cardiol* (2001) **87:** 320–3.

176. Whalley GA, Bagg W, Doughty RN et al, Pseudonormal diastolic filling unmasked with glyceryl trinitrate in patients with type 2 diabetes with poor metabolic control, *Diabetes Care* (2001) **24:** 1307–8.

177. Poirier P, Bogaty P, Garneau C et al, Diastolic dysfunction in normotensive men with well-controlled type 2 diabetes: importance of maneuvers in echocardiographic screening for preclinical diabetic cardiomyopathy, *Diabetes Care* (2001) **24:** 5–10.

178. Srivastava PM, Burrell LM, Jerums G et al, The prevalence of diabetic cardiomyopathy in patients with diabetes mellitus, *J Am Soc Echocardiogr* (2002) **15:** 533.

179. Valensi P, Sachs RN, Harfouche B et al, Predictive value of cardiac autonomic neuropathy in diabetic patients with or without silent myocardial ischemia, *Diabetes Care* (2001) **24:** 339–43.

180. Zellweger MJ, Pfisterer ME, Silent coronary artery disease in patients with diabetes mellitus, *Swiss Med Wkly* (2001) **131:** 427–32.

181. Cohn PF, Silent myocardial ischemia: classification, prevalence, and prognosis, *Am J Med* (1985) **79:** 2–6.

182. Rutter MK, Wahid ST, McComb JM et al, Significance of silent ischemia and microalbuminuria in predicting coronary events in asymptomatic patients with type 2 diabetes, *J Am Coll Cardiol* (2002) **40:** 56–61.

183. Langer A, Freeman MR, Josse RG et al, Detection of silent myocardial ischemia in diabetes mellitus, *Am J Cardiol* (1991) **67:** 1073–8.

184. Langer A, Freeman MR, Josse RG et al, Metaiodobenzylguanidine imaging in diabetes mellitus: assessment of cardiac sympathetic denervation and its relation to autonomic dysfunction and silent myocardial ischemia, *J Am Coll Cardiol* (1995) **25:** 610–18.

185. Ambepityia G, Kopelman PG, Ingram D et al, Exertional myocardial ischemia in diabetes: a quantitative analysis of anginal perceptual threshold and the influence of autonomic function, *J Am Coll Cardiol* (1990) **15:** 72–7.

186. Rosen SD, Paulesu E, Nihoyannopoulos P et al, Silent ischemia as a central problem: regional brain activation compared in silent and painful myocardial ischemia, *Ann Intern Med* (1996) **124:** 939–49.

187. Hikita H, Kurita A, Takase B et al, Usefulness of plasma beta-endorphin level, pain threshold and autonomic function in assessing silent myocardial ischemia in patients with and without diabetes mellitus, *Am J Cardiol* (1993) **72:** 140–3.

188. Weiner DA, Ryan TJ, Parsons L et al, Significance of silent myocardial ischemia during exercise testing in patients with diabetes mellitus: a report from the Coronary Artery Surgery Study (CASS) Registry, *Am J Cardiol* (1991) **68:** 729–34.

189. Pancholy SB, Schalet B, Kuhlmeier V et al, Prognostic significance of silent ischemia, *J Nucl Cardiol* (1994) **1**: 434–40.

190. O'Rourke RA, Brundage BH, Froelicher VF et al, American College of Cardiology/American Heart Association expert consensus document on electron-beam computed tomography for the diagnosis and prognosis of coronary artery disease, *Circulation* (2000) **102**: 126–40.

191. Roy TM, Peterson HR, Snider HL et al, Autonomic influence on cardiovascular performance in diabetic subjects, *Am J Med* (1989) **87**: 382–8.

192. Tristani FE, Kamper DG, McDermott DJ et al, Alterations of postural and Valsalva responses in coronary heart disease, *Am J Physiol* (1977) **233**: H694–9.

193. Airaksinen KE, Ikaheimo MJ, Linnaluoto MK et al, Impaired vagal heart rate control in coronary artery disease, *Br Heart J* (1987) **58**: 592–7.

194. Rothschild M, Rothschild A, Pfeifer M, Temporary decrease in cardiac parasympathetic tone after acute myocardial infarction, *Am J Cardiol* (1988) **62**: 637–9.

195. Eckberg DL, Drabinsky M, Braunwald E, Defective cardiac parasympathetic control in patients with heart disease, *N Engl J Med* (1971) **285**: 877–83.

196. Curb JD, Rodriguez BL, Burchfiel CM et al, Sudden death, impaired glucose tolerance, and diabetes in Japanese-American men, *Circulation* (1995) **91**: 2591–5.

197. Woo KS, White HD, Factors affecting outcome after recovery from myocardial infarction, *Annu Rev Med* (1994) **45**: 325–39.

198. van Ravenswaaij-Arts CM, Kollee LA, Hopman JC et al, Heart rate variability, *Ann Intern Med* (1993) **118**: 436–47.

199. Kleiger RE, Miller JP, Bigger JT, Jr et al, Decreased heart rate variability and its association with increased mortality after acute myocardial infarction, *Am J Cardiol* (1987) **59**: 256–62.

200. Fava S, Azzopardi J, Muscat HA et al, Factors that influence outcome in diabetic subjects with myocardial infarction, *Diabetes Care* (1993) **16**: 1615–18.

201. Zola B, Kahn JK, Juni JE et al, Abnormal cardiac function in diabetic patients with autonomic neuropathy in the absence of ischemic heart disease, *J Clin Endocrinol Metab* (1986) **63**: 208–14.

202. Consensus Statement, Standardizing measures in diabetic neuropathy, *Diabetes Care* (1995) **18**: 59–82.

203. Rollins MD, Jenkins JG, Carson DJ et al, Power spectral analysis of the electrocardiogram in diabetic children, *Diabetologia* (1992) **35**: 452–5.

204. Ziegler D, Dannehl K, Volksw D et al, Prevalence of cardiovascular autonomic dysfunction assessed by spectral analysis and standard tests of heart-rate variation in newly diagnosed IDDM patients, *Diabetes Care* (1992) **15**: 908–11.

205. Ewing DJ, Neilson JM, Shapiro CM et al, Twenty four hour heart rate variability: effects of posture, sleep, and time of day in healthy controls and comparison with bedside tests of autonomic function in diabetic patients, *Br Heart J* (1991) **65**: 239–44.

206. Pagani M, Malfatto G, Pierini S et al, Spectral analysis of heart rate variability in the assessment of autonomic diabetic neuropathy, *J Auton Nerv Syst* (1988) **23**: 143–53.

207. Standl E, Schnell O, A new look at the heart in diabetes mellitus: from ailing to failing, *Diabetologia* (2000) **43**: 1455–69.

208. Algra A, Tijssen JG, Roelandt JR et al, Heart rate variability from 24-hour electrocardiography and the 2-year risk for sudden death, *Circulation* (1993) **88**: 180–5.

209. Schwartz PJ, Randall WC, Anderson EA et al, Sudden cardiac death. Nonpharmacologic interventions, *Circulation* (1987) **76**: I215–19.

210. Schwartz PJ, La Rovere MT, Vanoli E, Autonomic nervous system and sudden cardiac death. Experimental basis and clinical observations for post-myocardial infarction risk stratification, *Circulation* (1992) **85**: I77–91.

211. Stevens MJ, Dayanikli F, Raffel DM et al, Scintigraphic assessment of regionalized defects in myocardial sympathetic innervation and blood flow regulation in diabetic patients with autonomic neuropathy, *J Am Coll Cardiol* (1998) **31**: 1575–84.

212. Stevens MJ, Raffel DM, Allman KC et al, Cardiac sympathetic dysinnervation in diabetes: implications for enhanced cardiovascular risk, *Circulation* (1998) **98**: 961–8.

213. Sima AA, Zhang W, Xu G et al, A comparison of diabetic polyneuropathy in type II diabetic BBZDR/Wor rats and in type I diabetic BB/Wor rats, *Diabetologia* (2000) **43**: 786–93.

214. Dyck PJ, Zimmerman BR, Vilen TH et al, Nerve glucose, fructose, sorbitol, myo-inositol, and fiber degeneration and regeneration in diabetic neuropathy, *N Engl J Med* (1988) **319**: 542–8.

215. Cameron NE, Cotter MA, Metabolic and vascular factors in the pathogenesis of diabetic neuropathy, *Diabetes* (1997) **46** (Suppl 2): S31–7.

216. Tomlinson DR, Mitogen-activated protein kinases as glucose transducers for diabetic complications, *Diabetologia* (1999) **42**: 1271–81.

217. Tesfaye S, Malik R, Ward JD, Vascular factors in diabetic neuropathy, *Diabetologia* (1994) **37**: 847–54.

218. Schnell O, Muhr D, Dresel S et al, Autoantibodies against sympathetic ganglia and evidence of cardiac sympathetic dysinnervation in newly diagnosed and long-term IDDM patients, *Diabetologia* (1996) **39**: 970–5.

219. Muhr D, Mollenhauer U, Ziegler AG et al, Autoantibodies to sympathetic ganglia, GAD, or tyrosine phosphatase in long-term IDDM with and without ECG-based cardiac autonomic neuropathy, *Diabetes Care* (1997) **20**: 1009–12.

220. Ejskjaer N, Arif S, Dodds W et al, Prevalence of autoantibodies to autonomic nervous tissue structures in Type 1 diabetes mellitus, *Diabet Med* (1999) **16**: 544–9.

221. Greene DA, Lattimer SA, Sima AA, Pathogenesis and prevention of diabetic neuropathy, *Diabetes Metab Rev* (1988) **4**: 201–21.

222. Greene DA, Lattimer SA, Sima AA, Sorbitol, phosphoinositides, and sodium-potassium-ATPase in the pathogenesis of diabetic complications, *N Engl J Med* (1987) **316**: 599–606.

223. Cameron NE, Cotter MA, Neurovascular dysfunction in diabetic rats. Potential contribution of autoxidation and free radicals examined using transition metal chelating agents, *J Clin Invest* (1995) **96**: 1159–63.

224. Low PA, Nickander KK, Oxygen free radical effects in sciatic nerve in experimental diabetes, *Diabetes* (1991) **40**: 873–7.

225. Tomlinson DR, Fernyhough P, Diemel LT, Role of neurotrophins in diabetic neuropathy and treatment with nerve growth factors, *Diabetes* (1997) **46** (Suppl 2): S43–9.

226. Hellweg R, Hartung HD, Endogenous levels of nerve growth factor (NGF) are altered in experimental diabetes mellitus: a possible role for NGF in the pathogenesis of diabetic neuropathy, *J Neurosci Res* (1990) **26**: 258–67.

227. Faradji V, Sotelo J, Low serum levels of nerve growth factor in diabetic neuropathy, *Acta Neurol Scand* (1990) **81**: 402–6.

228. Zanone MM, Banga JP, Peakman M et al, An investigation of antibodies to nerve growth factor in diabetic autonomic neuropathy, *Diabet Med* (1994) **11**: 378–83.

229. Schmid H, Forman LA, Cao X et al, Heterogeneous cardiac sympathetic denervation and decreased myocardial nerve growth factor in streptozotocin-induced diabetic rats: implications for cardiac sympathetic dysinnervation complicating diabetes, *Diabetes* (1999) **48**: 603–8.

230. Muhr-Becker D, Ziegler AG, Druschky A et al, Evidence for specific autoimmunity against sympathetic and parasympathetic nervous tissues in type 1 diabetes mellitus and the relation to cardiac autonomic dysfunction, *Diabet Med* (1998) **15**: 467–72.

231. Schnell O, Schwarz A, Muhr-Becker D et al, Autoantibodies against autonomic nervous tissues in type 2 diabetes mellitus: no association with cardiac autonomic dysfunction, *Exp Clin Endocrinol Diabetes* (2000) **108:** 181–6.

232. Kline RC, Swanson DP, Wieland DM et al, Myocardial imaging in man with I-123 meta-iodobenzylguanidine, *J Nucl Med* (1981) **22:** 129–32.

233. Sisson JC, Shapiro B, Meyers L et al, Metaiodobenzylguanidine to map scintigraphically the adrenergic nervous system in man, *J Nucl Med* (1987) **28:** 1625–36.

234. DeGrado TR, Hutchins GD, Toorongian SA et al, Myocardial kinetics of carbon-11-meta-hydroxyephedrine: retention mechanisms and effects of norepinephrine, *J Nucl Med* (1993) **34:** 1287–93.

235. Ziegler D, Diabetic cardiovascular autonomic neuropathy: prognosis, diagnosis and treatment, *Diabetes Metab Rev* (1994) **10:** 339–83.

236. Ewing DJ, Clarke BF, Diagnosis and management of diabetic autonomic neuropathy, *BMJ (Clin Res Edn)* (1982) **285:** 916–18.

237. Ewing DJ, Boland O, Neilson JM et al, Autonomic neuropathy, QT interval lengthening, and unexpected deaths in male diabetic patients, *Diabetologia* (1991) **34:** 182–5.

238. Gambardella S, Frontoni S, Spallone V et al, Increased left ventricular mass in normotensive diabetic patients with autonomic neuropathy, *Am J Hypertens* (1993) **6:** 97–102.

239. Ewing DJ, Diabetic autonomic neuropathy and the heart, *Diabetes Res Clin Pract* (1996) **30** (Suppl): 31–6.

240. Gregoratos G, Abrams J, Epstein AE et al, ACC/AHA/NASPE 2002 guideline update for implantation of cardiac pacemakers and antiarrhythmia devices. Summary article: a report of the American College of Cardiology/American Heart Association Task Force on Practice Guidelines (ACC/AHA/NASPE Committee To Update the 1998 Pacemaker Guidelines), *Circulation* (2002) **106:** 2145–61.

# 11

## Treatment of diabetic nephropathy: treatment of electrolyte and acid-base disturbances

Carol A Pollock

## INTRODUCTION

Diabetes mellitus is a chronic complex metabolic disorder that, in addition to the dysregulation of glucose, fat and protein metabolism, may be accompanied by disturbances in water, electrolyte and acid-base balance. Abnormalities in plasma electrolytes and acid-base homeostasis in diabetes mellitus may result from the following

1) hyperglycaemia
2) derangement in the normal tubular action of insulin
3) altered renal haemodynamics and perturbations in extracellular fluid volume, often associated with secondary abnormalities in glomerulotubular feedback
4) structural changes in the renal tubular cells, including thickening of the glomerular basement membrane, and accumulation of glycogen in the cytosol and lysosomes[1]
5) hyporeninaemic hypoaldosteronism
6) altered tubular function due to tubulointerstitial disease
7) drug therapy
8) decompensated diabetes mellitus, with ketosis or hyperosmolar states
9) renal failure.

It is known that in the absence of significant renal impairment, renal tubular abnormalities, rather than glomerular dysfunction, generally underlie persistent electrolyte and acid-base disturbances. Indeed, the incidence and prevalence of overt and incipient tubular dysfunction is increased in patients with diabetes mellitus.[2] The clinical significance of mild tubular dysfunction is generally limited. However, in the presence of associated hormonal abnormalities and concomitant drug therapy, specific electrolyte and acid-base disturbances characteristic of diabetes mellitus may develop. These will be discussed in this chapter.

In contrast to the derangement in electrolyte and acid-base homeostasis that may occur in stable patients with diabetes mellitus, decompensated diabetes mellitus is frequently accompanied by systemic metabolic abnormalities. Derangements of electrolytes and acid-base homeostasis specifically associated with ketosis or hyperosmolality will be briefly discussed. Abnormalities that uniformly arise as a consequence of a reduction in renal function independently of the cause of renal failure, and that are not specific to, or more common in, patients with diabetes mellitus, will not be addressed.

## ELECTROLYTE ABNORMALITIES

### Potassium

Aberrations in potassium homeostasis are the most clinically important electrolyte abnormality in both type 1 and type 2 diabetes mellitus. Acute derangements in glycaemic control (such as ketoacidosis or hyperosmolar states) may acutely influence potassium homeostasis, and in patients with a severe reduction in glomerular filtration rate a more chronic perturbation may be observed. However, even in the absence of these complications, patients with diabetes mellitus may have impaired potassium homeostatic mechanisms due to a multiplicity of factors.

These include hormonal derangements, renal tubular dysfunction, mild reduction in glomerular filtration rate, mild to moderate increases in blood-sugar levels and concomitant drug therapy. Hyperkalaemia, that is, an increase in the potassium concentration in the extracellular fluid compartment, is more commonly observed than hypokalaemia, and is not always reflected in parallel changes in the intracellular potassium concentration. The reasons for abnormalities in potassium homeostasis resulting in hyperkalaemia are explored in detail below.

### Insulin deficiency

The role of insulin in the regulation of potassium homeostasis within the physiological range in normal individuals is unclear. The effects of insulin on potassium are independent of its effects on blood glucose.[3] Insulin-deficient individuals are predisposed to hyperkalaemia, in part due to impaired insulin-mediated cellular potassium uptake.[4] It has been well demonstrated that insulin stimulates muscle membrane Na,K ATPase activity, and thereby the Na pump, resulting in sodium efflux and potassium influx.[5–8] The Na pump has recently been characterized; it consists of three distinct isoforms of the alpha (catalytic) and beta (glycosylated) subunits, which differ in tissue expression.[9] Expression of the alpha$_2$ isoform, which has a lower Na affinity than does the alpha$_1$ isoform, is restricted to muscle and adipose tissue. More recently, a direct stimulatory effect of insulin on the alpha$_2$ subunit of the pump, resulting in an increased translocation of pump units to the plasma membrane,[9] or an increased affinity of the pump for sodium[10] has been demonstrated. In addition, insulin-mediated activation of sodium–hydrogen exchange[11] and Na channel opening[12] leads to an increased intracellular Na concentration and secondary activation of the Na pump.

Thus, in the presence of insulin deficiency or insulin resistance, there is a reduced stimulus for cellular uptake of potassium, resulting in hyperkalaemia.

### Hyporeninaemic hypoaldosteronism

Aldosterone is responsible for potassium secretion by the distal nephron. It acts on intracellular steroid receptors located predominantly in the principal cells of the cortical and the medullary collecting duct.[13–17] Aldosterone is not known to have any effect on the intercalated cell, the other main cell observed in the cortical collecting duct.[18–20] Immediately following stimulation of the aldosterone receptors, sodium conductance of the apical membrane of the principal cells increases, depolarizing the membrane and increasing potassium secretion. Because of the increased intracellular Na concentration, secondary activation of the Na pump occurs, facilitating potassium influx into the cell and increasing its availability for excretion.[18,21–25] After prolonged stimulation by aldosterone (12–48 hr), the potassium conductance of the apical membrane is enhanced, and the activity and number of Na pumps inserted into the basolateral membrane of the principal cells increases.[14–17,24,25] Whether these latter effects are directly caused by aldosterone, or are secondary to the effects on apical sodium conductance is controversial.[14,26–28] One unconfirmed report has suggested that an increase in potassium conductance is due to intracellular alkalosis induced by aldosterone.[27] In addition to the effects of aldosterone on the secretion of potassium in the kidney, the adrenal secretion of aldosterone is enhanced when serum levels of potassium are elevated, and this constitutes a closed-loop feedback system for the regulation of serum potassium.[29,30]

Acquired hypoaldosteronism is observed in diabetes mellitus, manifesting as hyperkalaemia and hyperchloraemic metabolic acidosis (see below). This almost always occurs in the presence of subtle renal disease, often when the glomerular filtration rate is normal.[31–35]

Many alternative forms of tubulointerstitial renal disease are characterized by tubular resistance to the effects of aldosterone, resulting in hyperkalaemia and metabolic acidosis.[36–39] However, in the majority of patients, the reduced plasma aldosterone leads to a compensatory increase in plasma renin, which returns plasma aldosterone, and hence serum potassium, to normal. In patients with diabetes mellitus, and occasionally in some other forms of tubulointerstitial renal disease, a compensatory increase in plasma renin does not occur, resulting in the syndrome of hyporeninaemic hypoaldosteronism, characterized by persistent hyperkalaemia and acidosis.[40]

The reasons why a compensatory increase in plasma renin does not occur in patients with diabetes mellitus remain the subject of speculation. Several possibilities have been suggested and it is likely that different mechanisms co-exist in a single patient:

1) The structure or function of the juxtaglomerular apparatus may be specifically impaired.[32]
2) The conversion from pro-renin to renin is impaired.[33]
3) Associated autonomic insufficiency leads to decreased renin production.[34,41]
4) Reduced renal prostaglandin production results in decreased renin production mediated by the prostaglandin, particularly prostacyclin, path-

ways.[42] The reduction in renal prostaglandin production may be local, and associated with specific damage to the juxtaglomerular apparatus, or may be due to a specific defect in calcium- or noradrenaline-induced increases in prostacyclin pathways in diabetic patients.[43] Non-steroidal anti-inflammatory drugs and selective cyclo-oxygenase (COX-2) inhibitors both reduce intrarenal prostaglandin production, resulting in hyperkalaemia.[44,45]

5) There are direct inhibitory effects of hyperkalaemia on renin secretion.[35,38,46]
6) Elevated levels of antidiuretic hormone in diabetic patients inhibit renin secretion.[40]
7) Volume expansion in renal impairment directly suppresses renin secretion.[4]
8) Co-existent adrenal abnormality exists.

The diagnosis of hyporeninaemic hypoaldosteronism should be considered if the features listed in Table 11.1 are present. Salt wasting and hypotension are not commonly observed in hyporeninaemic hypoaldosteronism in diabetes mellitus, as the deficiency is not usually complete, and underlying renal disease is associated with sodium retention. If hyponatraemia or hypotension co-exists with hyperkalaemia and hyperchloraemic acidosis, primary adrenal insufficiency should be considered.

Hyperkalaemia may be associated with either hyporeninaemic hypoaldosteronism or primary tubular dysfunction. In both these circumstances, fractional potassium excretion is likely to be low, but should normalize with mineralocorticoid treatment if the primary cause is adrenal insufficiency.

## Hyperosmolality

An increase in plasma osmolality due to hyperglycaemia in insulin-deficient subjects results in an increased plasma potassium concentration due to the effects of tonicity on transcellular potassium distribution.[48–51] The mechanism involves movement of

---

**Table 11.1 Laboratory features of hyporeninaemic hypoaldosteronism.**

Unexplained hyperkalaemia (in the setting of normal, mild or moderate renal impairment)

Hyperchloraemic acidosis

Low urinary potassium excretion relative to the degree of hyperkalaemia

Normal plasma ratio of renin:aldosterone

---

both fluid and potassium (due to solvent drag) from the intracellular to the extracellular space.[52,53] In addition, the cellular dehydration that accompanies an increase in extracellular osmolality results in an increased cellular potassium concentration, activating potassium channels and causing a flux from the intracellular to the extracellular fluid.[54] This is unlikely to occur in normal subjects, as a parallel increase in plasma insulin occurs which stimulates cellular potassium uptake (see above). Although initial reports were of patients who had low aldosterone levels in addition, it is well recognized that hyperkalaemia can occur in diabetic subjects with normal renal function and normal aldosterone levels.[50,51,55]

## Sodium

Salt and water balance may be significantly deranged, usually dependent on the degree of glycaemic control and the concomitant hormonal and neurogenic responses inherent in diabetes mellitus. Hypertension in almost all hypertensive patients is sodium sensitive,[56,57] and a strong relationship exists between salt sensitivity and glomerular hypertension, which has been strongly implicated in the development of diabetic nephropathy.[56,58] Urinary sodium retention occurs early in the development of diabetes mellitus.[56,59,60] Sodium sensitivity of blood pressure appears before hypertension develops and is related to the degree of albuminuria.[61]

The state of activation of the sympathetic nervous system plays a key role in the regulation of renal salt and water excretion. In studies of children with insulin-dependent diabetes mellitus of up to 13 years' duration, the baseline level of sympathetic nervous system activation decreased with an increasing duration of disease. Conversely, physical stress induced an increased activation of the sympathetic nervous system, and sodium and water retention that was more marked with a longer duration of the disease.[62] Rarely does activation of the sympathetic nervous system, in the absence of change in antidiuretic hormone levels, induce any change in serum sodium levels.

Although serum sodium concentration is generally normal in diabetes mellitus, hyponatraemia may develop in the setting of acute hyperglycaemia as water is osmotically driven from the intracellular compartment to the extracellular fluids.[63] Although the relationship is not linear, the plasma sodium falls by approximately 1.6 mM/l for each 100 mg/dl (5.6 mmol/l) increase in plasma glucose.[64,65]

Generally, the hyponatraemia does not need specific treatment apart from correction of the blood glucose. In the presence of glycosuria, sodium and water loss accompany the osmotic losses and may result in either hypo- or hypernatraemia. The net effect depends upon the relative losses of salt and water, but also on the nature of the fluid replacement regimen.

## Calcium

Abnormalities in calcium and phosphate homeostasis are inherent in patients with impaired renal function, including those with diabetic nephropathy. However, in patients with normal renal function or incipient nephropathy, most studies have shown normal serum calcium concentrations and calcium–phosphate homeostasis.[66–68]

It is recognized that abnormalities in vitamin D and osteocalcin metabolism occur commonly in both adults and children with early-stage diabetic nephropathy, that is, in patients with microalbuminuria.[66,69–71] Although serum calcium, magnesium and parathyroid hormone are not directly affected in the early stages of diabetic renal disease,[67,68,72] longer-term follow-up is needed to gauge the effect of tubular dysfunction on electrolyte homeostasis. The relationship between diabetic nephropathy with significant renal impairment, and indeed other causes of end-stage renal failure with respect to calcium–phosphate homeostasis, and bone disease is well defined, and beyond the scope of this text.

In contrast to the generally normal serum calcium levels, accumulation in cytosolic free calcium has been documented in type 2 diabetes mellitus.[73] It is known that elevation of cytosolic free calcium, within the physiological range, participates in stimulus contraction coupling, and regulation of cardiac output and blood pressure, via indirect effects on vasomotor tone, and hormone and cytokine releases and responses.[74–76] After extreme noxious insults, increased intracellular calcium may lead to cell degeneration and cell death.[77,78] However, more moderate elevations in intracellular Ca concentrations enhance insulin resistance and reduce cellular glucose transport.[79] It has also been suggested that elevations in intracellular calcium in the presence of hyperglycaemia are associated with an increased risk of complications such as cardiac hypertrophy.[80] Cellular uptake of calcium into platelets is enhanced in patients with diabetes mellitus.[81] However, whether these changes have a causal relationship with vascular and metabolic disease, as suggested, is unknown.

## Magnesium

Magnesium depletion is a common feature of diabetes mellitus, usually in relation to poor glycaemic control. Its incidence varies from 25% to 39%.[82] It has been suggested that an impairment of magnesium metabolism may favour the onset and progression of diabetic complications, perhaps by affecting the activity of the Na,K-ATPase,[83] or phosphorylation of the insulin receptor.[76] The principal factors regulating magnesium homeostasis are unknown, but there is no evidence that reduced intake or gastrointestinal absorption of magnesium is responsible for the low serum levels observed. It is thus likely that an enhanced urinary loss occurs. Variations in insulin levels within the physiological range[84] and plasma glucose concentrations within the range observed in patients with diabetes mellitus[85] are known to influence renal magnesium excretion. Hyperglycaemia regulates renal magnesium excretion independent of diuresis or glycosuria, glomerular filtration and proximal tubular reabsorptive function as assessed by lithium clearance.[85] Glucose loading in itself may increase urinary magnesium excretion,[86] and may occur independently of any concomitant change in plasma insulin levels.[85] Similarly, variations in plasma insulin levels, independent of changes in glucose, are associated with alterations in renal magnesium excretion.[84]

Although insulin is known to increase renal magnesium excretion, enhanced magnesium excretion of between 24% and 88% is also observed in patients with insulin deficiency and hence type 1 diabetes mellitus.[87–92] Increased urinary magnesium losses are reflected in low muscle magnesium content in patients with both type 1 and type 2 diabetes.[87,88,91] Indeed, decreasing intracellular magnesium concentrations in vitro leads to cellular insulin resistance and inhibits insulin-mediated glucose transport, thus exacerbating the metabolic effects of diabetes mellitus.[76,79]

The degree of renal excretion of magnesium correlates with markers of poor glycaemic control such as retinopathy,[89] and as glycaemic control improves, so does renal magnesium loss.[88–90] As hyperinsulinaemia has also been shown to cause enhanced renal magnesium excretion,[84,93,94] it is not surprising that patients with type 2 diabetes have also been documented to have increased urinary magnesium excretion.[95,96] Osmotic diuresis is likely to play an important aetiological role, but a primary tubular defect has also been proposed.[97] The relative contribution of these parameters has not been delineated.

Elevations of serum ionized magnesium concentrations have been reported in patients with type 2 diabetes mellitus, independently of glycaemic control.[98] However, there are few studies assessing ionized magnesium, and the results are conflicting.[99,100]

Intracellular magnesium concentrations reflect physiologically active magnesium, and are decreased in patients with type 2 diabetes mellitus.[73,101] Intracellular magnesium plays an important physiological role in cellular biochemistry, being necessary for enzyme activation, nerve conduction, ion transport, ATP transfer and, importantly, regulation of glycolysis.[102–106] Low intracellular magnesium concentrations and indeed hypomagnesaemia are associated with increased oxygen free radical production,[107] and prior low serum magnesium concentration sensitizes cells to oxidative damage.[108] Magnesium itself has antioxidative properties, potentially mediated by an increased rate of spontaneous dismutation of the superoxide ion.[109] Hence, a low serum magnesium should be normalized.

## Phosphate

Normal individuals given a glucose load may develop hypophosphataemia due to the concomitant insulin-induced increase of cellular glucose uptake into muscle and liver. DeFronzo et al[110] demonstrated that induction of hyperinsulinaemia and maintenance of stable blood glucose resulted in enhanced proximal tubular reabsorption of phosphate. This insulin-induced increase in cellular phosphate uptake by the kidney is due to a direct effect of enhanced sodium–phosphate co-transport in the proximal tubule.[111]

Increased renal losses of phosphate are well described in glycosuria, ketoacidosis and polyuria. Serum phosphate levels may initially be normal, but as treatment with insulin is given, cellular uptake of phosphate occurs and hypophosphataemia ensues.[112] In the majority of cases, phosphate depletion is minimal, and specific replacement is not indicated. However, in a minority of cases with prolonged ketoacidosis, replacement of phosphate is required. In these cases of severe prolonged hypophosphataemia, renal glucose uptake is reduced, probably in relation to the fall in levels of renal tubular cytosolic nucleotides needed for glucose transport.[113]

Children with type 1 diabetes mellitus have a reversible decrease in renal tubular phosphate reabsorption, which manifests as a low fasting serum phosphate, an increased urinary phosphate excretion and a markedly lower tubular phosphate transport relative to the glomerular filtration rate.[114]

## METABOLIC ACIDOSIS

Patients with diabetes mellitus and good glycaemic control may develop metabolic acidosis in the absence of any significant decrease in renal excretory capacity. These patients have renal tubular acidosis, which has been attributed to the following:

1) hypoaldosteronism
2) hyperkalaemia
3) a primary tubular defect associated with diabetic nephropathy.

As discussed above, hypoaldosteronism results in the development of hyperchloraemic metabolic acidosis; it is termed type 4 renal tubular acidosis. Renal tubular acidosis arises as net acid excretion is decreased as a direct effect of lower aldosterone levels. As detailed previously, this results in decreased depolarization of the apical membrane, causing decreased potassium and hydrogen ion excretion. Thus, in contrast to type 1 and type 2 renal tubular acidosis, it is hyperkalaemia, rather than hypokalaemia, that leads to suppression of renal ammonia production, exacerbating the acidosis. In patients with hyporeninaemic hypoaldosteronism, including those with diabetes mellitus, the urinary pH can be reduced to lower than 5.5 if the plasma bicarbonate is lowered. This contrasts with patients with type 1 classical distal tubular acidosis, who are unable to acidify their urine under any circumstances.

It has been proposed that a primary tubular acidifying defect exists in patients with diabetes mellitus, since the acidosis may persist despite correction of the mineralocorticoid defect and normalization of the serum potassium.[115] However, in vivo microperfusion studies in diabetic animals, with and without renal impairment, demonstrate that distal tubular bicarbonate reabsorptive capacity is normal, and is not influenced by the presence of hyperglycaemia, changes in extracellular fluid volume, potassium homeostasis, renal insufficiency or the degree of acidosis.[116]

In patients with more advanced renal failure, metabolic acidosis occurs in parallel with progressive loss of renal excretory function. However, the degree of acidaemia has been reported to be less than in patients with non-diabetic renal failure and a similar loss of excretory function.[117,118] This is not explained by concomitant drug use, gastrointestinal hydrogen ion loss or reduced protein catabolic rate. Rather, it appears that an efficient extrarenal generation of buffers exists in patients with diabetes mellitus. It has been postulated that ketoacid anions may be the source of this extrarenal bicarbonate generation,[117] but this awaits confirmation. In patients with type 1 diabetes mellitus, an impaired ventilatory response in systemic acidosis has been reported.[119,120] This has been postulated to arise either from an abnormality in the medullary chemoreceptor,[121] or from respiratory muscle fatigue due to the acidosis.

## DRUG-INDUCED ABNORMALITIES IN ACID-BASE OR ELECTROLYTES IN PATIENTS WITH DIABETES MELLITUS

Patients with diabetes mellitus obviously have clear abnormalities in key metabolic pathways. However, in the absence of significant renal impairment, clinically significant alterations in the pharmacokinetic properties of drugs, leading to abnormalities in electrolyte and acid-base homeostasis, are uncommon. Drugs that have been reported to have an increased risk of inducing such abnormalities are discussed further.

### Metformin

Metformin hydrochloride is a biguanide that has been used with increasing frequency over the last few years in patients with type 2 diabetes mellitus. The glucose-lowering effects and clinical indications for the use of metformin are discussed elsewhere. One of the rare, but important, side effects of metformin therapy is the development of lactic acidosis.[122] The mortality rates in reported cases are up to 50%.[123,124] The exact mechanism whereby metformin therapy leads to acidosis is unknown. However, biguanides are thought to reduce gluconeogenesis from alanine, pyruvate and lactate. Thus, theoretically, lactic acid could accumulate unless an efficient mechanism for removal through renal excretion exists.[125] A related but chemically different biguanide, phenformin, was removed from the market because of an unacceptable incidence of lactic acidosis of 40–64 cases per 100 000 person years.[125,126] Unlike phenformin, metformin is reported to increase peripheral glucose utilization without enhancing lactate production.[127]

The exact incidence of lactic acidosis associated with metformin use is unknown, but population-based studies have estimated a rate of 2–9 cases per 100 000 person years.[125,128,129] Most of the reported cases have occurred in patients with co-morbid conditions, such as renal failure, that in themselves may have contributed to the acidosis. The incidence rates

of lactic acidosis in the USA before the introduction of metformin have been similarly estimated to be 9 per 100 000 years.[130] Thus, although the risk of developing lactic acidosis in patients taking metformin is likely to be small, it is recommended that it should be avoided in patients with a significant reduction in renal function or in patients with intercurrent illness that may disturb lactate metabolism.[131]

### Drug-induced hyperkalaemia

Because patients with diabetes mellitus have an increased tendency to hyperkalaemia (see above), drugs that alter potassium homeostasis have a more pronounced effect and, in general, increase the likelihood that overt hyperkalaemia will develop. Drugs induce hyperkalaemia by decreasing potassium excretion or by altering the distribution of potassium between intra- and extracellular compartments (Table 11.2). The more common drugs affecting potassium homeostasis are further discussed.

### Angiotensin-converting enzyme inhibitors and angiotensin II receptor antagonists

The prescription of medications designed to block the renin-angiotensin system is commonly used to control hypertension and to reduce the risk and rate of progression of complications related to diabetes mellitus.[132–134] In patients with hyporeninaemic hypoaldosteronism, hyperkalaemia may be precipitated, particularly when drugs that decrease potassium secretion are prescribed concomitantly. In clinical practice, this is relatively uncommon unless a significant decrease in glomerular filtration rate is present. In the studies that demonstrated a beneficial effect of irbesartan or losartan on the progression of renal disease in type 2 diabetes, 1.5–1.9% of patients developed hyperkalaemia, necessitating cessation of the drug.[132,133] In a case-control study of 1818 patients using angiotensin-converting enzyme inhibitors, 11% of patients developed hyperkalaemia (defined as greater than 5.1 mmol/l).[135] The risk of hyperkalaemia was increased in patients with renal impairment (serum creatinine greater than 0.136 mmol/l) and in patients with congestive cardiac failure, but was not increased in patients with diabetes in whom the serum creatinine was not raised. Thus, it is recommended that the serum potassium levels should be measured and monitored in patients with diabetes mellitus commencing ACE inhibitors or angiotensin II receptor antagonists,

| Table 11.2 Drugs precipitating hyperkalaemia in patients with diabetes mellitus. | |
|---|---|
| **Reduced potassium excretion** | **Redistribution of potassium between intracellular and extracellular compartments** |
| Angiotensin-converting enzyme inhibitors | Beta-blockers |
| Angiotensin II receptor blockers | Digitalis |
| Non-steroidal anti-inflammatory agents | Succinylcholine |
| Potassium-sparing diuretics | |
| Heparin | |
| Trimethoprim | |
| Cyclosporin | |

particularly when raised serum creatinine is present. If hyperkalaemia occurs, it may be modified by appropriate dietary modification, correction of acidosis with bicarbonate, the concurrent use of a thiazide or loop diuretic,[135] and, in some circumstances, the use of an anion exchanger such as resonium.

## Trimethoprim

Trimethoprim is known to elevate serum potassium levels in patients with clinical conditions, such as diabetes mellitus or concomitant drug therapy, that reduce potassium secretion in the kidney.

## Diuretics

Potassium secretion is blocked by two independent classes of diuretic. Spironolactone, a direct mineralocorticoid antagonist, binds competitively to the intracellular aldosterone receptor via the basolateral membrane of the distal tubule.[136] Amiloride and triamterene are mineralocorticoid-independent, binding reversibly to the luminal aspect of the tubular membrane, blocking reabsorption of filtered sodium. Due to the associated reduction in luminal negativity, potassium and hydrogen ion secretion is reduced. Potassium-sparing diuretics are more likely to precipitate hyperkalaemia in patients with diabetes mellitus. It has been recognized since the early 1960s that thiazide diuretics may have an adverse effect on insulin resistance and insulin release,[137,138] and may promote hypokalaemia in the hypertensive population. However, whether a differential elec-

trolyte profile occurs in patients with diabetes mellitus has not been reported.

## Cyclosporin A

Hyperkalaemia, attributed to cyclosporin A usage, has been described in solid organ transplantation.[139,140] This is reported to be disproportionate to any reduction in glomerular filtration rate, and associated with hyporeninaemic hypoaldosteronism, which may be amplified in patients with diabetes mellitus due to pre-existing hypoaldosteronism. In patients treated with concomitant beta-blockade, the hyporeninaemia may further attenuate a rise in aldosterone and compound the problem.

## Cyclo-oxygenase (COX) inhibitors

Non-steroidal anti-inflammatory agents may precipitate hyperkalaemia by a reduction in glomerular filtration rate and inhibition of the renin-angiotensin system.[141] Inhibition of prostaglandin $(PG)I_2$ and $PGE_2$ induces vasoconstriction, reducing renal perfusion and also glomerular filtration and distal sodium delivery, both of which may cause hyperkalaemia.[141,142] When biologically active, these prostaglandins stimulate the renin-angiotensin system and antagonize antidiuretic hormone. Their inhibition results in a state equivalent to hyporeninaemic hypoaldosteronism, which is exacerbated in the presence of diabetes mellitus, particularly in the presence of drugs that concomitantly affect the renin-angiotensin axis. Selective COX-2 and nonselective

COX inhibitors have the same propensity for renal effects, including the reduction in glomerular filtration and induction of hyperkalaemia.

## WATER HOMEOSTASIS AND DIABETES MELLITUS

Clearly, water homeostasis is acutely deranged with severe perturbations in glucose metabolism in diabetes mellitus. Urine flow rate and thirst are increased because of glucose- and ketone-induced diuresis. Plasma vasopressin levels are elevated in both type 1 and type 2 diabetes mellitus,[143–146] and this limits glucose-induced water loss by increasing the permeability of the collecting duct to water and urea, thereby promoting more intense water reabsorption in the renal medulla. The amount of water required for excretion of increased filtered osmoles is therefore limited, allowing the concentration of glucose in the urine to exceed by far that observed in the plasma. Hence, despite the increased urine flow rate and enhanced water loss observed in hyperglycaemia, the kidney has an enhanced concentrating ability. Animal studies have shown that the solute free water reabsorption, that is, the amount of free water that the kidney reabsorbs in order to excrete the actual load of osmoles at the observed osmolality, is four times higher in insulin-deficient diabetic rats than in normal animals.[147]

Perturbations in the relationship between osmotic and non-osmotic stimuli and vasopressin release are amplified in the presence of diabetes mellitus. Plasma vasopressin increases in response to hypertonic saline infusion[148] and cigarette smoking,[149] and falls in response to hypoglycaemia to a greater extent than would be observed in non-diabetic subjects. The hypersecretion of vasopressin results in a decreased vasopressin content in the neurohypophysis in patients with uncontrolled type 2 diabetes mellitus,[150] and the normal circadian rhythm associated with vasopressin release is lost in experimental models of poorly controlled type 1 diabetes mellitus.[151]

A resetting of the osmostat is suggested by the finding that, during hyperglycaemia, plasma vasopressin remains in the high range, despite low plasma sodium.[145,152] However, resetting of the osmostat does not appear to be a direct consequence of hyperglycaemia, as, in acute studies, infusion of hypertonic dextrose in diabetic and nondiabetic subjects did not induce an increase in plasma vasopressin.[153] An increased sensitivity of the osmostat is also suggested in animal studies, as the vasopressin release is exaggerated in response to the osmolality.[151] Conversely, abrupt insulin deficiency, induced by cessation of an insulin infusion in patients with diabetes mellitus, is associated with a reduced vasopressin rise, despite a rapid increase in glycaemia.[154]

It has been postulated that a chronic elevation in some plasma amino acids is responsible for the increase in plasma vasopressin observed in patients with diabetes mellitus.[146] Abnormal amino-acid homeostasis, due to the disturbances in insulin-induced cellular amino-acid uptake, is well known.[155] However, its relationship to the elevation in vasopressin observed in patients with diabetes mellitus is not confirmed.[156–159]

Because of the chronic elevation of vasopressin in patients with diabetes mellitus, several studies have examined the possibility that vasopressin receptors could be desensitized. The main receptors responsible for vasopressin action and degradation in the kidney are the V1a receptor, located on the luminal membrane of the principal cells in the collecting duct,[160] and the V2 receptor, located on the basolateral membrane. Binding of circulating vasopressin to the V2 receptor results in increased cyclic AMP, which mediates the vasopressin-induced increase in water reabsorption. Filtered vasopressin binds to the V1a receptor, and this diminishes the action of circulating vasopressin by accelerating the intracellular degradation of cAMP.[161] Studies assessing these receptors in rodent models[162–164] and man[165] have demonstrated a ubiquitous downregulation of V1a receptors in the kidney, liver and platelets, but no change in the V2 receptor density or affinity in the kidney.[162] Thus, these changes, together with the elevations in plasma vasopressin concentrations, enhance the conservation of water during osmotic diuresis.

Despite the beneficial effects of an elevation of plasma vasopressin on limiting the obligate water loss associated with glycosuria, concern exists that raised levels of vasopressin may contribute to the development of diabetic nephropathy. Although beyond the scope of the current discussion, chronic elevations in plasma vasopressin in non-diabetic animal models induce glomerular hyperfiltration,[164,166] albuminuria[167] and abnormalities in renal cell growth and function.[146,168] Conversely, a decrease in urinary concentrating activity reduces glomerulosclerosis and tubulointersitial injury in models of reduced renal mass.[169–171] Studies in diabetic models have shown that orally active V2 receptor blockade abrogates the hyperfiltration and albuminuria,[172] suggesting that the adverse effects in diabetes mellitus are mediated through the V2 receptor. As the V1a receptors are desensitized, there is unlikely to be any effect of an elevated plasma vasopressin on platelet aggregation, or vasopressin-mediated metabolic effects in the liver.

## FLUID AND ELECTROLYTE ABNORMALITIES IN DIABETIC KETOACIDOSIS

Ketoacidosis is a serious, acute, metabolic complication that may occur in patients with both type 1 and type 2 diabetes. The classical clinical picture includes polyuria, polydipsia, polyphagia, weight loss, vomiting and abdominal pain. It is usually characterized by significant increases in blood glucose and associated hyperosmolality. However, it is not uncommon for ketoacidosis to present with euglycaemia (defined as a blood sugar less than 16.7 mmol/l), and this has been reported with a frequency of up to 30%.[173] By definition, the patient will have systemic acidosis and associated electrolyte abnormalities. Acute derangements in specific electrolytes may occur due to fluid shifts, hypertonicity, insulin deficiency and/or acidaemia. Thus, the clinically important abnormalities in electrolytes occur in patients both with and without renal impairment, as, in general, the acute changes are independent of alterations in renal function

### Sodium

Hyponatraemia may occur as a result of the osmotic flux of water from the intracellular to the extracellular space due to hypertonicity. Less commonly, severe hypertriglyceridaemia may further exacerbate hyponatraemia. Generally, the presence of hyponatraemia requires no modification of the initial fluid therapy used in the acute resuscitation.

### Potassium

Hyperkalaemia initially occurs due to the shift of potassium into the extracellular space as a consequence of hypertonicity, insulin deficiency, acidaemia and the osmotic diuresis. If low, or even normal, potassium is evident, a severe total-body potassium deficit is present, and more aggressive potassium replacement is required as part of the acute resuscitation. Bolus insulin administration is likely to lower serum potassium acutely, and may induce a risk of hypokalaemia.[174] As hyperkalaemia may occur if renal dysfunction is present, it is recommended that potassium is withheld from the fluids initially used for resuscitation, but administered when renal function is ensured and a normal or low serum potassium is demonstrated. Potassium is administered in the form of potassium chloride, or in combination with potassium phosphate in a ratio of 2/3 potassium chloride and 1/3 potassium phosphate (see below).

### Phosphate

Whole-body phosphate deficits are common in diabetic ketoacidosis as a result of shifts in the intracellular and extracellular compartments due to hypertonicity, acidaemia and urinary losses from diuresis. Hence, serum phosphate levels may be initially normal and fall during treatment. The consequences of hypophosphataemia include respiratory and skeletal muscle weakness, cardiomyopathy, haemolytic anaemia, and decreased levels of 2,3-diphosphoglycerate that cause a leftward shift in the oxygen dissociation curve. Only a minority of patients with hypophosphataemia require replacement of phosphate during the acute treatment of diabetic ketoacidosis.

## REFERENCES

1. Ritchie S, Waugh D, The pathology of Armanni-Ebstein diabetic nephropathy. *Am J Pathol* 1957; **33**: 1035–57.
2. Kordonouri O, Kahl A, Jörres A et al, The prevalence of incipient tubular dysfunction, but not of glomerular dysfunction, is increased with diabetes onset in childhood. *J Diabetes Complications* 1999; **13**: 320–4.
3. Cohen P, Barzilai N, Lerman A et al, Insulin effects on glucose and potassium metabolism in vivo: evidence for selective insulin resistance in humans. *J Clin Endocrinol Metab* 1991; **73**: 564–8.
4. Bia MJ, DeFronzo RA, Extrarenal potassium homeostasis. *Am J Physiol* 1981; **240**: F257–68.
5. Gavryck WA, Moore RD, Thompson RC, Effect of insulin upon membrane-bound $(Na^+ + K^+)$-ATPase extracted from frog skeletal muscle. *J Physiol* 1975; **252**: 43–58.
6. Zierler K, Rogus EM, Rapid hyperpolarization of rat skeletal muscle induced by insulin. *Biochim Biophys Acta* 1981; **640**: 687–92.
7. Wu FS, Zierler K, Insulin stimulation of an electrogenic pump at high extracellular potassium concentration. *Am J Physiol* 1985; **249**: E12–16.
8. Zierler K, Rogus EM, Scherer RW et al, Insulin action on membrane potential and glucose uptake: effects of high potassium. *Am J Physiol* 1985; **249**: E17–25.
9. Marette A, Krischer J, Lavoie L et al, Insulin increases the $Na(+)$-$K(+)$-ATPase $\alpha_2$-subunit in the surface of rat skeletal muscle: morphological evidence. *Am J Physiol* 1993; **265**: C1716–22.
10. Lytton J, Insulin affects the sodium affinity of rat adipocyte $(Na^+, K^+)$-ATPase. *J Biol Chem* 1985; **260**: 10075–80.

11. Rosic NK, Standaert ML, Pollet RJ, The mechanism of insulin stimulation of $(Na^+,K^+)$-ATPase transport activity in muscle. *J Biol Chem* 1985; **260**: 6206–12.

12. McGeoch JEM, Guidotti G, An insulin-stimulated cation channel in skeletal muscle. Inhibition by calcium causes oscillation. *J Biol Chem* 1992; **267**: 832–41.

13. Farman N, Vandewalle A, Bonvalet JP, Aldosterone binding in isolated tubules. II. An autoradiographic study of concentration dependency in the rabbit nephron. *Am J Physiol* 1982; **242**: F69–77.

14. Petty KJ, Kokko JP, Marver D, Secondary effect of aldosterone on Na K ATPase activity in the rabbit cortical collecting tubule. *J Clin Invest* 1981; **68**: 1514–21.

15. Doucet A, Katz AI, Short-term effect of aldosterone on Na-K-ATPase in single nephron segments. *Am J Physiol* 1981; **241**: F273–8.

16. El Mernissi G, Chabardes D, Doucet A et al, Changes in tubular basement membrane markers after chronic DOCA treatment. *Am J Physiol* 1983; **245**: F100–9.

17. El Mernissi G, Doucet A, Short-term effects of aldosterone and dexamethasone on Na-K-ATPase along the rabbit nephron. *Pflugers Arch* 1983; **399**: 147–51.

18. O'Neil RG, Aldosterone regulation of sodium and potassium transport in the cortical collecting duct. *Semin Nephrol* 1990; **10**: 365–74.

19. Kashgarian M, Biemesderfer D, Caplan M et al, Monoclonal antibody to Na, K-ATPase: immunocytochemical localisation along nephron segments. *Kidney Int* 1985; **28**: 899–913.

20. Stanton B, Janzen A, Klein-Robbenhaar G et al, Ultrastructure of rabbit initial collecting tubule. Effect of adrenal corticosteroid treatment. *J Clin Invest* 1985; **75**: 1327–34.

21. Tomita K, Pisano JJ, Knepper MA, Control of sodium and potassium transport in the cortical collecting duct of the rat. Effects of bradykinin, vasopressin, and deoxycorticosterone. *J Clin Invest* 1985; **76**: 132–6.

22. Wingo CS, Kokko JP, Jacobson HR, Effects of in vitro aldosterone on the rabbit cortical collecting tubule. *Kidney Int* 1985; **28**: 51–7.

23. Stanton BA, Regulation by adrenal corticosteroids of sodium and potassium transport in loop of Henle and distal tubule of rat kidney. *J Clin Invest* 1986; **78**: 1612–20.

24. Sansom SC, O'Neil RG, Effects of mineralocorticoids on transport properties of cortical collecting duct basolateral membrane. *Am J Physiol* 1986; **251**: F743–57.

25. Koeppen B, Giebisch G, Cellular electrophysiology of potassium transport in the mammalian cortical collecting tubule. *Pflugers Arch* 1985; **405** (Suppl 1): S143–6.

26. Allen GG, Barratt LJ, Effect of aldosterone on the transepithelial potential difference of the rat distal tubule. *Kidney Int* 1981; **19**: 678–86.

27. Bastl CP, Hayslett JP, The cellular action of aldosterone in target epithelia. *Kidney Int* 1992; **42**: 250–64.

28. Horisberger JD, Rossier BC, Aldosterone regulation of gene transcription leading to control of ion transport. *Hypertension* 1992; **19**: 221–7.

29. McKenna TJ, Island DP, Nicholson WE et al, The effects of potassium on early and late steps of aldosterone biosynthesis in cells of the zona glomerulosa. *Endocrinology* 1978; **103**: 1411–16.

30. Douglas JG, Effects of high potassium diet on angiotensin II receptors and angiotensin-induced aldosterone production in rat adrenal glomerulosa cells. *Endocrinology* 1980; **106**: 983–90.

31. Schambelan M, Sebastian A, Hyporeninemic hypoaldosteronism. *Adv Intern Med* 1979; **24**: 385–405.

32. Schindler AM, Sommers SC, Diabetic sclerosis of the renal juxtaglomerular apparatus. *Lab Invest* 1966; **15**: 877–84.

33. deLeiva A, Christlieb AR, Melby JC et al, Big renin and biosynthetic defect of aldosterone in diabetes mellitus. *N Engl J Med* 1976; **295**: 639–43.

34. Christlieb AR, Munichoodappa C, Braaten JT, Decreased response of plasma renin activity to orthostasis in diabetic patients with orthostatic hypotension. *Diabetes* 1974; **23**: 834–40.

35. Schambelan M, Stockigt J, Biglieri E, Isolated hypoaldosteronism in adults. A renin deficiency syndrome. *N Engl J Med* 1972; **287**: 573–8.

36. Batlle DC, Arruda JA, Kurtzman NA, Hyperkalemic distal renal tubular acidosis associated with obstructive uropathy. *N Engl J Med* 1981; **304**: 373–80.

37. Batlle DC, Mozes MF, Manaligod J et al, The pathogenesis of hyperchloremic acidosis associated with kidney transplantation. *Am J Med* 1981; **70**: 786–96.

38. Sealey JE, Clark I, Bull MB et al, Potassium balance and the control of renin secretion. *J Clin Invest* 1970; **49**: 2119–27.

39. DeFronzo RA, Hyperkalaemia and hyporeninemic hypoaldosteronism. *Kidney Int* 1980; **17**: 118–34.

40. Williams GH, Hyporeninemic hypoaldosteronism. *N Engl J Med* 1986; **314**: 1041–2.

41. Tuck ML, Sambhi MP, Levin L, Hyporeninemic hypoaldosteronism in diabetes mellitus. Studies of the autonomic nervous system's control of renin release. *Diabetes* 1979; **28**: 237–41.

42. Henrich WL, Role of prostaglandins in renin secretion. *Kidney Int* 1981; **19**: 822–30.

43. Nadler JL, Lee FO, Hsueh E et al, Evidence of prostacyclin deficiency in the syndrome of hyporeninemic hypoaldosteronism. *N Engl J Med* 1986; **314**: 1015–20.

44. Ruilope LM, Garcia Robles R, Paya C et al, Effects of long-term treatment with indomethacin on renal function. *Hypertension* 1986; **8**: 677–84.

45. Zimran A, Kramer M, Plaskin M et al, Incidence of hyperkalaemia induced by indomethacin in a hospital population. *BMJ* 1985; **291**: 107–8.

46. Szylman P, Better OS, Chaimowitz C et al, Role of hyperkalemia in the metabolic acidosis of isolated hypoaldosteronism. *N Engl J Med* 1976; **294**: 361–5.

47. Oh MS, Carroll HJ, Clemmons JE et al, A mechanism for hyporeninemic hypoaldosteronism in chronic renal disease. *Metabolism* 1974; **23**: 1157–66.

48. Cox M, Sterns RH, Singer I, The defense against hyperkalemia: the roles of insulin and aldosterone. *N Engl J Med* 1978; **299**: 525–32.

49. Goldfarb S, Cox M, Singer I, Acute hyperkalemia induced by hyperglycemia: hormonal mechanisms. *Ann Intern Med* 1976; **84**: 426–32.

50. Ammon RA, May WS, Nightingale SD, Glucose-induced hyperkalemia with normal aldosterone levels: studies in a patient with diabetes mellitus. *Ann Intern Med* 1978; **89**: 349–51.

51. Nicolis GL, Kahn T, Sanchez A et al, Glucose-induced hyperkalemia in diabetic subjects. *Arch Intern Med* 1981; **141**: 49–53.

52. Makoff DL, da Silva JA, Rosenbaum BJ et al, Hypertonic expansion: acid-base and electrolyte changes. *Am J Physiol* 1970; **218**: 1201–7.

53. Moreno M, Murphy C, Goldsmith C, Increase in serum potassium resulting from the administration of hypertonic mannitol and other solutions. *J Lab Clin Med* 1969; **73**: 291–8.

54. Hirose M, Biphasic changes in plasma potassium concentration by mannitol infusion in rats. *Jpn J Physiol* 1992; **42**: 49–61.

55. Sunderlin FS Jr, Anderson GH Jr, Streeten DH et al, The renin-angiotensin-aldosterone system in diabetic patients with hyperkalemia. *Diabetes* 1981; **30**: 335–40.

56. Kimura G, Brenner BM, The renal basis for salt sensitivity in hypertension. In: *Hypertension: Pathophysiology, Diagnosis, and Management*, 2nd edn (Laragh JH, Brenner BM, eds). Raven

Press: New York, 1995; 1569–88.

57. Tuck M, Corry D, Trujillo A, Salt-sensitive blood pressure and exaggerated vascular reactivity in the hypertension of diabetes mellitus. *Am J Med* 1990; **88**: 210–16.

58. Kimura G, Brenner BM, Indirect assessment of glomerular capillary pressure from pressure-natriuresis relationship: comparison with direct measurements reported in rats. *Hypertens Res* 1997; **20**: 143–8.

59. Campese VM, Salt sensitivity in real hypertension: renal and cardiovascular implications. *Hypertension* 1994; **23**: 531–50.

60. Parving HH, Osterby R, Ritz E, Diabetic nephropathy. In: *Brenner & Rector's The Kidney*, 6th edn (Brenner BM, ed.). WB Saunders: Philadelphia, 1999; 1731–73.

61. Imanishi M, Yoshioka K, Okumura M et al, Sodium sensitivity related to albuminuria appearing before hypertension in type 2 diabetic patients. *Diabetes Care* 2001; **24**: 111–16.

62. Tulassay T, Yasar A, Madacsy L et al, The role of sympathetic-adrenergic activity in the regulation of acid-base homeostasis and renal sodium excretion under acute physical stress in type-I diabetic children (IDDM). *Acta Biomed Ateneo Parmense* 1992; **63**: 175–86.

63. Feig PU, McCurdy DK, The hypertonic state. *N Engl J Med* 1977; **297**: 1444–54.

64. Katz MA, Hyperglycemia-induced hyponatremia—calculation of expected serum sodium depression. *N Engl J Med* 1973; **289**: 843–4.

65. Moran SM, Jamison RL, The variable hyponatremic response to hyperglycaemia. *West J Med* 1985; **142**: 49–53.

66. Verrotti A, Basciani F, Carle F et al, Calcium metabolism in adolescents and young adults with type 1 diabetes mellitus without and with persistent microalbuminuria. *J Endocrinol Invest* 1999; **22**: 198–202.

67. Giacca A, Fassina A, Caviezel F et al, Bone mineral density in diabetes mellitus. *Bone* 1988; **9**: 29–36.

68. Hough FS, Alterations of bone and mineral metabolism in diabetes mellitus. II. Clinical studies in 206 patients with type 1 diabetes mellitus. *S Afr Med J* 1987; **72**: 120–6.

69. Storm TL, Sorensen OH, Lund B et al, Vitamin D metabolism in insulin-dependent diabetes mellitus. *Metab Bone Dis* 1983; **5**: 107–10.

70. Gregorio F, Cristallini S, Santeusiano F et al, Osteopenia associated with non-insulin-dependent diabetes mellitus: what are the causes? *Diabetes Res Clin Pract* 1994; **23**: 43–54.

71. Inukai T, Fujiwara Y, Tayama K et al, Alterations in serum levels of 1 alpha,25(OH)2D3 and osteocalcin in patients with early diabetic nephropathy. *Diabetes Res Clin Pract* 1997; **38**: 53–9.

72. Auwerx J, Dequeker J, Bouillon R et al, Mineral metabolism and bone mass at peripheral and axial skeleton in diabetes mellitus. *Diabetes* 1988; **37**: 8–12.

73. Barbagallo M, Gupta RK, Dominguez LJ et al, Cellular ionic alterations with age: relation to hypertension and diabetes. *J Am Geriatr Soc* 2000; **48**: 1111–16.

74. Rasmussen H, The calcium messenger system. *N Engl J Med* 1986; **314**: 1094–101.

75. Borle AB, Control, modulation and regulation of cell calcium. *Rev Physiol Biochem Pharmacol* 1981; **90**: 13–153.

76. Barbagallo M, Gupta RK, Bardicef O et al, Altered ionic effects of insulin in hypertension: role of basal ion levels in determining cellular responsiveness. *J Clin Endocrinol Metab* 1997; **82**: 1761–5.

77. Avioli LV, Calcium, cell function and cell death. *Am J Nephrol* 1986; **6** (Suppl 1): 151–4.

78. Orrenius S, McConkey DJ, Bellomo G et al, Role of $Ca^{2+}$ in toxic cell killing. *Trends Pharmacol Sci* 1989; **10**: 281–5.

79. Draznin B, Sussman KE, Kao M et al, The existence of an optimal range of cytosolic free calcium for insulin-stimulated glu-

cose transport in rat adipocytes. *J Biol Chem* 1987; **262**: 14385–8.

80. Barbagallo M, Gupta RK, Resnick LM, Cellular ions in NIDDM: relation of calcium to hyperglycemia and cardiac mass. *Diabetes Care* 1996; **19**: 1393–8.

81. Gill JK, Fonseca V, Dandona P et al, Differential alterations of spontaneous and stimulated $^{45}Ca^{(2+)}$ uptake by platelets from patients with type 1 and type 2 diabetes mellitus. *J Diabetes Complications* 1999; **13**: 271–6.

82. Nadler JL, Rude RK, Disorders of magnesium metabolism. *Endocrinol Metab Clin North Am* 1995; **24**: 623–41.

83. Winegard AI, Does a common mechanism induce the diverse complications of diabetes? *Diabetes* 1987; **36**: 396–406.

84. Djurhuus MS, Skott P, Hother-Nielsen O et al, Insulin increases renal magnesium excretion: a possible cause of magnesium depletion in hyperinsulinaemic states. *Diabetic Med* 1995; **12**: 664–9.

85. Djurhuus MS, Skott P, Vaag A et al, Hyperglycaemia enhances renal magnesium excretion in type 1 diabetic patients. *Scand J Clin Lab Invest* 2000; **60**: 403–9.

86. Ericsson Y, Angmar-Mansson B, Flores M, Urinary mineral ion loss after sugar ingestion. *Bone Miner* 1990; **9**: 233–7.

87. Sjogren A, Floren CH, Nilsson A, Magnesium deficiency in IDDM related to level of glycosylated hemoglobin. *Diabetes* 1986; **35**: 459–63.

88. Johansson G, Danielson BG, Ljunghall S et al, Evidence for a disturbed magnesium metabolism in diabetes mellitus. *Magnes Bull* 1981; **2**: 178–80.

89. McNair P, Christensen MS, Christiansen C et al, Renal hypomagnesaemia in human diabetes mellitus: its relation to glucose homeostasis. *Eur J Clin Invest* 1982; **12**: 81–5.

90. Fujii S, Takemura T, Wada M et al, Magnesium levels in plasma, erythrocyte and urine in patients with diabetes mellitus. *Horm Metab Res* 1982; **14**: 161–2.

91. Sjogren A, Floren CH, Nilsson A, Oral administration of magnesium hydroxide to subjects with insulin-dependent diabetes mellitus: effects on magnesium and potassium levels and on insulin requirements. *Magnesium* 1988; **7**: 117–22.

92. Ponder SW, Brouhard BH, Travis LB, Hyperphosphaturia and hypermagnesuria in children with IDDM. *Diabetes Care* 1990; **13**: 437–41.

93. Ocsenyi Z, Tulassay T, Miltenyi M, Effect of insulin on renal electrolyte handling. *Child Nephrol Urol* 1988; **9**: 16–20.

94. Lindeman RD, Adler S, Yiengst MJ et al, Influence of various nutrients on urinary divalent cation excretion. *J Lab Clin Med* 1967; **70**: 236–45.

95. Sjogren A, Floren CH, Nilsson A, Magnesium, potassium and zinc deficiency in subjects with type II diabetes mellitus. *Acta Med Scand* 1988; **224**: 461–6.

96. Chen MD, Li PY, Tsou CT et al, Selected metals status in patients with noninsulin-dependent diabetes mellitus. *Biol Trace Elem Res* 1995; **50**: 119–24.

97. Tosiello L, Hypomagnesemia and diabetes mellitus. A review of clinical implications. *Arch Intern Med* 1996; **156**: 1143–8.

98. Mikhail N, Ehsanipoor K, Ionized serum magnesium in type 2 diabetes mellitus: its correlation with total serum magnesium and hemoglobin A1c levels. *South Med J* 1999; **92**: 1162–6.

99. Corica F, Cucinotta D, Buemi M et al, Serum ionized magnesium in type 2 diabetes. *South Med J* 2000; **93**: 1038–40.

100. Corsonello A, Ientile R, Buemi M et al, Serum ionized magnesium levels in type 2 diabetic patients with microalbuminuria or clinical proteinuria. *Am J Nephrol* 2000; **20**: 187–92.

101. Resnick LM, Gupta RK, Bhargava KK et al, Cellular ions in hypertension, diabetes, and obesity: a nuclear magnetic resonance spectroscopic study. *Hypertension* 1991; **17**: 951–7.

102. Wacker WEC, Parisi AF, Magnesium metabolism. *N Engl J Med* 1968; **278**: 658–63.

103. Altura BM, Altura BT, Magnesium ions and contraction of vascular smooth muscles: relationship to some vascular diseases. *Fed Proc* 1981; **40**: 2672–9.

104. Barbagallo M, Resnick LM, Calcium and magnesium in the regulation of smooth muscle function and blood pressure: the ionic hypothesis of cardiovascular and metabolic disease and vascular ageing. In: *Endocrinology of the Vasculature* (Sowers JR, ed.). Humana Press: Totawa, NJ, 1996; 283–300.

105. Laughlin MR, Thompson D, The regulatory role for magnesium in glycolytic flux of the human erythrocyte. *J Biol Chem* 1996; **271**: 28977–83.

106. Paolisso G, Barbagallo M, Hypertension, diabetes mellitus and insulin resistance: the role of intracellular magnesium. *Am J Hypertens* 1997; **10**: 346–55.

107. Weglicki WB, Bloom S, Cassidy MM et al, Antioxidants and the cardiomyopathy of Mg-deficiency. *Am J Cardiovasc Pathol* 1992; **4**: 210–15.

108. Freedman AM, Mak IT, Stafford RE et al, Erythrocytes from magnesium-deficient hamsters display an enhanced susceptibility to oxidative stress. *Am J Physiol* 1992; **262**: C1371–5.

109. Afanas'ev IB, Suslova TB, Cheremisina ZP et al, Study of antioxidant properties of metal aspartates. *Analyst* 1995; **120**: 859–62.

110. DeFronzo RA, Goldberg M, Agus ZS, The effects of glucose and insulin on renal electrolyte transport. *J Clin Invest* 1976; **58**: 83–90.

111. Hammerman MR, Rogers S, Hansen VA et al, Insulin stimulates Pi transport in brush border vesicles from proximal tubular segments. *Am J Physiol* 1984; **247**: E616–24.

112. Knochel JP, Jacobsen HR, Renal handling of phosphorus, clinical hypophosphatemia and phosphorus depletion. In: *The Kidney*, 3rd edn (Brenner BM, Rector FC Jr, eds.). WB Saunders: Philadelphia, 1986; 619–62.

113. Gold LW, Massry SG, Friedler RM, Effect of phosphate depletion on renal tubular reabsorption of glucose. *J Lab Clin Med* 1977; **89**: 554–9.

114. Ditzel J, Brochner-Mortensen J, Kawahara R, Dysfunction of tubular phosphate reabsorption related to glomerular filtration and blood glucose control in diabetic children. *Diabetologia* 1982; **23**: 406–10.

115. Perez GO, Oster JR, Vaamonde CA, Renal acidosis and renal potassium handling in selective hypoaldosteronism. *Am J Med* 1974; **57**: 809–16.

116. Levine DZ, Iacovitti M, Burns KD, Distal tubule bicarbonate reabsorption in intact and remnant diabetic kidneys. *Kidney Int* 2000; **57**: 544–9.

117. Caravaca F, Arrobas M, Pizarro JL et al, Metabolic acidosis in advanced renal failure: differences between diabetic and non-diabetic patients. *Am J Kidney Dis* 1999; **33**: 892–8.

118. Wallia R, Greenberg A, Piraino B et al, Serum electrolyte patterns in end-stage renal disease. *Am J Kidney Dis* 1986; **8**: 98–104.

119. Ikegaya N, Yonemura K, Suzuki T et al, Impairment of ventilatory response to metabolic acidosis in insulin-dependent diabetic patients with advanced nephropathy. *Renal Failure* 1999; **21**: 495–8.

120. Guh JY, Lai YH, Yu LK et al, Evaluation of ventilatory responses in severe acidemia in diabetic ketoacidosis. *Am J Nephrol* 1997; **17**: 36–41.

121. Wanke T, Abrahamian H, Lahrmann H et al, No effect of naloxone on ventilatory responses to progressive hypercapnia in IDDM patients. *Diabetes* 1993; **42**: 282–7.

122. Lalau JD, Lacroix C, de Cagny B et al, Metformin-associated lactic acidosis in diabetic patients with acute renal failure. *Nephrol Dial Transplant* 1994; **9** (Suppl 4): 1126–9.

123. Bailey CJ, Turner RC, Metformin. *N Engl J Med* 1996; **334**: 574–9.

124. Misbin RI, Green L, Stadel BV et al, Lactic acidosis in patients with diabetes treated with metformin. *N Engl J Med* 1998; **338**: 265–6.

125. Stang MR, Wysowski DK, Butler-Jones D, Incidence of lactic acidosis in metformin users. *Diabetes Care* 1999; **22**: 925–7.

126. Defronzo RA, Pharmacologic therapy for type 2 diabetes mellitus. *Ann Intern Med* 1999; **131**: 281–303.

127. Cusi K, Consoli A, DeFronzo RA, Metabolic effects of metformin on glucose and lactate metabolism in noninsulin-dependent diabetes mellitus. *J Clin Endocrinol Metab* 1996; **81**: 4059–67.

128. Campbell IW, Metformin and the sulfonylureas: the comparative risk. *Horm Metab Res Suppl* 1985; **15**: 105–11.

129. Wiholm BE, Myrhed M, Metformin-associated lactic acidosis in Sweden 1977–1991. *Eur J Clin Pharmacol* 1993; **44**: 589–91.

130. Brown JB, Pedula K, Barzilay J et al, Lactic acidosis rates in type 2 diabetes. *Diabetes Care* 1998; **21**: 1659–63.

131. Sulkin TV, Bosman D, Krentz AJ, Contraindications to metformin therapy in patients with NIDDM. *Diabetes Care* 1997; **20**: 925–8.

132. Lewis EJ, Hunsicker LG, Clarke WR et al, Collaborative Study Group. Renoprotective effect of the angiotensin-receptor antagonist irbesartan in patients with nephropathy due to type 2 diabetes. *N Engl J Med* 2001; **345**: 851–60.

133. Brenner BM, Cooper ME, de Zeeuw D et al, Effects of losartan on renal and cardiovascular outcomes in patients with type 2 diabetes and nephropathy. *N Engl J Med* 2001; **345**: 861–86.

134. Lewis EJ, Hunsicker LG, Bain RP et al, The effect of angiotensin-converting-enzyme inhibition on diabetic nephropathy. The Collaborative Study Group. *N Engl J Med* 1993; **329**: 1456–62.

135. Reardon LC, Macpherson DS, Hyperkalemia in outpatients using angiotensin-converting enzyme inhibitors. How much should we worry? *Arch Intern Med* 1998; **158**: 26–32.

136. Ramsay LE, Hettiarachchi J, Fraser R et al, Amiloride, spironolactone and potassium chloride in thiazide-treated hypertensive patients. *Clin Pharmacol Ther* 1980; **27**: 533–43.

137. Shapiro AP, Benedik TG, Small JL, Effect of thiazides on carbohydrate metabolism in patients with hypertension. *N Engl J Med* 1961; **265**: 1028–33.

138. Pollare T, Lithell H, Berne C, A comparison of the effects of hydrochlorothiazide and captopril on glucose and lipid metabolism in patients with hypertension. *N Engl J Med* 1989; **321**: 868–73.

139. Adu D, Michael J, Turney J et al, Hyperkalaemia in cyclosporin treated renal allograft recipients. *Lancet* 1983; **ii**: 370–2.

140. Bantle JP, Nath KA, Sutherland DE et al, Effects of cyclosporine on the renin-angiotensin-aldosterone system and potassium excretion in renal transplant recipients. *Arch Intern Med* 1985; **145**: 505–8.

141. Garella S, Matarese RA, Renal effects of prostaglandins and clinical adverse effects of nonsteroidal anti-inflammatory agents. *Medicine* 1984; **63**: 165–81.

142. Clive DM, Stoff JS, Renal syndromes associated with nonsteroidal anti-inflammatory drugs. *N Engl J Med* 1984; **310**: 563–72.

143. Zerbe RL, Vinicor F, Robertson GL, Plasma vasopressin in uncontrolled diabetes mellitus. *Diabetes* 1979; **28**: 503–8.

144. Kamoi K, Ishibashi M, Yamaji T, Thirst and plasma levels of vasopressin, angiotensin II and atrial natriuretic peptide in patients with non-insulin-dependent diabetes mellitus. *Diabetes Res Clin Pract* 1991; **11**: 195–202.

145. Iwasaki Y, Kondo K, Murase T et al, Osmoregulation of plasma vasopressin in diabetes mellitus with sustained hyperglycemia. *J Neuroendocrinol* 1996; **8**: 755–60.

146. Bankir L, Bardoux P, Ahloulay M, Vasopressin and diabetes mellitus. *Nephron* 2001; **87**: 8–18.

147. Ahloulay M, Schmitt F, Dechaux M et al, Vasopressin and urinary concentrating activity in diabetes mellitus. *Diabetes Metab* 1999; **25**: 213–22.

148. Van Itallie CM, Fernstrom JD, Osmolal effects on vasopressin secretion in the streptozotocin-diabetic rat. *Am J Physiol* 1982; **242**: E411–17.

149. Chiodera P, Volpi R, Capretti L et al, Abnormal effect of cigarette smoking on pituitary hormone secretions in insulin-dependent diabetes mellitus. *Clin Endocrinol* 1997; **46**: 351–7.

150. Fujisawa I, Murakami N, Furuto-Kato S et al, Plasma and neurohypophyseal content of vasopressin in diabetes mellitus. *J Clin Endocrinol Metab* 1996; **81**: 2805–9.

151. Granda TG, Velasco A, Rausch A, Variations and interrelation between vasopressin and plasma osmolality in diabetic rats with insulin treatment. *Life Sci* 1998; **63**: 1305–13.

152. Zerbe RL, Vinicor F, Robertson GL, Regulation of plasma vasopressin in insulin dependent diabetes mellitus. *Am J Physiol* 1985; **249**: E317–25.

153. Thompson CJ, Davis SN, Butler PC et al, Osmoregulation of thirst and vasopressin secretion in insulin dependent diabetes mellitus. *Clin Sci* 1988; **74**: 599–606.

154. Vokes TP, Aycinena PR, Robertson GL, Effect of insulin on osmoregulation of vasopressin. *Am J Physiol* 1987; **252**: E538–48.

155. Berger M, Zimmermann-Telschow H, Berchtold P et al, Blood amine acid levels in patients with insulin excess (functioning insulinoma) and insulin deficiency (diabetic ketosis). *Metabolism* 1978; **27**: 793–9.

156. Zinneman HH, Nuttall FQ, Goetz FC, Effect of endogenous insulin on human amino acid metabolism. *Diabetes* 1966; **15**: 5–8.

157. Rosenlund BL, Effects of insulin on free amino acids in plasma and the role of the amino acid metabolism in the etiology of diabetic microangiopathy. *Biochem Med Metab Biol* 1993; **49**: 375–91.

158. Pijl H, Potter van Loon BJ, Toornvliet AC et al, Insulin-induced decline of plasma amino acid concentrations in obese subjects with and without non-insulin-dependent diabetes. *Metabolism* 1994; **43**: 640–6.

159. Hadj-Aissa A, Bankir L, Fraysse M et al, Influence of the level of hydration on the renal response to a protein meal. *Kidney Int* 1992; **42**: 1207–16.

160. Ikeda M, Yoshitomi K, Imai M et al, Cell $Ca^{2+}$ response to luminal vasopressin in cortical collecting tubule principal cells. *Kidney Int* 1994; **45**: 811–16.

161. Conrad KP, Dunn MJ, Renal prostaglandins and other eicosanoids. In: *Renal Physiology* (Windhager EE, ed.). Oxford University Press: Oxford, 1992; 1707–57.

162. Trinder D, Phillips PA, Stephenson JM et al, Vasopressin V1 and V2 receptors in diabetes mellitus. *Am J Physiol* 1994; **266**: E217–23.

163. Phillips PA, Risvanis J, Hutchins AM et al, Down-regulation of vasopressin V1a receptor mRNA in diabetes mellitus in the rat. *Clin Sci* 1995; **88**: 671–4.

164. Gellai M, Silverstein JH, Hwang JC et al, Influence of vasopressin on renal hemodynamics in conscious Brattleboro rats. *Am J Physiol* 1984; **246**: F819–27.

165. Thibonnier M, Woloschak M, Platelet aggregation and vasopressin receptors in patients with diabetes mellitus. *Exp Biol Med* 1988; **188**: 149–52.

166. Bouby N, Ahloulay M, Nsegbe E et al, Vasopressin increases glomerular filtration rate in conscious rats through its antidiuretic action. *J Am Soc Nephrol* 1996; **7**: 842–51.

167. Bardoux P, Martin H, Ahloulay M et al, Vasopressin contributes to hyperfiltration, albuminuria, and renal hypertrophy in diabetes mellitus: study in vasopressin-deficient Brattleboro rats. *Proc Natl Acad Sci USA* 1999; **96**: 10397–402.

168. Bankir L, Kriz W, Adaptation of the kidney to protein intake and to urine concentrating activity: similar consequences in health and CRF. *Kidney Int* 1995; **47**: 7–24.

169. Bouby N, Bachmann S, Bichet D et al, Effect of water intake on the progression of chronic renal failure in the 5/6 nephrectomized rat. *Am J Physiol* 1990; **258**: F973–9.

170. Bouby N, Hassler C, Bankir L, Contribution of vasopressin to progression of chronic renal failure: study in Brattleboro rats. *Life Sci* 1999; **65**: 991–1004.

171. Sugiura T, Yamauchi A, Kitamura H et al, High water intake ameliorates tubulointerstitial injury in rats with subtotal nephrectomy: possible role of TGF-beta. *Kidney Int* 1999; **55**: 1800–10.

172. Bardoux P, Bouby N, Bankir L, L'albuminurie du diabète de type 1 est réduite par l'administration chronique d'un antagoniste des récepteurs V2 de la vasopressine chez le rat (abst). *Diabetes Metab* 2000; **26** (Suppl 1): R31.

173. Munro JF, Campbell IW, McCuish AC et al, Euglycaemic diabetic ketoacidosis. *BMJ* 1973; **2**: 578–80.

174. Schade DS, Eaton RP, Dose response to insulin in man. Differential effects on glucose and ketone body regulation. *J Endocrinol Metab* 1977; **44**: 1038–53.

# 12

# Novel approaches to the treatment of diabetic nephropathy

Robyn G Langham, Darren J Kelly and Richard E Gilbert

## INTRODUCTION

While strategies to achieve good glycaemic control, antihypertensive therapy and the use of agents which block the renin-angiotensin system (RAS) have provided major advances in the therapy of diabetic renal disease, the response is incomplete and the incidence of end-stage renal failure (ESRF) due to diabetes continues to rise.[1]

This chapter focuses on new agents that modulate the pathogenetic pathways underlying the development of diabetic nephropathy, as well as new therapies to provide simultaneously more effective treatment of hypertension with blockade of the RAS. These include drugs that modulate the formation and action of advanced-glycation end products (AGEs), agents that target the activity of protein kinase C (PKC) and compounds which alter the activities of various vasoactive hormone systems.

## ADVANCED-GLYCATION END PRODUCTS (AGES)

Chronic hyperglycaemia leads to the formation of long-lived non-enzymatically glycated proteins referred to as AGEs, a heterogeneous group of molecules that have been implicated not only in the complications of diabetes, but also in non-diabetic renal disease and the consequences of normal ageing, such as loss of renal function, cognitive decline, skin changes, and cataracts.[2]

### AGE formation

The formation of AGEs occurs from the non-enzymatic condensation of a sugar-derived carbonyl group with a reactive amino group, resulting in the formation of an unstable Schiff base (aldimine) with subsequent Amadori rearrangement to form a more stable ketoamine. Over time, these intermediates undergo further modification to produce a range of poorly characterized compound products, termed AGEs (Figure 12.1). These AGEs produce irreversible changes in macromolecules, covalently cross-linking amino groups and leading to significant structural alterations in long-lived molecules such as collagen. In addition to the structural consequences of AGE accumulation, a number of pathophysiological changes have been attributed to the binding of AGE to receptors. In particular, these include activation of PKC and increased expression of a range of pathogenetic growth factors including transforming growth factor-β (TGF-β), platelet-derived growth factor (PDGF) and vascular endothelial growth factor (VEGF).

### AGE receptors

Several binding sites and receptors for AGEs have been identified. These include the macrophage scavenge receptor (types I and II), the receptor for AGE (RAGE), oligosaccharide transferase-48 (AGE-R1), 80K-H phosphoprotein (AGE-R2) and galaectin-3 (AGE-R3).[3] The best characterized is RAGE, a multiligand member of the immunoglobulin superfamily of cell-surface receptors.[4] Binding of AGEs to RAGE initiates a transduction pathway that includes mitogen-activated protein (MAP) kinase,[5] NF-κB activation,[6] and subsequent generation of proinflammatory molecules (such as IL-1α and TNF-α), as well as development of a procoagulant state, vasoconstriction and enhanced adhesion molecule expression.

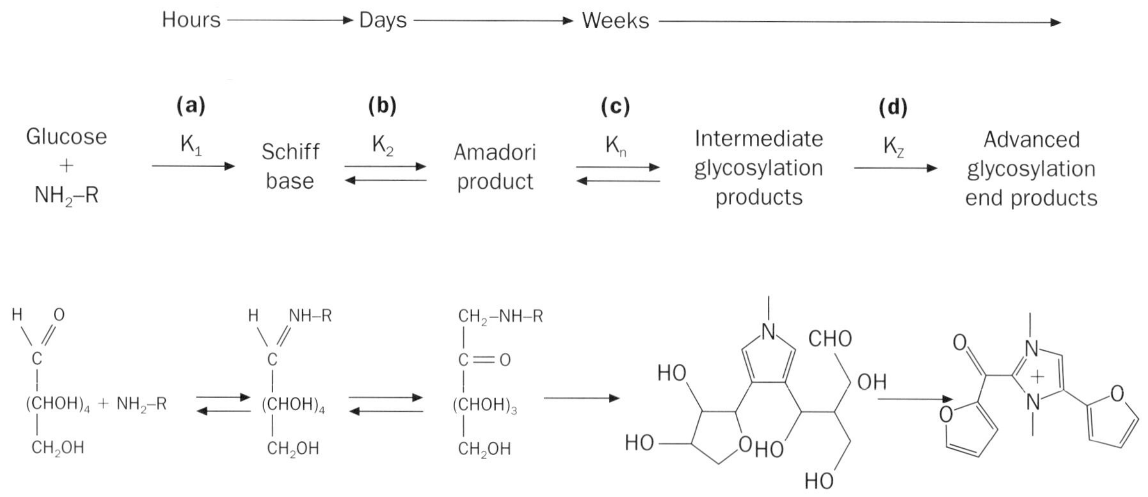

**Figure 12.1** AGE formation. Amino groups react with carbonyl groups of reducing sugars to form **(a)** an unstable Schiff base, which then rearranges to yield **(b)** a more stable Amadori product or ketoamine. **(c)** Intermediate glycation end products then form from progressive modification, including oxidation, dehydration and cyclization, and further modification occurs with time to give rise to **(d)** AGEs. K1: conceptual reaction rate constant (reproduced with permission from *American Journal of Kidney Disease*[2]).

## Strategies for blocking AGE formation

There are a number of potential strategies for blocking the AGE pathway. Most of the therapies developed thus far have been directed at inhibition of AGE formation. Aminoguanidine, the most extensively studied of the AGE formation inhibitors, is a small nucleophilic compound that interacts with intermediate glycation products and prevents cross-link formation.[7] Several animal studies have demonstrated attenuation of the structural, functional, growth factor overexpression and signal transduction pathway activation in experimental diabetic nephropathy.[8–10] The results of a phase II/III clinical trial aimed at assessing the efficacy of aminoguanidine in human diabetic nephropathy with the acronym ACTION (A Clinical Trial in Overt Nephropathy) have concluded. While the details of the study outcomes have not yet been published, Alteon, the pharmaceutical company responsible for these studies, has indicated that aminoguanidine therapy was associated with a statistically significant reduction of urinary protein excretion, over and above the effect of ACE inhibition as standard medical care.[11] However, a trend to reduced progression of declining glomerular filtration rate (GFR) failed to achieve statistical significance. Other AGE formation inhibitors, such as ALT 486,[12] NNC39–0028[13] and OPB 9195,[14] await clinical evaluation.

## Cross-link breakers

Cleavage of the covalent AGE cross-links is also a target for drug therapies following the discovery that N-phenacylthiazolium bromide (PTB) can cleave covalent AGE-derived protein cross-links.[15] However, studies in diabetic rats have failed to demonstrate beneficial effects in experimental diabetic nephropathy,[13] although other 'cross-link breakers', such as ALT 711 (a stable derivative of PTB), have been shown to improve age-related myocardial stiffness.[16] Indeed, ALT711, is currently in phase II clinical trials examining vascular compliance and isolated systolic hypertension.[17]

## Receptor blockade

Another strategy for inhibition of AGE action is by inhibition of its interaction with its cognate receptor, RAGE. This has been accomplished by Schmidt and colleagues by the administration of the soluble, extracellular domain of RAGE (sRAGE).[4] This moiety blocks AGE-induced gene activation in vascular tissue as well as reducing diabetes-associated hyperpermeability and vasculopathy.[18,19] These findings suggest that RAGE may be an important therapeutic target for drug discovery programmes seeking to identify new treatments for diabetic nephropathy.

# PROTEIN KINASE C (PKC)

Hyperglycaemia is the central aetiological factor in the pathogenesis of the long-term complications of diabetes. Detailed examination of glucose-induced intracellular biochemical pathways has not only led to a greater understanding of the underlying pathophysiological processes but has also yielded specifically targeted new therapeutic agents.

## PKC activation in diabetes

Following its transport into the cell, glucose may undergo further metabolism by both anabolic and catabolic pathways. In most cells, the majority of intracellular glucose is catabolized by glycolysis. Thus, in the diabetic setting, high levels of extracellular glucose lead to increased glycolytic flux in those cells that do not require insulin for glucose entry. This in turn leads to increased *de novo* synthesis of diacylglycerol (DAG), an activating cofactor for the key intracellular enzyme, PKC. Furthermore, other pathways leading to PKC activation may also be increased in the diabetic state including receptor-mediated DAG generation by phospholipase C, cleavage of phosphatidylcholine and phospholipase $A_2$-dependent lipid catabolism.

## PKC isoenzymes

Rather than a single enzyme, PKCs are a family of serine/threonine kinases with wide-ranging effects on the extracellular signal transduction pathway. Thus, PKC activation may lead to a myriad of effects on cell proliferation, differentiation, expression profile, contractility and permeability.[20] At the present time, 12 isoforms of PKC have been identified and classified into three categories: classical, novel, and atypical, according to their calcium and phospholipid dependence.[21] The classical or conventional PKCs (cPKCs) are activated by DAG, phosphatidylserine and calcium, and include isoforms α, two β splice variants (βI and βII) and γ. The cPKCs consist of two cysteine-rich C1 domains, which bind DAG/phorbol ester, and a calcium-binding C2 domain. The structurally similar, novel PKCs (nPKCs) (isoforms δ, ε, η, θ and μ) also require DAG for activation, but, as they lack a functional C2 domain, do not require calcium. The atypical PKCs (aPKCs) (isoforms ζ, ι and λ) are dissimilar structurally to both the cPKCs and aPKCs, and are activated neither by calcium nor by DAG.

## Effects of PKC activation

A number of key pathogenetic pathways of direct relevance to diabetic nephropathy are activated by PKC.[22,23] These include the expression of a number of growth factors such as the major profibrotic growth factor implicated in diabetic nephropathy, transforming growth factor-β (TGF-β)[24] and other relevant growth factors, including platelet-derived growth factor (PDGF),[25] insulin-like growth factor-I (IGF-I) and vascular endothelial growth factor (VEGF)[26] (Figure 12.2).

However, despite its numerous isoforms and the multiple pathways that may lead to its activation, studies by George King and colleagues have suggested that diabetes is associated with a preferential activation of the β isoform of PKC.[27] This finding has important therapeutic implications, as, given its ubiquitous presence and diverse physiological functions, inhibition of all PKC isoforms would likely be toxic, while specific isoform inhibition may not. Indeed, this concept has led to drug discovery programmes seeking to develop PKC isoform-specific inhibitors. The largest group of such selective kinase inhibitors are

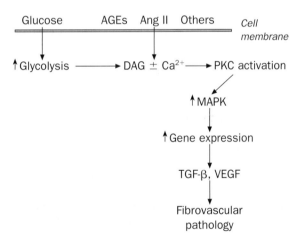

**Figure 12.2** Activation and effects of PKC. Classical or conventional PKC is activated by DAG, which can be generated by the *de novo* pathway **(a)** from glycolytic intermediates, or via the ligand-receptor pathway **(b)**. In the latter, DAG is generated from the hydrolysis of membrane-associated phosphoinositide-containing phospholipids through the activity of phospholipases C and D (PLC, PLD). The activation of PKC results in a myriad of downstream effects, including increased gene expression of vascular endothelial growth factor (VEGF) and transforming growth factor-β (TGF-β). Ang II: angiotensin II; IL-1: interleukin 1; LDL: low-density lipoprotein; PDGF: platelet-derived growth factor; TX: thromboxane.

those that compete for ATP-binding sites.[28] To date, the one most studied in renal disease is LY333531 (Eli-Lilly and Co., Indianapolis, IN, USA), an orally active, non-toxic inhibitor with PKC-β specificity. In preclinical studies on diabetic rats, treatment with LY333531 resulted in improved GFR, and reduction in urinary albumin compared with untreated diabetic rats.[29] Furthermore, these effects were accompanied by attenuation in mesangial expansion[30] with a reduction in TGF-β and collagen expression.[27] In addition, recent studies have demonstrated LY333531 treatment led to a reduction in albuminuria, structural injury, and TGF-β expression in the diabetic Ren-2 rat, despite continued hypertension and hyperglycaemia.[31] Phase II clinical studies with this compound are currently in progress for the treatment of diabetic complications in the USA and in Europe.[28]

## HYPERTENSION AND DIABETIC RENAL DISEASE

The most important target in attempting to slow the rate of progression of renal disease, regardless of aetiology, is control of hypertension. Current recommendations of the Joint National Committee on Prevention, Detection, Evaluation and Treatment of High Blood Pressure (JNC-VI) endorse a target blood pressure of 130/85 mmHg in diabetic patients with lowering of this target to 125/75 in the presence of >1 g/day proteinuria.[32] These targets are evidence-based supported by the findings of major randomized prospective, long-term clinical trials examining the progression of diabetic nephropathy or of cardiovascular events.[33] However, despite these recommendations, and comparable targets established by the World Health Organization–International Society of Hypertension (WHO–ISH), the realization of these BP targets is uncommon. A recent study has shown that achievement of a blood pressure <140/90 mmHg occurs in only 27% of hypertensive patients in the USA and only 6% of those in the UK.[32] Intervention studies in diabetic renal disease have highlighted the importance of RAS blockade with angiotensin-converting enzyme inhibitors (ACEIs) in type 1 diabetes[34] and angiotensin receptor blockers (ARBs) in type 2 diabetes;[35,36] this action has beneficial effects on both proteinuria and the rate of decline of renal function exceeding those obtained by control of blood pressure alone. However, despite the efficacy of ACEIs and ARBs in lowering systemic blood pressure, an average of 3.2 different medications is still required to achieve recommended blood pressure targets.[33] Agents that provide improved blood

pressure control and subsequent renoprotection are needed. The topic of hypertension and diabetic renal disease is discussed in more depth in Chapter 7.

## Vasopeptidase inhibition

Several interrelated vasoactive hormone systems contribute to blood pressure homeostasis in normal and pathological situations. These include the RAS, the kallikrein-kinin system (KKS) and the natriuretic peptide system (NPS). Together, these three systems modulate vascular tone and sodium/water balance as well as having growth-factor like actions. The interrelationship between these systems may be important, not only in the pathogenesis of hypertension but also in progressive renal and cardiac failure (Figure 12.3). Both ACE (EC 3.4.15.1) and neutral endopeptidase (NEP) (EC 3.4.24.11) are zinc-containing cell-surface peptidases that share structural similarities at their active sites permitting a series of dual ACE–NEP inhibitors, referred to as vasopeptidase inhibitors (VPIs) to be developed.[37] By simultaneously affecting the activity of both the natriuretic system and the RAS, VPIs result in a range of potentially favourable changes in vasoactive peptides, leading to better blood pressure control independent of plasma renin activity and $Na^+$ status. In addition, other vasoactive peptides are affected by blockade of the ACE/NEP systems. For example, ACE inhibitors prevent the degradation of bradykinin and lower circulating levels of endothelin (ET), antidiuretic hormone and norepinephrine, while NEP inhibitors have been shown to reduce ET and to potentiate the natriuretic effects of adrenomedullin.[37]

## Dual vasopeptidase inhibitors in development

There are a number of dual ACE/NEP VPIs currently the subject of preclinical and clinical studies. Omapatrilat (Bristol-Myers Squibb, Princeton, NJ, USA) is the furthest advanced in clinical development, as phase II/III studies in hypertension and cardiac failure have recently been completed.[38] Other ACE/NEP VPIs, which vary in their $IC_{50}$ for ACE and NEP, include SA 7060, MDL 100240, MDL 100173, fasidotril, sampatrilat, alatriopril, CGS 30440 and S 21402.[39] Other dual VPIs, agents that inhibit NEP and endothelin-converting enzyme (ECE), are less advanced, as are triple VPIs that inhibit ACE, NEP and ECE.

A number of animal studies of renal disease have examined the relative efficacy of VPIs and ACE inhibitors. In a study of diabetic spontaneously

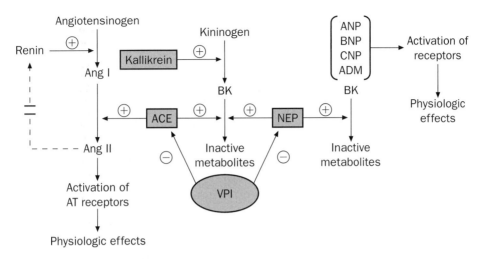

**Figure 12.3** Interactions and major components of the renin-angiotensin, natriuretic peptide and kinin-kallikrein systems. The effects of VPIs are mediated by inhibiting angiotensin-converting enzyme (ACE) and neutral endopeptidase (NEP). This results in decreased formation of angiotensin II (Ang II) and decreased degradation of natriuretic peptides. ADM: adrenomedullin; ANP: atrial natriuretic peptide; BNP: brain natriuretic peptide; CNP: C-type natriuretic peptide (reproduced with permission from poster presentation by Kostis JB, et al. In: *Vasopeptidase Inhibition: Scientific Presentations and Abstracts*, vol. II; August 2000 (Bristol-Myers Squibb: Princeton, NJ)).

hypertensive rats (SHR), the dual NEP/ACE inhibitor S 21402 was found to be more effective at lowering blood pressure than the ACE inhibitor captopril, although the effect of both drugs on albuminuria was similar.[40] In the subtotally nephrectomized rat, a preclinical model with some similarities to diabetic nephropathy, two studies have indicated that the VPIs omapatrilat and CGS 30440 provide a greater reduction in proteinuria, despite similar blood pressure lowering.[41,42] Furthermore, in addition to superior preservation of renal function, omapatrilat treatment was also associated with increased survival. Others have, however, suggested that this increased renoprotective effect of omapatrilat may be secondary to a better hypotensive effect.[10] Nevertheless, the ability of the VPIs to lower blood pressure and to provide renoprotection, highlights the potential of these agents, possibly as monotherapy, in the management of patients with hypertension and nephropathy. While similar in efficacy to ACE inhibition in congestive heart failure,[43] whether the VPIs provide greater reno-protection in patients with progressive diabetic nephropathy remain uncertain.

## CONCLUSIONS

The understanding of the importance of both glucose-dependent and independent pathways in the patho-genesis of diabetic nephropathy has resulted in the development of important new therapies that focus more precisely on the underlying pathophysiological mechanisms. Emerging data from both preclinical studies and early clinical trials are keenly awaited.

## REFERENCES

1. Ritz E, Rychlik I, Locatelli F, et al, End-stage renal failure in type 2 diabetes: a medical catastrophe of worldwide dimensions, *Am J Kidney Dis* (1999) **34:**795–808.
2. Raj DS, Choudhury D, Welbourne TC, et al, Advanced glycation end products: a nephrologist's perspective, *Am J Kidney Dis* (2000) **35:**365–80.
3. He CJ, Zheng F, Stitt A, et al, Differential expression of renal AGE-receptor genes in NOD mice: possible role in nonobese diabetic renal disease, *Kidney Int* (2000) **58:**1931–40.
4. Schmidt AM, Stern DM, RAGE: a new target for the prevention and treatment of the vascular and inflammatory complications of diabetes, *Trends Endocrinol Metab* (2000) **11:**368–75.
5. Lander HM, Tauras JM, Ogiste JS, et al, Activation of the receptor for advanced glycation end products triggers a p21(ras)-dependent mitogen-activated protein kinase pathway regulated by oxidant stress, *J Biol Chem* (1997) **272:**17810–14.
6. Huttunen HJ, Fages C, Rauvala H, Receptor for advanced glycation end products (RAGE)-mediated neurite outgrowth and activation of NF-kappaB require the cytoplasmic domain of the receptor but different downstream signaling pathways, *J Biol Chem* (1999) **274:**19919–24.
7. Brownlee M, Vlassara H, Kooney A, et al, Aminoguanidine prevents diabetes-induced arterial wall protein cross-linking, *Science* (1986) **232** (4758):1629–32.
8. Soulis-Liparota T, Cooper M, Papazoglou D, et al, Retardation

by aminoguanidine of development of albuminuria, mesangial expansion, and tissue fluorescence in streptozocin-induced diabetic rat, *Diabetes* (1991) **40**:1328–34.

9. Osicka TM, Yu Y, Panagiotopoulos S, et al, Prevention of albuminuria by aminoguanidine or ramipril in streptozotocin-induced diabetic rats is associated with the normalization of glomerular protein kinase C, *Diabetes* (2000) **49**:87–93.

10. Cao Z, Burrell LM, Tikkanen I, et al, Vasopeptidase inhibition attenuates the progression of renal injury in subtotal nephrectomized rats, *Kidney Int* (2001) **60**:715–21.

11. http://www.alteonpharma.com. Alteon Pharmaceuticals.

12. Kochakian M, Manjula BN, Egan JJ, Chronic dosing with aminoguanidine and novel advanced glycosylation end product-formation inhibitors ameliorates cross-linking of tail tendon collagen in STZ-induced diabetic rats, *Diabetes* (1996) **45**:1694–700.

13. Oturai PS, Christensen M, Rolin B, et al, Effects of advanced glycation end-product inhibition and cross-link breakage in diabetic rats, *Metabolism* (2000) **49**:996–1000.

14. Tsuchida K, Makita Z, Yamagishi S, et al, Suppression of transforming growth factor beta and vascular endothelial growth factor in diabetic nephropathy in rats by a novel advanced glycation end product inhibitor, OPB-9195, *Diabetologia* (1999) **42**:579–88.

15. Vasan S, Zhang X, Kapurniotu A, et al, An agent cleaving glucose-derived protein crosslinks in vitro and in vivo, *Nature* (1996) **382** (6588):275–8.

16. Asif M, Egan J, Vasan S, et al, An advanced glycation endproduct cross-link breaker can reverse age-related increases in myocardial stiffness, *Proc Natl Acad Sci USA* (2000) **97**:2809–13.

17. Kass DA, Shapiro EP, Kawaguchi M, et al, Improved arterial compliance by a novel advanced glycation end-product crosslink breaker, *Circulation* (2001) **104**:1464–70.

18. Schmidt AM, Hasu M, Popov D, et al, Receptor for advanced glycation end products (AGEs) has a central role in vessel wall interactions and gene activation in response to circulating AGE proteins, *Proc Natl Acad Sci USA* (1994) **91**:8807–11.

19. Wautier JL, Zoukourian C, Chappey O, et al, Receptor-mediated endothelial cell dysfunction in diabetic vasculopathy. Soluble receptor for advanced glycation end products blocks hyperpermeability in diabetic rats, *J Clin Invest* (1996) **97**:238–43.

20. Meier M, King GL, Protein kinase C activation and its pharmacological inhibition in vascular disease, *Vasc Med* (2000) **5**:173–85.

21. Newton AC, Protein kinase C: structure, function, and regulation, *J Biol Chem* (1995) **270**:28495–8.

22. Koya D, King GL, Protein kinase C activation and the development of diabetic complications, *Diabetes* (1998) **47**:859–66.

23. Aiello LP, Bursell S-E, Clermont A, et al, Vascular endothelial growth factor-induced retinal permeability is mediated by protein kinase C in vivo and suppressed by an effective orally active β-isoform-selective inhibitor. *Diabetes* (1997) **46**:1473–80.

24. Ziyadeh FN, Role of transforming growth factor beta in diabetic nephropathy, *Exp Nephrol* (1994) **2**:137.

25. Rui L, Archer SF, Argetsinger LS, et al, Platelet-derived growth factor and lysophosphatidic acid inhibit growth hormone binding and signaling via a protein kinase C-dependent pathway, *J Biol Chem* (2000) **275**:2885–92.

26. Xia P, Aiello LP, Ishii H, et al, Characterization of vascular endothelial growth factor's effect on the activation of protein kinase C, its isoforms, and endothelial cell growth, *J Clin Invest* (1996) **98**:2018–26.

27. Koya D, Jirousek MR, You-Wei L, et al, Characterization of pro-

tein kinase C β isoform activation on gene expression of transforming growth factor-β, extracellular matrix components, and prostanoids in the glomeruli of diabetic rats, *J Clin Invest* (1997) **100**:115–26.

28. Goekjian PG, Jirousek MR, Protein kinase C in the treatment of disease: signal transduction pathways, inhibitors, and agents in development, *Curr Med Chem* (1999) **6**:877–903.

29. Ishii H, Jirousek MR, Koya D, et al, Amelioration of vascular dysfunction in diabetic rats by an oral PKC β inhibitor. *Science* (1996) **272**:728–31.

30. Koya D, Haneda M, Nakagawa H, et al, Amelioration of accelerated diabetic mesangial expansion by treatment with a PKC beta inhibitor in diabetic db/db mice, a rodent model for type 2 diabetes. *FASEB J* (2000) **14**:439–47.

31. Kelly DJ, Zhang Y, Hepper C, et al, Protein kinase C beta inhibition attenuates the progression of experimental diabetic nephropathy in the presence of continued hypertension. *Diabetes* (2003) **52**:512–18.

32. Joint National Committee on Prevention, Detection, Evaluation, and Treatment of High Blood Pressure. The sixth report of the Joint National Committee on Prevention, Detection, Evaluation, and Treatment of High Blood Pressure, *Arch Intern Med* (1997) **157**:2413–45.

33. Bakris GL, Williams M, Dworkin L, et al, Preserving renal function in adults with hypertension and diabetes: a consensus approach. National Kidney Foundation Hypertension and Diabetes Executive Committees Working Group, *Am J Kidney Dis* (2000) **36**:646–61.

34. Lewis EJ, Hunsicker LG, Bain RP, et al for the Collaborative Study Group, The effect of angiotensin-converting-enzyme inhibition on diabetic nephropathy, *N Engl J Med* (1993) **329**:1456–62.

35. Lewis EJ, Hunsicker LG, Clarke WR, et al, Renoprotective effect of the angiotensin-receptor antagonist irbesartan in patients with nephropathy due to type 2 diabetes, *N Engl J Med* (2001) **345**:851–60.

36. Brenner BM, Cooper ME, de Zeeuw D, et al, Effects of losartan on renal and cardiovascular outcomes in patients with type 2 diabetes and nephropathy, *N Engl J Med* (2001) **345**:861–9.

37. Burnett JC Jr, Vasopeptidase inhibition: a new concept in blood pressure management, *J Hypertens Suppl* (1999) **17**:S37–43.

38. Rouleau JL, Pfeffer MA, Stewart DJ, et al, Comparison of vasopeptidase inhibitor, omapatrilat, and lisinopril on exercise tolerance and morbidity in patients with heart failure: IMPRESS randomised trial, *Lancet* (2000) **356** (9230):615–20.

39. Gilbert RE, Kelly DJ, Atkins RC, Novel approaches to the treatment of progressive renal disease, *Curr Opin Pharmacol* (2001) **1**:183–9.

40. Tikkanen T, Tikkanen I, Rockell MD, et al, Dual inhibition of neutral endopeptidase and angiotensin-converting enzyme in rats with hypertension and diabetes mellitus, *Hypertension* (1998) **32**:778–85.

41. Cohen DS, Mathis JE, Dotson RA, et al, Protective effects of Cgs 30440, a combined angiotensin-converting enzyme inhibitor and neutral endopeptidase inhibitor, in a model of chronic renal failure. *J Cardiovasc Pharmacol* (1998) **32**:87–95.

42. Taal MW, Nenov VD, Wong W, et al, Vasopeptidase inhibition affords greater renoprotection than angiotensin-converting enzyme inhibition alone, *J Am Soc Nephrol* (2001) **12**:2051–9.

43. Packer M, Califf RM, Konstam MA, et al, Comparison of omapatrilat and enalapril in patients with chronic heart failure: the Omapatrilat Versus Enalapril Randomized Trial of Utility in Reducing Events (OVERTURE). *Circulation* (2002) **106**:920–6.

# 13

# Summary of the management of the patient with diabetic nephropathy: mild to moderate renal involvement

Rudolf Bilous and Steve Jones

The essential elements of the management of early diabetic kidney disease are primary prevention and, if microalbuminuria becomes established, secondary prevention in order to halt or at least reduce the rate of progression to more advanced forms of diabetic kidney disease. In addition, cardiovascular mortality rates are particularly high in patients with diabetic nephropathy, and attention should be paid to risk factors. The main treatment modalities that have been demonstrated to prevent and/or reduce the rate of progression of diabetic nephropathy in randomized controlled trials (RCTs) are as follows:

1) maintaining good long-term glycaemic control
2) effective early treatment with antihypertensive agents
3) dietary protein restriction.

## DIAGNOSING MICROALBUMINURIA

Microalbuminuria is the first clinically apparent manifestation of diabetic kidney disease. At a consensus meeting in 1985, microalbuminuria was defined as a urinary albumin excretion rate (UAER) of 20–200 μg/min on timed urine collections. A UAER in this range was known to be highly predictive of the subsequent development of 'clinical nephropathy',[1] defined by the presence of dipstick-positive proteinuria. Timed urine collections are now largely reserved for research protocols. In clinical practice, microalbuminuria is detected by measuring the urinary albumin concentration, usually expressed as a ratio to urinary creatinine concentration (Table 13.1). As intraindividual variation in albumin:creatinine ratio (ACR) is high, with reported

coefficients of variation of up to 30–60%,[2] several measures over a period of months are required to make a diagnosis of microalbuminuria. At least two out of three values in the microalbuminuric range are required to confirm the presence of microalbuminuria.

## DIAGNOSIS OF DIABETIC NEPHROPATHY

Non-diabetic renal disease may occur in 3–28% of diabetic patients with proteinuria.[3] These apparently high rates are derived from biopsy series and probably reflect the fact that only unusual patients undergo renal biopsy. It is important to identify such patients, as they may require specific treatment. The diagnosis of diabetic nephropathy is usually made on clinical grounds, and biopsy is reserved for patients with features described in Table 13.2.

## GENETIC PREDISPOSITION

Sib-pair studies[4,5] and familial clustering in the Diabetes Control and Complications Trial (DCCT) have suggested that diabetic nephropathy occurs in those with an inherited predisposition. However, the precise nature of the responsible genetic abnormality, possibly several abnormalities, is poorly defined. As there is currently no test that is useful at the individual level, all patients with newly diagnosed diabetes have to be regarded as at equal risk of developing diabetic nephropathy and managed accordingly.

**Table 13.1 Definitions of microalbuminuria.**

| | Normoalbuminuria | Microalbuminuria | Overt nephropathy (Macroalbuminuria) |
|---|---|---|---|
| **Timed overnight collection** | <20 µg/min | 20–199 µg/min | ≥ 200 µg/min (dipstick-positive if >300 µg/min) |
| **24-hr collection** | <30 mg/24 hr | 30–299 mg/24 hr | ≥300 mg/24 hr |
| **Albumin:creatinine ratio (ACR)** | Men <br> <2 mg/mmol <br> <20 mg/gm <br> Women <br> <3 mg/mmol <br> <30 mg/gm | Men <br> 2–20 mg/mmol <br> 20–300 mg/gm <br> Women <br> 3–30 mg/mmol <br> 30–300 mg/gm | Men <br> >20 mg/mmol <br> >300 mg/gm <br> Women <br> >30 mg/mmol <br> >300 mg/gm |

**Table 13.2 Renal biopsy may be considered if there are features suggesting non-diabetic kidney disease.**

**Features that suggest non-diabetic kidney disease**

Rapid deterioration in renal function

Sudden development of nephrotic syndrome

Heavy haematuria

Absence of diabetic retinopathy

Short duration of type 1 diabetes

Clinical or laboratory evidence of non-diabetic systemic disease

## MAINTAINING GOOD GLYCAEMIC CONTROL

### Primary prevention of microalbuminuria

The maintenance of good glycaemic control, in both type 1 and type 2 diabetes, has been shown to reduce the cumulative incidence of microalbuminuria.[6–8] Some authors have suggested that there is a 'glycaemic threshold' in type 1 diabetes below which microalbuminuria does not occur.[9] Although this is disputed, the relationship between glycaemic control and microvascular complications in type 1 diabetes appears to be curvilinear, with the risk of developing microalbuminuria rising markedly as $HbA_{1c}$ increases above 8–8.5%.[9,10] In type 2 diabetes, there is a linear reduction in risk as $HbA_{1c}$ is reduced to 7%, with no evidence of a glycaemic threshold for the development of microvascular complications.[11] A threshold for intervention to improve glycaemic control is therefore recommended at an $HbA_{1c}$ value of 8%. Ideally, $HbA_{1c}$ should be reduced to and maintained at 7% or less.

### Secondary prevention of the development of 'overt' diabetic nephropathy

Observational studies have suggested that the rate of progression from microalbuminuria to dipstick-positive proteinuria is associated with poor glycaemic control. A recent observational study in people with type 1 diabetes has suggested that progression can be reduced if $HbA_{1c}$ is maintained below 8.5%.[12] However, randomized controlled trials have failed to demonstrate that improved glycaemic control can reduce the rate of progression, possibly because of type 2 error and relatively short periods of follow-up.[13] Nevertheless, an intervention threshold for $HbA_{1c}$ of 8% and a goal of 7% has been recommended in microalbuminuric patients with type 1 and type 2 diabetes in order to prevent the progression of other microvascular complications such as retinopathy.

## Reducing the rate of decline of renal function

There is no evidence from RCTs to suggest that good glycaemic control can slow progression of diabetic nephropathy once renal function starts to decline. However, in an observational study of people with type 1 diabetes, good glycaemic control (HbA$_{1c}$ < 8%) was associated with a slower rate of decline in renal function.[14] Good glycaemic control is also important in reducing the rate of progression of other microvascular complications.

Achieving and maintaining tight glycaemic control requires intensive input from the patient and health-care professionals. Targets may be modified in specific circumstances such as in the very young, the very old and those with hypoglycaemic unawareness. It is now clear that type 2 diabetes is a progressive condition and that a high proportion of patients will require insulin therapy to maintain good long-term glycaemic control.

## EFFECTIVE EARLY TREATMENT WITH ANTIHYPERTENSIVE AGENTS

### Primary prevention of microalbuminuria

In normotensive, normoalbuminuric patients with type 1 diabetes, there is no convincing evidence that antihypertensive treatment prevents or delays the onset of microalbuminuria. The EUCLID study suggested that ACE inhibition may reduce the rate of change of UAER within the normoalbuminuric range, in people with type 1 diabetes.[15] However, the rate of progression to microalbuminuria in this study was not significantly reduced as a result of treatment with lisinopril. Normoalbuminuric, normotensive patients with type 1 diabetes are therefore not routinely treated with antihypertensive agents in an attempt to prevent the development of microalbuminuria.

In patients with type 1 diabetes, blood pressure rises as UAER enters the microalbuminuric range, and continues to rise thereafter.[16] The presence of either hypertension or microalbuminuria should prompt screening for the other. Both require treatment in their own right to prevent progression to more advanced forms of diabetic nephropathy. Details of the therapeutic strategies are described in the section below relating to secondary prevention.

In type 2 diabetes, hypertension commonly precedes microalbuminuria. In the United Kingdom Prospective Diabetes Study (UKPDS), hypertension was present in 38% of the cohort at diagnosis, but only 21% of these individuals had a raised UAER.[8] Treatment with beta-blockers or angiotensin-converting enzyme inhibitors (ACEIs) appears to be effective in reducing the development of microalbuminuria in type 2 diabetes. There does not appear to be a 'blood-pressure threshold' below which there is no risk of developing the microvascular complications of type 2 diabetes.[17]

## Secondary prevention of the development of 'overt' diabetic nephropathy

Treatment with antihypertensive agents, particularly those which modulate the renin-angiotensin axis, are of proven benefit in reducing the rate of progression from microalbuminuria to proteinuria. In patients with type 1 diabetes, there appears to be an advantage in using ACEIs, even if blood pressure is within the normal range.[18] In type 2 diabetes, a recent study has shown a similar effect with the angiotensin II receptor blocker (AIIRB) irbesartan.[19] A low-sodium diet (less then 50 mmol/day) increases the efficacy of ACEIs and should be recommended.[20] In addition to preventing progression of microalbuminuria, ACEIs appear to have a beneficial effect on cardiovascular mortality and morbidity in diabetic patients with a raised UAER.[21]

Treatment with ACEIs or AIIRBs should therefore be commenced once microalbuminuria is detected. Blood pressure should ideally be maintained at or below 130/80 mmHg.[22,23] This requires intensive effort on the part of the patient and physician. While such agents are recommended as first-line treatment, combination therapy with beta-blockers, calcium-channel blockers, diuretics and α-blockers, and possibly angiotensin II receptor blockers is often required.

## Reducing the rate of decline in renal function

Antihypertensive agents, especially those which modulate the renin-angiotensin axis, are essential and are of proven benefit in reducing the rate of decline in glomerular filtration rate (GFR) in diabetic patients with established nephropathy.[24-26] ACEIs may exert a specific renal protective effect and appear to be more effective in reducing UAER than dihydropiridine calcium-channel blockers, though this reduction in albuminuria has not always been associated with a difference in the rate of decline of GFR.[27]

Treatment with ACE inhibitors or AIIRBs is recommended in all diabetic patients with proteinuria, even if blood pressure is not elevated. Ideally, most patients should have started such therapy at the microalbuminuric stage. An initial blood-pressure target of 130/80 mmHg has been recommended in patients with proteinuria. Once renal function starts to decline and protein excretion reaches 1 g in 24 hr, even more stringent blood-pressure targets of less than 125/75 mmHg have been suggested.[22] Meeting such targets in patients with declining renal function invariably requires combination therapy, often including a loop diuretic. The latter are particularly important should the patient develop peripheral oedema as part of the nephrotic syndrome.

Blood-pressure targets for all people with diabetes usually reflect consensus opinion and are often aimed at reducing cardiovascular events rather than renal outcome. Such targets are generally determined by balancing aspiration against what can be achieved in practice. An intervention threshold for hypertension in normoalbuminuric patients, initially with non-pharmacological measures, is recommended if blood pressure exceeds 140/90 mmHg. If antihypertensive agents are required, treatment with an ACEI is usually recommended in the first instance, although other agents including beta-blockers, diuretics, calcium-channel blockers, angiotensin II receptor blockers and α-blockers may be equally effective. Ideally, blood pressure should be maintained at or below 130/80 mmHg in all people with diabetes.[23] However, in the UKPDS, 29% of patients in the intensively treated arm required three or more agents to achieve a mean blood pressure of 142/82 mmHg, falling well short of the targets described above.[8]

## DIETARY PROTEIN RESTRICTION

There does not appear to be a role for dietary protein restriction until the stage of overt nephropathy has been reached and possibly renal function (GFR) has begun to decline. Even at this stage, the role of protein restriction is controversial; however, there does appear to be a benefit of a modest reduction in dietary protein intake. The general consensus is to restrict protein intake to approximately that of the adult recommended dietary allowance of 0.8 g/kg per day, approximately 10% of daily calories, with a further reduction to 0.6 g/kg per day once GFR begins to fall.[28]

## OTHER MEASURES

### Smoking cessation

There is some evidence to suggest that smoking can hasten the progression of microalbuminuria to proteinuria.[29] In addition, as patients with diabetic nephropathy are at increased risk of premature death from cardiovascular disease, smoking should be strongly discouraged.

### Monitoring renal function

Once proteinuria is established, the aim of treatment is to prevent or at least reduce the rate of decline in renal function. Historically, the rate of decline of GFR has been in the order of 10 ml/min per year. This rate of decline can be modified by aggressive antihypertensive therapy, as described above, and can be monitored clinically by plotting the reciprocal serum creatinine against time. Such a plot enables the clinician to determine the impact of therapy, detect sudden changes in renal function that might require additional investigation and specific treatment, and estimate when individual patients are likely to require renal replacement therapy.

### Early referral to nephrology services

Patients with diabetic nephropathy and declining renal function should be referred to nephrology services at an early stage and certainly by the time creatinine levels have risen to 2.3 mg/dl (220 μmol/l). This is to ensure optimization of treatment and early consideration for renal replacement therapy.

### Management of cardiovascular risk factors and cardiovascular disease

Patients with diabetic nephropathy are at particularly high risk of cardiovascular disease and premature death. As such, they need to be screened carefully for cardiovascular risk factors which, if detected, should be treated aggressively. Treatments such as cholesterol-lowering therapies and antihypertensive regimens, particularly with ACEIs, and smoking cessation may have the twin benefits of reducing the risk of cardiovascular events and preventing progression to diabetic nephropathy.

## Multidisciplinary approach

As diabetic kidney disease progresses, treatment becomes increasingly complicated and involves multiple therapies, lifestyle modifications and a large number of health-care professionals (Table 13.3). The latter is likely to include all members of the diabetes team, ophthalmologists, cardiologists and nephrologists. An important task for the diabetologist is the co-ordination of these services to ensure that treatment of one part of the condition does not occur at the expense of other elements.

**Table 13.3   Summary of the management of diabetic nephropathy.**

|  | Stage of diabetic nephropathy | | |
| --- | --- | --- | --- |
|  | **Normal UAER** | **Microalbuminuria** | **Proteinuria** |
| Key features | UAER normal<br>Blood pressure may be raised (type 2 diabetes) | UAER raised<br>BP increased<br>CV risk increased | UAER raised<br>BP increased<br>GFR declines<br>CV risk increased<br>Other complications of diabetes likely |
| Main aim | Primary prevention | Prevent progression | Prevent decline in renal function |
| Glycaemic control | Intervention threshold:<br>$HbA_{1c} > 8\%$<br>Ideal: $< 7\%$ | Intervention threshold:<br>$HbA_{1c} > 8\%$<br>Ideal: $< 7\%$ | (Prevent non-renal complications) |
| Antihypertensive therapy | Intervention threshold:<br>140/90 mmHg<br>Ideal: 130/80 mmHg<br><br>ACEI first line | Intervention threshold:<br>140/90 mmHg<br>Ideal: 130/80 mmHg<br><br>ACEI or AIIRB first line | Intervention threshold:<br>140/90 mmHg<br>125/75 mm Hg if protein excretion $\geq 1$ g/24 hr<br>ACEI or AIIRB first line |
| Lifestyle modification | Carbohydrate restriction<br>Smoking cessation<br>Modest salt intake | Carbohydrate restriction<br>Smoking cessation<br>Modest salt intake | Carbohydrate restriction<br>Smoking cessation<br>Modest salt intake<br>Protein restriction<br>Low-fat diet |
| Agencies involved | Diabetes team* | Diabetes team*<br>Possibly:<br>Ophthalmologist<br>Cardiologist | Diabetes team*<br>Nephrologist<br>Probably:<br>Ophthalmologist<br>Cardiologist<br>Possibly:<br>Vascular surgeon<br>Radiologist |
| Additional aims |  | Reduce CV risk | Reduce CV risk |

*Diabetes team includes physician, diabetes specialist nurse, dietitian, retinal screener, podiatrist. UAER: urinary albumin excretion rate; CV risk: cardiovascular risk; ACEI: angiotensin-converting enzyme inhibitor; AIIRB: angiotensin type 2 receptor blocker.

## REFERENCES

1. Mogensen CE, Chachati A, Cristiensen CK et al, Microalbuminuria: an early marker of renal involvement in diabetes. *Uraemia Invest* 1985; **9:** 89–95.

2. Winocour P, Marshall S, Measurement and expression of microalbuminuria. In: *Microalbuminuria*. Cambridge University Press: Cambridge, 1998; 11–39.

3. Grenfell A, Management of nephropathy. In: *Textbook of Diabetes* (Pickup J, Williams G, eds.). Oxford: Blackwell Science, 1997; 54.1–54.19.

4. Quinn M, Angelico MC, Warram JH et al, Familial factors determine the development of diabetic nephropathy in patients with IDDM. *Diabetologia* 1996; **39:** 940–5.

5. Diabetes Control and Complications Trial Research Group, Clustering of long-term complications in families with diabetes in the diabetes control and complications trial. *Diabetes* 1997; **46:** 1829–39.

6. Diabetes Control and Complications Trial Research Group, The effect of intensive treatment of diabetes on the development and progression of long-term complications in insulin-dependent diabetes mellitus. *N Engl J Med* 1993; **329:** 977–86.

7. Diabetes Control and Complications Trial Research Group, Effect of intensive therapy on the development and progression of diabetic nephropathy in the Diabetes Control and Complications Trial. *Kidney Int* 1995; **47:** 1703–20.

8. UK Prospective Diabetes Study Group, Tight blood pressure control and risk of macrovascular and microvascular complications in type 2 diabetes: UKPDS 38. *BMJ* 1998; **317:** 703–13.

9. Krolewski AS, Laffel LM, Krolewski M et al, Glycosylated hemoglobin and the risk of microalbuminuria in patients with insulin-dependent diabetes mellitus. *N Engl J Med* 1995; **332:** 1251–5.

10. Diabetes Control and Complications Trial Research Group, The absence of a glycemic threshold for the development of long-term complications: the perspective of the Diabetes Control and Complications Trial. *Diabetes* 1996; **45:** 1289–98.

11. Stratton IM, Adler AI, Neil HA et al, Association of glycaemia with macrovascular and microvascular complications of type 2 diabetes (UKPDS 35): prospective observational study. *BMJ* 2000; **321:** 405–12.

12. Warram JH, Scott LJ, Hanna LS et al, Progression of microalbuminuria to proteinuria in type 1 diabetes: nonlinear relationship with hyperglycemia. *Diabetes* 2000; **49:** 94–100.

13. Microalbuminuria collaborative study group. Intensive therapy and progression to clinical albuminuria in patients with insulin dependent diabetes mellitus and microalbuminuria. *BMJ* 1995; **311:** 973–7.

14. Mulec H, Blohme G, Grande B et al, The effect of metabolic control on rate of decline in renal function in insulin-dependent diabetes mellitus with overt diabetic nephropathy. *Nephrol Dial Transplant* 1998; **13:** 651–5.

15. EUCLID Study Group. Randomised placebo-controlled trial of lisinopril in normotensive patients with insulin-dependent diabetes and normoalbuminuria or microalbuminuria. *Lancet* 1997; **349:** 1787–92.

16. Hansen WH, Poulsen PL, Ebbehoj E, Blood pressure elevation in diabetes: the results from 24-h ambulatory blood pressure recordings. In: *The Kidney and Hypertension in Diabetes Mellitus*, 5th edn (Mogensen CE, ed.). Kluwer: Norwell, 2000; 339–62.

17. Adler AI, Stratton IM, Neil HA et al, Association of systolic blood pressure with macrovascular and microvascular complications of type 2 diabetes (UKPDS 36): prospective observational study. *BMJ* 2000; **321:** 412–19.

18. Viberti G, Mogensen CE, Groop LC et al, Effect of captopril on progression to clinical proteinuria in patients with insulin-dependent diabetes mellitus and microalbuminuria. European Microalbuminuria Captopril Study Group. *JAMA* 1994; **271:** 275–9.

19. Parving HH, Lehnert H, Brochner-Mortensen J et al, The effect of irbesartan on the development of diabetic nephropathy in patients with type 2 diabetes. *N Engl J Med* 2001; **345:** 870–8.

20. Heeg JE, de Jong PE, van der Hem GK et al, Efficacy and variability of the antiproteinuric effect of ACE inhibition by lisinopril. *Kidney Int* 1989; **36:** 272–9.

21. Heart Outcomes Prevention Evaluation Study Investigators, Effects of ramipril on cardiovascular and microvascular outcomes in people with diabetes mellitus: results of the HOPE study and MICRO-HOPE substudy. *Lancet* 2000; **355:** 253–9.

22. Joint National Committee on Prevention, Evaluation and Treatment of High Blood Pressure, The National High Blood Pressure Education Program Coordinating Committee, Sixth Report of the Joint National Committee on Prevention, Detection, Evaluation and Treatment of High Blood Pressure. *Arch Intern Med* 1997; **157:** 2413–46.

23. American Diabetes Association, Clinical practice recommendations 2001. *Diabetes Care* 2001; **24**(S1): S3.

24. Lewis EJ, Hunsicker LG, Bain RP et al, The effect of angiotensin-converting-enzyme inhibition on diabetic nephropathy. Collaborative Study Group. *N Engl J Med* 1993; **329:** 1456–62.

25. Lewis EJ, Hunsicker LG, Clarke WR et al, Renoprotective effect of the angiotensin-receptor antagonist irbesartan in patients with nephropathy due to type 2 diabetes. *N Engl J Med* 2001; **345:** 851–60.

26. Brenner BM, Cooper ME, de Zeeuw D et al, Effects of losartan on renal and cardiovascular outcomes in patients with type 2 diabetes and nephropathy. *N Engl J Med* 2001; **345:** 861–9.

27. Tarnow L, Rossing P, Jensen C et al, Long-term renoprotective effect of nisoldipine and lisinopril in type 1 diabetic patients with diabetic nephropathy. *Diabetes Care* 2000; **23:** 1725–30.

28. Walker J, Non-glycaemic intervention in diabetic nephropathy: the role of dietary protein intake. In: *The Kidney and Hypertension in Diabetes Mellitus*, 5th edn (Mogensen C, ed.). Kluwer: Boston, 2000; 473–85

29. Sawicki P, Didjugeit U, Mulhauser I et al, Smoking is associated with progression of diabetic nephropathy. *Diabetes Care* 1994; **17:** 126–31.

# 14

# The treatment of diabetic patients with advanced renal involvement

David Jonathan van Dijk and Geoffrey Boner

## INTRODUCTION

Advanced renal involvement in the diabetic patient may be defined as a major decrease in glomerular filtration rate (GFR) to below 30 ml/min and/or urinary excretion of protein within the nephrotic range (>3.5 g/day). At this stage, there is inexorable progression of renal disease, and the patient will reach end-stage renal disease (ESRD) within a relatively short period (months to a few years). Treatment of these patients should be aimed at reducing the progression of the renal disease, at preventing or treating comorbid conditions, and at preparing the patient for renal replacement therapy (RRT).

Patients with diabetic nephropathy should be referred to a nephrologist early in the course of their disease. It is essential that patients with advanced disease who have not been followed by a nephrologist be referred to one as soon as possible. There have been reports from both Europe and the USA showing that a high proportion of patients with diabetic nephropathy were referred to a nephrologist late in the course of their disease, and that the treatment, which they had received was often suboptimal.[1,2] The approach to treatment should then be multidisciplinary, and the team should include a nephrologist, a diabetologist, an ophthalmologist, a dietician, a cardiologist, a neurologist and other specialists, where necessary. Cooperation with the primary-care physician, a social worker and a specialist nurse is invaluable.

Intensive and comprehensive treatment may delay the deterioration of renal function even at this stage of the disease. Such a delay in the rate of progression of the renal involvement will postpone commencement of RRT, with subsequent preservation of quality of life and reduction in the cost of treatment. Moreover, prevention and treatment of comorbid conditions will reduce morbidity and mortality, and improve the prognosis for patients with ESRD.

The factors that affect the progression of the renal disease in patients with diabetic nephropathy have been reviewed by several authors.[3–6] These factors include ethnic origin, hereditary factors, age, control of hyperglycemia, control of hypertension, presence of proteinuria, presence of hyperlipidemia and smoking. Treatment of some of these factors even in patients with advanced renal disease may result in a decrease in the rate of deterioration of renal function and thus delay onset of ESRD. These factors may also play a role in the initiation of comorbid conditions such as atherosclerotic heart disease, heart failure and peripheral vascular disease.

In this chapter, we will describe the putative effect of treating hypertension, maintaining strict metabolic control of diabetes, control of smoking and the use of a low-protein diet on progression in those patients with advanced renal disease. We will then discuss the treatment of anemia associated with renal disease. This will be followed by discussion of comorbid conditions, namely, cardiovascular disease and hyperlipidemia. Factors involved in the pathogenesis and treatment of renal osteodystrophy and metabolic acidosis, two important complications of advanced renal disease, will also be described. Monitoring and adjustment of medications and their dosages is of the utmost importance in the treatment of patients with severely reduced renal function. Finally, there will be a short discussion on preparing the patient for RRT.

## HYPERTENSION

It is now several years since the treatment of hypertension has been considered to be the cornerstone in the preservation of renal function in patients with advanced renal disease.[7–9] In these early studies, the various investigators used conventional antihypertensive therapy, which did not include angiotensin-converting enzyme inhibitors (ACE-I). Reduction in blood pressure has been shown to affect both the progression of renal disease and the development of cardiac disease.[10] It is well established that the goal in treatment of blood pressure in both type 1 and type 2 diabetes mellitus should be a blood pressure not exceeding 130/80 mmHg in the absence of significant proteinuria and not exceeding 125/75 mmHg if accompanied by proteinuria in excess of 1.0 g/24 hr.[11,12] The first line of treatment in patients even with advanced diabetic nephropathy should be ACE-I inhibitors or angiotensin II receptor antagonists (AIIR).[11,12] Reduction of blood pressure even in relatively advanced diabetic nephropathy may still have a beneficial effect on the deterioration in GFR.[13,14] These studies have shown prolongation of the time to initiation of RRT, after starting treatment with ACE-I or AIIR, even in the presence of advanced disease.

In 1985, Taguma et al showed that treatment with ACE-I even in advanced diabetic nephropathy resulted in a decrease in proteinuria and stabilization of renal function.[13] In other studies including patients with less advanced disease but with overt proteinuria, ACE-I treatment resulted in a decrease in proteinuria.[15,16] In 1993, Lewis et al showed the beneficial effect of captopril treatment in patients with mild to moderate renal impairment and proteinuria due to type 1 diabetes mellitus, in a large, randomized, double-blind study.[17] In fact, these investigators were able to show a 50% reduction in the risk of doubling of serum creatinine as well as in the combined risk of ESRD or death during the study. The beneficial effect of captopril treatment was achieved mainly in patients who had an initial serum creatinine of ≥1.5 mg/dl. The decrease in proteinuria remained stable throughout the study period.

No similar randomized, controlled trials have been performed to show the effects of ACE-I in type 2 diabetes mellitus patients with mild to moderate renal impairment. However, there is evidence showing that treatment with ACE-I reduces proteinuria and may thus have a similar protective effect on nephropathy in patients with type 2 diabetes mellitus.[18–20] Two large randomized studies recently published have shown that the use of AIIR in the treatment of type 2 diabetic patients with moderate to advanced diabetic nephropathy resulted in a significant reduction in the risk of developing ESRD or death.[21,22] In fact, in one of the studies, there was a significant decrease in the rate of progression even in those patients who had doubled their serum creatinine during the study.[14] This beneficial effect on the progression of diabetic nephropathy was independent of blood pressure control, as the patients in both the control and treatment groups received conventional antihypertensive treatment in addition to the study medication, resulting in similar mean blood pressures in both groups.[21]

It is likely that all ACE-I and AIIR agents, which interrupt the renin-angiotensin system, have similar effects. Treatment with ACE-I or AIIR not only causes a decrease in proteinuria but also has a beneficial effect on cardiovascular complications.[21–24] Even in patients who have lost up to 50% of their renal function, a significant reduction in proteinuria correlated with a reduction in the rate of loss of renal function. Cardiovascular complications are significantly reduced in those patients when treated with these medications. In most patients with advanced renal disease, it is impossible to reduce the blood pressure to target values by monotherapy with either ACE-I or AIIR.[25] Thus, other antihypertensive agents, such as diuretics, calcium-channel blockers, preferably of the nondihydropyridine type but also of the dihydropyridine group, β-blockers and centrally acting agents, should be added. The treatment of hypertension in patients with diabetic nephropathy is discussed extensively in Chapter 7. The various agents should be added to the therapeutic regimen, and the dose should be titrated until the desired blood-pressure levels are achieved. Initiation of treatment with ACE-I may result in an increase of up to 30% in serum creatinine during the first 4 months in some of the patients. This increase in serum creatinine is generally not considered to be a reason for discontinuing the treatment.[25] These compounds may also cause hyperkalemia. Consequently, serum potassium should be measured at regular intervals, and potassium-lowering medication, such as furosemide and/or sodium polystyrene sulfonate, should be added in order to keep the serum potassium levels within normal limits. AIIR do not generally cause either hyperkalemia or increase in serum creatinine.[21] Blood chemistry should thus be monitored frequently.

## METABOLIC CONTROL OF DIABETES MELLITUS

Very few data are available at present on a possible beneficial effect of strict metabolic control of diabetes on the progression of advanced renal disease. Strict control of glucose is fully discussed in Chapter 6. The DCCT trial, which examined the effect of intensive control of diabetes in type 1 patients as opposed to conventional treatment, showed a significant reduction in proteinuria in patients with normal renal function.[26] As this study included a relatively small number of patients with reduced renal function, the authors were unable to show a significant effect in this group of patients.[26] Neither Mulec et al nor the UKPDS study addressed this issue in advanced renal failure.[27,28] Despite this relative lack of data, metabolic control should be improved in order to minimize the risk of metabolic complications and other microvascular and possibly macrovascular complications of diabetes mellitus, such as diabetic ketoacidosis, diabetic retinopathy, diabetic neuropathy and cardiovascular disorders.[29]

## SMOKING

Smoking has been shown to have significant detrimental effects, including increased proteinuria and increased mortality in patients with diabetic nephropathy.[30–39] Recently, Chuahirun and Wesson showed that type 2 diabetic patients who smoked had a faster decline of renal function than non-smokers.[40] In addition to its renal effects, smoking causes an immediate increase in blood pressure, and has a synergistic effect with other risk factors for cardiovascular complications, such as diabetes mellitus, hypertension, hypercholesterolemia, hyperuricemia, the presence of the nephrotic syndrome and other causes of hypercoagulability. This is in addition to the well-established role of smoking in the etiology of chronic lung disease and pulmonary carcinoma. It is thus imperative that every patient be made to understand the importance of quitting this habit.

## DIETARY PROTEIN RESTRICTION

Protein restriction (see Chapter 8) may have a beneficial effect on the progression of renal disease even in patients with advanced involvement.[41–46] Walker et al and Barsotti et al showed that protein restriction in both type 1 and type 2 diabetic patients slowed progression.[41,42] In a large study, Klahr et al showed that dietary protein restriction in nondiabetic renal disease may delay the rate of progression of renal disease.[43] Two meta-analyses, one combining five studies by Pedrini et al and another combining 13 studies by Kasiske et al, showed that dietary protein restriction was also effective in retarding the progression of renal disease in diabetes.[44,45] It has been suggested that the optimal amount of protein in the diet is 0.8 g of high biological value protein/kg body weight per day. However, as most of these patients are restricted in their intake of carbohydrates and proteins, they require a well-planned diet in order to prevent protein malnutrition. These patients should be closely followed in order to ensure compliance and prevent malnutrition.

## ANEMIA

In 1836, Richard Bright showed that anemia could appear as a complication of renal disease. The major cause of this anemia is the decrease in production and release of erythropoietin by the diseased kidney.[47] Other causes of anemia in the patient with renal failure include a shortening of erythrocyte survival, resistance of the bone marrow to erythropoietin, iron deficiency and folic acid deficiency.[48–50] Diabetic patients with renal failure have a greater degree of anemia than nondiabetic patients with the same degree of renal failure.[51] This difference is due to a greater decrease in the production of erythropoietin in patients with diabetic nephropathy than in patients with nondiabetic renal disease.[52] The presence of anemia may be an important element in the uremic syndrome. Treatment of anemia with human recombinant erythropoietin has been shown to result in less symptomatology, more physical activity and better cognitive function.[52] It has even been suggested that the treatment of anemia in patients with reduced renal function may improve cardiac function and decrease the incidence of heart failure.[53] Thus, therapy with human recombinant erythropoietin should be started early in the course of the disease. The target hemoglobin level should be approximately 12 g/dl. Other causes of anemia such as occult hemorrhage, hemolysis, iron deficiency or vitamin $B_{12}$ deficiency should be excluded and treated, when present, before commencing therapy with erythropoietin. Treatment with erythropoietin includes one to three subcutaneous or intravenous injections per week with adjustment of the dose according to response.[54] The hemoglobin concentration should be monitored at regular intervals and the dosage of erythropoietin adjusted according to the results. Increased erythropoiesis following erythropoietin treatment results in increased utilization of available iron. Patients receiving erythropoietin should thus be monitored for iron availability. The tests should include regular assessment of serum iron, ferritin, transferrin and percentage of hypochromic erythrocytes. An oral iron supplement should be prescribed and intravenous iron should be administered in patients with a severe or nonresponsive iron deficiency.

## CARDIOVASCULAR DISEASE

Macrovascular disease is much more prevalent in diabetic patients and even more so in patients with diabetic nephropathy than in nondiabetic subjects.[55–58] According to the data of the USRDS, almost 40% of patients entering RRT programs have evidence of arteriosclerotic cardiovascular disease; in diabetic patients, this percentage is higher at approximately 60%.[59] Cardiovascular disease is the most frequent cause of morbidity and mortality in patients with diabetic nephropathy both before and after progression to ESRD (a more detailed description of cardiac complications and their treatment is found in Chapter 10).[59,60] The prevalence of atherosclerotic heart disease is about 45% and the incidence of peripheral vascular disease (PVD) about 65%. Treatment with ACE-I resulted in a reduction in cardiovascular and microvascular events in diabetic patients in the HOPE and MICRO-HOPE studies.[61,62] The HOT study and the UKPDS trial showed that tight blood-pressure control in diabetic patients significantly decreased cardiovascular events.[63,64] Thus, when treating the patient with advanced diabetic nephropathy, the utmost importance must be attached to the prevention and treatment of cardiovascular disease. Prophylactic measures should be aimed at metabolic control of diabetes, strict control of blood pressure, cessation of smoking, treatment of hyperlipidemia, treatment of anemia and the encouragement of regular physical activity. Early recognition of the signs of these complications is mandatory for timely diagnosis and therapeutic intervention.

## HYPERLIPIDEMIA

Hyperlipidemia is an independent risk factor for the progression of diabetic nephropathy in both the animal model and human type 1 and type 2 diabetes mellitus (see Chapter 9).[63–65] Therapeutic agents from the statin group have mainly been used to reduce serum cholesterol levels, whereas fibrates are used to decrease the serum levels of triglycerides. In addition to the effects of these agents on the serum lipid profile and thus protection against cardiovascular disease, several reports have shown that treatment of diabetic patients with renal involvement with these agents may cause a decrease in albuminuria, and one

study even described an attenuation of the rate of decline in renal function during treatment with a statin.[66–74] However, there are no unequivocal data as to the beneficial effect of HMG Co-A reductase inhibitors on preservation of renal function.[66–74] Moreover, treatment with fibrates may cause a further reduction in renal function.[75] Except for gemfibrozil, these compounds should be prescribed at reduced dosages or not be given at all.[76] Thus, the preferred treatment of hyperlipidemia in patients with renal disease should be a statin. However, these medications should be used with caution, and the dose should be adjusted according to renal function. Both fibrates and statins may cause muscle damage as expressed by an increase in serum creatine phosphokinase (CPK) levels and liver-function disturbances, such as increases in the serum concentrations of liver enzymes. These biochemical side effects may necessitate cessation of treatment with these medications. Therefore, regular measurement of these laboratory parameters is recommended.

## RENAL OSTEODYSTROPHY

Renal osteodystrophy develops early in the progression of renal disease. A decrease in serum calcium concentration causes an increase in PTH secretion. This change in serum calcium concentration is due to decreased production of calcitriol, the active form of vitamin D, due to decreased hydroxylation of 25-hydroxycalciferol by the diseased kidney, a decreased number of vitamin D receptors and resistance of these receptors to vitamin D.[77,78] Retention of phosphorus also plays an important role in the pathogenesis of secondary hyperparathyroidism.[77–82] Other factors that may play a role include aluminum toxicity, metabolic acidosis and increased catecholamine levels.[83,84] This secondary hyperparathyroidism is one of the factors in the development of renal osteodystrophy. This condition progresses with a further decrease in renal function. The control of hyperphosphatemia is thus of utmost importance in preventing the development of this condition. An adequate diet, with restricted intake of phosphorus and protein, should be prescribed when the creatinine clearance is 30–40 ml/min.[85] Phosphate binders are widely prescribed in order to prevent intestinal absorption of phosphorus salts. However, these agents are not without side effects. Aluminum-containing binders may cause microcytic anemia, osteomalacia and encephalopathy.[86] Calcium-containing salts may cause hypercalcemia and extraosseous calcification, including increased stiffness of the arterial wall.[87,88] Recently, Sevelamer hydrochloride, a nonabsorbable polymer, not containing calcium or aluminum, has been introduced as a phosphate-binder.[89–94] This agent has also been shown to attenuate the progression of coronary and aortic calcification in patients on hemodialyis.[95] In addition, low-dose calcium and calcitriol or other active analogs of vitamin D may be helpful in preventing secondary hyperparathyroidism.[96] The product of serum calcium and phosphorus (mg/dl) should be kept below 55 (arbitrary units). Therefore, regular measurement of serum calcium and phosphorus should be performed and treatment adjusted according to the results.

## METABOLIC ACIDOSIS

A high anion-gap metabolic acidosis is a common feature in advanced renal disease (see Chapter 11). This acidosis is the result of a decrease in the renal excretion of inorganic and organic acids, decreased production of ammonia and decreased production of bicarbonate by the kidney with a resultant decrease in the buffering capacity of the body. The bone may act as an additional source of buffer, the release of bicarbonate, calcium and phosphate from the bone resulting in loss of bone mineral content.[97,98] The metabolic acidosis has various systemic effects, namely, cardiovascular (reduced contractility and arrhythmia), pulmonary (Kussmaul respiration), gastrointestinal, renal (sodium and potassium wasting, uric acid retention and hypercalciuria), electrolyte disturbances (potassium, calcium and magnesium), and metabolic and hormonal (protein wasting, catecholamines, aldosterone secretion, parathyroid hormone, vitamin D, and organic acid synthesis). These effects may be deleterious, although in most patients they are not severe and often do not require treatment.[99] Strict control of diabetes mellitus may be effective in the correction of the metabolic disturbance. Treatment with oral bicarbonate may be used where necessary.

## CHOICE OF MEDICATIONS AND ADJUSTMENT OF DOSAGES

Most diabetic patients with advanced renal failure receive multiple medications. These include mainly medications for the treatment of diabetes (insulin and/or oral hypoglycemic drugs), hypertension and dyslipidemia. The dosage of many of these medications requires adjustment in order to prevent accumulation and toxic side effects—for example, certain ACE-I, oral hypoglycemic agents and antibiotics.[76,100] Adjustment of dosage must take into account the degree of renal impairment and the pathways responsible for the metabolism and clearance of the respective drugs, that is, hepatic or renal. Absolute or relative contraindications exist for certain compounds in patients with advanced renal failure. For example, treatment with metformin should be stopped as soon as serum creatinine is greater than 1.5 mg/dl in male and above 1.4 mg/dl in female patients. Continued treatment with this drug may lead to the development of lactic acidosis, especially in diabetic patients with congestive heart failure.[101]

Interaction of drugs taken concomitantly is much more frequent in patients with decreased renal function. Nonsteroidal anti-inflammatory drugs (NSAIDs), including the COX-2 inhibitors should not be prescribed in these patients. Numerous reports have shown the deleterious effects of NSAIDs on renal function in patients with renal impairment. The new generation of COX-2 inhibitors have similar effects of the traditional NSAIDs on the kidney, as the COX-2 enzyme is expressed within the kidney, but not in all body tissues.[102–105] As some of these compounds are available as over-the-counter (OTC) drugs in many countries, and as they may be more likely to result in severe side effects if taken simultaneously with ACE-I or AIIR, special attention should be paid with respect to this issue, with patients being warned for their danger. In any event, renal function should be estimated before prescribing medications in this category of patients. As serum creatinine is a poor marker of renal function, creatinine clearance should be determined by a 24-hr urine collection or by estimating the creatinine clearance with the Cockcroft–Gault formula, which expresses creatinine clearance as follows:

$$\text{creatinine clearance (ml/min)} = ([140-age] \times BW) \div (SCr \times 72) \text{ in males and} \times 0.85 \text{ in females.}$$

Age is given in years, BW (body weight) in kg and SCr (serum creatinine) in mg/dl.[106] The MDRD formula has also been proposed as a good estimate of GFR.[107] The renal function should be estimated by one of these equations before deciding on the adjustment of the dosage of a medication.

## PREPARATION OF THE DIABETIC PATIENT FOR RRT

RRT is usually initiated when the GFR is below 10

---

**Table 14.1. Preparation of the diabetic patient for renal replacement therapy (RRT).**

1. Regular clinic visits in order to assess the patient's condition, renal function and blood-pressure control
2. Strict control of blood pressure (preferably ACE-I or AIIR) and treatment to slow progression
3. Prevention of malnutrition—assessment and adjustment of diet
4. Prevention of cardiovascular disease—treatment of hypertension, anemia, hyperlipidemia and/or other factors causing cardiovascular disease
5. Routine monitoring for anemia, metabolic acidosis, renal osteodystrophy, side effects of medications, and the treatment of these conditions
6. Routine monitoring for presence of viral diseases, such as hepatitis B, hepatitis C or AIDS
7. Monitoring the presence of other chronic infectious conditions, such as tuberculosis
8. Active immunization against pneumococcal pneumonia and hepatitis B
9. Counseling the patient and deciding on the therapeutic modality
10. Early preparation of the patient according to the modality of RRT

---

ml/min in patients with nondiabetic renal disease. Diabetic patients tend to have more frequent complications when the GFR falls below 15 ml/min. Thus, it is suggested that dialysis or transplantation should be implemented in the diabetic patient when the GFR is about 15 ml/min. Indications for early initiation of RRT include cachexia and malnutrition, metabolic acidosis, fluid overload and hyperkalemia, which are nonresponsive to treatment and signs or symptoms of uremia such as uremic pericarditis, severe nausea and vomiting and significant weakness.[108,109]

Table 14.1 summarizes how to prepare the diabetic patient for RRT. The use of dialysis is described in Chapter 16 and of transplantation in Chapter 20.

A multidisciplinary team should counsel the patients, giving them all the relevant information on the use of the various modalities of RRT. This should be done when the GFR is 20–30 ml/min. The patients are then able to decide on their treatment modality. If it is decided to treat the patient with hemodialysis, an arteriovenous fistula should be created as soon as possible, leaving sufficient time for the access to mature before use (at least 1 month). If the patient decides on peritoneal dialysis, a peritoneal catheter should be inserted as soon as possible and at least 1 month should elapse before the catheter can be used. During this waiting period, the patient should be followed routinely for conditions such as heart failure, fluid overload, uremic pericarditis, uremic symptoms, hyperkalemia and acidosis, which would require early initiation of treatment. If the permanent access has not matured, a temporary access may be used to treat the patient where acute treatment is indicated.

# REFERENCES

1. Pommer W, Bressel F, Chen F et al, There is room for improvement of preterminal care in diabetic patients with end-stage renal failure—the epidemiological evidence in Germany, *Nephrol Dial Transplant* (1997) **12:** 1318–20.
2. Crook ED, Harris J, Oliver B et al, End-stage renal disease owing to diabetic nephropathy in Mississippi: an examination of factors influencing renal survival in a population prone to late referral, *J Investig Med* (2001) **49:** 284–91.
3. Marcantoni C, Ortalda V, Lupo A et al, Progression of renal failure in diabetic nephropathy, *Nephrol Dial Transpl* (1998) **13**(Suppl 8):16–19.
4. Rossing P, Promotion, prediction and prevention of progression of nephropathy in type 1 diabetes mellitus, *Diabet Med* (1998) **15:** 900–19.
5. Ritz E, Orth SR, Nephropathy in patients with type 2 diabetes mellitus, *N Engl J Med* (1999) **341:** 1127–33.
6. Vora JP, Ibrahim HAA, Bakris GL, Responding to the challenge of diabetic nephropathy: the historic evolution of detection, prevention and management, *J Hum Hypertens* (2000) **14:** 667–85.
7. Mogensen CE, Progression of nephropathy in long-term diabetics with proteinuria and effect of initial anti-hypertensive treatment, *Scand J Clin Invest* (1976) **36:** 383–8.
8. Christensen CK, Mogensen CE, Effect of antihypertensive treatment on progression of incipient diabetic nephropathy, *Hypertension* (1985) **7:** 109–13.
9. Parving HH, Andersen AR, Smidt UM et al, Early aggressive antihypertensive treatment reduces rate of decline in kidney function in diabetic nephropathy, *Lancet* (1983) **1:** 1175–9.
10. Psaty BM, Smith NL, Siscovick DS et al, Health outcomes associated with antihypertensive therapies used as first-line agents. A systematic review and meta-analysis, *JAMA* (1997) **277:** 739–45.
11. The Sixth Report of the Joint National Committee on Prevention, Detection, Evaluation and Treatment of High Blood Pressure, *Arch Intern Med* (1997) **157:** 2413–46.
12. World Health Organization–International Society of Hypertension Guidelines for the Management of Hypertension. Guidelines Subcommittee, *J Hypertens* (1999) **17:** 151–83.
13. Taguma Y, Kitamoto Y, Futaki G et al, Effect of captopril on heavy proteinuria in azotemic diabetics, *N Eng J Med* (1985) **313:** 1617–20.

14. The Reduction of Endpoints in NIDDM with the Angiotensin II Antagonist Losartan Study (RENAAL), unpublished data.

15. Parving H-H, Hommel E, Nielsen MD et al, Effect of captopril on blood pressure and kidney function in normotensive insulin-dependent diabetics with nephropathy, *BMJ* (1989) **299:** 533–636.

16. Hommel C, Parving H-H, Mathiesen E et al, Effect of captopril on kidney function in insulin-dependent diabetic patients with nephropathy, *BMJ* (1986) **293:** 467–70.

17. Lewis EJ, Hunsicker LG, Bain RP et al, The effect of angiotensin-converting-enzyme inhibition on diabetic nephropathy. The Collaborative Study Group, *N Engl J Med* (1993) **329:** 1456–62.

18. Ravid M, Savin H, Jutrin I et al, Long term stabilizing effect of angiotensin-converting enzyme inhibition on plasma creatinine and on proteinuria in normotensive type II diabetic patients, *Ann Intern Med* (1993) **118:** 577–81.

19. Ravid M, Savin H, Lishner M, Long-term renoprotective effect of angiotensin-converting enzyme inhibition in non-insulin-dependent diabetes mellitus. A 7-year follow-up study, *Arch Intern Med* (1996) **156:** 286–9.

20. Lebovitz HE, Wiegmann TB, Cnaan A et al, Renal protective effects of enalapril in hypertensive NIDDM: role of baseline albuminuria, *Kidney Int* (1994) (Suppl 45): 150–5.

21. Brenner BM, Cooper M, de Zeeuw D et al, for the RENAAL Study Investigators, effects of losartan on renal and cardiovascular outcomes in patients with type 2 diabetes and nephropathy, *N Engl J Med* (2001) **345:** 861–9.

22. Lewis EJ, Hunsicker LG, Clarke WR et al for the Collaborative Study Group. Renoprotective effect of the angiotensin-receptor antagonist irbesartan in patients with nephropathy due to type 2 diabetes, *N Engl J Med* (2001) **345:** 851–60.

23. Keane WF, Eknoyan G, Proteinuria, albuminuria, risk assessment, detection, elimination (PARADE): a position paper of the National Kidney Foundation, *Am J Kidney Dis* (1999) **33:** 1004–10.

24. Heart Outcomes Prevention Evaluation (HOPE) Study Investigators, Effects of ramipril on cardiovascular and microvascular outcomes in people with diabetes mellitus: results of the HOPE study and MICRO-HOPE substudy, *Lancet* (2000) **355:** 253–9.

25. Bakris GL, Williams M, Dworkin L et al, for the National Kidney Foundation Hypertension and Diabetes Executive Committee's Working Group, Preserving renal function in adults with hypertension and diabetes: a consensus approach, *Am J Kidney Dis* (2000) **36:** 646–61.

26. The effect of intensive treatment of diabetes on the development and progression of long-term complications in insulin-dependent diabetes mellitus. The Diabetes Control and Complications Trial Research Group, *N Engl J Med* (1993) **329:** 977–86.

27. Mulec H, Blohmé G, Gründe B et al, The effect of metabolic control on rate of decline in renal function in insulin-dependent diabetes mellitus with overt diabetic nephropathy, *Nephrol Dial Transplant* (1998) **13:** 651–5.

28. Stratton IM, Adler AI, Neil HAW et al, on behalf of the UK Prospective Diabetes Study Group, Association of glycemia with macrovascular and microvascular complications of type 2 diabetes (UKPDS 35): prospective observational study, *BMJ* (2000) **321:** 405–12.

29. Intensive blood-glucose control with sulphonylureas or insulin compared with conventional treatment and risk of complications in patients with type 2 diabetes (UKPDS 33). UK Prospective Diabetes Study, (UKPDS) Group, *Lancet* (1998) **352:** 837–53.

30. Chase HP, Garg SK, Marshall G et al, Cigarette smoking increases the risk of albuminuria among subjects with type 1 diabetes, *J Am Med Assoc* (1991) **256:** 614–17.

31. Gambara V, Ruggenenti P, Perna A, Smoking is the strongest predictor of mortality in non-insulin dependent diabetes, *J Am Soc Nephrol* (1997) **8:** 137A.

32. Howard G, Wagenknecht LE, Burke GL et al, Cigarette smoking and progression of atherosclerosis: The Atherosclerosis Risk in Communities (ARIC) Study, *JAMA* (1998) **279:** 119–24.

33. Sawicki PT, Didjurgeit U, Mülhauser I et al, Smoking is associated with progression of diabetic nephropathy, *Diabetes Care* (1994) **17:** 126–31.

34. Klein R, Klein BEK, Moss SE et al, Ten-year incidence of gross proteinuria in people with diabetes, *Diabetes* (1995) **44:** 916–23.

35. Bruno G, Cavallo-Perin P, Bargero G et al, Prevalence and risk factors for micro- and macroalbuminuria in an Italian population-based cohort of NIDDM subjects, *Diabetes Care* (1996) **19:** 43–7.

36. Yokoyama H, Tomonaga O, Hirayama M et al, Predictors of the progression of diabetic nephropathy and the beneficial effect of angiotensin-converting enzyme inhibitors in NIDDM patients, *Diabetologia* (1997) **40:** 405–11.

37. Orth SR, Ritz E, Schrier RW, The renal risks of smoking, *Kidney Int* (1997) **51:** 1669–77.

38. Bonora E, Targher G, Zenere M-B et al, Relationship of uric acid concentration to cardiovascular risk factors in young men. Role of obesity and central fat distribution. The Verona Young Men Atherosclerosis Risk Factors Study, *Int J Obes Relat Metab Disord* (1996) **20:** 975–80.

39. Brown WV, Risk factors for vascular disease in patients with diabetes, *Diab Obes Metab* (2000) **2**(Suppl 2): S11–18.

40. Chuahirun T, Wesson DE, Cigarette smoking predicts faster progression of type 2 established diabetic nephropathy despite ACE inhibition, *Am J Kidney Dis* (2002) **39:** 376–82.

41. Walker JD, Bending JJ, Dodds RA et al, Restriction of dietary protein and progression of renal failure in diabetic nephropathy, *Lancet* (1989) **2:** 1411–15.

42. Barsotti G, Cupisti A, Barsotti M et al, Dietary treatment of diabetic nephropathy with chronic renal failure, *Nephrol Dial Transplant* (1998) **13**(Suppl 8): 49–52.

43. Klahr S, Levey AS, Beck GJ et al, for the Modification of Diet in Renal Disease Study Group, The effects of dietary protein restriction and blood pressure control on the progression of chronic renal disease, *N Engl J Med* (1994) **330:** 877–84.

44. Pedrini MT, Levey AS, Lau J et al, The effect of dietary protein restriction on the progression of diabetic and nondiabetic renal diseases: a meta-analysis, *Ann Intern Med* (1996) **124:** 627–32.

45. Kasiske BL, Lakatua JDA, Ma JZ et al, A meta-analysis of the effects of dietary protein restriction on the rate of decline in renal function, *Am J Kidney Dis* (1998) **31:** 954–61.

46. Hebert LE, Wilmer WA, Falkenhain ME et al, Renoprotection: one or many therapies? *Kidney Int* (2001) **59:** 1211–26.

47. Caro J, Brown S, Miller O et al, Erythropoietin levels in uremic and anephric patients, *J Lab Clin Med* (1979) **93:** 449–58.

48. Eschbach JW, Korn D, Finch C-A, $^{14}$C cyanate as a tag for red cell survival in normal and uremic man, *J Lab Clin Med* (1977) **89:** 823–8.

49. Fisher JW, Mechanism of the anemia of chronic renal failure, *Nephron* (1980) **25:** 106–11.

50. Livio M, Gotti E, Marchesi D et al, Uraemic bleeding: role of anaemia and beneficial effect of red cell transfusions, *Lancet* (1982) **2:** 1013–15.

51. Bosman DR, Winkler AS, Marsden JT et al, Anemia with erythropoietin deficiency occurs early in diabetic nephropathy, *Diabetes Care* (2001) **24:** 495–9.

52. Eschbach JW, The anemia of chronic renal failure: pathophysiology and the effects of recombinant erythropoietin, *Kidney Int* (1989) **35:** 134–48.

53. Silverberg DS, Wexler D, Blum M et al, The use of subcutaneous erythropoietin and intravenous iron for the treatment of the anemia of severe, resistant congestive heart failure improves cardiac and renal function and functional cardiac class, and markedly reduces hospitalizations, *J Am Coll Cardiol* (2000) **35**: 1737–44.

54. Eschbach JW, Adamson JW, Anemia in renal disease. In: Schrier RW, Gottschalk CW, eds, *Diseases of the Kidney*, 5th edn (Little, Brown: Boston, MA, 1993) 2743–58.

55. Culleton BF, Larson MG, Wilson PW et al, Cardiovascular disease and mortality in a community-based cohort with mild renal insufficiency, *Kidney Int* (1999) **56**: 2214–19.

56. Parving HH, Diabetic hypertensive patients. Is this a group in need of particular care and attention? *Diabetes Care* (1999) **22**(Suppl 2B): 76–9.

57. Morgan CL, Currie CJ, Stott NC et al, The prevalence of multiple diabetes-related complications, *Diabet Med* (2000) **17**: 146–51.

58. Tight blood pressure control and risk of macrovascular and microvascular complications in type 2 diabetes: UKPDS 38. UK Prospective Diabetes Study Group, *BMJ* (1998) **317**: 703–13.

59. US Renal Data System, USRDS 2001 Annual Data Report: Atlas of End-Stage Renal Disease in the United States, National Institutes of Health, National Institute of Diabetes and Digestive and Kidney Diseases, Bethesda, MD (2001).

60. Garcia MJ, McNamara PM, Gordon T et al, Morbidity and mortality in diabetics in the Framingham population. Sixteen year follow-up study, *Diabetes* (1974) **23**: 105–11.

61. Yusuf S, Sleight P, Pogue J et al, The Heart Outcomes Prevention Evaluation Study Investigators. Effects of an angiotensin-converting-enzyme inhibitor, ramipril, on cardiovascular events in high-risk patients, *N Engl J Med* (2000) **342**: 145–53.

62. The Heart Outcomes Prevention Evaluation (HOPE) Study Investigators. Effects of ramipril on cardiovascular and microvascular outcomes in people with diabetes mellitus: results of the HOPE and MICRO-HOPE study, *Lancet* (2000) **355**: 253–9.

63. Keane WF, The role of lipids in renal disease: future challenges, *Kidney Int Suppl* (2000) **75**: S27–31.

64. Jandeleit-Dahm K, Cao Z, Cox AJ et al, Role of hyperlipidemia in progressive renal disease: focus on diabetic nephropathy, *Kidney Int Suppl* (1999) **71**: S31–6.

65. Ravid M, Brosh D, Ravid-Safran D et al, Main risk factors for nephropathy in type 2 diabetes mellitus are plasma cholesterol levels, mean blood pressure, and hyperglycemia, *Arch Intern Med* (1998) **158**: 998–1004.

66. Hommel E, Andersen P, Gall MA et al, Plasma lipoproteins and renal function during simvastatin treatment in diabetic nephropathy, *Diabetologia* (1992) **35**: 447–51.

67. Zhang A, Vertommen J, Van Gaal L et al, Effects of pravastatin on lipid levels, in vitro oxidizability of non-HDL lipoproteins and microalbuminuria in IDDM patients, *Diabetes Res Clin Pract* (1995) **29**: 189–94.

68. Biesenbach G, Zazgornik J, Lovastatin in the treatment of hypercholesterolemia in nephrotic syndrome due to diabetic nephropathy stages IV–V, *Clin Nephrol* (1992) **37**: 274–9.

69. Nielsen S, Schmitz O, Moller N et al, Renal function and insulin sensitivity during simvastatin treatment in type 2 (non-insulin-dependent) diabetic patients with microalbuminuria, *Diabetologia* (1993) **36**: 1079–86.

70. Lam KS, Cheng IK, Janus ED et al, Cholesterol-lowering therapy may retard the progression of diabetic nephropathy, *Diabetologia* (1995) **38**: 604–9.

71. Bender RSO, The effect of cholesterol-lowering therapy on the progression of diabetic nephropathy is unproved, *Diabetologia* (1996) **39**: 368–70.

72. Parving HH, Cholesterol-lowering therapy may retard the progression of diabetic nephropathy, *Diabetologia* (1996) **39**: 367–8.

73. Tonolo G, Ciccarese M, Brizzi P et al, Reduction of albumin excretion rate in normotensive microalbuminuric type 2 diabetic patients during long-term simvastatin treatment, *Diabetes Care* (1997) **20**: 1891–5.

74. Barnes DJ, Stephens EG, Mattock MB et al, The effect of simvastatin on the progression of renal disease in IDDM patients with elevated urinary albumin excretion. *Proceedings of the European Diabetic Nephropathy Study Group, 11th Meeting* (Rennes, France, 29–30 May, 1998).

75. Broeders N, Knoop C, Antoine M et al, Fibrate-induced increase in blood urea and creatinine: is gemfibrozil the only innocuous agent? *Nephrol Dial Transplant* (2000) **15**: 1993–9.

76. Aronoff GR, Berns JS, Brier ME et al, *Drug Prescribing in Renal Failure*, 4th edn (American College of Physicians: Philadelphia, 1999) 85–6.

77. Slatopolsky E, The role of calcium, phosphorus and vitamin D metabolism in the development of secondary hyperparathyroidism, *Nephrol Dial Transplant* (1998) **3**: 3–8.

78. Drüeke TB, The pathogenesis of parathyroid gland hyperplasia in chronic renal failure, *Kidney Int* (1995) **48**: 259–72.

79. Silver J, Molecular mechanisms of secondary hyperparathyroidism, *Nephrol Dial Transplant* (2000) **15**(Suppl 5):S2–S7.

80. Almaden Y, Hernandez A, Torregrosa V et al, High phosphate level directly stimulates parathyroid secretion and synthesis by human parathyroid tissue *in vitro, J Am Soc Nephrol* (1998) **9**: 1845–52.

81. Slatopolsky E, Finch J, Denda M et al, Phosphorus restriction prevents parathyroid gland growth. High phosphorus directly stimulates PTH secretion in vitro, *J Clin Invest* (1996) **97**: 2534–40.

82. Roussanne MC, Lieberherr M, Souberbielle JC et al, Human parathyroid cell proliferation in response to calcium, NPS R-467, calcitriol and phosphate, *Eur J Clin Invest* (2001) **31**: 610–16.

83. Cannata JB, Hypokinetic azotemic osteodystrophy, *Kidney Int* (1998) **54**: 1000–16.

84. Cannata JB, Adynamic bone and chronic renal failure: an overview, *Am J Med Sci* (2000) **320**: 81–4.

85. Martinez I, Saracho R, Montenegro J et al, The importance of dietary calcium and phosphorus in the secondary hyperparathyroidism of patients with early renal failure, *Am J Kidney Dis* (1997) **29**: 496–502.

86. Parkinson IS, Ward MK, Feest RWP et al, Fracturing dialysis osteodystrophy and dialysis encephalopathy, *Lancet* (1979) **1**: 406–9.

87. Guerin AP, London GM, Marchais SJ et al, Arterial stiffening and vascular calcifications in end-stage renal disease, *Nephrol Dial Transplant* (2000) **15**: 1014–21.

88. Goodman WG, Goldin J, Kuizon BD et al, Coronary-artery calcification in young adults with end-stage renal disease who are undergoing dialysis, *N Engl J Med* (2000) **342**: 1478–83.

89. Chertow GM, Burke SK, Lazarus JM et al, Poly[allylamine hydrochloride] (RenaGel): a noncalcemic phosphate binder for the treatment of hyperphosphatemia in chronic renal failure, *Am J Kidney Dis* (1997) **29**: 66–71.

90. Burke SK, Slatopolsky EA, Goldberg DI, RenaGel, a novel calcium- and aluminium-free phosphate binder, inhibits phosphate absorption in normal volunteers, *Nephrol Dial Transplant* (1997) **12**: 1640–4.

91. Rosenbaum DP, Holmes-Farley SR, Mandeville WH et al, Effect of RenaGel, a non-absorbable, cross-linked, polymeric phosphate binder, on urinary phosphorus excretion in rats, *Nephrol Dial Transplant* (1997) **12**: 961–4.

92. Goldberg DI, Dillon MA, Slatopolsky EA et al, Effect of RenaGel, a non-absorbed, calcium- and aluminium-free phos-

phate binder, on serum phosphorus, calcium, and intact parathyroid hormone in end-stage renal disease patients, *Nephrol Dial Transplant* (1998) **13:** 2303–10.

93. Slatopolsky EA, Burke SK, Dillon MA, RenaGel, a nonabsorbed calcium- and aluminum-free phosphate binder, lowers serum phosphorus and parathyroid hormone. The RenaGel Study Group, *Kidney Int* (1999) **55:** 299–307.

94. Bleyer AJ, Burke SK, Dillon M et al, A comparison of the calcium-free phosphate binder sevelamer hydrochloride with calcium acetate in the treatment of hyperphosphatemia in hemodialysis patients, *Am J Kidney Dis* (1999) **33:** 694–701.

95. Chertow GM, Burke SK, Raggi P, Treat to Goal Working Group, Sevelamer attenuates the progression of coronary and aortic calcifications in hemodialysis patients, *Kidney Int* (2002) **62:** 245–52.

96. Locatelli F, Cannata-Andia JB, Drüeke TB et al, Management of disturbances of calcium and phosphate metabolism in chronic renal insufficiency, with emphasis on the control of hyperphoshatemia, *Nephrol Dial Transplant* (2002) **17:** 723–31.

97. Narins RG, Gopal Krishma G, Yee J et al, The metabolic acidosis. In: Narins RG, ed., *Maxwell and Kleeman's Clinical Disorders of Fluid and Electrolyte Metabolism*, 5th edn (McGraw-Hill: New York, 1994) 769–825.

98. Kussmaul A, Concerning a peculiar mode of death in diabetics, concerning acetonemia, the glycerin treatment of diabetes and the injection of diastase into the blood in this disease, *Dtsch Arch F Klin Med* (1874) **14:** 1.

99. Bailey JL, Mitch WE, Metabolic acidosis as a uremic toxin, *Semin Nephrol* (1996) **16:** 160–6.

100. Gambertoglio JG, Aweeka FT, Blythe WB, Use of drugs in patients with renal failure. In: Schrier RW Gottschalk CW, eds, *Diseases of the Kidney*, 5th edn (Little, Brown: Boston, MA, 1993) 3211–68.

101. Connolly V, Kesson CM, Metformin treatment in NIDDM patients with mild renal impairment, *Postgrad Med J* (1996) **72:** 352–4.

102. Brater DC, Harris C, Redfern JS et al, Renal effects of COX-2-selective inhibitors, *Am J Nephrol* (2001) **21:** 1–15.

103. Harris RC Jr, Cyclooxygenase-2 inhibition and renal physiology, *Am J Cardiol* (2002) **89:** 10D–17D.

104. Ahmad SR, Kortepeter C, Brinker A et al, Renal failure associated with the use of celecoxib and rofecoxib, *Drug Saf* (2002) **25:** 537–44.

105. Noroian G, Clive D, Cyclo-oxygenase-2 inhibitors and the kidney: a case for caution, *Drug Saf* (2002) **25:** 165–72.

106. Cockcroft DW, Gault MH, Prediction of creatinine clearance from serum creatinine, *Nephron* (1976) **16:** 31–41.

107. Manjunath G, Sarnak MJ, Levey AS, Prediction equations to estimate glomerular filtration rate: an update, *Curr Opin Nephrol Hypertens* (2001) **10:** 785–92.

108. Iseki K, Uehara H, Nishime K et al, Impact of the initial levels of laboratory variables on survival in chronic dialysis patients, *Am J Kidney Dis* (1996) **28:** 541–8.

109. Stenvinkel P, Barany P, Chung SH et al, A comparative analysis of nutritional parameters as predictors of outcome in male and female ESRD patients, *Nephrol Dial Transplant* (2002) **17:** 1266–74.

# 15

# Pregnancy and therapeutic measures in the patient with diabetic nephropathy

Claudia Ferrier and Eileen Gallery

## PREGNANCY ALTERATIONS IN RENAL FUNCTION AND GLUCOSE HOMEOSTASIS

In normal pregnancy, blood sugar remains within tightly controlled limits, while insulin secretion doubles between the first and the third trimester.[1] The reason for this relative insulin resistance is uncertain, but it is likely that many pregnancy hormones, some of which are known to be insulin antagonists, including human placental lactogen, glucagon and cortisol, play a role.[2] If insulin secretion cannot increase sufficiently to offset the increase in peripheral insulin resistance, gestational diabetes can develop. This abnormality may be confined to pregnancy or may represent the first manifestation of type 2 diabetes.[3]

In normal pregnancy, many anatomical and functional changes occur in the urinary tract,[4] changes which have an impact on many underlying renal disorders, including diabetic renal disease. There is ureteric dilatation and an increase in urinary dead space, both of which increase the risk of ascending infection in the 6–8% of all pregnant women who have asymptomatic bacteriuria.[4,5] The normal pregnancy increase of ~30% in glomerular filtration rate (GFR) is due to an increase in renal blood flow with no change in glomerular capillary pressure.[6,7] Glomerulotubular balance also changes in pregnancy to allow reabsorption of almost 99% of glomerular filtrate, but there is commonly a net increase in glucose excretion, with demonstrable glycosuria in the presence of a normal blood sugar in most women at some stage of pregnancy.[8] Glycosuria is even more common in women with diabetes, even with acceptable control of blood-sugar levels. This adds to their increased risk of ascending urinary tract infection and pyelonephritis.

It is generally accepted that increased glomerular capillary pressure is an early event causing hyperfiltration in a diabetic nephropathy.[9] In a diabetic woman, the pregnancy-related increase in GFR[7] could therefore potentiate the underlying hyperfiltration and potentially accelerate the progression of diabetic nephropathy. Moreover, in the presence of impaired renal function, hypertension and/or proteinuria, the functional decline in renal function after pregnancy could be even faster.

Over the past half-century, the chance of successful pregnancy in the patient with pre-existing diabetes mellitus has increased from 50% to nearly 100%. This has been due to recognition of the importance of tight blood-sugar control from preconception and throughout pregnancy. While perinatal mortality is now rare, there is still significant morbidity.[10] Congenital malformation is related to poor control of diabetes at preconception and during the period of organogenesis in early pregnancy, while neonatal macrosomia, respiratory problems, jaundice and hypoglycaemia are related to poor control in later pregnancy.[11] Even with the best care, maternal and perinatal complications are more frequent in women with diabetes than in the general antenatal population. Women with end-organ damage from either microvascular or macrovascular disease are at particular risk. While this review focuses primarily on diabetic renal disease, brief consideration is given to other manifestations of both microvascular and macrovascular disease (retinopathy and coronary artery disease), as these are also of great clinical significance and pregnancy may have an impact on their development and progression. Areas which are specifically addressed below are (a) the potential effects of underlying diabetes on pregnancy, and (b) the effect of pregnancy on the potential progression of diabetic renal and vascular disease.

## Significance of diabetes for pregnancy

The woman with pre-existing diabetes carries several risks into pregnancy. Chronic hypertension is common, and may be exacerbated during pregnancy, as may pre-existing proteinuria.[12] In the woman who already has hypertension and proteinuria, a diagnosis of superimposed pre-eclampsia is difficult to confirm, and often relies on additional biochemical evidence such as disproportionate hyperuricaemia, or additional features such as coagulopathy or hepatic functional abnormality.[13] The extremely variable rate reported for this complication (15–50%) (reviewed in reference 14) reflects this uncertainty in clinical diagnosis. Pyelonephritis, encountered in 1–2% of the antenatal population overall, has been reported in over 10% of women with diabetes.[15]

Although perinatal mortality is now rare in women with diabetes, morbidity is still increased significantly for a number of reasons. The incidence of congenital abnormalities is increased in diabetic pregnancy. In a recent ultrasound study,[16] an incidence of over 7% for major, and 2% for minor abnormalities was reported, 60% of them central nervous system or cardiovascular, a relative risk of almost six fold. Major abnormalities were associated not with nephropathy but with poor glycaemic control and with maternal obesity, which also resulted in an increased incidence of antepartum detection of congenital abnormalities. Even in those without congenital abnormalities, there are long-term sequelae of fetal development in a diabetic intrauterine environment. These include reduced insulin secretion and insulin resistance, both of importance in the development of type 2 diabetes in a subsequent generation.[17]

Premature delivery is common. While fetal macrosomia is a risk for women with poorly controlled diabetes, the presence of established hypertension, of renal disease and renal functional impairment, and of superimposed pre-eclampsia are all risk factors for intrauterine fetal growth restriction and the occurrence of acute fetal distress. There are few follow-up data for this group of patients, but at least one group[18] has described a high incidence of developmental and/or psychomotor retardation in children born prematurely to women with diabetic nephropathy.

## Significance of pregnancy for diabetes

### Nephropathy: renal disease outcome

Although there are descriptions of pregnancy outcome in women with microalbuminuria (urinary albumin excretion rate of 20–200 µg/min) in early gestation,[19] there is a dearth of information on the effects of pregnancy on long-term renal prognosis in diabetic women with preconception microalbuminuria. It is well recognized that in primary renal disease the degree of renal functional impairment prior to conception, rather than proteinuria, may influence the natural course of the disease.[20] Moreover, the physiological increase in urinary protein excretion during pregnancy may be markedly pronounced in women with underlying renal disease, independently of renal haemodynamic changes.[21] Women with underlying diabetic nephropathy, even those with only microalbuminuria, can expect an increase in the severity of proteinuria, which usually resolves, postpartum, to levels similar to those prior to pregnancy.

Several studies, mostly cross-sectional or retrospective, have addressed the issue of the longer term effect of pregnancy on the progression of established diabetic nephropathy.[21–25] In general, they indicate that pregnancy does not significantly alter the rate of decline in renal function in the woman with early nephropathy. The question of progression in women with more severe renal disease is vexed. There are anecdotal reports of accelerated progression in some patients, but whether this is a true effect of pregnancy, or an effect of suspension of renoprotective therapy (such as ACE inhibition) for a prolonged period of time is unclear.[26]

There are a few reports dealing with a limited number of pregnancies in women with *mildly impaired* renal function (plasma creatinine of <125 µmol/l) (Table 15.1). Several authors showed no acceleration in the progression of diabetic nephropathy.[27–32] They concluded that pregnancy does not affect the underlying disease and that end-stage renal disease (ESRD) in ~5% of women reflects the natural course of the disease rather than an adverse effect of pregnancy.

By contrast, the outcome of diabetic nephropathy is more guarded in women with significantly impaired renal function prior to pregnancy. The severity of complications is related to the degree of pre-existing renal functional impairment (Table 15.1). In *mild to moderate* renal failure (plasma creatinine of ≥125 µmol/l and <250 µmol/L) two out of five studies[25,31,33–35] showed an accelerated decline in renal function, accounting for 40% of risk, and 20% of patients reached ESRD earlier than non-pregnant women with diabetic nephropathy of similar severity. In *moderate to severe* renal failure (plasma creatinine of ≥250 µmol/l), Biesenbach and Purdy[36,37] reported not only an accelerated progression but also

**Table 15.1 Influence of pregnancy on progression of diabetic nephropathy.**

| Prepregnancy serum creatinine | Subjects *n* | Follow-up (months) | Accelerated progression | Irreversible ESRD |
|---|---|---|---|---|
| **<125 µmol/l** | | | | |
| Kitzmiller, 1981[27] | 23 | 9–35 | No | 3 |
| Dicker, 1986[28] | 5 | 6–12 | No | 0 |
| Grenfell, 1986[29] | 20 | 6–120 | No | 2 |
| Reece, 1988[30] | 31 | 1–86 | No | 6 |
| Miodovnik, 1996[31] | 136 | 36 | No | 1 |
| Bar, 2000[32] | 24 | 24 | No | 0 |
| **Total** | **239** | | **0/6 (0%)** | **12/239 (5%)** |
| | | | | |
| **125–249 µmol/l** | | | | |
| Reece, 1990[33] | 11 | 48 | No | 0 |
| Kimmerle, 1995[34] | 29 | 4–108 | No | 8 |
| Gordon, 1996[25] | 34 | 36 | Yes | 3 |
| Miodovnik, 1996[31] | 46 | Median 6 | Yes | 12 |
| Mackie, 1996[35] | 6 | 6–96 | No | 3 |
| **Total** | **126** | | **2/5 (40%)** | **26/126 (21%)** |
| | | | | |
| **≥250 µmol/l** | | | | |
| Biesenbach, 1992[36] | 5 | 13–42 | Yes | 5 |
| Purdy, 1996[37] | 11 | 6–138 | Yes | 7 |
| **Total** | **16** | | **2/2 (100%)** | **12/16 (75%)** |

ESRD = end-stage renal disease.

a premature decline to ESRD in 75% of the 16 patients studied.

The relationship of nephropathy outcome to renal-function impairment prior to pregnancy is not confined to diabetic women.[32,38–43] Data obtained from pregnancies in women suffering from renal diseases other than diabetes, show a similar trend (Figure 15.1). This suggests that prepregnancy renal impairment, rather than histological diagnosis, is associated with accelerated progression of underlying nephropathy.

In any nephropathy, uncontrolled hypertension adversely influences the natural course of the disease.[44] Several authors have reported that pregnancy per se in women with primary glomerulonephritis and chronic hypertension adversely affects long-term renal prognosis.[39,45,46] In contrast, Jungers et al[42] showed a similar renal survival in pregnant and non-pregnant women with various forms of renal disease accompanied by hypertension, suggesting that hypertension, rather than pregnancy, adversely affects the course of the disease. This is not surpris-

ing, since pregnancy extends over a limited period of time compared to long-standing hypertensive disorders.

Retardation of progression of proteinuric renal disease in non-pregnant individuals has been documented with both ACE inhibitors (for review, see reference 47) and angiotensin II receptor antagonists.[48,49] ACE inhibitors reduce intraglomerular pressure and improve proteinuria in non-pregnant diabetic patients.[50] Both ACE inhibitors and angiotensin II receptor blockers, however, should be avoided in pregnancy because they interfere with the fetal renin-angiotensin system and may also be teratogenic.[51]

### Nephropathy: maternal and fetal outcome

Pregnant women with an underlying renal disease are at higher risk of the development of maternal hypertensive complications, premature deliveries and intrauterine fetal growth restriction.[52] Because hypertension and proteinuria during pregnancy are common problems in women with underlying renal

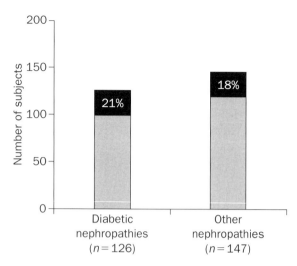

**Figure 15.1** Effects of pregnancy on progression of nephropathy in women with pre-existing moderate renal failure. ■ Percentage of patients who reached end-stage renal disease. Data from References 31, 33–36.

disease, it is not always easy to make or exclude a diagnosis of pre-eclampsia. However, there is some histological evidence that worsening of hypertension combined with increased proteinuria may be regarded as superimposed pre-eclampsia.[53] Gestational hypertension tends to occur more often in women with elevated blood pressure prior to pregnancy, though normotensive women with underlying renal disease also have a higher risk of the development of superimposed pre-eclampsia than women without renal disease.[45]

As in other renal diseases, the occurrence of increased proteinuria, hypertension and impaired renal function in diabetic nephropathy may necessitate early delivery. Cumulative data[25,27,29,30,32,54–57] show that in diabetic nephropathy the prevalence of *pre-eclampsia* may reach 44% (Figure 15.2). Since the incidence of pre-eclampsia increases with the degree of pre-existing renal functional impairment, the rate of pre-eclampsia varies between 15% and 80%. The variability also depends on the somewhat unclear definition and distinction between hypertension and/or superimposed pre-eclampsia.

Fetal complications are more common if there is significant proteinuria, hypertension or overt renal insufficiency prior to conception,[52] and the prematurity rate increases with progressive decline of the glomerular filtration rate.[58] *Prematurity* may also result from worsening of maternal complications such as pre-eclampsia or uncontrolled hypertension, thus requiring early delivery. As shown in Figure

15.2, the fetal outcome of women with diabetic nephropathy is characterized by a 48% prematurity rate, with deliveries before 34 weeks' gestation in 26% of pregnancies.[25,27,29,30,32,54–57] These rates are comparable to those reported by Jones et al[40] in primary renal diseases with moderate or severe renal impairment and are higher than the 10% rate reported in the general antenatal population. *Intrauterine fetal growth restriction (IUGR)* may occur alone or combined with pre-eclampsia. As depicted in Figure 15.2, the average IUGR rate is 14%, ranging from 9% to 22% and is comparable to the 12% rate reported in women with non-diabetic renal disease and normal renal function.[59]

Despite the increased fetomaternal complication rates, overall infant survival in women with diabetic nephropathy is close to 100%.[14] However, a high prematurity rate may be associated with long-term sequelae in the children of diabetic mothers. Therefore, these patients need close follow-up during and after pregnancy by an expert multidisciplinary team.

## Microvascular disease—Retinopathy
Diabetic retinopathy progresses with pregnancy, the risk related to the severity of baseline retinopathy, particularly proliferative disease.[60] It is not clear to what extent the pregnancy is causally involved in long-term progression, or whether it reflects the natural history of an underlying progressive disease. Surprisingly few studies appear to have addressed this specific question. Chaturvedi et al[61] reported, in a cross-sectional survey of type 1 diabetic women, a lower prevalence of retinopathy in parous (8%) than in nulliparous (16%) women, which persisted after correction for glycaemic control. A smaller prospective study of diabetic women during a 4-year follow-up period showed the same incidence of proliferative retinopathy (35%) in nulliparous women and those who had been pregnant.[62]

## Macrovascular disease—Coronary artery disease
Diabetic women have a significantly increased risk of atherosclerosis and associated myocardial infarction. Pregnancy is associated with fluid retention, increased cardiac output, decreased peripheral vascular resistance and acute fluid shifts during labour and delivery, all of which constitute cardiac workloads necessitating increased myocardial oxygen consumption. These factors combine to increase the risk of myocardial ischaemia, which is further exacerbated in the presence of underlying renal disease and/or hypertension.[63] There is a particular risk in

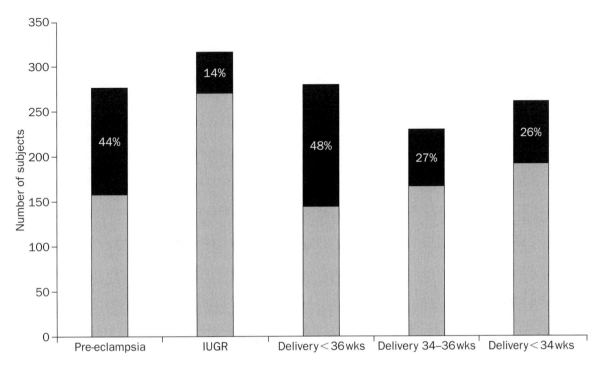

**Figure 15.2** Maternal and fetal outcome in pregnancies with diabetic nephropathy. Cumulative data from References 25, 27, 29, 30, 32, 54–57. ■ Percentage of patients who developed the complication. IUGR: intrauterine fetal growth restriction.

the early postpartum period because of fluid redistribution. Hypoglycaemia may increase the risk of significant myocardial damage.

## Strategies to optimize pregnancy outcome in diabetic nephropathy

Since the majority of women with diabetes, even those with diabetic nephropathy, can have successful pregnancy outcomes, it should rarely be necessary to counsel them against pregnancy. Planning for pregnancy should begin well before conception, and care during pregnancy is best accomplished by a multidisciplinary team including obstetrician, physician and neonatologist.

### Control of blood sugar
There should be frank discussion of the potential risks of congenital abnormality, and the advisability of achieving tight control of the blood sugar with normalization of $HbA_{1c}$ levels should be stressed. The patient should work towards this degree of control prior to conception, and it should then be maintained throughout gestation. This not only reduces

the risk of congenital abnormality, but also minimizes the glomerular hyperfiltration and is therefore renoprotective.

### Control of blood pressure
Hypertension is a common feature of diabetic nephropathy, and strict control of blood pressure is of value in slowing progression of renal damage. In the non-pregnant state, most patients are treated with angiotensin-converting enzyme inhibitors or angiotensin II receptor-blocking agents. Neither of these drugs is suitable for use in pregnancy, because of their adverse fetal effects, but alternative agents can be used safely. These include centrally acting drugs (alpha methyl DOPA and clonidine), calcium channel-blocking drugs (verapamil and nifedipine) and vasodilators (hydralazine), alone or in combination. The usual aim is to lower the blood pressure to 130/80 mmHg or below. Therapy with agents suitable for use in pregnancy should be stabilized prior to conception.

### Regular monitoring in pregnancy
Women with diabetes should undergo their antenatal care, labour and delivery in a specialist perinatal

unit familiar with the management of diabetic pregnancy. Frequent antenatal review is of value to measure blood pressure and check glycaemic control. In addition, because 6–8% of all sexually active women have asymptomatic bacilluria, patients should be screened for this intermittently during pregnancy, and infections treated promptly. Proteinuria should be measured serially, and fluid balance assessed clinically. Since there is likely to be an increase in pre-existing proteinuria, this should not cause undue concern. Dietary restriction of salt may be necessary in some patients with nephrotic range proteinuria, but is not advised routinely, because of the physiological need for fluid accumulation in pregnancy. Similarly, dietary protein restriction is not routinely advised in the pregnant woman whose glomerular filtration rate is normal. Fetal growth and well-being should also be serially monitored during pregnancy, clinically, by uterine ultrasound, and the fetal heart rate should be monitored.

*Planned delivery*
Because of an increased incidence of late intrauterine fetal death, traditional management of the diabetic pregnant woman included elective delivery between 36 and 38 weeks' gestation. This, together with delayed fetal pulmonary maturation in the fetuses of women with diabetes[64] resulted in a relatively high incidence of hyaline membrane disease in the newborns.[65] Improved control of blood sugar and blood pressure, and close monitoring of fetal well-being has diminished the need for premature delivery. Provided that control is tight and the pregnancy is uncomplicated, the onset of spontaneous labour can be awaited in the majority of diabetic women (even those with early diabetic nephropathy), as first demonstrated by Drury and colleagues in Dublin.[66] Both mother and baby should be closely monitored during labour and delivery, and close supervision should be continued in the early puerperium.

*Postpartum care*
A return to prepregnancy levels of insulin therapy, and adjustment of antihypertensives and dietary recommendations should occur under close supervision in the early postpartum period. The question of appropriate methods of contraception should be addressed at this time.

## CONCLUSION

Diabetic women without microvascular or macrovascular disease in general do well in pregnancy,

although the fetus still faces a high risk of problems, including congenital abnormality, unless there is careful planning and tight control of diabetes. In those with early microvascular disease, there is little evidence for a deleterious effect of pregnancy on the underlying pathophysiology, although the situation is much less clear for those with more advanced disease. Because of the increased risk of disorders such as premature labour and superimposed pre-eclampsia, the pre-existing diabetes and its complications have a relative adverse effect on the fetus, although perinatal mortality has become a rare event, and morbidity is less severe than a decade ago. The presence of macrovascular disease such as coronary artery disease constitutes a significant risk factor for maternal welfare when exposed to the haemodynamic and cardiovascular challenge of pregnancy.

The diabetic woman with these underlying complications should be counselled, both about the risks of pregnancy to her ongoing health and about the risk of the underlying disease to the contemplated pregnancy. Should a decision to attempt pregnancy be undertaken, careful planning and therapy should be instituted prior to pregnancy, and continued throughout gestation and into the postpartum period. Both mother and fetus should be closely monitored by a skilled multidisciplinary team throughout this period of time.

## REFERENCES

1. Lind T, Billewicz WZ, Brown G, A serial study of changes occurring in the oral glucose tolerance test during pregnancy, *J Obstet Gynaecol Br Cwlth* (1973) **80:** 1033–9.
2. Ryan EA, Enns L, Role of gestational hormones in the induction of insulin resistance, *J Clin Endocrinol Metab* (1988) **67:** 341–7.
3. Kuehl C, Insulin secretion and insulin resistance in pregnancy and GDM. Implications for diagnosis and management, *Diabetes* (1991) **40**(Suppl 2): 18–24.
4. Bailey RR, Rolleston GL, Kidney length and ureteric dilatation in the puerperium, *J Obstet Gynaecol Br Cwlth* (1971) **78:** 55–61.
5. Charles D, *Infections in Obstetrics and Gynaecology* (WB Saunders: Philadelphia, 1980) 103–82.
6. Davison JM, Overview: Kidney function in pregnant women. *Am J Kidney Dis* (1987) **9:** 248–52.
7. Dunlop W. Serial changes in renal haemodynamics during normal human pregnancy, *Br J Obstet Gynaecol* (1981) **88:** 1–9.
8. Davison JM, Dunlop W, Changes in renal hemodynamics and tubular function induced by normal human pregnancy, *Semin Nephrol* (1984) **4:** 198–207.
9. Vora JP, Anderson S, Brenner BM, Pathogenesis of diabetic glomerulopathy: the role of glomerular hemodynamic factors. In: Mogensen CE, ed. *The Kidney and Hypertension in Diabetes Mellitus*, 2nd edn. (Kluwer Academic: Boston, 1994) 223–32.
10. Landon MB, Gabbe SG, Diabetes mellitus. In: Barron WM, Lindheimer MD, eds, *Medical Disorders During Pregnancy*, 3rd edn (Mosby: St Louis, 2000) 71–100.
11. Roversi GD, Gargiulo M, A new approach to treatment of dia-

betic pregnant women, *Am J Obstet Gynecol* (1979) **135**: 567–76.

12. Sobczak M, Pertynska M, Wilczynski J, Arterial hypertension during pregnancy complicated by type 1 diabetes—clinical aspects, *Ginekol Pol* (2001) **72**: 1247–54.

13. Brown M, Pregnancy-induced hypertension: pathogenesis and management, *Aust N Z J Med* (1991) **21**: 257–73.

14. Rosenn BM, Miodovnik M, Medical complications of diabetes mellitus in pregnancy, *Clin Obstet Gynecol* (2000) **43**: 17–31.

15. Cunningham FK, Lucas MJ, Urinary tract infections complicating pregnancy, *Baillieres Clin Obstet Gynaecol* (1994) **8**: 353–73.

16. Wong SF, Chan FY, Cincotta RB et al, Routine ultrasound screening in diabetic pregnancies, *Ultrasound Obstet Gynecol* (2002) **19**: 171–6.

17. van Assche FA, Holemans K, Aerts L, Long term consequences for offspring of diabetes during pregnancy, *Br Med Bull* (2001) **60**: 173–82.

18. Kimmerle R, Zass RP, Cupisti S et al, Pregnancies in women with diabetic nephropathy: long term outcome for mother and child, *Diabetologia* (1995) **38**: 227–35.

19. Mogensen CE, Klebe JG, Microalbuminuria and diabetic pregnancy. In: Morgensen CE, ed., *The Kidney and Hypertension in Diabetes Mellitus* (Martinus Nijhoff: Boston, MA, 1988) 223–44.

20. Jungers P, Forget D, Henry-Amar M et al, Chronic kidney disease and pregnancy. In: Grünfeld JP, Maxwell MH, Bach JF, Crosnier J, Funck-Brentano JL, eds., *Advances in Nephrology*. (Year Book Medical Publishers: Chicago, 1986) 103–41.

21. Katz AI, Davison JM, Hayslett JP et al, Pregnancy in women with renal disease, *Kidney Int* (1980) **18**: 192–206.

22. Rosenn B, Miodovnik M, Kranias G et al, Does pregnancy increase the risk for development and progression of benign diabetic retinopathy? *Am J Obstet Gynecol* (1981) **141**: 741–51.

23. Chaturvedi N, Stephenson JM, Fuller JH, The relationship between pregnancy and long term maternal complications in the EURODIAB IDDM Complications Study, *Diabet Med* (1995) **12**: 494–9.

24. Hemachandra A, Ellis D, Lloyd CE et al, The influence of pregnancy on IDDM complications, *Diabetes Care* (1995) **18**: 950–4.

25. Gordon M, Landon MB, Samuel P et al, Perinatal outcome and long term follow-up associated with modern management of diabetic nephropathy, *Obstet Gynecol* (1996) **87**: 401–9.

26. Bar J, Chen R, Schonfeld A et al, Pregnancy outcome in patients with insulin dependent diabetes mellitus and diabetic nephropathy treated with ACE inhibitors before pregnancy, *J Pediatr Endocrinol Metab* (1999) **12**: 659–65.

27. Kitzmiller JL, Brown ER, Philippe M et al, Diabetic nephropathy and perinatal outcome, *Am J Obstet Gynecol* (1981) **141**: 741–51.

28. Dicker D, Feldberg D, Peleg D et al, Pregnancy complicated by diabetic nephropathy, *J Perinat Med* (1986) **14**: 299–307.

29. Grenfell A, Brudenell JM, Doddrige MC et al, Pregnancy in diabetic women who have proteinuria, *Q J Med* (1986) **59**: 379–86.

30. Reece EA, Coustan DR, Hayslett JP et al, Diabetic nephropathy: pregnancy performance and fetomaternal outcome, *Am J Obstet Gynecol* (1988) **159**: 56–66.

31. Miodovnik M, Rosenn B, Khoury J et al, Does pregnancy increase the risk of development and progression of diabetic nephropathy? *Am J Obstet Gynecol* (1996) **174**: 1180–9.

32. Bar J, Ben-Rafael Z, Padoa A et al, Prediction of pregnancy outcome in subgroups of women with renal disease, *Clin Nephrol* (2000) **53**: 437–44.

33. Reece EA, Winn N, Hayslett JP et al, Does pregnancy alter the rate of progression of diabetic nephropathy? *Am J Perinatol* (1990) **7**: 193–7.

34. Kimmerle R, Zass RP, Cupisti S et al, Pregnancies in women with diabetic nephropathy: long-term outcome for mother and child, *Diabetologica* (1995) **38**: 227–35.

35. Mackie AD, Doddrige MC, Gamsu HR et al, Outcome of pregnancy in patients with insulin-dependent diabetes mellitus and nephropathy with moderate renal impairment, *Diabetes Med* (1996) **13**: 90–6.

36. Biesenbach G, Stoger H, Zazgornik J, Influence of pregnancy on progression of diabetic nephropathy and subsequent requirement of renal replacement therapy in female type 1 diabetic patient with impaired renal function, *Nephrol Dial Transplant* (1992) **7**: 105–9.

37. Purdy LP, Hantsch CE, Molitch ME et al, Effect of pregnancy on renal function in patients with moderate-to-severe diabetic renal insufficiency, *Diabetes Care* (1996) **19**: 1067–74.

38. Hou SH, Grosssman SD, Madias NE, Pregnancy in women with renal disease and moderate renal insufficiency, *Am J Med* (1985) **78**: 185–94.

39. Imbasciati E, Pardi G, Capetta P et al, Pregnancy in women with chronic renal failure, *Am J Nephrol* (1986) **6**: 193–8.

40. Jones DC, Hayslett JP, Outcome of pregnancy in women with moderate or severe insufficiency, *N Engl J Med* (1996) **335**: 226–32.

41. Becker GJ, Ihle BU, Fairley KA et al, Effect of pregnancy on moderate renal failure in reflux nephropathy, *BMJ* (1986) **292**: 796–8.

42. Jungers P, Houillier P, Forget D et al, Influence of pregnancy on the course of primary chronic glomerulonephritis, *Lancet* (1995) **346**: 1122–4.

43. Cunningham GF, Cox SM, Harstad TW et al, Chronic renal disease and pregnancy outcome, *Am J Obstet Gynecol* (1990) **163**: 453–9.

44. Nenov VD, Taal MW, Sakharova OV et al, Multi-hit nature of chronic renal disease, *Curr Opin Nephrol Hypertens* (2000) **9**: 85–97.

45. Packham DK, Fairley KF, Ihle BU et al, Comparison of pregnancy outcome between normotensive and hypertensive women with primary glomerulonephritis, *Clin Exp Hypertens* (1988) **B6**: 387–99.

46. Surian M, Imbasciati E, Cosci P et al, Glomerular disease in pregnancy. A study of 123 pregnancies in patients with primary and secondary glomerular diseases, *Nephron* (1984) **36**: 101–5.

47. Ruggenenti P, Schieppati A, Remuzzi G, Progression, remission, regression of renal diseases, *Lancet* (2001) **357**: 1601–8.

48. Brenner BM, Cooper ME, de Zeew D et al, Effects of losartan on renal and cardiovascular outcomes in patients with type 2 diabetes and nephropathy, *N Engl J Med* (2001) **345**: 870–8.

49. Nakao N, Yoshimura A, Morita H et al, Combination treatment of angiotensin-II receptor blocker and angiotensin-converting-enzyme inhibitor in non-diabetic renal disease (COOPERATE): a randomised controlled trial, *Lancet* (2003) **361**: 117–24.

50. Bjork S, Mulec H, Johnsen SA et al, Renal protective effect of enalapril in diabetic nephropathy, *BMJ* (1992) **304**: 339–43.

51. Mastrobattista JM, Angiotensin converting enzyme inhibitors in pregnancy, *Semin Perinatol* (1997) **21**: 124–34.

52. Hou S, Pregnancy in women with chronic renal disease, *N Engl J Med* (1985) **312**: 836–9.

53. Kincaid-Smith PS, Fairley KF, Hypertensive disorders of pregnancy. In: Dilys J, ed., *The Kidney and Hypertension in Pregnancy* (Churchill Livingstone: Edinburgh, 1993) 37–55.

54. Ferrier C, Taminelli L, Wauters JP. Pregnancy in renal disease. Experience of a single Swiss center. Proceedings of the Annual Meeting of the Swiss Society of Nephrology. Lausanne, Switzerland, 7–8 December, 1995.

55. Reece EA, Leguizamon G, Homko C, Stringent control in diabetic nephropathy associated with optimisation of pregnancy outcomes, *J Matern Fetal Med* (1998) **7**: 213–16.

56. Pierce J, California Diabetes and Pregnancy Program data system report, 1992, *Clin Perinatol* (1993) **20**: 565–6.

57. Rosenn BM, Miodovnik M, Khoury JC et al, Outcome of pregnancy in women with diabetic nephropathy, *Am J Obstet Gynecol* (1997) **176:** S179.

58. Davison J, Baylis C, Renal disease. In: De Swiet M, ed., *Medical Disorders in Obstetric Practice* (Blackwell Scientific: London, 1989) 226–305.

59. Ferrier C, North RA, Becker G et al, Uterine artery waveform as a predictor of pregnancy outcome in women with underlying renal disease, *Clin Nephrol* (1994) **42:** 362–8.

60. Rosenn B, Miodovnik M, Kranias G et al, Does pregnancy increase the risk for development and progression of benign diabetic retinopathy? *Am J Obstet Gynecol* (1981) **141:** 741–51.

61. Chaturvedi N, Stephenson JM, Fuller JH, The relationship between pregnancy and long term maternal complications in the EURODIAB IDDM Complications Study, *Diabet Med* (1995) **12:** 494–9.

62. Hemachandra A, Ellis D, Lloyd CE et al, The influence of pregnancy on IDDM complications, *Diabetes Care* (1995) **18:** 950–4.

63. Gordon MC, Landon MB, Boyle J et al, Coronary artery disease in insulin-dependent diabetes mellitus of pregnancy (class H): a review of the literature, *Obstet Gynecol Surv* (1996) **51:** 437–44.

64. Gluck L, Kulovich MV, Lecithin-sphyngomyelin ratios in amniotic fluid in normal and abnormal pregnancy, *Am J Obstet Gynecol* (1973) **115:** 539–46.

65. Usher RM, Allen AC, MacLean FH, Risk of respiratory distress syndrome related to gestational age, route of delivery and maternal diabetes, *Am J Obstet Gynecol* (1971) **111:** 826–9.

66. Drury MI, Management of the pregnant diabetic—are the pundits right? *Diabetologia* (1986) **29:** 10–12.

# 16

# The use of dialysis in the treatment of diabetic patients with end-stage renal disease

Yalemzewd Woredekal and Eli A Friedman

Diabetic nephropathy is the leading cause of end-stage renal disease (ESRD) in the USA, Japan, and industrialized Europe. Despite a modest advance in slowing progression of renal disease in diabetic patients, the number of new diabetic patients accepted for renal replacement therapy has been increasing steadily for the last decade. The United States Renal Data System (USRDS) in 2001 reported that of 340 261 US patients receiving either dialytic therapy or a kidney transplant in 1999, 33.6% had diabetes.[1] Furthermore, during 1999, of 82 692 new cases of ESRD, 46.2% were listed as having diabetes (Figure 16.1). Much of the increase in diabetic ESRD is in older people with type 2 diabetes. The mean age of new diabetic patients accepted for renal replacement therapy in the USA is 60 years,[1] and the majority of these patients have more than one comorbid condition at the start of renal replacement therapy. Management of diabetic patients with progressive renal insufficiency is a challenge because of comorbid conditions that accompany the nephropathy. Diabetic azotemic patients have greater mortality than nondiabetic patients with equivalent renal insufficiency, usually due to cardiovascular disease, cerebrovascular disease, and sepsis. Illustrating the role of extrarenal disease over time, Schleiffer et al[2] screened 565 hospitalized type 2 diabetic patients for nephropathy and associated extrarenal disease between 1988 and 1992. Of these, 280 patients had no clinical nephropathy, 38 had microalbuminuria, 105 had overt proteinuria, 55 were azotemic, and 87 had ESRD on dialytic therapy. When patients with no clinical sign of nephropathy were compared with those on dialytic therapy, the prevalence of extrarenal disease was several times greater in the latter group during the course of the development of nephropathy: hypertension (53–89%), left ventricular hypertrophy (39–81%), myocardial infarction

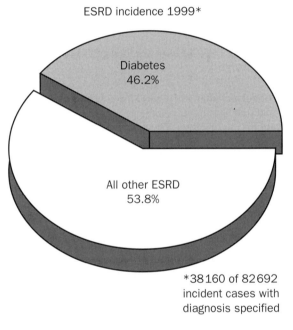

ESRD incidence 1999*

Diabetes 46.2%

All other ESRD 53.8%

*38 160 of 82 692 incident cases with diagnosis specified

**Figure 16.1** Extracted from USRDS 2001 report demonstrating that of 82 692 new cases of ESRD patients, 46.2% were diagnosed to have diabetes mellitus.

(14–36%), peripheral vascular disease (27–77%), proliferative retinopathy (6–46%), and internal carotid artery stenosis (15–36%). Pre-existing comorbid conditions play a major role in the genesis of the lower survival rate of diabetic patients on renal replacement therapy. Therefore, a proactive rather than reactive management strategy is required for the diabetic patients with renal insufficiency. In view of the exceptionally high rate of comorbid extrarenal complications that are probable during treatment for kidney failure, detection before irretrievable injury should be incorporated into all planning. By defining collaborative measures with key support services (Figure 16.2), particularly cardiology, ophthalmology, and podiatry, an overall plan for conserving patient time, energy, and finances should be constructed for each patient. Thus, for example, three-monthly visits to a podiatrist, annual retinal examinations, and annual dobutamine stress tests might be appropriate for one asymptomatic diabetic dialysis patient, while bimonthly visits to a podiatrist, three-monthly visits to a cardiologist, and monthly laser photocoagulation treatments might be advisable for another patient beset by complications. All patients in a program should be entered into a 'comorbidity grid' that prompts needed consultations and underscores their omission.

## OPTIONS FOR RENAL REPLACEMENT THERAPY

Diabetic patients with ESRD have similar options for renal replacement therapy, as do nondiabetic patients. Apart from detection and treatment of risk factors for progression of renal disease and monitoring the course of comorbid conditions, it is important to explore various modalities of renal replacement therapy to determine which option best suits the patient. The different types of renal replacement therapy available for diabetic ESRD patients include hemodialysis, peritoneal dialysis, kidney transplant alone, and a combined pancreas and kidney transplant, which is unique to diabetic patients (Table 16.1). This chapter focuses on dialytic therapy. Before

a specific patient is assigned to dialysis, it is important that patients and their families are properly informed about the advantages and disadvantages of each modality of treatment.

Which treatment is best for a particular patient is determined by considering the patient's age, level of education, severity of comorbid conditions, social and family support, and geographical location (Table 16.2). For example, a patient with severe cardiomyopathy may be restricted to continuous ambulatory peritoneal dialysis (CAPD) because the stress of extracorporeal blood circulation in hemodialysis might precipitate cardiac decompensation. However, young, motivated, and independent diabetic patients can choose from a menu of available modalities of treatment, preferably selecting kidney transplant.

## PREPARATION OF THE DIABETIC PATIENT FOR RENAL REPLACEMENT THERAPY

Although normalizing blood pressure, tightly controlling blood glucose, low-protein diet, and cessation of smoking may retard the development and progression of diabetic nephropathy, many patients will still progress to ESRD.[3–10] Under the guidance of a nephrologist, a team of specialists is required to optimize management of diabetic azotemic patients during the pre-ESRD period (Figure 16.2). Patient education concerning the complex regimen outlined above should be started once diabetic nephropathy is diagnosed. Regular scheduled meetings with both a nurse educator and nutritionist, coupled with participation in patient support groups, can play a vital role in guiding ESRD patients to make appropriate choices of treatment.

The option of kidney transplantation must be explored early and repeatedly. Age up to 75 years is not an exclusion criterion, especially when multiple healthy sibling donors are available; referral to a transplant team is in the patient's interest. Long-term

---

**Table 16.1  Treatment options for diabetic azotemic patients.**

1. Hemodialysis
   Home hemodialysis
   In-center hemodialysis
   Daily hemodialysis
2. Peritoneal dialysis
   Continuous ambulatory peritoneal dialysis (CAPD)
   Continuous cycling peritoneal dialysis (CCPD)
3. Transplantation
   Kidney alone (living related, unrelated donor or
   cadaver donor)
   Combined pancreas and kidney (cadaver donor)

---

**Table 16.2  Factors determining choice of renal replacement therapy**

Age
Level of education
Severity of comorbid condition
Social and family support
Geographical location

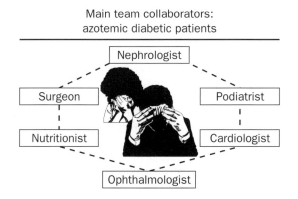

Main team collaborators:
azotemic diabetic patients

**Figure 16.2** Collaboration of specialists guided by a nephrologist is required to optimize care for azotemic diabetic patients.

survival is greatly superior with a kidney transplant than in any dialytic regimen (Figure 16.3).

Depending upon the choice of treatment, there are specific preparatory steps that should be initiated. For example, for those electing hemodialysis, it is important to establish vascular access in the non-dominant arm when creatinine clearance is around 25 ml/min. It is of immense importance that the veins in the forearm are properly protected. This is often a problem in diabetic patients under the care of non-nephrologists lacking understanding of the life-line importance attached to the patency of forearm veins. Education regarding vascular access should begin when the serum creatinine exceeds 3 mg/dl.[11] Predialysis management includes preserving fore-arm cutaneous veins by avoiding venous punctures, intravenous catheters, and maintaining good nutritional status while sustaining an hematocrit above 33%, as necessary, by administration of erythropoietin and supplemental iron. Metabolic bone disease due to secondary hyperparathyroidism should be minimized by the use of intestinal phosphate binders along with synthetic vitamin D (Table 16.3).

## TIMING TO INITIATE RENAL REPLACEMENT THERAPY

Although evidence from prospective, controlled, clinical trials is lacking, there is a widespread consensus among nephrologists that diabetic individuals develop uremic symptoms at a higher level of residual

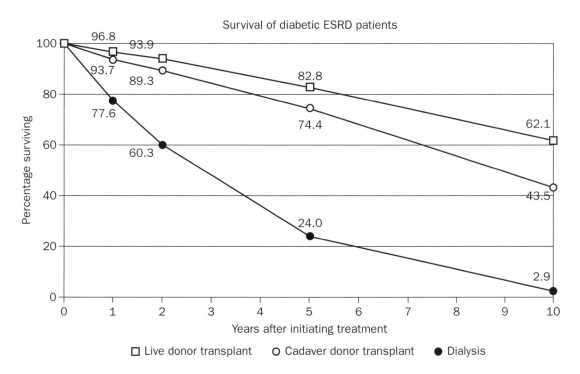

Survival of diabetic ESRD patients

□ Live donor transplant   O Cadaver donor transplant   ● Dialysis

**Figure 16.3** Extracted from USRDS 2001 report demonstrating the superior survival of transplantation as compared to dialytic therapy.

**Table 16.3    Pre-ESRD care for diabetic azotemic patients.**

Adequate blood-pressure control

Adequate glycemic control

Preserving cutaneous vein for vascular access

Correction of anemia

Maintenance of calcium and phosphate balance

renal function, and that dialysis should be initiated earlier than in nondiabetics.[12-15] As renal failure progresses, the diabetic kidney is progressively less able to compensate for hypoalbuminemia by regulation of volume and sodium balance; and as a result, hypertension and fluid overload may become refractory at a relatively high glomerular filtration rate (GFR). Concomitant gastroparesis and nephrotic syndrome may exacerbate protein–calorie malnutrition, and retinopathy may progress more rapidly as GFR falls close to 15 ml/min.[16] Many nephrologists believe that early initiation of dialysis protects against malnutrition during the pre-ESRD period and might prevent the increased morbidity and early mortality related to malnutrition among dialysis patients. The Canada-USA (CANUSA) study of peritoneal dialysis showed that nutritional status at initiation of dialytic therapy is correlated with residual renal function at its initiation.[17] In general, it is advisable to start dialytic therapy for diabetic patients when the creatinine clearance is between 10 and 15 ml/min.

## MAINTENANCE HEMODIALYSIS

The USRDS 2001 registry reported that 74.7% of all prevalent diabetic ESRD patients are treated by hemodialysis and 7% by peritoneal dialysis, while 17.5% had a functioning kidney transplant.[1] Hemodialysis treatment for diabetics is similar to that for nondiabetic patients. An ideal hemodialysis regimen consists of at least thrice-weekly dialysis, lasting for 4–5 hr, during which extracorporeal blood flow is maintained at 300–500 ml/min. The preferred vascular access is an arteriovenous fistula, because it leads to less infection or thrombosis than prosthetic grafts. Some investigators have found that access-related morbidity and hospital admission are increased,[18] and duration of access patency is reduced in diabetics,[19-21] while others discerned little or no difference compared with nondiabetic ESRD patients.[22-24] Patients with long-standing diabetes,

however, often have pre-existing vascular disease, and a fistula cannot be created or does not mature sufficiently to allow for adequate dialysis, necessitating surgical insertion of a prosthetic vascular graft.

Following creation of an arteriovenous fistula, it is necessary to wait 12–36 weeks for its maturation. While a synthetic graft can be used as early as 2 weeks after insertion, it is usually advisable to wait 8 weeks or longer, because wound healing is delayed in uremic diabetic patients. Therefore, it is important that diabetic patients with nephropathy be referred early to a nephrologist so that preparation, including vascular access, can be effected before any urgent need for dialysis.

When the timing is precise, it is noted that diabetic hemodialysis patients actually receive a lower dialysis dose than nondiabetics because of the interruption of dialysis due to either dialysis-related complications or inadequate access blood flow.[25]

## COMPLICATIONS RELATED TO HEMODIALYSIS

### Thrombosis and infection of vascular access

Nearly 90% of graft thromboses are associated with stenosis of venous outflow.[22,26,27] A minority of graft thromboses occur in the absence of an identifiable anatomic lesion, hypotension, intravascular volume depletion, and graft compression during sleep, or as a result of dialysis staff attempting to achieve hemostasis. Vascular thrombosis can be prevented by frequent surveillance of the access by a nephrologist and dialysis staff, allowing elective surgical revisions or angioplasty.[28]

Access-related infections are a major source of morbidity and mortality among diabetic dialysis patients. The incidence of vascular access-related infection is highest when central venous dialysis catheters are used; native arteriovenous fistulas carry the lowest risk of infection. A high proportion of infections related to vascular access are caused by staphylococcus organisms; these infections carry high rates of mortality, and recurrent, metastatic complications. Bacteremia should be suspected in febrile diabetic patients on hemodialysis, and the vascular access should be promptly inspected. If the source of infection is suspected to be the vascular access, empiric antibiotic therapy, guided by demographic data and severity of illness, should be administered promptly and continued until the causative organism is identified, and then a specific antimicrobial regimen can be applied. Prolonged parenteral administration of an antibiotic is recommended to minimize complications of infection, especially in cases of staphylococcal bacteremia.

Ischemic pain in the hand following vascular access placement is common in diabetic patients, and may be caused by obstructive arterial disease and/or graft steal, or by ischemic monomelic neuropathy.[29–31] Hand gangrene in dialysis patients is almost always restricted to diabetic patients, and can lead to severe local infection and the need for emergency amputation.[32,33] Interventions such as percutaneous angioplasty of stenotic arteries,[30] ligation of the vascular access, or transposition grafting may be used to increase blood flow to the compromised area.

## Intradialytic hypotension

Intradialytic hypotension is a common adverse event seen mostly in diabetic patients on hemodialysis. Although the incidence of intradialytic hypotension has been reduced since bicarbonate replaced acetate in dialysate for standard hemodialysis, it remains a problem for diabetic patients. Prolonged hypotensive episodes may precipitate angina pectoris and myocardial infarction, or even access thrombosis.

The major contributors to recurrent intradialytic hypotension in diabetic hemodialysis patients are reduced myocardial contractility related to ischemic heart disease,[34] diastolic dysfunction related to diabetic cardiomyopathy with resultant decreased left ventricular compliance and filling, and autonomic neuropathy (diabetic and uremic), which results in the abolition of the reflex, increase in heart rate and increased peripheral vascular resistance that usually occur to prevent hypotension before interstitial fluid is mobilized into the intravascular compartment.[35–37]

Measures to reduce dialysis-related hypotension are listed in Table 16.4. A combination of midodrine (an oral alpha-1 adrenergic agonist) and lowering dialysate temperature by 2°C will decrease the incidence of intradialytic hypotension.[38,39] Anand et al have also found that administering dobutamine

intradialytically in those with reduced cardiac function (systolic function $<40\%$) significantly reduces intradialytic hypotension.[40]

## Hypertension

Almost all diabetic patients are hypertensive at the start of dialysis therapy and are taking antihypertensive medication.[41] Diabetics with nephropathy are prone to derangements in sodium/volume homeostasis even before reaching ESRD.[42,43] There is a general consensus that the principal pathogenetic mechanism for hypertension in dialysis patients is volume expansion.[44,45] Diabetic patients, for undetermined reasons, which may include stimulation of thirst by hyperglycemia and high plasma osmolality, gain more weight between dialysis than nondiabetics,[46,47] expanding their extracellular volume and contributing to hypertension. Fluid overload not only contributes to the high prevalence of hypertension, but also explains the higher incidence of pulmonary edema in diabetic dialysis patients. In a prospective, observational, multicenter study, Kimmel et al found that increased interdialytic weight gain is associated with a significant increase in relative mortality risk in diabetic ESRD patients.[48]

Normalization of body weight (dry weight) is the most efficient way to control blood pressure in dialysis patients. Under maintenance hemodialysis therapy, optimal fluid removal in diabetic patients is a crucial unsolved problem.[49] Accelerated arteriosclerosis and autonomic neuropathy make it difficult to attain an optimal dry weight. Nevertheless, intensive efforts should be made to strive for optimal dry weight. Intradialytic cramps and hypotension are less prevalent with continuous fluid removal during long dialysis sessions. Alternatively, frequent dialysis should be considered in diabetic patients. Kjellstrand and Ting found better quality of life in nondiabetic patients with various cardiac problems when subjected to frequent dialysis—fluid removal was better tolerated, and fluid overload was reduced.[50]

## Malnutrition

A low serum albumin level is typical in diabetic patients at the start of renal replacement therapy as well as during long-term maintenance hemodialysis.[41,51] Protein restriction during the predialysis period, persistent urinary protein loss, poor appetite, and gastroparesis contribute to protein malnutrition

---

**Table 16.4   Measures to minimize intradialytic hypotension**

Use of bicarbonate bath
Cooling of dialysate fluid by 2°C
Longer dialysis with slow ultrafiltration rate
Midodrine hydrochloride 2.5–5 mg before dialysis

in diabetic patients. Furthermore, suboptimal chronic inflammation may explain the lower albumin level seen in diabetic dialysis patients.[51] Impaired gastric emptying (gastroparesis), a manifestation of autonomic neuropathy, afflicts about one-half of all diabetic patients,[52,53] and is present in the majority of azotemic diabetic patients when initially evaluated for renal replacement therapy.[54]

Intensive dietary education and intense dialysis therapy are required to improve appetite and consequently calorie and protein intake in diabetic patients undergoing dialysis. For those with autonomic neuropathy (nausea, vomiting and gastroparesis), prokinetic drugs such as metoclopromide or erythromycin are used to increase intestinal motility.

## PERITONEAL DIALYSIS

Peritoneal dialysis (PD) is an alternative mode of dialytic therapy available for diabetic ESRD patients. In the USA, peritoneal dialysis is selected by only 7% of all diabetic patients on renal replacement therapy.[1] As is true for hemodialysis, preparation of patients for CAPD requires patient education and advance planning for placement of an intraperitoneal catheter. Most centers wait at least 2 weeks after catheter insertion before starting training for CAPD and catheter use to allow for ingrowth of fibroblasts into the cuff. This reduces the chance of leakage of peritoneal fluid once treatment is initiated. Motivated patients can learn the technique of fluid exchange in about 1 week, though the usual training range is 10–30 days. Volume exchange of 2–3l of sterile dialysate containing different concentrations of glucose 4–6 times daily is prescribed according to the patient's size and residual renal function. Another alternative to manual exchange of dialysate is the use of a mechanical cycling device in a regimen termed continuous cyclic peritoneal dialysis (CCPD). To achieve good glycemic control, when patients are continuously exposed to glucose-rich dialysate fluid, regular insulin in large doses (30–130 units/day) is added to each dialysate bag.[55] If the insulin requirement exceeds 100 units per exchange as guided by finger-stick glucose measurements, additional subcutaneous injection of long-acting insulin is usually beneficial. Diabetic patients have to be taught the impact of a glucose-rich dialysate on control of blood glucose, and should be monitored closely after initiation of therapy until the problem of insulin dosage is mastered.

Some nephrologists view peritoneal dialysis as the preferred choice of treatment for diabetic ESRD patients.[56] Indeed, there are specific indications for CAPD or CCPD when vascular access sites have been exhausted or in those with severe congestive heart failure or angina, or severe dialysis-related hypotension. Peritoneal dialysis offers lower vascular stress because of its relatively slow ultrafiltration rate coupled with less rapid solute removal, resulting in smaller shifts in serum osmolality, and causing fewer hypotensive episodes.

## COMPLICATIONS RELATED TO PERITONEAL DIALYSIS

### Peritonitis

Peritonitis is the main complication of peritoneal dialysis, and accounts for 30–50% of all hospital admissions in CAPD patients.[57] It is also the main reason for technique failure resulting in discontinuation of CAPD and switching to hemodialysis.[58] Surprisingly, despite the longer duration required for treatment of each episode, the overall risk of contracting peritonitis is no greater in diabetic than nondiabetic ESRD patients.[59]

Chronic carriers of *Staphylococcus aureus* are at increased risk of peritonitis. The treatment for peritonitis is similar for both diabetic and nondiabetic patients. When peritonitis is suspected, a sample of the dialysate effluent should be obtained for laboratory evaluation, including cell count with differential, Gram's stain, and culture. An elevated white cell count in the peritoneal fluid of more than $100/mm^3$ of which at least 50% are polymorphonuclear neutrophils, indicates microbial peritonitis, and mandates prompt initiation of antimicrobial therapy.

If Gram's stain shows either Gram-positive or Gram-negative organisms, a single antimicrobial agent should be administered. If the Gram's stain shows both Gram-positive and Gram-negative organisms, or no organism is seen in the presence of increased cell count, prompt initiation of antibiotic treatment is indicated. The current empiric antibiotic treatment for PD-related peritonitis is to use a combination of first-generation cephalosporin and ceftazidime.[60] This combination therapy has a good antibacterial efficacy for both Gram-positive and Gram-negative organisms.

The increased prevalence of vancomycin-resistant organisms worldwide has prompted physicians to discourage routine use of vancomycin for empiric treatment of peritonitis. Vancomycin is reserved for true methicillin-resistant organisms. The routine use of aminoglycosides is also avoided because of the concern to preserve residual renal function for those with urine volume >100 ml/day.

Both the first-generation cephalosporin and ceftazidime can be mixed in the same dialysate bag and can be administered as a single daily dose, which has an advantage of ease of use by patient and staff, both in hospital or at home.

The duration of antibiotic treatment varies depending upon the type of organism isolated from PD fluid culture. For example, in patients with an uncomplicated, coagulase-negative staphylococcus, 10–14 days of appropriate antibiotic treatment is adequate. However, in patients with *S. aureus* peritonitis or with a single, Gram-negative organism, a 3-week antibiotic treatment is recommended.

Most patients with PD-related peritonitis show considerable clinical improvement within 48–72 hr after initiation of antibiotic treatment. If no significant clinical improvement is observed after 96 hr of antibiotic treatment, evaluation of the patient for possible mycobacterial or fungal infection and removal of the catheter should be considered.

Although many physicians feel that catheter removal is indicated immediately in fungal peritonitis, recent experience with the newer antifungal agents (flucytosine and fluconazole) suggests that these agents may also be effective treatment.[61,62] If clinical improvement is seen, the treatment should continue for 4–6 weeks; however, if no clinical response is seen after 4–7 days of therapy, the catheter should be removed immediately.

## Malnutrition

The prevalence of malnutrition in patients undergoing CAPD is higher than with hemodialysis. Large protein loss (8–10 g per day) in dialysate fluid,[63] early satiety due to increased intra-abdominal pressure, gastroparesis, anorexia caused by underdialysis, and the loss of residual renal function are believed to contribute to malnutrition in diabetic CAPD patients.

To maintain protein balance, peritoneal dialysis patients should ingest at least 1.5 g protein per kg of body weight per day, and are advised to eat small and frequent meals. Although impractical, because of the high cost, malnourished peritoneal dialysis patients reportedly gain nutritional benefit from dialysate containing essential amino acids.[64]

## Metabolic abnormalities

Diabetic patients undergoing CAPD have an increased level of total cholesterol, triglyceride, and apolipoprotein B, and a decreased level of high-density lipoprotein;[65,66] hyperlipidemia is greater in such patients than in patients undergoing hemodialysis.[67] Little et al plotted longitudinal changes in lipid profile in relation to weight gain, comorbidity, and dialysis treatment in patients treated with CAPD, and found that the strongest predictors of worsening lipid profiles were weight gain and pre-existing cardiovascular comorbidity, with no association with glucose load or protein losses.[68]

Lipoprotein (LP(a)) is increasingly being recognized as an independent cardiovascular risk factor, and patients undergoing CAPD have a higher serum level of LP(a).[69,70] Misra et al noted that the increased plasma concentration of LP(a) in CAPD patients is not due to decreased catabolism, but is caused by increased synthesis.[71] Hypoalbuminemia may be an important factor, in the elevation of plasma LP(a) in CAPD patients.

Many studies have shown that the lipid-lowering drugs, especially HMO-reductase inhibitors, are effective and well tolerated in the treatment of dyslipidemia in CAPD patients.[72,73] Aggressive nutritional and pharmacological treatment of dyslipidemia is essential in diabetic CAPD patients in order to reduce the incidence of vascular diseases.

## SURVIVAL AND REHABILITATION

Although the survival of diabetics on renal replacement therapy has steadily improved in the last decade (Figure 16.4), it remains lower than in nondiabetic ESRD patients. Myocardial infarction, sepsis, and stroke are the most common cause of death.[1] The comorbid conditions, including blindness, amputation, cardiovascular disease, and stroke, that accompany diabetic nephropathy have an impact on rehabilitation and survival.[74] In 1986, Lowder et al reported that of 232 diabetic patients on hemodialysis in Brooklyn, New York, only seven were employed, while 65% were unable to conduct routine daily activities without assistance.[75] This finding was reaffirmed by an identical result in a survey conducted in 1999.[76]

Collins et al reported excellent survival in diabetic patients who received a high dose of hemodialysis.[77] In diabetics, dialysis delivery may be more frequently interrupted because of hypotensive episodes, intradialytic symptoms, or malfunction of vascular access. Therefore, special attention should be given to adequacy of dialysis, and every attempt should be made to achieve and maintain a KT/V

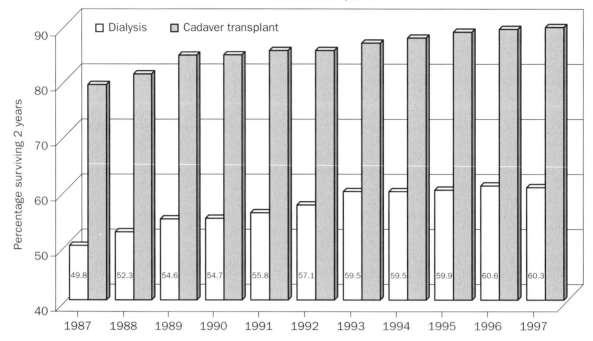

**Figure 16.4** Extracted from USRDS 2001 report demonstrating improvement in 2-year survival in diabetic ESRD patients in 1987–97.

>1.3 for diabetic ESRD patients, a policy that may offer an opportunity to improve overall survival in this group of patients.

## REFERENCES

1. United States Renal Data System (USRDS) 2001 Annual Data Report. The National Institute of Health, National Institute of Diabetes and Digestive and Kidney Disease, Bethesda, MD, 2001.
2. Schleiffer T, Holken H, Brass H, Morbidity in 565 type 2 diabetic patients according to stage of nephropathy. *J Diabetes Complications* 1998; **12:** 103–9.
3. Deedwania PC, Hypertension and diabetes: new therapeutic options. *Arch Intern Med* 2000; **160:** 1585–94.
4. Chantrel F, Bouiller M, Kolb I et al, Antihypertensive treatment in type 2 diabetes and diabetic nephropathy. *Nephrologie* 2000; **21:** 47–52.
5. Chan JC, Ko GT, Leung DH et al, Long term effects of angiotensin-converting enzyme inhibition and metabolic control in hypertensive type 2 diabetic patients. *Kidney Int* 2000; **57:** 590–600.
6. Diabetic Control Complication Trial Research Group. The effect of intensive treatment of diabetes on the development and progression of long-term complication. *N Engl J Med* 1993; **329:** 977–86.
7. United Kingdom Prospective Diabetes Study Group. Intensive glucose control with sulphonylureas or insulin compared with conventional treatment and risk of complication in patients with type 2 diabetes mellitus. *Lancet* 1998; **352:** 837–53.
8. Ohkibo Y, Kishikawa H, Araki E, Intensive insulin therapy prevents the progression of diabetic microvascular complications in Japanese patients with non-insulin dependent diabetes mellitus: a randomized prospective 6 year study. *Diabetes Res Clin Pract* 1995; **28:** 103–17.
9. Pijls LT, de Vries H, Donker AJ et al, The effect of protein restriction on albuminuria in patients with type 2 diabetes mellitus: a randomized trial. *Nephrol Dial Transplant* 1999; **14:** 1445–53.
10. Hansen HP, Christensen PK, Tauber-Lassen E et al, Low protein diet and kidney function in insulin dependent diabetic patients with nephropathy. *Kidney Int* 1999; **55:** 621–8.
11. NKF-DOQI: Clinical Practice Guidelines for Vascular Access. *Am J Kidney Dis* 1997; **30** (Suppl 3): S150–90.
12. Malagone JM, Abuelo JG, Pezzullo JC et al, Clinical and laboratory features of patients with chronic renal disease at the start of dialysis. *Clin Nephrol* 1989; **31:** 77–87.
13. Tzamaloukas AH, Diabetes. In: *Handbook of Dialysis*, 2nd edn (Daugirdas JT, Ing TS, eds). Little Brown: Boston, 1994; 422–32.
14. Markell MS, Hemodialysis for end-stage diabetic nephropathy. In: *Dialysis Therapy*, 2nd ed. (Nissenson AR, Fine RN, eds).Hanley & Belfus: Philadelphia, 1993; 319–22.
15. Friedman EA, Miles AMV, Dialytic management of diabetic uremic patients. In: *Replacement of Renal Function by Dialysis*, 4th edn (Winchester JF, Jacobs C, Kjellstrand CM et al, eds).

Kluwer: Dordrecht, 1996; 935–53.

16. Kjellstrand CM, Simmons RI, Goetz FC et al, Mortality and morbidity in diabetic patients accepted for renal transplantation. *Proc Eur Transplant* 1997; **9**: 345–58.

17. Churchill DN, Taylor DW, Keshaviah PR et al, Adequacy of dialysis and nutrition in continuous peritoneal dialysis; association with clinical outcome. *J Am Soc Nephrol* 1996; **7**: 198–207.

18. Feldman HI, Held PJ, Hutchinson JT et al, Hemodialysis vascular access morbidity in the United States. *Kidney Int* 1993; **43**: 1091–6.

19. Roy-Chaudhury P, Kelly BS, Miller MA et al, Venous neointimal hyperplasia in polytetrafluroethylene dialysis graft. *Kidney Int* 2001; **59**: 2325–34.

20. Goldwasser P, Avram MM, Collier JT et al, Correlates of vascular access occlusion in hemodialysis. *Am J Kidney Dis* 1994; **24**: 785–94.

21. Windus DW, Jendrisak MD, Delmez JA, Prosthetic fistula survival and complications in hemodialysis patients—effects of diabetes and age. *Am J Kidney Dis* 1992; **19**: 448–52.

22. Lay JP, Ashleigh RJ, Tranconi L et al, Result of angioplasty of Brescia-Cimino haemodialysis fistulae. *Clin Radiol* 1998; **53**: 608–11.

23. Mayers JD, Markell MS, Cohen LS et al, Vascular access surgery for maintenance hemodialysis. Variables in hospital stay. *ASAIO J* 1992; **38**: 113–15.

24. Chazan JA, London MR, Pono LM, Long term survival of vascular access in a large chronic hemodialysis population. *Nephron* 1995; **69**: 228–33.

25. Cheigh J, Raghavan J, Sullivan J et al, Is insufficient dialysis a cause for high morbidity in diabetic patients? *J Am Soc Nephrol* 1991; **2**: 317.

26. Beathard GA, Settle SM, Shields MW, Salvage of the nonfunctioning arteriovenous fistula. *Am J Kidney Dis* 1999; **33**: 977–9.

27. Schwab SJ, Improving access patency: pre-end stage renal disease strategies. *J Am Soc Nephrol* 1998; **9** (Suppl): S124–9.

28. Windus DW, Audrain J, Vanderson R et al, Optimization of high efficiency hemodialysis by detection and correction of fistula dysfunction. *Kidney Int* 1990; **38**: 337–41.

29. Hye RJ, Wolf YG, Ischemic monomelic neuropathy. An underrecognized complication of hemodialysis access. *Ann Vasc Surgery* 1994; **8**: 578–82.

30. Valji K, Hye RJ, Roberts AC et al, Hand ischemia in patients with hemodialysis access graft. Angiographic diagnosis and treatment. *Radiology* 1995; **196**: 697–701.

31. Riggs JE, Moss AH, Labosky DA et al, Upper extremity ischemic monomelic neuropathy: a complication of vascular access procedures in uremic diabetic patients. *Neurology* 1989; **39**: 997–8.

32. Caroll LL, Tzamaloukas AH, Scremin AE et al, Hand dysfunction in patients on chronic hemodialysis. *Int J Artif Organs* 1993; **16**: 694–9.

33. Tzamaloukas AH, Murata GH, Harford AM et al, Hand gangrene in diabetic patients on chronic dialysis. *ASAIO Trans* 1991; **37**: 638–43.

34. Nakamoto M, The mechanism of intradialytic hypotension in diabetic patients. *Nippon Jinzo Gakkai Shi/Jpn J Nephrol* 1994; **36**: 374–81.

35. Hampl H, Berweck S, Ludat K et al, How can hemodialysis associated hypotension and dialysis induced symptoms be explained and controlled, particularly in diabetic atherosclerotic patients? *Clin Nephrol* 2000; **53** (Suppl): S69–79.

36. Pelosi G, Emdin M, Carpeggiani C et al, Impaired sympathetic response before intradialytic hypotension: a study based on spectral analysis of heart rate and pressure variability. *Clin Sci* 1999; **96**: 23–31.

37. Straver B, de Vries PM, ten Voorde BJ et al, Intradialytic hypotension in relation to pre-existed autonomic dysfunction in

hemodialysis patients. *Int J Artif Organs* 1998; **21**: 794–801.

38. Cruz DN, Mahnensmith RL, Brickel HM et al, Midodrine and cool dialysate are effective therapies for symptomatic intradialytic hypotension. *Am J Kidney Dis* 1999; **33**: 920–6.

39. Maggiore Q, Pizzarelli F, Zoccalli C et al, Effects of extracorporeal blood cooling on dialytic arterial hypotension. *Proc Eur Dial Transplant Assoc* 1981; **28**: 686–9.

40. Anand V, Bastani B, Dhanraj JP et al, Intradialytic dobutamine therapy in hemodialysis patient with hypotension. *Am J Nephrol* 1999; **19**: 459–63.

41. Chantrel F, Enache I, Bouiller M et al, Abysmal prognosis of patients with type 2 diabetes entering dialysis. *Nephrol Dial Transplant* 1999; **14**: 129–36.

42. Weidmann P, Beretta-Piccoli C, Trost BN, Pressor factor and responsiveness in hypertension accompanying diabetes mellitus. *Hypertension* 1985; **7**: 1133–42.

43. Ditzel J, Lervang HH, Brochner-Mortensen J, Renal sodium metabolism in relation to hypertension in diabetes. *Diabete Metab* 1989; **15**(3 pt 2): 292–5.

44. Cheigh JS, Milite C, Sullivan JF et al, Hypertension is not adequately controlled in hemodialysis patients. *Am J Kidney Dis* 1992; **19**: 453–9.

45. Fishbane S, Natke E, Maesaka JK, Role of volume overload in dialysis-refractory hypertension. *Am J Kidney Dis* 1996; **28**: 257–61.

46. Woredekal Y, Berlyne BM, Barth RH, High interdialytic weight gain in diabetics on hemodialysis (HD): in search of causes. *J Am Soc Nephrol* 1994; **5**: 506 (abst).

47. Ifudu O, Dulin AL, Friedman EA, Interdialytic weight gain correlates with glycosylated hemoglobin in diabetic hemodialysis patients. *Am J Kidney Dis* 1994; **23**: 686–91.

48. Kimmel PL, Varela MP, Peterson RA et al, Interdialytic weight gain and survival in hemodialysis patients. Effects of duration of ESRD and diabetes mellitus. *Kidney Int* 2000; **57**: 1141–51.

49. Jaeger JQ, Mehta R, Assessment of dry weight in hemodialysis. An overview. *J Am Soc Nephrol* 1999; **10**: 392–403.

50. Kjellstrand C, Ting G, Daily hemodialysis: dialysis for next century. *Adv Renal Replace Ther* 1998; **5**: 267–74.

51. Biesenbach G, Debska-Slizien A, Zagomik J, Nutritional status in type 2 diabetic patients requiring hemodialysis. *Nephrol Dial Transplant* 1999; **14**: 655–8.

52. Horowitz M, Fraser R, Disordered gastric motor function in diabetes mellitus. *Diabetologia* 1994; **37**: 543–51.

53. Annese V, Bassotti G, Caruso N et al, Gastrointestinal motor dysfunction symptoms, and neuropathy in non-insulin dependent diabetes mellitus. *J Clin Gastroenterol* 1999; **29**: 171–7.

54. Clark DW, Nowak TV, Diabetic gastroparesis. What to do when gastric emptying is delayed. *Postgrad Med* 1994; **95**: 195–8.

55. Flynn CT, Nanson JA, Intraperitoneal insulin with CAPD. An artificial pancreas. *Trans Am Soc Artif Organs* 1979; **25**: 114–17.

56. Legrain M, Rottenbourg J, Bentchikou A et al, Dialysis treatment of insulin dependent diabetic patients. Ten years' experience. *Clin Nephrol* 1984; **21**: 72–81.

57. Rottenbourg J, Peritoneal dialysis in diabetics. In: *Peritoneal Dialysis* (Nolph KD, ed.). Martinus Nejhoff: Boston, 1985; 363–79.

58. Port FK, Wolfe RA, Mauger EA et al, Comparison of survival probabilities for dialysis patients versus cadaveric renal transplant recipients. *JAMA* 1993; **270**: 1339–43.

59. Maiorca R, Vonesh E, Cancarini GC et al, A six year comparison of patients and technique survival in CAPD and hemodialysis. *Kidney Int* 1988; **34**: 518–22.

60. Keane WF, Bailie GR, Boeschoten E et al, Adult Peritoneal Dialysis-Related Peritonitis Treatment Recommendations 2000 Update. *Perit Dial Int* 2000; **20**: 396–411.

61. Kameoka H, Dumakawa K, Matuoka T et al, Intraperitoneal flu-

conazole for fungal peritonitis in CAPD: report of two cases. *Perit Dial Int* 1999; **19:** 481–3.

62. Wang AY, Yu AW, Li PK et al, Factors predicting outcome of fungal peritonitis in peritoneal dialysis: analysis of a 9-year experience of fungal peritonitis in a single center. *Am J Kidney Dis* 2000; **36:** 183–92.

63. Blumenkrantz MJ, Gahl GM, Kopple JD et al, Diagnosis of protein calorie malnutrition in diabetic patients on hemodialysis and peritoneal dialysis. *Nephron* 1986; **42:** 133–40.

64. Held PJ, Port FK, Blagg CR et al, The United States Renal Data System Annual Data Report. *Am J Kidney Dis* 1990; **16** (Suppl 2): 34–43.

65. Siamopoulos KC, Elisaf MS, Bairaktari HT et al, Lipid parameters including lipoprotein (a) in patients undergoing CAPD and hemodialysis. *Perit Dial Int* 1995; **15:** 342–7.

66. Kimak E, Solski J, Janicka L et al, Concentration of Lp(a) and other apolipoproteins in predialysis, hemodialysis, continuous ambulatory peritoneal dialysis and post-transplant patients. *Clin Chem Lab Med* 2000; **38:** 421–5.

67. Attman PO, Samuelsson OG, Moberly J, Apolipoprotein B-containing lipoproteins in renal failure: the relation to mode of dialysis. *Kidney Int* 1999; **55:** 1536–42.

68. Little J, Phillips L, Russell L et al, Longitudinal lipid profiles on CAPD: their relationship to weight gain, comorbidity, and dialysis factors. *J Am Soc Nephrol* 1998; **9:** 1931–9.

69. Misra M, Webb AT, Reaveley DA et al, The effect of change of renal replacement therapy on serum lipoprotein (a) concentration. *Adv Perit Dial* 1997; **13:** 168–73.

70. Avram MM, Sreedhara R, Patel N et al, Is an elevated level of serum lipoprotein (a) a risk factor for cardiovascular disease in CAPD patients? *Adv Perit Dial* 1996; **12:** 266–71.

71. Misra M, Reaveley DA, Cooper C et al, Mechanism for elevated plasma lipoprotein (a) in patients on dialysis: turnover studies. *Adv Perit Dial* 1998; **14:** 223–7.

72. Akcicek F, Ok E, Duman S et al, Lipid-lowering effects of simvastatin and gemfibrozil in CAPD patients: a prospective crossover study. *Adv Perit Dial* 1996; **12:** 261–5.

73. Li PK, Mak TW, Lam CW et al, Lovastatin treatment of dyslipoproteinemia in patients on continuous ambulatory peritoneal dialysis. *Perit Dial Int* 1993; **13** (Suppl 2): S428–30.

74. Blake C, Codd MB, Cassidy A et al, Physical function, employment and quality of life in end stage renal disease. *J Nephrol* 2000; **13:** 142–9.

75. Lowder CM, Perri NA, Friedman EA, Demographics, diabetes type, and degree of rehabilitation in diabetic patients on maintenance hemodialysis in Brooklyn. *J Diabetes Complications* 1988; **2:** 227–32.

76. Delano BG, Suresh U, Feldman J et al, Dismal rehabilitation in predominantly type 2 diabetics on dialysis in inner city Brooklyn. *Clin Nephrol* 2000; **54:** 94–104.

77. Collins AL, Liao A, Umen A et al, Diabetic hemodialysis patients treated with a high KT/V have a lower risk of death than standard KT/V. *J Am Soc Nephrol* 1991; **2:** 318.

# 17

# Treatment of diabetic retinopathy in the patient with diabetic nephropathy

Ruth Axer-Siegel and Gad Dotan

## ASSOCIATION OF DIABETIC RETINOPATHY AND DIABETIC NEPHROPATHY

Diabetic retinopathy is the leading cause of new cases of blindness in persons aged 20–74 years in the USA.[1] It is present to some degree in nearly all patients who have type 1 (insulin-dependent) diabetes mellitus (DM) and in more than 60% of patients who have type 2 (non-insulin-dependent) DM for 20 years or more.[2,3] In the Wisconsin Epidemiologic Study of Diabetic Retinopathy (WESDR), at the 4-year follow-up of patients with older-onset diabetes, diabetic retinopathy was the sole or contributing cause of impaired vision in 69% of eyes in patients taking insulin and in 26% of eyes in the patients not taking insulin.[4]

Diabetes mellitus is also the leading underlying cause of end-stage renal disease (ESRD) in the USA.[5] Diabetic nephropathy develops in 35–45% of patients with type 1 DM, with peak occurence between 10 and 15 years after onset of the disease. The risk in patients who do not have proteinuria after 20–25 years is only about 1% per year. The rate of diabetic nephropathy in type 2 DM is 20–34%. Patients with type 2 DM and microalbuminuria are at a 20–40% risk of clinical proteinuria after 10–15 years, often with deterioration to ESRD. Overall, 20–40% of patients with type 1 DM and 10–20% with type 2 DM will develop ESRD.[5]

Diabetic patients with renal disease, as evidenced by proteinuria, elevated blood urea nitrogen, and elevated blood creatinine, nearly always present with retinopathy. Even patients with microalbuminuria are at high risk. However, only 35% of patients with symptomatic retinopathy have signs of renal disease. Severe retinopathy is associated with cardiovascular disease, stroke, diabetic nephropathy, and amputation.[6]

The physiological factors that govern the development of diabetic retinopathy include increased intravascular hydrostatic pressure with altered autoregulation of vascular flow, and impairment of the blood-retinal barrier, which leads to increased vascular permeability. These hemodynamic abnormalities in the retina are analogous to those that occur in the kidney in an earlier stage of diabetes; that is, increased renal blood flow and increased glomerular permeability with resultant albuminuria.[7] Moreover, vascular endothelial growth factor (VEGF), which induces vascular endothelial cell proliferation, migration, and vasopermeability in many cells and tissues, has been identified as a primary initiator of proliferative diabetic retinopathy (PDR) and is a potential mediator of nonproliferative retinopathy (NPDR). VEGF has also been implicated in the development of neuropathy and nephropathy in the diabetic patient.[8]

## RISK FACTORS FOR RETINOPATHY

Age at diagnosis, puberty, duration of diabetes, quality of metabolic control, serum lipid level, hypertension, and proteinuria and nephropathy are risk factors for the development and progression of diabetic retinopathy.

### Patient age and duration of disease

The frequency and severity of retinopathy increase with the duration of diabetes in populations with both younger and older onset of disease.[2,3] In a cohort of 10 709 patients with diabetes, coronary heart disease was present in 25.2%, cerebrovascular disease in 9.6%, complications of diabetic foot in

18.1%, retinopathy in 16.5%, and nephropathy in 2.0%. All complications were related to both patient age and duration of diabetes, although duration was particularly predictive of the microvascular complications (retinopathy and nephropathy).[9]

Long-standing diabetes, irrespective of type, is a high risk factor for the development of diabetic maculopathy. The close association of maculopathy with diabetic nephropathy and neuropathy, and with several atherosclerotic risk factors, suggests that these may play a role in its pathogenesis.[10]

## Hyperglycemia and quality of metabolic control

Data from epidemiological studies demonstrate a strong relationship between hyperglycemia and the development or progression of diabetic retinopathy. In the WESDR, the glycosylated hemoglobin ($HbA_{1c}$) level at baseline was found to be a significant predictor of the 4- and 10-year incidence of the development and progression of retinopathy, the progression to PDR, and the incidence of macular edema in patients with younger-onset DM (diagnosis before 30 years of age) and in patients with older-onset DM, taking or not taking insulin.[11,12] Other studies have shown that both retinopathy and nephropathy were directly related to higher fasting or 2-hr plasma glucose, and that fasting plasma glucose can predict both microvascular disease and mortality.[13]

The insulin resistance of type 2 DM was found to be closely associated with the progression of the microangiopathies. Advanced retinopathy (preproliferative and proliferative) was observed more frequently in insulin-resistant than insulin-sensitive patients (p < 0.02), as were also proteinuria and nephropathy (p < 0.01). Furthermore, insulin resistance was significantly more severe in patients with both retinopathy and nephropathy than in patients free of these microangiopathies (p < 0.01).[14]

The relationship between stringent glycemic control, expressed as $HbA_{1c}$ level, and the risk of development and progression of retinopathy or nephropathy in patients with type 1 DM was demonstrated in the Diabetes Control and Complications Trial (DCCT).[15–17] The reduced risk of progression persisted for at least 4 years, despite increasing hyperglycemia.[18] Accordingly, the United Kingdom Prospective Diabetes Study (UKPDS) reported a significantly reduced risk of progression of retinopathy also in patients with type 2 DM who received intensive treatment with either a sulfonylurea or insulin.[19] The Kumamoto study reported that the risk of both types of microvascular complications in patients with type 2 DM increased dramatically as $HbA_{1c}$ levels exceeded 8%.[20] Finally, in a meta-analysis of 16 clinical trials, Wand et al[21] showed that the risk of retinopathy progression was higher in the first 6–12 months of intensive glycemic control, but then decreased significantly after 2 years or more. Therefore, patients maintaining tight glycemic control should be followed very closely.

## Serum lipids

Data from epidemiological studies suggest a relationship between serum lipids and the presence, development, or progression of diabetic retinopathy. Patients with elevated total cholesterol and low-density lipoprotein cholesterol are much more likely to have severe, hard exudates in the macula,[22,23] and this correlates strongly with visual loss. High levels of triglycerides were also associated with increased progression of retinopathy and greater risk of developing PDR.[22]

## Hypertension

Hypertension significantly accelerates the onset of proliferative retinopathy and may result in hypertensive retinopathy superimposed on diabetic retinopathy. Apparently, the increased blood pressure, through its effect on blood flow, damages the retinal capillary endothelial cells. Even minor elevations in blood pressure increase the risk of hemorrhage and exudates in NPDR.[24] In the WESDR, diastolic blood pressure was a significant predictor of the 14-year progression of diabetic retinopathy and incidence of PDR in patients with younger-onset type 1 DM.[25]

The UKPDS found that in hypertensive patients with type 2 DM, tight control of blood pressure with either the angiotensin-converting enzyme (ACE) inhibitor captopril or the beta-blocker atenolol resulted in a 35% reduction in retinal photocoagulation compared to conventional controls.[26] At the 7.5-year follow-up, there was a 34% reduction in the rate of progression of retinopathy and a 47% reduction in the deterioration of visual acuity by three lines or more. The effect was largely due to a reduction in the incidence of diabetic macular edema. These findings strongly support tight blood-pressure control in patients with type 2 DM to prevent visual loss.[26] While atenolol and captopril were equally effective in the UKPDS in reducing the risk of developing these microvascular complications in persons with newly diagnosed type 2 DM,[26] other clinical trials have shown that the type of antihypertensive drug may be important in patients with type 1 DM.

Data from the EURODIAB Controlled Trial of Lisinopril in Insulin-Dependent Diabetes Mellitus (EUCLID) showed that lisinopril decreased the progression of retinopathy by two or more grades, and the progression to proliferative retinopathy.[27] Retinopathy progressed by at least one level in 13.2% of the 150 patients receiving lisinopril compared to 23.4% of the 166 patients receiving placebo. This 50% reduction remained constant even when controlling for center and glycemic control. Progression was not associated with albuminuric status at baseline, and there was no increase in hyperglycemic status. However, patients with better glycemic control benefited more. Lisinopril may also decrease the progression of the renal disease in normotensive patients with type 1 DM and little or no nephropathy. These findings suggest that ACE inhibitors are a powerful tool to prevent progression of microalbuminuria in diabetes, and that they may prove useful as an adjunctive therapy to intensified insulin in preventing the development of microalbuminuria and the progression of retinopathy in type 1 DM.[27]

## Proteinuria and nephropathy

Data from most studies suggest an association between the prevalence of diabetic nephropathy, as manifested by microalbuminuria or gross proteinuria, and retinopathy.[28,29] Patients with increased albumin secretion were found to have a statistically significant increase in frequency of retinopathy—PDR in particular—with increasing levels of urinary albumin excretion.[30]

Rheologic, lipid and platelet abnormalities associated with nephropathy may be involved in the pathogenesis of retinopathy. Moreover, the elevated fibrinogen level which exists at the early stage of microangiopathy has been shown to be significantly associated with diabetic retinopathy and nephropathy.[31]

## DIALYSIS IN PATIENTS WITH DIABETIC RETINOPATHY

Data from case series show that visual function can be preserved in most patients with type 1 DM treated by hemodialysis. In a study by El Shahat et al,[32] of 46 eyes of 23 patients with preserved vision at the start

of hemodialysis, stabilization was achieved in 74% and improvement in 7%; two patients became blind. The aggravation of visual function was related mainly to the development of PDR, and not to the hemodialysis. In another study, visual function was prospectively compared in 112 patients with type 1 DM, studied chronologically, of whom 63% were treated with hemodialysis and 37% with peritoneal dialysis.[33] Preservation of vision correlated well with overall control of blood pressure in both groups. Loss of vision was independent of the dialysis modality, glucose control, and time of onset (young/old) of diabetes.

In a prospective fluorescein angiography study of 40 eyes of 22 patients with diabetic macular edema and ESRD, at 4 weeks after initiation of hemodialysis, macular leakage was unchanged in 70%, decreased in 10% and increased in 20% from baseline. These results indicate that hemodialysis does not benefit macular leakage in diabetic patients with ESRD.[34]

Regarding vitreoretinal surgery, studies show that renal failure and hemodialysis apparently have no deteriorative influence on the outcome of vitrectomy for PDR. In a series of 76 eyes of 66 patients, no uncontrollable hemorrhage occurred either during or immediately after surgery. Final visual acuity after surgery was the same as the preoperative visual acuity in 31.5% of eyes; improvement was seen in 60.5% of eyes.[35]

Together, these data indicate that careful ophthalmic follow-up, together with close control of diabetes, blood pressure and uremia, can promote preservation of vision in most insulin-dependent diabetic patients treated by dialysis.

## RENAL AND PANCREAS TRANSPLANTATION IN PATIENTS WITH DIABETIC RETINOPATHY

Patients with uremia due to diabetic nephropathy have a high prevalence of severe PDR and blindness at the time of presentation for kidney and pancreas transplantation. In most diabetic patients, retinopathy remains stable or improves after kidney transplantation, but regular ophthalmologic follow-up is important to detect eyes in which further laser treatment may be indicated.[36] Patients with renal failure may benefit from combined pancreatic and kidney transplantation (SPK). A high proportion of patients managed with SPK have advanced diabetic retinopathy as a consequence of long duration of type 1 DM and the presence of ESRD. In a series of 54 patients, Chow et al[37] found that uremic patients with diabetic nephropathy had a high prevalence of severe proliferative diabetic retinopathy and blindness at the time of presentation for SPK, but these subsequently stabilized to inactive PDR with appropriate laser therapy and the metabolic control achieved by the transplant. Similarly, Pearce et al[38] reported that more than 90% of their 20 patients after SPK had stable diabetic retinopathy.

The impact of SPK on the progression of advanced diabetic retinopathy was evaluated by Wang et al.[39] Fifty-one patients with type 1 DM after SPK were compared with 21 patients after kidney transplantation only. After 1 year, the combined transplantation group showed a nonsignificant benefit in overall progression of the retinopathy. In a similar study, Koznarova et al[40] reported that in the SPK group ($n = 45$), funduscopic findings at the end of follow-up were improved in 21.3%, stabilized in 61.7% or worsened in 17.0%. The respective figures for the kidney-transplant group were 6.1%, 48.8%, and 45.1% ($p < 0.001$). These differences were maintained even at 3 years after transplantation. Furthermore, before transplantation, 78% of the SPK group and 81% of the kidney-transplant group had been treated by laser. The need for additional laser therapy after transplantation was significantly lower in the SPK group (31% vs 58%, $p < 0.001$). The authors concluded that pancreas transplantation exerts a beneficial effect on the course of diabetic retinopathy even in its late stage.

## OCULAR COMPLICATIONS OF RENAL FAILURE, HEMODIALYSIS, AND RENAL TRANSPLANTATION

### Vascular lesions

Diabetic patients with renal failure on renal dialysis or after renal transplantation are at risk of developing additional ocular complications owing to the chronic hypertension and hyperlipidemia associated with kidney disease. These patients are also at risk of drug-induced side effects and complications of dialysis and kidney transplantation.

In addition to the previously discussed complications of hypertensive retinopathy or aggravation of diabetic retinopathy, macular edema, and PDR, in patients with malignant hypertension, ischemic changes may occur in the retina, choroid, and optic nerve, producing cotton-wool spots, flame-shaped hemorrhages, hard exudates, exudative retinal detachment, papilledema, or optic atrophy. In patients with severe and long-standing hypertension,

a sudden relative drop in arterial pressure may cause infarction of the optic nerve and blindness. Anterior ischemic optic neuropathy and retinal infarction have also been described as complications of hemodialysis-associated hypertension.[41]

Uremia, anemia, and papilledema of intracranial hypertension are other risk factors for optic neuropathy in patients with chronic renal diseases. In addition, patients with chronic hypertension are predisposed to retinal arterial and venous obstructive diseases.

Sudden blindness due to Purtscher's-like vaso-occlusive retinopathy, with or without central nervous symptoms, may occur in patients with chronic renal failure, in patients receiving hemodialysis and in renal transplant recipients after allograft rejection.[42]

### Serous retinal detachment

Serous retinal detachment, resembling central serous chorioretinopathy, may occur after organ transplantation or during hemodialysis.[43] In the severe form, bilateral bullous retinal detachment, multiple retinal pigment epithelial detachments, and yellow fibrin-like subretinal exudates beneath the sensory retinal detachment may be observed. Precipitating factors include impaired fluid and electrolyte balance, choroidopathy associated with systemic hypertension, thrombotic microangiopathy, immune complex vasculitis, and dysfunction of the overlying retinal pigment epithelium, which may be influenced by stress and immunosuppressive therapy. In some cases, treatment with photocoagulation is successful. In most patients, the detachments resolve with normalization of visual acuity at the time of remission of the thrombotic microangiopathy, but blindness may rarely occur due to ischemic ocular changes.[44]

### Glaucoma and cataract

Intraocular pressure may rise during hemodialysis and cause acute glaucoma in susceptible patients with increased resistance of aqueous outflow. Corticosteroids can also induce glaucoma, and corticosteroid-induced posterior subcapsular cataract is common in renal transplant patients.

## Infectious and neoplastic processes

Both infectious and neoplastic processes are more common in renal transplant recipients and other immunocompromised patients, and may affect the ocular and periocular tissues. Necrotizing retinitis is the most frequent severe ocular complication and is usually caused by cytomegalovirus, and rarely by herpes simplex or herpes zoster with or without associated keratitis. In addition to viral infections, numerous bacterial and fungal organisms have been associated with endophthalmitis in renal transplant patients.[45]

## TREATMENT

Patients with diabetic nephropathy should be examined by an ophthalmologist at least once a year, and more frequently in the presence of severe hypertension and albuminuria, because of the risk of diabetic retinopathy. Laser photocoagulation is warranted for diabetic retinopathy. Patients with clinically significant macular edema should receive focal laser treatment, and patients with severe NPDR or PDR should be treated by panretinal photocoagulation. Photocoagulation is not contraindicated in patients who take anticoagulants and is safe in dialyzed patients with well-controlled blood pressure.

Despite preventive measures and timely treatment, a substantial number of patients still develop complications of progressive retinopathy and may become candidates for vitrectomy. The indications for vitrectomy are mainly nonclearing vitreous and premacular hemorrhage and retinal detachment. Renal failure and hemodialysis do not appear to have deteriorative influence on the outcome of vitrectomy for proliferative diabetic retinopathy.

Because of their efficacy as antihypertensive agents and demonstrated benefit in retarding the progression of diabetic nephropathy, ACE inhibitors are recommended as the primary treatment for all hypertensive diabetic patients with microalbuminuria, overt albuminuria, or diabetic nephropathy. In normotensive patients with type 1 DM, the optimal time to initiate treatment with an ACE inhibitor is not clear, although some researchers recommend doing so when microalbuminuria is evident. In patients with type 2 DM, the benefits of ACE inhibitors have not been completely established. However, on the basis of the results in patients with type 1 DM or other types of chronic renal insufficiency, their use in patients with type 2 DM is reasonable.

Since PDR is an important indicator for increased risk of ischemic heart disease, stroke, diabetic nephropathy and amputation, affected patients should be monitored for heart disease. Overall, maintenance of euglycemia, and blood pressure of at least 130/85 mmHg, use of ACE inhibitors in patients with microalbuminuria, close management of hyperlipidemia, and education of patients to stop smoking will most likely prevent or slow the progression of diabetic nephropathy, and can reduce extrarenal vascular injury as well.

Patients treated with dialysis should receive careful ophthalmic follow-up together with close control of diabetes, blood pressure and uremia in order to ensure preservation of vision. Advanced diabetic retinopathy is present in a high proportion of cases managed with kidney transplantation or SPK as a consequence of the duration of type 1 DM and the presence of ESRD. In most diabetic patients, retinopathy remains stable or improves after kidney transplantation and SPK. However, regular ophthalmological follow-up is important for early detection of eyes which need further laser treatment or vitreoretinal surgery, as well as the timely diagnosis of possible complications such as glaucoma, cataract, retinitis and other opportunistic infections.

## REFERENCES

1. Klein R, Klein BEK, Vision disorders in diabetes. In: National Diabetes Data Group. *Diabetes in America: Diabetes Data Compiled 1984* (NIH Publ No 85–1468). US Department of Health and Human Services: Bethesda, MD, 1985; 1-2.
2. Klein R, Klein BEK, Moss SE et al, The Wisconsin Epidemiologic Study of Diabetic Retinopathy. II. Prevalence and risk of diabetic retinopathy when age at diagnosis is less than 30 years. *Arch Ophthalmol* 1984; **102**: 520–6.
3. Klein R, Klein BEK, Moss SE et al, The Wisconsin Epidemiologic Study of Diabetic Retinopathy. III. Prevalence and risk of diabetic retinopathy when age at diagnosis is 30 or more years. *Arch Ophthalmol* 1984; **102**: 527–32.
4. Moss SE, Klein R, Klein BEK, The incidence of vision loss in a diabetic population. *Ophthalmology* 1988; **95**: 1340–8.
5. FitzSimmons SC, Newman JM, Katz PP et al, The natural history and epidemiology of diabetic nephropathy. Implications for prevention and control. *JAMA* 1990; **263**: 1954–60.
6. Klein R, Moss SE, Klein BEK et al, Relation of ocular and systemic factors to survival in diabetes. *Arch Intern Med* 1989; **149**: 266–72.
7. Gardner TW, Leith E, Antonetti DA et al, A new hypothesis on mechanisms of retinal vascular permeability in diabetes. In: *The Diabetic Renal-Retinal Syndrome*, 6th edn (Friedman EA, L'Esperance FA, eds.). Kluwer: Dordrecht, Netherlands, 1998; 169–79.
8. Aiello LP, Wong JS, Role of vascular endothelial growth factor in diabetic vascular complications. *Kidney Int* 2000; **58**: S113–19.

9. Morgan CL, Currie CJ, Stott NC et al, The prevalence of multiple diabetes-related complications. *Diabetic Med* 2000; **17:** 146–51.

10. Zander E, Herfurth S, Bohl B et al, Maculopathy in patients with diabetes mellitus type 1 and type 2: associations with risk factors. *Br J Ophthalmol* 2000; **84:** 871–6.

11. Klein R, Moss SE, Klein BEK et al, The Wisconsin Epidemiologic Study of Diabetic Retinopathy. XI. The incidence of macular edema. *Ophthalmology* 1989; **96:** 1501–10.

12. Klein R, Klein BEK, Moss SE et al, Relationship of hyperglycemia to the long-term incidence and progression of diabetic retinopathy. *Arch Intern Med* 1994; **154:** 2169–78.

13. Gabir MM, Hanson RL, Dabelea D et al, Plasma glucose and prediction of microvascular disease and mortality: evaluation of 1997 American Diabetes Association and 1999 World Health Organization criteria for diagnosis of diabetes. *Diabetes Care* 2000; **23:** 1113–18.

14. Suzuki M, Kanazawa A, Shiba M et al, Insulin resistance in diabetic microangiopathies. *J Diabetes Complications* 2000; **14:** 40–5.

15. Diabetes Control and Complications Trial Research Group, The effect of intensive treatment of diabetes on the development and progression of long-term complications in insulin-dependent diabetes mellitus. *N Engl J Med* 1993; **329:** 977–86.

16. Diabetes Control and Complications Trial Research Group, Effect of intensive therapy on the development and progression of diabetic nephropathy in the Diabetes Control and Complications Trial. *Kidney Int* 1995; **47:** 1703–20.

17. Diabetes Control and Complications Trial Research Group, Effect of intensive diabetes treatment on nerve conduction in the Diabetes Control and Complications Trial. *Ann Neurol* 1995; **38:** 869–80.

18. The Diabetes Control and Complications Trial/Epidemiology of Diabetes Interventions and Complications Research Group, Retinopathy and nephropathy in patients with type 1 diabetes four years after trial of intensive therapy. *N Engl J Med* 2000; **342:** 381–9.

19. UK Prospective Diabetes Study Group, Intensive blood-glucose control with sulfonyl-ureas or insulin compared with conventional treatment and risk of complications in patients with type 2 diabetes, UKPDS 33. *Lancet* 1998; **352:** 837–53.

20. Ohkubo Y, Kishikawa H, Araki E et al, Intensive insulin therapy prevents the progression of diabetic microvascular complications in Japanese patients with non-insulin-dependent diabetes mellitus: a randomized prospective 6-year study. *Diabetes Res Clin Pract* 1995; **28:** 103–17.

21. Wand PH, Lau J, Chalmers TC, Meta-analysis of effects of intensive blood-glucose control on late complications of type I diabetes. *Lancet* 1993; **341:** 1306–9.

22. Chew EY, Klein ML, Ferris FL III et al, Association of elevated serum lipid levels with retinal hard exudate in diabetic retinopathy, ETDRS Report No. 22. *Arch Ophthalmol* 1996; **114:** 1079–84.

23. Klein BEK, Moss SE, Klein R et al, The Wisconsin Epidemiologic Study of Diabetic Retinopathy. XIII. Relationship of serum cholesterol to retinopathy and hard exudate. *Ophthalmology* 1991; **98:** 1261–5.

24. Knowler WC, Bennett PH, Ballintine EJ, Increased incidence of retinopathy in diabetes with elevated blood pressure. *N Engl J Med* 1980; **302:** 645–50.

25. Klein R, Klein BEK, Moss SE et al, The Wisconsin Epidemiologic Study of Diabetic Retinopathy. XVII. The 14-year incidence and progression of diabetic retinopathy and associated risk factors in type 1 diabetes. *Ophthalmology* 1998; **105:** 1801–15.

26. UK Prospective Diabetes Study Group, Tight blood pressure control and risk of macrovascular and microvascular complications in type 2 diabetes. UKPDS38. *BMJ* 1998; **317:** 703–13.

27. Chaturvedi N, Sjolie AK, Stephenson JM et al, Effect of lisinopril on progression of retinopathy in normotensive people with type 1 diabetes: The EUCLID Study Group, EURODIAB Controlled Trial of Lisinopril in Insulin-Dependent Diabetes Mellitus. *Lancet* 1997; **351:** 28–31.

28. Cruikshanks KJ, Ritter LL, Klein R et al, The association of microalbuminuria with diabetic retinopathy: the Wisconsin Epidemiologic Study of Diabetic Retinopathy. *Ophthalmology* 1993; **100:** 862–7.

29. Klein R, Moss SE, Klein BEK, Is gross proteinuria a risk factor for the incidence of proliferative retinopathy? *Ophthalmology* 1993; **100:** 1140–6.

30. Johansen J, Sjokie AK, Exhoj O, The relation between retinopathy and albumin excretion rate in insulin-dependent diabetes mellitus. From the Funene County Epidemiology of Type 1 Diabetes Complications Survey. *Acta Ophthalmologica* 1994; **72:** 347–51.

31. Asakawa H, Tokunaga K, Kawakami F, Elevation of fibrinogen and thrombin-antithrombin III complex levels of type 2 diabetes mellitus patients with retinopathy and nephropathy. *J Diabetes Complications* 2000; **14:** 121–6.

32. El Shahat Y, Rottembourg J, Bellio P et al, Visual function can be preserved in insulin-dependent diabetic patients treated by maintenance haemodialysis. *Proc Eur Dial Transplant Assoc* 1980; **17:** 167–72.

33. Diaz-Buxo JA, Burgess WP, Greenman M et al, Visual function in diabetic patients undergoing dialysis: comparison of peritoneal and hemodialysis. *Int J Artif Organs* 1984; **7:** 257–62.

34. Tokuyama T, Ikeda T, Sato K, Effects of haemodialysis on diabetic macular leakage. *Br J Ophthalmol* 2000; **84:** 1397–1400.

35. Hayashi H, Kurata Y, Imanaga Y et al, Vitrectomy for diabetic retinopathy in patients undergoing hemodialysis for associated end-stage renal failure. *Retina* 1998; **18:** 156–9.

36. Laatikainen L, Summanen P, Ekstrand A et al, Ophthalmological follow-up of diabetic patients after kidney transplantation. *Ger J Ophthalmol* 1993; **2:** 24–7.

37. Chow VC, Pai RP, Chapman JR et al, Diabetic retinopathy after combined kidney-pancreas transplantation. *Clin Transplant* 1999; **13:** 356–62.

38. Pearce IA, Ilango B, Sells RA et al, Stabilisation of diabetic retinopathy following simultaneous pancreas and kidney transplant. *Br J Ophthalmol* 2000; **84:** 736–40.

39. Wang Q, Klein R, Moss SE et al, The influence of combined kidney-pancreas transplantation on the progression of diabetic retinopathy. A case series. *Ophthalmology* 1994; **101:** 1071–6.

40. Koznarova R, Saudek F, Sosna T et al, Beneficial effect of pancreas and kidney transplantation on advanced diabetic retinopathy. *Cell Transplant* 2000; **9:** 903–8.

41. Hamed LM, Winward KE, Glaser JS et al, Optic neuropathy in uremia. *Am J Ophthalmol* 1989; **108:** 30–5.

42. Stoumbos VD, Klein ML, Goodman S, Purtscher's-like retinopathy in chronic renal failure. *Ophthalmology* 1992; **99:** 1833–9.

43. Friberg TR, Eller AW, Serous retinal detachment resembling central serous chorioretinopathy following organ transplantation. *Graefes Arch Clin Exp Ophthalmol* 1990; **228:** 305–9.

44. Gass JDM, Bullous retinal detachment and multiple retinal pigment epithelial detachments in patients receiving hemodialysis. *Graefes Arch Clin Exp Ophthalmol* 1992; 230:454–8.

45. Leys AM, The eye and renal diseases. In: *Duane's Clinical Ophthalmology*. Lippincott Williams and Wilkins: Philadelphia, PA, 1999; 1–10.

# 18

# Treatment of diabetic foot and peripheral vascular disease in patients with diabetic nephropathy

Paul G McNally and Nick London

## INTRODUCTION

Diabetes mellitus is a common cause of end-stage renal failure, and by the time renal disease develops, most patients invariably have evidence of neuropathy, foot ulceration, peripheral vascular disease and small and large vessel vascular injury elsewhere. Attention to lower limb arterial disease and the presence of neuropathy is often neglected, and particularly so in asymptomatic patients. It should be remembered that by the time diabetic nephropathy develops, peripheral neuropathy and peripheral vascular disease are already advanced in many patients. Assessing the contribution made by neuropathy or ischaemia is vitally important because their management strategies differ.[1,2] All patients with renal disease secondary to diabetes should be examined on a regular and thorough basis with regard to potential lower limb and foot complications. For many patients, swift identification of the foot at risk will prevent significant morbidity and mortality in the future and will help to maintain their quality of life, in terms of a lower risk of foot ulceration and amputation procedures. Unfortunately, a significant number of amputations are either unnecessary or unnecessarily aggressive, but the establishment of multidisciplinary foot clinics has helped reduce the number of major amputations by more than half.[3,4] This chapter will discuss a practical approach to identifying patients with diabetic renal disease at risk of these complications.

## EPIDEMIOLOGY

Foot ulceration and lower limb amputation are leading causes of morbidity and mortality for all patients with diabetes. More days are spent in hospital as a direct consequence of foot problems than for any other complication associated with diabetes, and this complication carries a heavy economic burden for both patients and health-care systems. The incidence of diabetic foot ulcers is up to 5% per annum, with a prevalence of up to 10%.[5–7] The cumulative incidence of amputations in type 1 and type 2 patients with diabetes is in the region of 15%,[8,9] with approximately three-quarters of all diabetes-related amputations being preceded by an ulcer.[1–3] For patients with diabetes and end-stage renal failure, the incidence of foot complications (including amputations) is considerably higher (25%) than in those without end-stage renal failure (10%).[10] In patients with type 2 diabetes undergoing haemodialysis, the figures are rather more depressing. A German study reported that 16% of patients with type 2 diabetes undergoing haemodialysis had a prior history of amputation, while 44% were found to have evidence of peripheral vascular disease.[11] Other groups have shown that up to two-thirds of patients with diabetes entering renal replacement programmes have clinical evidence of peripheral neuropathy.[12] Pugh et al recorded a diagnosis of peripheral neuropathy in 84% of patients with type 1 diabetes and in 60% of those with type 2 diabetes at the start of renal replacement therapy. Evidence of peripheral neuropathy was found also in two-thirds of patients with established nephropathy (mean serum creatinine of 178 μmol/l) secondary to type 1 diabetes.[13]

Various risk factors contribute to the development of diabetic foot ulcers, including long duration of diabetes, peripheral neuropathy (sensory, motor and autonomic), peripheral vascular disease, glycaemic control, foot deformity, limited joint mobility, increased plantar foot pressure, prior foot ulceration, prior amputation, higher body weight, poor vision and minor trauma.[1,2,10,14–20] Recurrent ulceration is generally found in patients with worsening peripheral sensory neuropathy, poor diabetes control, delayed presentation to carers and a tendency to consume more alcohol.[21] Risk factors for amputation are similar and include long duration of diabetes, neuropathy and peripheral vascular disease, poor diabetes control, a history of ulceration or prior amputation, retinopathy and inadequate patient education.[15–17,22,23] Despite the presence of these known risk factors, the outcomes for patients with diabetes and foot complications vary across centres. For example, there is a wide variation in age-adjusted amputation rates for non-traumatic lower limb amputation in diabetes.[24–28] These studies show a six-fold difference in amputation rates, ranging from 2.1/1000 to 13.7/1000 patients. The disparity in amputation rates is more than likely to indicate differences in clinical practice rather than intrinsic differences in the nature of the disease. There is no doubt that preventative measures and a multidisciplinary approach to the management of diabetic foot problems improve outcome. Protective factors identified include provision of diabetes education for patients,[29] the use of aspirin[17] and multidisciplinary foot services.[3,4]

## FACTORS ASSOCIATED WITH DIABETIC FOOT PROBLEMS AND PERIPHERAL VASCULAR DISEASE

### Neuropathy

Loss of protective sensation as a consequence of peripheral neuropathy is the most important factor leading to foot ulceration and amputation. Neuropathy presents in many ways, but the most common pattern is a chronic, distal, symmetrical sensorimotor polyneuropathy. Up to half of older type 2 patients with diabetes have significant sensory impairment.[1,30–32] Chronic sensorimotor neuropathy is often unnoticed by the patient, but in the early stages symptoms may be present, including paraesthesia, numbness, and sharp, stabbing, shooting and burning pains, which are often worst at night. The absence of symptoms may be associated with severe sensory loss. Sensory neuropathy often involves both sides in a symmetrical distribution, affecting feet more than hands. Motor neuropathy may result in muscle loss or wasting, and foot deformities, which precipitate abnormally high plantar foot pressures.[33] Abnormally high pressures are frequently transmitted through the metatarsal heads, and patients with neuropathy have significantly higher foot pressures than those without neuropathy.[34] The presence of autonomic neuropathy compounds matters by leading to the development of arterial shunts on the plantar surface of the foot, resulting in a redirection of blood flow away from the nutrient capillaries and the skin, and a decrease in transcutaneous oxygen concentration.[35] Loss of autonomic control also affects pseudomotor function, leading to the foot's becoming dry, cracked and fissured, a condition which may act as a portal for infective bacteria. Other causes of neuropathy may occur in patients with diabetes and need to be considered, including alcohol abuse, renal failure, drugs and vitamin B deficiency.

Loss of protective sensation predisposes the feet to repeated episodes of unnoticed trauma, formation of callus, and blisters. Damaging tight footwear may not be perceived as so by the patient, who tolerates badly fitted shoes. Puncture wounds may develop due to walking barefoot and stepping on drawing pins or nails. Foreign objects are extremely common in shoes, and it is imperative that patients keenly inspect their footwear prior to daily wearing. Burns are common in patients with insensitive feet who use hot-water bottles or rest their feet against radiators or close to open fires (Figure 18.1). Painless mechanical trauma and high plantar pressure are the most common reasons for developing ulceration in diabetic foot problems. Callus develops over areas of high pressure, and typically, in these areas, ulcer formation follows (Figure 18.2). Poorly fitting shoes may accelerate the build-up of callus, which may undergo ischaemic pressure necrosis and ulceration. Removal of callus is associated with around a 35–40% reduction in peak plantar pressures.[36]

### Foot deformity and Charcot's arthropathy

Foot deformities are common and develop for a variety of reasons. Motor neuropathy leads to an imbalance of the intrinsic muscles of the foot, which allows the development of claw toe. The dorsal surface of the claw toe often rubs against the under-surface toe area of the shoe, causing ulceration, or else the protective fat pad beneath the metatarsophalangeal joint

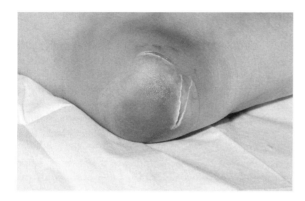

**Figure 18.1** Hot-water bottle heel injury in a patient with neuropathic feet.

ple joints. This deformity is better known as Charcot's foot or Charcot's arthropathy.

In the early stages, the patient often presents with a markedly swollen foot, crammed into ordinary footwear. This acute Charcot's arthropathy typically presents as a hot, erythematous and swollen foot, which may not be abnormally shaped or grossly deformed. This presentation makes acute Charcot's arthropathy difficult to differentiate from cellulitis. Although the foot is neuropathic and pulses are generally easily palpable, acute Charcot's arthropathy may be painful or uncomfortable. The foot typically feels warm and appears erythematous and dry to touch. Measurement of skin temperature may reveal a gradient of 2–5° compared to the contralateral foot.[37] Radiology in the acute stages may reveal no bony abnormality but later may show gross changes.

In time, the arthropathy will progress to chronic Charcot's foot, which is typically painless and grossly deformed (Figure 18.3). Ulceration develops

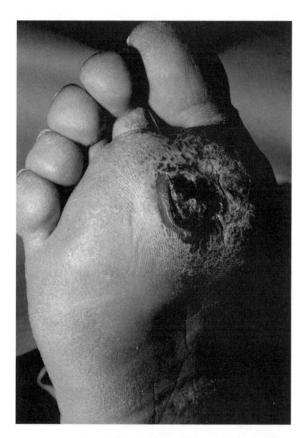

**Figure 18.2** Marked callus formation over metatarsal heads in a patient with neuropathic feet.

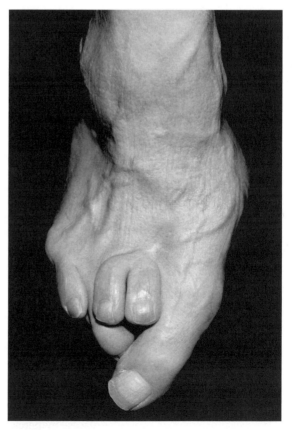

**Figure 18.3** Typical Charcot's arthropathy showing a grossly deformed and painless foot.

is pulled out of position, exposing this area to high plantar pressures and ulceration. Other patients develop progressive and destructive arthropathy, which is typically painless, affecting single or multi-

over areas of high pressure as a consequence of the abnormally shaped foot, or else as a complication of mild trauma due to footwear or puncture wounds. The pathogenesis of this arthropathy is attributable to neuropathy and repeated trauma. Not only is there loss of peripheral sensation and motor function, but also damage to the autonomic peripheral nerves leads to bone arteriovenous shunting, hypovascularity and demineralization.[38,39] The demineralization is assumed to lead to weakening of the bone, and the foot is at high risk of fracture injury and further joint distortion. Insensitive joints are subjected to their extreme ranges of motions, leading to joint effusions and instability. In the early stages, minimal deformity is present, but with time, mid-talar joint collapse with developing rocker bottom deformity becomes evident. Ankle neuroarthropathy may lead to gross deformity with joint fusions, subluxations and crepitus.

## Arterial disease

Diabetes accelerates the initiation and propagation of vascular disease such that 84% of diabetic patients who live for longer than 20 years after the diagnosis will have some form of vascular disease, and peripheral vascular disease is up to three times more common than in non-diabetics.[40] The basic pathophysiology of atherosclerosis in diabetes is probably no different from that in non-diabetic patients; however, some of the risk factors are more prevalent in the diabetic population. It has been shown that, compared to non-diabetics with peripheral vascular disease, diabetic patients with peripheral vascular disease are twice as likely to have disease of the distal popliteal or tibial vessels.[41] However, there is no evidence that diabetic patients suffer from more macrovascular disease of the pedal vessels. Indeed, Conrad[42] demonstrated that the pedal vessels of diabetic patients were less frequently affected with atheroma than those of non-diabetics. Nor is there any evidence to support the widely held concept of obliterative microvascular or 'small vessel' disease of the diabetic foot. There is evidence, however, for reduced microvascular hyperaemia, impaired, posturally induced vasoconstriction and maldistribution of cutaneous blood flow. These functional microvascular abnormalities are thought to result from neuropathy and/or proximal macrovascular disease. Importantly, it has been shown that these functional microvascular abnormalities can improve after correction of proximal macrovascular disease by percutaneous transluminal angioplasty or bypass surgery.[43]

## Infection

Foot infections commonly occur in association with neuropathy and ischaemia and are often a precursor to amputation.[44] More days are spent as hospital inpatients for foot complications than for any other diabetes-related complications. Clinical studies have reported that 25–50% of diabetic foot infections lead to a minor amputation, with up to 40% requiring major amputation. Nonetheless, the presence of bacteria does not necessarily indicate that it is a major factor in the development of the ulcer or its failure to heal. Troublesome infection is a clinical diagnosis and should be based on signs of erythema, discharge, odour or frank cellulitis (Figure 18.4). Many patients will have evidence of peripheral vascular disease (up to two-thirds), and 80% will have lost protective sensation as assessed neurologically.

Bacteria gain entry via breaks in the skin, ingrowing toenails, callus which has fissured, and neuropathic and ischaemic ulcers. Foot ulcers are a haven for bacterial growth, and a number of organisms are commonly encountered (Table 18.1). Mild infections occurring in patients who have not previously received antibiotic therapy are usually caused by only one or two species of bacteria, almost invariably aerobic, Gram-positive cocci. *Staphylococcus aureus* is by far the most important pathogen in diabetic foot infections.[45] Gram-negative bacilli, mainly Enterobacteriaceae, are found in many patients with chronic or previously treated infections. *Pseudomonas* species are often isolated from wounds that have

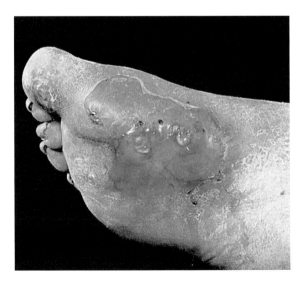

**Figure 18.4** Forefoot cellulitis showing erythema and purulent discharge extending up the foot.

**Table 18.1** Commonly encountered bacteria isolated from diabetic foot ulcers.

| Gram-positive | Gram-negative | Anaerobes |
| --- | --- | --- |
| *Staphylococcus aureus* | *Enterobacter* | *Bacteroides* |
| *Enterococcus* spp. | *Proteus* | *Clostridium* |
| *Streptococcus* spp. | *Pseudomonas aeruginosa* | |
| Methicillin Resistant Staphylococcus Aureus (MRSA) | *Klebsiella* | |
| | *Escherichia coli* | |

been soaked or treated with wet dressings. Anaerobic species are more frequent in ischaemic wounds with necrosis or deep-seated infections. Antibiotic-resistant organisms, especially MRSA, are common in patients who have received antibiotic therapy, and in recent years they have proved a major problem.[46,47] Often these latter infections have been acquired during previous hospitalization. In cases of localized mild cellulitis that is not limb threatening, infection is likely to be caused by Gram-positive cocci of the *Staphylococcus* or *Streptococcus* genus.[48] More extensive and deep-seated infection of the lower leg and foot is associated with a high risk of amputation.[28,49] Severe infections may present as extensive cellulitis spreading from a foot wound or ulcer and up the leg. Localized abscess formation and underlying osteomyelitis may be found and may evolve into limb- or life-threatening events. Deeper infection is a major concern, as it may precipitate amputation. Spread of infection to ligaments and bones may develop rapidly, and extensive cellulitis may develop in association with necrotizing fasciitis, localized abscess formation, septicaemia and osteomyelitis (Figure 18.5). Early aggressive antibiotic management and surgical intervention may preserve the affected limb. In many cases, the extent of the infection is greater than expected, and is found to track along tendon sheaths and into muscle. The patient is generally systemically unwell and the condition life-threatening. Gram-positive cocci (*S. aureus* and streptococci), anaerobic bacteria (*Bacteroides fragilis*) and Gram-negative bacilli (*Escherichia coli*) are often implicated. The diagnosis of osteomyelitis can be difficult, particularly from acute Charcot's arthropathy, as both induce a red, warm and swollen foot. Radiology in the early stages may appear normal, and complex radiological diagnostic procedures may be required.[50] Some centres have used magnetic resonance scanning with a high specificity and sensitivity. However, the simple technique of being able to probe to bone carries a high positive predictive value, confirming a diagnosis in up to 85% of cases.[51]

## ASSESSMENT OF FOOT PROBLEMS AND PERIPHERAL VASCULAR DISEASE

### Assessment of neuropathy

Examination of the feet in patients with diabetes is often the most neglected aspect of the clinical examination.[52] The feet should be examined at least annually in all patients and more frequently in those patients identified as high risk. Visual inspection of the lower legs and feet may throw light on the underlying aetiology of diabetic foot problems. Ulcers secondary to neuropathy tend to occur on the plantar aspect of the feet under areas of high plantar

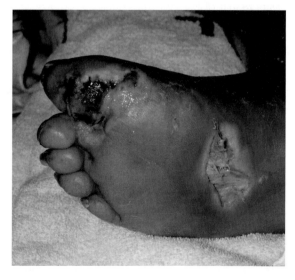

**Figure 18.5** Deep infection tracking throughout the forefoot, leading to abscess formation and necrotizing fasciitis.

pressure (metatarsal heads especially), while ischaemic ulcers tend to affect the toes and dorsum of the foot. Evidence of neuropathy may include dry and cracked skin as a consequence of autonomic neuropathy. Significant ischaemia will manifest as loss of hair on the dorsum of the foot and toes, tight and shiny skin around the toes, and a dusky red appearance (Figure 18.6 and Table 18.2). Obvious ulceration should be noted, but smaller ulcers between the toes may be missed unless routinely assessed.

A wide variety of techniques are used to assess neurological integrity. A simple clinical examination may involve the use of a tuning fork (128 Hz) to assess vibration sense. This should be carried out at the tips of the toes, the first metatarsophalangeal joint and the ankle in a progressive manner. Pinprick sensation is often used to assess the protective

sensation associated with pain. However, this assessment is prone to interinvestigator variation due to the pressure applied to the pin. There is also a danger of puncture wounds, and only dedicated neurological testing pins must be used. In recent years, the ability to perceive, or protective perception, may be more reliably assessed with the Semmes-Weinstein monofilaments.[53] These monofilaments are placed against the skin and pressure is applied until the monofilament buckles. The monofilament should be applied to the skin for a couple of seconds and should not slide across the skin or make repeated contact. The thicker the monofilament, the more force is required to buckle. The patient should perceive this sensation and identify the area being touched at the time of the monofilament buckles. A 10-g force (5.07 monofilament) is the upper limit deemed to confer adequate protection. If a patient is unable to feel this monofilament at any of the tested areas, significant neuropathy is present and protected pain sensation is lost.[54] Monofilaments equivalent to 1 g of linear pressure or higher are considered consistent with neuropathy. Specialist footwear should be considered in patients demonstrated to have loss of protective sensation. The inability to feel the tuning vibrating at the base of the great toenail carries the same significance as the inability to feel a 10-g force of monofilament, and such a patient should be considered for specialist footwear. The feet should be examined for foot deformities, areas of callus, fissures or cracked skin, dryness and ulceration, and the state of the toenails assessed. Structural deformities such as hammer toes, bunions, calluses and Charcot's arthropathy increase the risk of ulceration and should be documented. Light touch sensa-

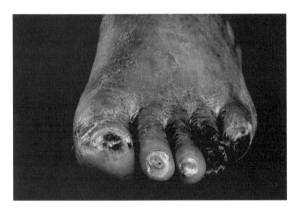

**Figure 18.6** Typical ischaemic foot showing dusky red appearance, dry skin, loss of hair and gangrene of the toes.

**Table 18.2** Comparison of neuropathic and ischaemic characteristics.

| Neuropathic | Ischaemic |
| --- | --- |
| Reduced sensation | Lesions often painful |
| Painless | Claudication |
| Foot pulses present | Skin shiny and without hair |
| Foot warm and well perfused | Atrophy of subcutaneous tissue |
| Callus | Foot cold, pale or dusky red; absent foot pulses |
| Ulcers typically plantar | Buerger's test positive |
| Skin dry and cracked | Ulcers or gangrene affecting dorsum of foot or toes |
| Claw toes | |
| Charcot's arthropathy | |

tion can be assessed with a cotton wool wisp on the dorsum of the foot. Motor nerve function may be assessed by documenting the Achilles tendon reflexes. This assessment provides information of large motor nerve function. In distal symmetrical polyneuropathy, the more distal reflexes will be affected more than the upper extremities.

## Assessment of vascular disease

A history of claudication, or rest pain, indicates peripheral vascular disease. The classic history of vascular claudication is pain in the calf produced by exercise that is relieved within 2–3 min by standing still. Patients may also suffer pain in the thigh and/or buttock. The pain is often described as 'cramping', 'aching' or 'tight'. The classic history of rest pain consists of pain in the foot brought on by going to bed at night and relieved by dangling the foot out of bed. Some patients are afraid to go to bed and sleep upright in a chair. The pain is severe and usually described as 'agonizing' or 'burning'. As the ischaemia progresses, the pain may become continuous and resistant to even opiate analgesia.

In addition to pulse palpation, examination of the lower limb should include looking for areas of gangrene and/or ulceration. Paradoxically, the affected foot may be bright red due to the accumulation of vasodilator metabolites. Buerger's test is useful for the assessment of critical ischaemia—when it is elevated, an ischaemic foot becomes deathly pale (Figure 18.7). There are two fundamental questions to be answered with respect to the vascular assessment of the diabetic foot. First, is the blood supply to the limb impaired? If it is, the second question is, where is the location of the disease? The global vascular status of the lower limb can be assessed by measurement of the ankle brachial pressure index (ABPI), by measuring toe pressures or by the pole test. The specific advantage of toe pressures and the pole test is that they allow an accurate assessment of distal arterial perfusion in diabetic patients with calcified calf arteries when the ABPI may be falsely raised. The localization of disease is best achieved by colour duplex scanning or arteriography. Colour duplex scanning has revolutionized the localization of lower limb vascular disease in recent years; in many centres, it has displaced diagnostic arteriography.[55]

The ABPI (Figure 18.8) is measured by placing a standard blood-pressure cuff around the ankle just above the malleoli, and the cuff is inflated above systolic pressure, causing the pedal Doppler signals to

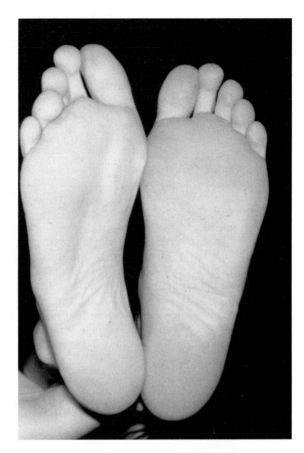

**Figure 18.7** Buerger's test. On elevation, this patient's critically ischaemic right foot becomes deathly pale.

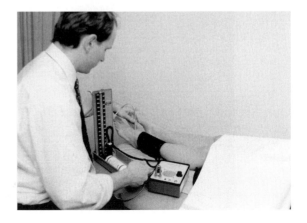

**Figure 18.8** Measurement of the ABPI. The patient should be supine and rested for at least 10 min.

disappear. The point at which the Doppler signal first returns on gradually lowering cuff pressure, marks the systolic pressure at ankle level. A similar systolic blood-pressure measurement is taken from the brachial artery in the arm as an estimate of systemic/central aortic pressure. The ratio of the highest recorded systolic blood pressure at the ankle to the brachial systolic blood pressure at the arm forms the ABPI. Normal limbs without proximal arterial disease record indices of 1 and above. Indices below 0.5 are suggestive of severe arterial disease, and the patient may suffer from rest pain, ulceration or gangrene.[56]

A potential difficulty arises with incompressible vessels. Spuriously high pressures are recorded, and, even at maximum cuff pressure, it may be impossible to eliminate the pedal Doppler signals. This is caused by medial calcification, a condition to which diabetic patients are particularly prone (Figure 18.9). In this situation, the alternatives are the measurement of toe pressures or the pole test. To measure toe pressures (Figure 18.10), an occlusion cuff 2–3 cm in diameter is placed around the proximal phalanx of the great toe,

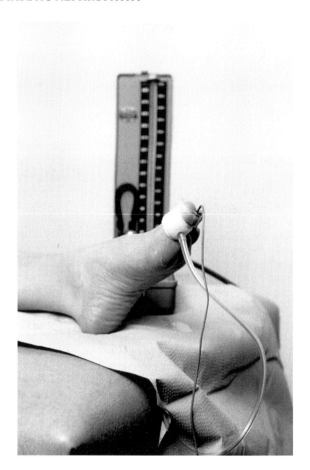

**Figure 18.10** Measurement of toe pressure.

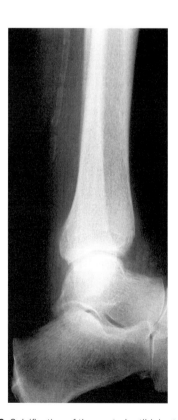

**Figure 18.9** Calcification of the posterior tibial artery in a patient with diabetes.

and the alterations in digital artery pulses during the inflation and deflation of this cuff are detected by a photoelectric cell placed on the toe. The cuff is inflated until the pulses in the digital arteries disappear, and the cuff is then deflated and the point at which the signals reappear is the systolic pressure measurement of the toe. Toe pressures are normally lower than those found in either the brachial arteries or the tibial arteries at the ankle. This is probably because of the high resistance created by small digital arteries. Toe pressures in patients with no arterial symptoms are 90–100 mmHg, whereas in the presence of critical ischaemia the pressure drops to below 30 mmHg. The pole test[57] involves listening to the pedal pulse by Doppler ultrasound while the patient's leg is raised alongside a pole (Figure 18.11). The height at which the Doppler signal disappears is translated into a pressure by use of an appropriately calibrated pole. A maximum pressure of 60–70 mmHg can be recorded, because this test is

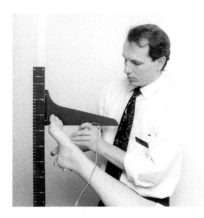

**Figure 18.11** Pole test. A pedal artery is insonated with a pencil Doppler while the leg is raised alongside a pole calibrated in mmHg. The height at which the signal disappears is the pedal artery pressure.

limited by how high a patient can lift the leg. The pole test provides a pedal pressure measurement which can be compared to the brachial pressure measurement in the same way as the conventional ABPI.

Colour duplex ultrasonography of the lower limb arteries involves tracing the vessels in both B-mode and colour, while frequently switching to the Doppler spectra to ensure that no changes in blood-flow haemodynamics have been missed. A twofold increase in velocity across a stenosis equates to a 50% diameter-reducing stenosis seen on arteriography.[58] The results of lower limb colour duplex scans are best expressed in the form of a diagram of the lower limb arteries, on which areas that contain a peak velocity ratio of >2, or are occluded, are clearly marked. If arteriography is required, digital subtraction arteriography is performed by a transfemoral approach. This allows excellent images to be obtained from the infrarenal aorta to the forefoot, under local anaesthesia with little patient discomfort. Intravascular, iodinated contrast media is potentially nephrotoxic, an effect which is transient (reaching a maximum at approximately 48 hr) and usually of no clinical significance in patients with normal renal function. All patients should have their serum creatinine measured prior to angiography. If their creatinine is raised, but below 300 μmol/l, the angiogram should not be performed as a day case, and intravenous fluids should be commenced at least 6 hr before the investigation. Non-steroidal anti-inflammatory drugs (with the exception of aspirin) should also be stopped. If the patient's creatinine is

in excess of 300 μmol/l (3.3 mg/dl), serious consideration should be given as to gleaning the relevant information by alternative imaging techniques or by the use of other contrast media (such as gadolinium or carbon dioxide). Attention has recently been focused on the risk of an interaction between iodinated contrast media and metformin.[59] If there is a transient impairment of renal function induced by the contrast medium, this can cause a reduction in the renal excretion of metformin, and lactic acidosis may result. This situation carries a high (approximately 50%) mortality rate. Recent recommendations from a systematic review[59] indicate that as long as the patient has normal renal function, contrast angiography can be performed safely. If the patient has a high creatinine, the metformin should be stopped prior to contrast injection.

## Assessment of infection

The majority of ulcers and skin lesions harbour bacteria, but they may not necessarily have contributed to the onset of the ulceration or skin lesion. Infection is likely in the presence of purulent discharge or signs of inflammation (swelling, redness or pain). Infections most often affect the forefoot—in particular, the toes and metatarsal heads—often on the plantar aspect of the foot (Figure 18.4). Deeper infections leading to osteomyelitis generally develop from the contiguous spread of a deeper tissue infection through the cortex of the bone. Deep-seated infections are often complicated by osteomyelitis, and a diagnosis can be made in most cases by a simple demonstration of probing to bone with a sterile metal probe. All patients with a deep or long-standing ulcer or infection, particularly if located over a bony prominence, should be assessed for possible osteomyelitis. Radiology of the affected area should be undertaken, but in the early stages no changes may be apparent. Nonetheless, typical changes develop in up to three-quarters of patients with long-standing bony involvement, leading to cortical erosions, periosteal reactions or bony collapse. More sensitive radiological procedures have been reported, including technetium-99 bone scans, indium-111 leucocytes scan, and the MRI and PET techniques.[60,61] Obtaining bone fragments for culture and antibiotic sensitivity is helpful and may be performed in the outpatient setting. Palpation of the infected area may reveal crepitus, a finding that indicates soft tissue gas and necrosis. Forefoot infections may drain with the aid of gravity within the tissues of the foot, leading to aggressive necrotizing fasciitis

**Table 18.3** Comparison of the low- and high-risk diabetic feet.

| Low-risk | High-risk |
| --- | --- |
| Intact protective sensation | Loss of protective sensation |
| Foot pulses present | Absent foot pulses |
| No foot deformity | Foot deformity |
| No history of ulceration or amputation | Previous ulceration or amputation |
| Appropriate footwear | Inappropriate footwear |
| No callus | Excess callus |

(Figure 18.5). The true extent of the suppuration may not become apparent until the area is surgically debrided. These types of infections may progress very rapidly in patients with diabetes, and aggressive intravenous therapy should be introduced early. The finding of deep-seated infections is an indication to admit the patient to hospital for aggressive antibiotic therapy and multidisciplinary assessment of the infection. Close collaboration with vascular and orthopaedic colleagues is paramount.

Table 18.3 details the features associated with low and high-risk diabetic feet

## MANAGEMENT OF DIABETIC FOOT PROBLEMS AND PERIPHERAL VASCULAR DISEASE

After identification of the high-risk foot, it is important that efforts are made to prevent ulceration or worse complications from developing. The cornerstones of management include protection of the at-risk foot by appropriate footwear, education of the patient with regard to foot care, optimizing vascular supply to the lower leg and foot, and maintaining control of vascular risk factors and diabetes. Evidence from clinical studies has provided evidence that preventative strategies reduce the prevalence of diabetic foot ulcers and amputations.[3,4] As a general rule, ulcers will not heal in the presence of ischaemia. Non-weight bearing is vitally important for the ulcerated foot not only because the feet are insensitive and neuropathic ulcers are painless, but also because continued mobility without adequate protection leads to increased pressure necrosis, forcing bacteria deeper into the tissue. The use of crutches and wheelchairs is seldom successful in achieving total and consistent non-weight bearing.

One of the best techniques to ensure non-weight bearing in appropriately selected patients is the use of a contact cast.[62] There are many methods available to reduce plantar pressure and provide protection to the area. Various forms of casts may be provided, including the Scotchcast boot[63] (Figure 18.12). This boot is individually fitted and moulded to the shape of the patient's foot. It is made from fibreglass tape and is lined with felt and soft bandaging. The boot is removable, allowing regular inspection of the ulcer for debridement and other local wound care. These lightweight casts allow the patient to remain ambulatory and in some cases to continue working. Infrequently encountered problems include the development of iatrogenic lesions due to rubbing or other pressure ulcers developing, making inspection of the foot and boot within the following week vitally important. Elderly patients are more prone to problems principally because of the limited mobility and balance when they wear one or two boots. Plantar ulcers that fail to respond to Scotchcast boots may be encased in a total-contact cast. This is a close-fitting plaster of Paris and fibreglass cast that holds the foot and lower leg to prevent slipping and rubbing. Care must be exercised, in making the cast, not to fashion a boot that is too tight. Skill in preparation of these casts is of utmost importance, and the casts should be removed weekly to permit wound inspection and to check for areas of rubbing.

A variety of other manufactured casts are available and in use. The foot is protected by a cast until the ulcer has completely healed. Most neuropathic plantar ulcers heal within a period of 6–12 weeks within these casts. Once the cast is removed, the feet should be placed in specialist pressure-relieving footwear to prevent future ulceration and other complications. This may involve the manufacture of custom-made leather footwear that is made from one piece of material. The shoes should allow plenty of space for the depth and width of the foot, have no

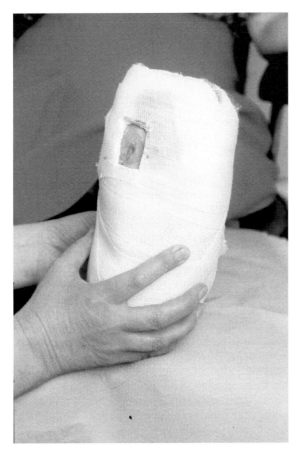

**Figure 18.12** A Scotchcast boot is made to protect the ulcer from pressure over the ulcer site, with a small window through which the ulcer can be seen.

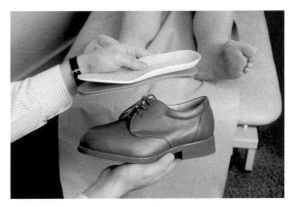

**Figure 18.13** Specialist footwear and insoles help reduce the risk of further ulceration by allowing space for the foot and by reducing pressure over parts of the foot with abnormally high pressures.

internal seams which may precipitate rubbing and be velcro-fastened or have lace-ups to prevent sliding within the footwear (Figure 18.13). Additional techniques to reduce abnormally high plantar pressures include specialist insoles contoured to the shape of the sole, and rocker bottom-soled shoes to alleviate pressure over the metatarsal heads. The inclusion of a specialist orthotist as part of the multidisciplinary foot team is a prerequisite.

Refractory ulcers occur frequently despite aggressive management protocols. In ulcers that are not showing signs of infection, new techniques to replace the patients' own damaged or destroyed dermis have been developed. Therapy consists of neonatal dermal fibroblasts cultured in vitro on bioabsorbable mesh to produce a living, metabolically active tissue containing the normal dermal matrix protein and cytokines. The manufactured graft is cut to the wound size and placed in the wound bed. The embedded fibroblasts within the tissue mesh secrete a variety of growth factors that are pivotal to neo-vascularization, epithelial migration and differentiation. Thus, a healthy dermal base is rebuilt over which the patient's epidermis can migrate and close the wound. Experience with these newer agents is limited, but accumulating data support a role for these novel techniques.[64,65]

## Peripheral vascular disease

The treatment of peripheral vascular disease in diabetic patients is by either percutaneous transluminal angioplasty or bypass grafting. Although the amputation rate in diabetics is up to five times higher than in non-diabetics,[66] recent studies comparing patency rates after percutaneous transluminal angioplasty or bypass grafting have not shown significant differences between the two groups.[67] This would suggest that part of the reason for the higher amputation rate in diabetic patients is delay in initiating treatment. Recent advances in catheter technology have allowed percutaneous transluminal angioplasty of tibial arteries (Figure 18.14), and refinements in surgical technique have allowed bypass grafting to pedal vessels. Both these advances are of particular benefit to diabetic patients.

Minor amputation of the foot in diabetic patients may be required for ischaemia, infection or a combination of the two. If ischaemia is present, it must be corrected prior to amputation, at which time all necrotic and/or infected tissue must be excised. The

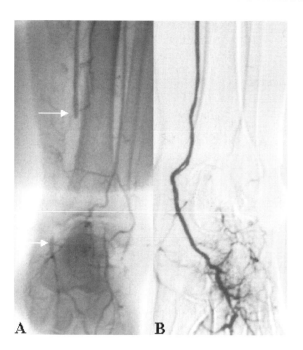

**Figure 18.14** An occlusion (between arrows) of the posterior tibial artery before (A) and after (B) angioplasty.

resulting wound is usually allowed to heal by secondary intention, or a skin graft is used (Figure 18.15). If infection/gangrene is extensive, a major amputation may be required. Twice as many below-

knee amputees as above-knee amputees are mobile around the home,[68] and a below-knee amputation is therefore greatly preferred.

## Infection

Infections that often appear to be minor and localized may very rapidly become limb- or life-threatening.[69] A bacterial culture should be taken from all ulcers, even if not clinically infected, as many ulcers harbour significant organisms, such as methicillin-resistant *S. aureus*. A positive bacterial diagnosis will assist in management by guiding appropriate antibiotic therapy. Although most patients with diabetic foot ulcers will receive antibiotic therapy, this practice remains contentious, with some studies showing that antibiotic therapy did not improve the outcome of uninfected lesions.[70] Other groups have suggested that all patients with open, uninfected foot ulcers should receive antibiotic therapy, with evidence showing an increased likelihood of healing, less infection, and less hospitalization and amputation. Most patients can be treated with oral antibiotics, but intravenous antibiotics are required for those patients who are systemically unwell or have deep-seated infection, purulent discharge, cellulitis or osteomyelitis. Many infections that respond to intravenous antibiotics over a 2–3-day period can be subsequently switched to oral antibiotics. Initially, antibiotic therapy should cover common pathogens

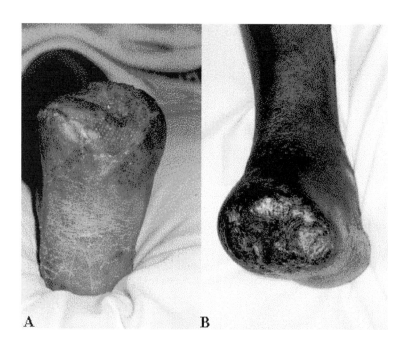

**Figure 18.15** A forefoot amputation in a diabetic patient before (A) and 3 weeks after (B) skin grafting.

and may become more focused once bacterial cultures are available. Initial treatment should incorporate an antibiotic acting against staphylococci and streptococci. However, multiple organisms are often present, requiring combination therapy. Recommended oral antibiotics for localized infection or mild cellulitis include flucloxacillin or augmentin in combination with metronidazole if Gram-negative bacteria are suspected. Deep-seated infections requiring intravenous antibiotics are generally treated with combination therapy incorporating flucloxacillin, penicillin and metronidazole, or a cephalosporin and metronidazole. Penicillin-sensitive patients may be treated with erythromycin. MRSA infections require intravenous vancomycin or teicoplanin. Antibiotic therapy for osteomyelitis should be based on bone culture results where possible. Prolonged therapy is generally required in combination with debridement to remove infected bone if possible; in many cases this therapy may prevent amputation.[71,72]

A wide variety of sterile dressings have been advocated to protect the ulcer site or lesion, although there is little evidence from clinical studies that one particular dressing is superior to another. Dressings that are applied over ulcers should in principle be sterile and non-adherent, covering all open lesions to protect them from further trauma, and to help absorb exudate and promote healing. Dressings need to be changed every 1–2 days. In our unit, the majority of ulcers are covered with a sterile, dry or saline-soaked, non-adherent dressing.

Infected foot ulcers and lesions (excluding cellulitis) should be debrided where possible.[73] Debridement allows removal of dead or necrotic tissue, foreign material and surrounding callus. This allows the wound to be inspected and its extent quantified. This form of debridement is usually undertaken by podiatrists but may be undertaken by other appropriately trained health-care professionals. Material is removed with a scalpel, scissors or more robust tissue clippers. The last-named often allow bone tissue protruding through an open wound to be removed. Frequent debridement is a prerequisite every 1–2 weeks in the early stages to assist healing. As an alternative to manual debridement, larval therapy has been tried in diabetic foot ulcers.[74,75] The maggots used are the larvae of *Lucilia sericata* (the adult insect is green in colour; its common name is greenbottle fly). These larvae remove the dead tissue by the production of powerful enzymes that break dead tissue down to the liquid form, which is then ingested. The larvae are applied until the wound looks clean, and the practice seems to be acceptable for most patients.

More deep-seated infections will require collaboration with surgical colleagues, as aggressive surgical debridement may reduce the risk of major amputation.[49] Abscess formation requires drainage of pus. Soft tissue necrosis or necrotizing fasciitis requires urgent debridement.[76] Hidden and deep-seated infections are generally associated with a systemically ill patient who is unlikely to improve until radical debridement has taken place, regardless of antibiotic therapy.

# REFERENCES

1. Pecoraro RE, Reiber GE, Burgess EM, Pathways to diabetic limb amputation. Basis for prevention. *Diabetes Care* 1990; **13**: 513–21.
2. Caputo GM, Cavanagh R, Ulbrecht JS et al, Assessment and management of foot disease in patients with diabetes. *N Engl J Med* 1994; **331**: 854–60.
3. Larsson J, Apelqvist J, Agardh CD et al, Decreasing incidence of major amputation in diabetic patients: a consequence of a multi-disciplinary foot care team approach? *Diabetic Med* 1995: **12**: 770–6.
4. Edmonds ME, Maelor Thomas EM, Blundell MP et al, Improved survival of the diabetic foot: the role of a specialised foot clinic. *Q J Med* 1986; **232**: 763–71.
5. Kumar S, Ashe HA, Fernando DJ et al, The prevalence of foot ulceration and its correlates in type 2 diabetic patients: a population-based study. *Diabetic Med* 1994; **11**: 480–4.
6. Walters DP, Gattling W, Mullee MA et al, The distribution and severity of diabetic foot disease: a community study with comparison to a non-diabetic group. *Diabetic Med* 1992; **9**: 354–8.
7. Moss SE, Klein R, Klein BE, The prevalence and incidence of lower extremity amputation in a diabetic population. *Arch Intern Med* 1992; **152**: 610–16.
8. Moss SE, Klein R, Klein BE, Long-term incidence of lower extremity amputations in a diabetic population. *Arch Intern Med* 1999; **5**: 391–8.
9. Eggers PW, Gohdes D, Pugh J, Non-traumatic lower extremity amputations in the Medicare end-stage renal disease population. *Kidney Int* 1999; **56**: 1524–33.
10. Hill MN, Feldman HI, Hilton SC et al, Risk of foot complications in long-term diabetic patients with and without ESRD: a preliminary study. *ANNA J* 1996; **23**: 381–6.
11. Wannner C, Krane V, Ruf G et al, for Die Deutsch Diabetes Dialyse Studie Investigators. Rationale and design of a trial improving outcome of type 2 diabetes on haemodialysis. *Kidney Int* 1999; **56** (Suppl 71): S222–6.
12. Pugh JA, Medina R, Ramirez M, Comparisons of the course to end-stage renal disease of type 1 and type 2 diabetic nephropathy. *Diabetologia* 1993; **36**: 1094–8.
13. Shaw JE, Gokal R, Hollis S et al, Does peripheral neuropathy invariably accompany nephropathy in type 1 diabetes mellitus? *Diabetes Res Clin Pract* 1998; **39**: 56–61.
14. Rith-Najarian SJ, Stolusky T, Gohdes DM et al, Identifying diabetic patients at high risk for lower-extremity amputation in a primary healthcare setting. *Diabetes Care* 1992; **15**: 1386–9.
15. Boyko E, Ahroni JH, Stensel V et al, A prospective study of risk factors for diabetic foot ulcer: the Seattle Diabetic Foot Study. *Diabetes Care* 1999; **22**: 1036–42.
16. Armstrong DG, Lavery LA, Vela SA et al, Choosing a practical screening instrument to identify patients at risk for diabetic foot ulceration. *Arch Intern Med* 1998; **158**: 289–92.

17. Veves A, Sarnow MR, Giurini JM et al, Differences in joint mobility and foot pressures between black and white diabetic patients. *Diabetic Med* 1995; **12**: 585–9.

18. Stess RM, Jensen SR, Mirmiran R, The role of dynamic plantar pressures in diabetic foot ulcers. *Diabetes Care* 1997; **20**: 855–8.

19. Moss SE, Klein R, Klein BE, The prevalence and incidence of lower extremity amputation in a diabetic population. *Arch Intern Med* 1992; **152**: 610–16.

20. Reiber G, Vileikyte L, Boyko EJ et al, Causal pathways for incident lower-extremity ulcers in patients with diabetes from two settings. *Diabetes Care* 1999; **22**: 157–62.

21. Mantey I, Foster A, Spencer S et al, Why do foot ulcers occur in diabetic patients? *Diabetic Med* 1999; **16**: 245–9.

22. Adler AI, Boyko EJ, Ahroni JH et al, Lower-extremity amputation in diabetes: the independent effects of peripheral vascular disease, sensory neuropathy, and foot ulcers. *Diabetes Care* 1999; **22**: 1029–35.

23. Mayfield JA, Reiber GE, Nelson RG et al, A foot risk classification system to predict diabetic amputations in Pima Indians. *Diabetes Care* 1996; **19**: 704–9.

24. Morris AD, McAlpine R, Steinke D et al, Diabetes and lower-limb amputation in the community. *Diabetes Care* 1998; **21**: 738–43.

25. Nelson R, Gohdes D, Everhart J et al, Lower-extremity amputations in NIDDM: 12-year follow-up study in Pima Indians. *Diabetes Care* 1988; **11**: 8–16.

26. Gujral J, McNally PG, O'Malley BP et al, Ethnic variations in the incidence of lower extremity amputation. *Diabetic Med* 1993; **10**: 271–4.

27. Lehto S, Pyorala K, Ronnemaa T et al, Risk factors predicting lower extremity amputations in patients with NIDDM. *Diabetes Care* 1996; **19**: 607–12.

28. Moss S, Klein R, Klein BE, The 14 year incidence of lower-extremity amputations in a diabetic population. *Diabetes Care* 1999; **22**: 951–9.

29. Reiber GE, Pecoraro RE, Koepsell TD, Risk factors for amputation in patients with diabetes mellitus. *Ann Intern Med* 1992; **117**: 97–105.

30. Partanen J, Niskanen L, Lehtinen J et al, Natural history of peripheral neuropathy in patients with non-insulin dependent diabetes. *N Engl J Med* 1995; **333**: 89–94.

31. Young MJ, Boulton GM, Mcleod AF et al, A multicentre study of the prevalence of diabetic peripheral neuropathy in the UK hospital clinic population. Diabetologia 1993; **36**: 150–4.

32. Tesfaye S, Stevens LR, Stephenson JM et al, Prevalence of diabetic peripheral neuropathy and its relation to glycaemic control and potential risk factors: the Eurodiab IDDM Complications Study. *Diabetologia* 1996; **39**: 1377–84.

33. Boulton AJM, Hardisty CA, Betts RP et al, Dynamic foot pressure and other studies as diagnostic and management aids in diabetic neuropathy. *Diabetes Care* 1983; **6**: 26–33.

34. Veves A, Fernando DJ, Walewski P et al, A study of foot pressures in a diabetic clinic population. *Foot* 1991; **1**: 89–92.

35. Boulton GM, Scarpello JH, Ward JD, Venous oxygenation in the diabetic neuropathic foot: evidence of arteriovenous shunting? *Diabetologia* 1982; **22**: 6–8.

36. Young MJ, Cavanagh PR, Thomas G et al, The effect of callus removal on dynamic plantar foot pressures in diabetic patients. *Diabetic Med* 1992; **9**: 55–7.

37. Armstrong DG, Todd WF, Lavery LA et al, The natural history of acute Charcot's arthropathy in a diabetic foot speciality clinic. *J Am Podiatr Assoc* 1997; **87**: 272–8.

38. Cundy TF, Edmonds ME, Watkins PJ, Osteopenia and metatarsal fractures in diabetic neuropathy. *Diabetic Med* 1985; **2**: 461–4.

39. Young MJ, Marshall A, Adams JE et al, Osteopenia, neurologi-

40. Beks PJ, Mackay AJ, De Neeling JN et al, Peripheral arterial disease in relation to glycaemic control in an elderly Caucasian population. The Hoorn Study. *Diabetologia* 1995; **38**: 86–96.

41. Haimovici H, Patterns of arteriosclerotic lesions of the lower extremity. *Arch Surg* 1967; **95**: 918–33.

42. Conrad MC, Large and small artery occlusion in diabetics and nondiabetics with severe vascular disease. *Diabetes* 1964; **13**: 366–72.

43. Jacobs MJ, Beches RC, Jorning PJ et al, Microvascular haemodynamics before and after vascular surgery in severe limb ischaemia. *Eur J Vasc Surg* 1990; **4**: 525–9.

44. Eneroth M, Apelqvist J, Stenstrom A, Clinical characteristics and outcome in 223 diabetic patients with deep foot infections. *Foot Ankle Int* 1997; **18**: 716–22.

45. Lipski BA, Pecoraro RE, Wheat LT, The diabetic foot: soft tissue and bone infection. *Infect Dis Clin North Am* 1990; **4**: 409–32.

46. Goldstein EJ, Citron DM, Nesbit CA, Diabetic foot infections: bacteriology and activity of 10 oral antimicrobial agents against bacteria isolated from consecutive cases. *Diabetes Care* 1996; **19**: 638–41.

47. Tentolouris N, Jude EB, Smirnof I et al, Methicillin-resistant *Staphylococcus aureus*: an increasing problem in a diabetic foot clinic. *Diabetic Med* 1999; **16**: 767–71.

48. Lipski BA, Pecorarore E, Larsen SA et al, Outpatient management of uncomplicated lower-extremity infections in diabetic patients. *Arch Intern Med* 1990; **150**: 790–7.

49. Tan JS, Friedman NM, Hazelton-Miller C et al, Can aggressive treatment of diabetic foot infections reduce the need for above-ankle amputations? *Clin Infect Dis* 1996; **23**: 286–91.

50. Newman LG, Waller J, Palestro CJ et al, Unsuspected osteomyelitis in diabetic foot ulcers: diagnosing and monitoring by leucocyte scanning with indium. *JAMA* 1991; **266**: 1246–51.

51. Grayson ML, Gibbons GW, Balogh K et al, Probing to bone in infected pedal ulcers. A clinical sign of underlying osteomyelitis in diabetic patients. *JAMA* 1995; **273**: 721–3.

52. Martin TL, Selby JV, Zhang D, Physician and patient prevention practices in NIDDM in a large urban managed-care organisation. *Diabetes Care* 1995; **18**: 1124–32.

53. Klenerman L, McCabe CJ, Cogley D et al, Screening for patients at risk of diabetic foot ulceration in a general diabetic outpatient clinic. *Diabetic Med* 1996; **13**: 561–3.

54. McNeely MJ, Boyko EJ, Ahroni JH et al, The independent contributions of diabetic neuropathy and vasculopathy in foot ulceration. How great are the risks? *Diabetes Care* 1995; **18**: 216–19.

55. Pemberton M, London NJM, Colour flow duplex imaging of occlusive arterial disease of the lower limb. *Br J Surg* 1997; **84**: 912–19.

56. London NJM, Cleveland TJ, Assessment of chronic lower limb ischaemia. In: *Vascular and Endovascular Surgery*, 2nd edn (JD Beard, PA Gaines, eds.). WB Saunders: Philadelphia, 2001; 27–54.

57. Smith FCT, Shearman CP, Simms MH et al, Falsely elevated ankle pressures in severe leg ischaemia: the pole test—an alternative approach. *Eur J Vasc Surg* 1994; **8**: 408–12.

58. Sensier Y, Hartshorne T, Thrush A et al, A prospective comparison of lower limb colour-coded duplex scanning with arteriography. *Eur J Vasc Endovasc Surg* 1996; **11**: 170–5.

59. McCartney MM, Gilbert FJ, Murchinson LE et al, Metformin and contrast media: a dangerous combination? *Clin Radiol* 1999; **54**: 29–33.

60. Lipsky BA, Osteomyelitis of the foot in diabetic patients. *Clin Infect Dis* 1997; **25**: 1318–26.

cal dysfunction and the development of Charcot neuroarthropathy. *Diabetes Care* 1995; **18**: 34–8.

61. Craig JG, Amin MB, Wu K et al, Osteomyelitis of the diabetic foot; MR imaging—pathological correlation. *Radiology* 1997; **203**: 849–55.

62. Armstrong DG, Lavery LA, Bushman TR, Peak foot pressures influence the healing time of diabetic foot ulcers treated with total contact casts. *J Rehab Res Dev* 1998; **35**: 1–5.

63. Burden AC, Jones GR, Jones R et al, Use of the 'Scotchcast boot' in treating diabetic foot ulcers. *BMJ* 1983; **286**: 1555–7.

64. Gentzkow G, Iwasaki S, Hershon K et al, Use of Dermagraft, a cultured human dermis, to treat a diabetic foot ulcer. *Diabetes Care* 1996; **19**: 350–4.

65. Naughton G, Mansbridge J, Gentzkow G, A metabolically active human dermal replacement for the treatment of diabetic foot ulcers. *Artif Organs* 1997; **21**: 1203–10.

66. Melliere D, Berrahal D, Desgranges P et al, Influence of diabetes on revascularisation procedures of the aorta and lower limb arteries: early results. *Eur J Vasc Endovasc Surg* 1999; **17**: 438–41.

67. Stephenson BM, Shute K, Shandall AA, Diabetic tibial disease: the case for revascularisation. *Ann R Coll Surg Engl* 1993; **75**: 133–6.

68. Houghton AD, Taylor PR, Thurlow S et al, Success rate for rehabilitation of vascular amputees: implications for preoperative assessment and amputation level. *Br J Surg* 1992; **79**: 753–5.

69. Cavanagh PR, Buse JB, Frykberg RG et al for the American Diabetes Association: Diabetic foot wound care. Consensus development conference. *Diabetes Care* 1999; **22**: 1354–60.

70. Chantelau E, Tanudjaja T, Altenhofer F et al, Antibiotic treatment for uncomplicated neuropathic forefoot ulcers in diabetes: a controlled trial. *Diabetic Med* 1996; **13**: 156–9.

71. Pittet D, Wyssa B, Herter-Clavel C et al, Outcome of diabetic foot infections treated conservatively. A retrospective cohort study with long-term follow-up. *Arch Intern Med* 1999; **159**: 851–6.

72. Venkatesan P, Lawn S, Mcfarland RM et al. Conservative management of osteomyelitis in the feet of diabetic patients. *Diabetic Med* 1997; **14**: 487–90.

73. Jones V, Debridement of diabetic foot lesions. *Diabet Foot* 1998; **3**: 88–94.

74. Thomas S, Jones M, Shutler S et al, Using larvae in modern wound management. *J Wound Care* 1996; **5**: 60–9.

75. Rayman A, Stansfield G, Woolard T et al, Use of larvae in the treatment of the diabetic necrotic foot. *Diabet Foot* 1998; **1**: 7–13.

76. Gibbons GW, Habershaw GM, Diabetic foot infections. Anatomy and surgery. *Infect Dis Clin North Am* 1995; **9**: 131–42.

# 19

# Practical aspects of nutritional management of patients with diabetic renal disease

Marianne Vennegoor

## INTRODUCTION

Diabetes mellitus is one of the most common forms of chronic disease, affecting millions of people around the world. The incidence and prevalence of this disease are increasing. A relatively high proportion of diabetic patients develop chronic renal disease consequently leading to morbidity often requiring expensive therapies. It would seem to be advantageous to develop therapeutic regimens that could change the disease process or prevent the development of complications.

Poor glycaemic control and uncontrolled hypertension contribute to macro- and microvascular disease and represent the two major risk factors for developing cardiovascular disease (CVD), nephropathy, retinopathy and neuropathy. Improving the treatment of hyperglycaemia (see Chapter 6), hypertension (see Chapter 7) and hyperlipidaemia (see Chapter 9) plays a role in the prevention of complications. Dietary management is essential in treating patients with either type 1 or type 2 diabetes. It is advantageous to refer those patients with renal involvement to specialized centres that provide combined diabetes and renal care with access to experienced support staff including dietitians.

It is now accepted that, in addition to a genetic predisposition, changes in lifestyle, excess food consumption and a reduction in physical activity contribute to the development of type 2 diabetes. In fact, the prevalence of type 2 diabetes among US adults is six times greater in subjects classified as obese class 2 than in those who are defined as overweight.[1] Treatment and prevention of obesity may help to reduce the number of people developing type 2 diabetes, and at the same time improve the control of hypertension and thus prevent or attenuate the development of proteinuria and glomerulosclerosis.[2]

## NUTRITIONAL MANAGEMENT OF DIABETIC PATIENTS WITHOUT RENAL INVOLVEMENT

During the past 10 years, nutritional guidelines, based on recommendations for the non-diabetic population, with specific recommendations for the nutritional care of diabetic patients, have been developed and implemented. These are regularly reviewed. An example is 'Recommendations for the nutritional management of patients with diabetes mellitus', which was prepared by the Nutrition and Diabetes Study Group (NDSG) of the European Association for the Study of Diabetes (EASD).[3,4] The American Diabetes Association released its updated guidelines in 2001.[5] Furthermore, national associations for diabetes care provide advice directly to patients on their own specialized internet sites.

The major objective of all these recommendations is to treat and prevent obesity and manage body weight. Thus, the aim of nutritional education should be to maintain an acceptable weight for height. This can be achieved by reducing the patient's energy intake if he or she is found to be overweight, and by increasing physical activity. The patient should be advised to maintain healthy eating habits, moderate alcohol consumption and cease smoking.

## CURRENT GUIDELINES FOR NUTRITIONAL TREATMENT OF DIABETICS (TABLE 19.1)

### Energy intake

*Patients with normal body-mass index (BMI) — 18.5–24.9*

There is no need for specific recommendations for energy intake, but BMI should be monitored at each

**Table 19.1  Recommendations for healthy eating and lifestyle.**

1. Sources of energy
   a. Protein: 10–15% of energy requirements
   b. Carbohydrate: 50–55% of total energy intake, mainly polysaccharides with a high fibre content
   c. Fat: 30–35% of total energy intake
      • Reduce intake of saturated fats
      • Increase intake of mono- and polyunsaturated types of fat (such as olive oil-based products)
   Avoid fats with a high *trans*-fatty acid content (found in manufactured/processed foods)
2. Increase in fibre and vitamins
   Increase intake of vegetables and fruits to at least five portions daily with potassium restriction in patients with hyperkalaemia
3. Intake of salt
   Reduce the intake to 6 g salt daily (100 mmol)
4. Recommendations for lifestyle changes
   a. Reduce alcohol consumption
      • Follow national recommendations
      • Do not drink on an empty stomach
   b. Increase exercise
      Level depends on physical fitness; 20–30 min walking 5 days a week may be sufficient
   c. Smoking
   Patients who smoke should be advised to stop smoking

clinic visit to prevent gradual weight gain over many years.

### *Overweight (BMI 25–29.9) and obese patients (BMI > 30)*

A conventional low-energy diet with exercise seems to provide better sustained weight loss than a diet with a very low energy content.[5,6] Very-low-calorie diets should be prescribed only to very obese patients with a BMI of >35 and should be implemented under medical supervision. Fad diets that restrict entire food groups, such as high-protein (also high in fat), low-carbohydrate diets, have not been proven to be safe and are not effective over a long period of time.

## Source of energy

### *Protein*

The amount of energy provided by protein should not exceed 10–15%, and should include a mixture of animal and vegetable protein.[4] The previous recommendation that protein intake should provide 10–20% of energy requires revision, as this quantity was based on the actual intake of the general population, and this is often twice the required amount. Many patients with type I diabetes in the EURODIAB IDDM Complication Study had an average protein intake of 1.5 g/kg per day. Reducing the amount of protein has been shown to cause a decrease in urinary albumin excretion rate in patients with type 1 diabetes and microalbuminuria, and this is a risk factor for the development of overt diabetic nephropathy.[7]

### *Fat*

The amount of energy derived from fat should not exceed 30% of total requirement. The source of most of this fat should be mono- and polyunsaturated types of fat such as sunflower oil and olive oil products. Manufactured foods containing *trans*-fatty acids, such as some types of margarine, biscuits and cakes, should be avoided.

### *Carbohydrate*

The amount of energy obtained from carbohydrate should be 50–60%, and should come mostly from polysaccharides with a high-fibre content such as high fibre cereal products, pulses, potatoes, wholegrain rice, wholewheat pasta and fruit.

## Concepts of healthy eating

Concepts of healthy eating include an increase in the intake of vegetables and fruit to at least five portions daily to supply sufficient water-soluble vitamins and antioxidants in addition to fibre. Furthermore, reduction in the intake of salt (NaCl) to 5–6 g salt (80–110 mmol Na) daily should be considered. Finally, patients should drink 2–3 litres of sugar-free liquids. Fruit juices contain fructose. Therefore, suitable alternative choices are water, tea and coffee without sugar, mineral water and other low-calorie drinks.

## Alcohol consumption

Men are advised to drink no more than 2 units and women no more than 1 unit per day (1 unit equals

500–600 ml beer or cider, 150 ml wine, 100 ml fortified wine or 30 ml of 40% proof spirits). One should avoid taking alcoholic drinks on an empty stomach, but instead should drink during a meal. Binge drinking should be avoided.

## Physical exercise

Recommendations vary from 20–30 min daily to several times per week. Examples of recommended exercise are brisk walking, cycling, rowing and swimming depending on age and level of fitness. Medical advice on taking exercise may be required.

## Smoking

Patients may need counselling to reduce and ultimately give up smoking.

## The role of the multidisciplinary diabetes care team

The dietitian and all renal healthcare support staff have a major role to play in developing suitable educational programmes backed up with written or taped information. A large proportion of patients from different ethnic backgrounds will require special consideration in respect of religious beliefs and cultural food habits that may affect their dietary intake. Educational materials will need to be adapted and translated into several languages. Audiotapes should be prepared for patients whose vision is compromised. The needs of elderly patients with diabetes must not be forgotten. In addition to the complications of diabetes, sight, hearing and mental capacity may be affected by the ageing process and this, in addition to psychosocial and economic factors, is likely to affect their nutritional intake.

Regular auditing of the provision of all types of services is essential to provide the most cost-effective care.

## Practical aspects in the nutritional management of diabetic patients at increased risk of chronic kidney disease (CKD) (Table 19.2)

Treatment is aimed at metabolic control of diabetes at all stages of CKD. Nutritional recommendations change as kidney function deteriorates. In fact, there

| Table 19.2 Goals of dietary treatment. |
| --- |
| • Treatment of overweight or obese patients prior to or early in development of chronic kidney disease<br>• Maintenance of optimal nutrition and prevention of macro- and micronutrient deficiencies at every stage of the disease<br>• Prevention of the development of renal osteodystrophy<br>• Promotion of a healthy diet and lifestyle<br>• Adjustment of patients' diet according to their usual intake in an effort to promote compliance<br>• Promotion of compliance by educating patients, their family and friends, and renal health-care professionals<br>• Regular follow-up in order to assess nutritional status, compliance and implement changes in accordance with progression of kidney disease |

are specific recommendations for each renal stage and each mode of renal replacement therapy (RRT).

Patients who develop CKD require specialist care and the contributions of an appropriately trained renal dietitian are paramount in order to improve the overall outcome of patient care. Early referral for dietary assessment and correction or adaptation of the patient's diet play an essential role.

### Stages of CKD (Table 19.3)
As part of its Kidney Disease Outcomes Quality Initiative (K/DOQI), the American National Kidney Foundation has recently published Clinical Practice Guidelines for Chronic Kidney Disease. This divides CKD into five stages depending on glomerular filtration rate (GFR) expressed as ml/min per 1.73 m² body surface area.[8]

### Protein intake

*Treatment of diabetic patients with CKD and normal or mildly reduced renal function (Table 19.4).* Patients with microalbuminuria should be monitored frequently to assess dietary and medical compliance. Protein is an important nutrient for repair and maintenance of tissue and growth. The prescribed dietary protein and energy intake should be sufficient to maintain nitrogen balance. Individual calculations should be based on the ideal body weight (within the patient's acceptable BMI range).

During the early stages of CKD, small to moderate changes in dietary protein may have a positive effect

**Table 19.3  Stages of chronic kidney disease (see reference 8).**

| Stage | Description | GFR (ml/min per 1.73 m²) |
|---|---|---|
| 1 | Kidney damage with normal or raised GFR | >90 |
| 2 | Kidney damage with mild decrease in GFR | 60–89 |
| 3 | Moderate decrease in GFR | 30–59 |
| 4 | Severe decrease in GFR | 15–29 |
| 5 | Kidney failure | <15 (or dialysis) |

GFR: glomerular filtration rate.

**Table 19.4  Nutritional management of diabetic patients with stages 1 and 2 chronic kidney disease.**

**Recommended daily intake**

| Nutrient | Amount | Comment |
|---|---|---|
| Protein | 0.8–1.0 g/kg ibw | No more than 10–15% of energy intake |
| Energy | 30–35 kcal/kg per day | Reduce to treat obesity |
| Sodium | 80–110 mmol per day | Equals 5–6 g salt |
| Phosphorus | Not restricted | |
| Potassium | Not restricted | |

ibw: ideal body weight.

on urinary albumin excretion rate, as has been shown in several studies in patients with type 1 and type 2 diabetes.[9] It should be noted that patients with micro- or macroalbuminuria tended to increase their protein intake.[7] In a randomized trial in patients with type 2 diabetes, small adjustments in protein intake resulted in a reduction in urinary albumin excretion.[9] The amount of protein, energy and sodium should be tailored to the personal needs of each individual patient, taking into consideration the level of kidney function.

*Diabetic patients with moderate or severe CKD (Tables 19.5 and 19.6).* Patients with progressive renal involvement should be monitored frequently in order to assess their nutritional status and compliance with the instructions for dietary and drug treatment. It is advisable to decrease the protein intake to 0.8–1.0 g/kg per day in patients with moderate loss of renal function (stage 3) and

0.6–0.8 g/kg ideal body weight (ibw)/day in those patients with severe loss of renal function (stage 4). However, patients need frequent monitoring for nutritional status and dietary compliance, and this may affect dietetic staffing levels. Kopple et al have suggested in the K/DOQI guideline no. 24 that patients with a GFR of <35 ml/min should be given a protein intake of 0.6–0.75 g/kg per day, at least 50% of which should be of high biological value.[10] But Waugh and Robertson have shown in a Cochrane review that protein restrictions of 0.3–0.8 g/kg per day appear to slow progression of kidney disease in insulin-dependent diabetic patients.[11] The very-low-protein diets are, however, difficult to follow for a long period of time and need close monitoring.

It is important to remember that an unplanned weight loss during the predialysis phase may be due to a spontaneous reduction in protein and energy intake, caused by changes in appetite and to the

**Table 19.5  Nutritional management of diabetic patients with stage 3 chronic kidney disease.**

**Recommended daily intake**

| Nutrient | Amount | Comment |
|---|---|---|
| Protein | 0.8–1.0 g/kg ibw per day | |
| Energy | 30–35 kcal/kg per day | |
| Sodium | 80–100 mmol/day | According to national recommendations |
| Phosphorus | 8–12 mg/kg per day | 600–700 mg/day (19–32 mmol/day) |
| Potassium | Reduce where necessary | Note should be made of medications, such as ACE inhibitors, which suppress urinary excretion of potassium |

ibw: ideal body weight.

**Table 19.6  Nutritional management of diabetic patients with stage 4 chronic kidney disease.**

**Recommended daily intake**

| Nutrient | Amount | Comments |
|---|---|---|
| Protein | 0.6–0.8 g/kg ibw per day | 50% of high biological value |
| Energy | 35 kcal/kg ibw per day | For patients under 60 years |
| | 30–35 kcal/kg ibw per day | For patients over 60 years and sedentary patients |
| Sodium | 80–100 mmol/day | 5–6 g salt/day |
| Phosphorus | 8–12 mg/kg per day | 600–700 mg (19–32 mmol/day) |
| Potassium | 1 mmol/kg per day | 2–3 g potassium/day |

ibw: ideal body weight.

development of nausea, leading to protein and energy malnutrition (PEM). This spontaneous reduction in protein intake with protein malnutrition could adversely affect prognosis of patients treated by dialysis.[12]

*Protein requirements for patients on dialysis (Table 19.7).* The K/DOQI guideline no. 15 recommends a dietary protein intake of 1.2 g/kg per day for clinically stable haemodialysis patients and 1.2–1.3 g/kg per day for peritoneal dialysis patients.[10] This level of protein intake takes into account dialytic losses. At least 50% of this protein should be of high biological value. Persistent proteinuria may result in significant protein loss and hypoalbuminaemia, even in patients on dialysis.

*Protein requirements of transplanted patients (Table 19.8).* The protein requirement for stable patients with a good functioning transplant is 1.0 g/kg per day, but this may have to be reduced in patients with reduced function of the graft.[13]

*Energy requirements (Tables 19.4–19.7)*

*Predialysis and dialytic phase of treatment.* The amount of energy required for maintaining metabolic balance is just as important as protein intake. Insufficient energy intake will lead to protein catabolism, negative nitrogen balance and unplanned weight loss. The recommendations for diabetic patients are the same as for non-diabetic patients with CKD. The K/DOQI guideline no. 17 for

**Table 19.7** Nutritional management of diabetic patients on dialysis (stage 5).

**Recommended daily intake**

| Nutrient | Mode of treatment | Amount | Comments |
|---|---|---|---|
| Protein | HD | 1.2 g/kg per day | At least 50% HBV |
| | PD | 1.2–1.3 g/kg per day | |
| Energy | HD + PD | 35 kcal/kg per day | Patients <60 years |
| | | 30 kcal/kg per day | Patients >60 years |
| | | | (In PD patients, calculate energy from absorbed glucose) |
| Phosphorus | HD + PD | 17 mg/kg per day | Total of 550 mg/day |
| Potassium | HD + PD | 1 mmol/kg per day | Total of 2–3 g/day |
| Sodium | HD + PD | 80–110 mmol/day | 5–6 g salt |
| Fluid | HD | 500–750 ml/day | In addition to daily urine output |
| | PD | 750 ml/day | Depending on fluid removal |
| Vitamins | HD + PD | Water-soluble only | Assess individual requirements |

HD: haemodialysis; PD: peritoneal dialysis; HBV: high biological value.

**Table 19.8** Nutritional management of diabetic patients following kidney transplantation.

**Recommended daily intake**

| Nutrient | Amount | Comments |
|---|---|---|
| Protein | 1.0 g/kg per day | Reduce to 0.8 g/kg per day with reduction in graft function; see Tables 19.4–19.6 |
| Energy | 30–35 kcal/kg per day | Reduce in presence of obesity |
| Sodium | 80–110 mmol/day | |
| Phosphorus | Not restricted | Restrict according to function; see Tables 19.4–19.6 |
| Potassium | Not restricted | Restrict according to function; see Tables 19.4–19.6 |

predialysis patients and no. 25 for patients on dialysis, suggest that those under 60 years of age and those 60 or older require 35 and 30 kcal/kg per day, respectively, to maintain nitrogen balance.[10] The energy provided by glucose absorption during peritoneal dialysis should be taken into account in calculating energy intake in peritoneal dialysis patients.

*After renal transplantation (Table 19.8).* Obesity is one of the major problems after a successful transplant and is multifactorial.[13] These factors include the following:

- increase in appetite, dietary freedom and steroid treatment
- poor glycaemic control associated with immunosuppressive drug therapy
- lack of exercise.

## How to calculate individual protein and energy requirements

Ideal body weight (ibw) is estimated with standard tables (weight and frame size) or the body-mass index (BMI). The BMI is calculated by dividing body weight (kg) by height in metres squared ($m^2$). A BMI of 18.5–25 is within normal range, while a BMI of <18.5 is indicative of malnutrition and a BMI of >30 of obesity. A waist circumference of >94 cm in men and > 80 cm in women is indicative of central obesity. If a patient has a BMI of 18.5–25, the actual weight should be used for calculation of energy and protein intake. If the BMI is greater than 25, one should use ibw.

## Recommended sources of energy (Table 19.1).

## Carbohydrates (1 g equals 4 kcal or 18 kJ).
Ideally, 50–55% of dietary energy should be obtained from carbohydrates containing unrefined fibre, such as unsweetened wholegrain breakfast cereals, wholemeal bread and breakfast cereals, wholegrain rice, whole-wheat pasta, and pulses such as lentils and dried beans.

## Fat (1 g = 9 kcal (38 kJ).
Fat is a concentrated form of energy, contributes to the palatability of a meal and provides a feeling of satiety. Ideally 30–35% of dietary energy should be obtained from fat. It is suggested that one increases the amount of food products with a high content of monosaturated or polyunsaturated fats. Examples of monosaturated fat sources are olive oil and olive oil-based margarine. Examples of polyunsaturated fat sources are sunflower, corn oil and margarines containing these types of oil. Manufactured foods with a high *trans*-fatty acid content such as certain types of margarine, biscuits, and cakes should be avoided.

## Management of protein-energy malnutrition (PEM) (Table 19.9)

The aetiology of PEM is often multifactorial. The reasons for this development include a reduced dietary intake, drug interactions, increased nutritional losses and altered metabolism. PEM is associated with increased risks, including delayed wound healing, decreased resistance to infection, electrolyte imbalance, prolonged hospitalization and even death.

In 1996, the Canada–USA Peritoneal Dialysis Study Group published the results of a large prospective multicentre study, also referred to as the CANUSA Study. This study showed that the relative risk of death increased with age; insulin-dependent diabetes mellitus; cardiovascular disease; low serum albumin, a possible marker of malnutrition; and worsening

nutritional status. Malnutrition estimated by subjective global assessment had a strong correlation with increased hospitalization.[14] A reduction in serum albumin may be due to a decrease in albumin synthesis, a marker of inflammation with a corresponding increase in acute phase C-reactive protein (CRP) levels, persistent albumin losses due to proteinuria and/or dialysis, and overhydration.[15] It should be noted that different assay methods may cause differences in the results of serum albumin concentrations. Prevention and treatment of PEM should start as soon as possible, even during the predialysis phase of treating CKD.

## Assessing nutritional status

Nutritional status should be assessed and documented by one of the following methods.

**BMI.** The BAPEN Malnutrition Advisory Group in the UK published a screening tool to help identify adult malnourished patients, based on height, weight and recent weight loss; it consists of three categories.[16]

1. BMI < 18.5: chronic protein-energy undernutrition probable
2. BMI 18.5–20.0: chronic protein-energy undernutrition possible
3. BMI > 20.0: chronic protein-energy undernutrition unlikely

**Classification of obesity**
4. BMI 25–29.9: pre-obese state
5. BMI 30–34.9: obesity class I
6. BMI 35–39.9: obesity class II (obese)
7. BMI 40–60: obesity class III (very obese).

*Nutritional assessment.* Nutritional assessment is done as follows:

1. estimation of dietary intake by a 24-hr dietary re-call
2. estimation of dietary intake by a 3-day food diary, including a weekend day and one haemodialysis day
3. in predialysis patients, a 24-hr urine sample used to assess protein/nitrogen losses (PNA) and proteinuria; calculation of PNA: g nitrogen in urine collection × 6.25 = g protein
4. collection of PD dialysate to estimate protein losses.

*Body composition (state of hydration may affect results).* The best-known techniques are as follows:

1. *Anthropometry* measures midarm/mid-upper arm muscle circumference and skinfold thickness.

| Table 19.9   Causes of protein–energy malnutrition in the dialysis patient. |
| --- |
| Reduced dietary intake |
|    Lack of appetite, nausea |
|    Pre-existing malnutrition |
|    Inadequate dietary nutrient intake |
|    Conflicting dietary advice (such as the need to increase protein intake, but lower the phosphorus content) |
|    Coexisting gastrointestinal disorders such as gastroparesis |
|    Comorbid conditions such as cardiac failure, cancer or other medical conditions compromising nutritional intake |
|    Inadequate provision of food in hospitals and nursing homes |
| Reduced appetite |
|    Raised serum leptin levels in CKD |
|    Poor leptin removal by dialysis |
|    Body fat mass, plasma insulin levels and incompatible dialysis membranes also contribute to hyperleptinaemia[27,28] |
| Inadequate dialysis treatment (persistent uraemic symptoms) |
|    Suppression of appetite due to glucose absorption, intra-abdominal compression and severe constipation in patients receiving PD treatment |
| Increased nutritional losses |
|    The loss of water-soluble nutrients during dialysis such as albumin, amino acids and water-soluble vitamins |
|    Persistent proteinuria |
|    Gastrointestinal losses in patients with accompanying enteropathies |
| Altered metabolism |
|    Protein degradation as a result of the dialysis process (HD) |
|    Untreated metabolic acidosis (protein catabolism) |
|    Decreased physical activity |
|    Intercurrent illness |
|    Hyperparathyroidism |
| Multiple drug regimens (also called polypharmacia) |
| Socio-economic limitations, illiteracy |
| Chronic depression, old age |

This is easy to perform and is non-invasive, but is influenced by hydration status, is sensitive to observer error and is less sensitive to change over time.

2. *Bioelectric impedance* is quick and non-invasive, but it is an indirect method and is influenced by hydration status and electrode sites.

3. *Dual energy X-ray absorptiometry* (DEXA) is a direct measurement of bone mineral, lean body mass and other compartments. DEXA is also influenced by hydration status, is costly and is not widely available.

*Subjective global assessment (SGA) in dialysis patients.* SGA is based on the patient's medical and nutritional history and physical examination. A trained nurse, a dietitian or a member of the medical team is required to complete a simple questionnaire, which includes the following categories: history of weight changes, dietary intake, gastrointestinal symptoms, functional status and metabolic stress, and disease state/comorbid disease, as well as a physical examination in order to assess loss of subcutaneous tissue, muscle wasting, oedema and ascites.[17] The overall rating then depends on the score for each item. The classification, rating from 7 to 1, is as follows:

6 or 7 in most categories—mild degree of malnutrition or normal

3, 4 or 5 in most categories—mild to moderate malnutrition

1 or 2 in most categories—severe malnutrition.

The CANUSA study showed that a one-unit

increase on the seven-point scale of SGA rating was associated with a 25% decline in relative risk of death.[17]

## Nutritional support

Methods of nutritional support are as follows.

- Oral or sip feeding is used for patients who are able to eat and drink normally. Flavoured energy-dense products with a high fat, protein and carbohydrate content may be used for sip feeding and need to be sipped slowly. Glucose monitoring and a review of the patient's drug regimen may be needed.
- Nasogastric or gastrostomy feeding is used for patients who are unable to eat or drink normally. Nocturnal tube feeding can be combined with normal oral intake during the day. Percutaneous enteral gastrostomy tubes are now widely used for long-term feeding in hospital and outpatient settings. There are several types of formulas with 1, 1.5 and 2 kcal per ml; the energy content is made up from fat, carbohydrate and protein. Tube feeding is generally well tolerated, but needs monitoring for glucose and insulin, and should be introduced slowly to avoid hyperosmolar diarrhoea. Dialysis regimens will also require reassessment to accommodate fluid removal.
- Intraperitoneal amino acids (IPAA) are used in patients on PD, whereby a 2-litre 1.1% amino acid-containing dialysate exchange replaces a 2-litre dextrose-containing dialysate, resulting in a net gain of 18 g amino acids. Patients must also take a high-energy meal or nutritional supplement when IPAA is used to facilitate protein utilization.

- Intradialytic parenteral nutrition (IDPN) is used in patients on haemodialysis. Approximately 1000 kcal in 1.5 litre fluid can be infused during HD, supplying 70 g protein as amino acids. This type of solution, made up from amino acid, emulsified fat and dextrose sources, can be manufactured by the hospital pharmacy or purchased from commercial pharmaceutical companies. There is, however, very little evidence that this expensive form of nutritional support, 10 times the cost of tube feeding, improves nutritional status and outcome of treatment.
- Total parenteral nutrition (TPN) is used for patients who are unable to receive oral/sip or enteral modes of nutrition support. As with IDPN, the administration of TPN requires the expertise of a nutritional support team and work with the renal team to implement the most effective form of nutritional support and adjust drug and dialysis regimens accordingly.

## Monitoring nutritional support

Monitoring changes in dietary intake, body composition and biochemistry after initiating nutritional support is an important element in auditing the quality of treatment.

### Electrolyte and water balance

#### Sodium* and water balance (Table 19.10).
*Na+, 1 mmol = 23 mg Na+ and 1 g salt contains 17 mmol Na+

A high sodium intake is considered by some investigators to be associated with the development of hypertension in the general population. As much as 80% of our salt intake is obtained from processed

---

**Table 19.10  How to reduce salt intake.**

- Prepare meals from fresh ingredients.
- Use little or no salt in the preparation of meals.
- Use herbs and spices, which do not contain salt, to add flavour to food.
- Avoid adding salt to food after preparation.
- Avoid excessive amounts of salty foods such as cured and processed foods, including takeaway meals.
- Avoid using salt substitutes containing potassium salts such as potassium chloride (potassium salts are now added to manufactured foods such as bread and other processed and cured foods).
- Avoid meals prepared with monosodium glutamate (MSG). Chinese, Thai, Indonesian and Japanese meals may all be prepared with MSG, which is an essential ingredient of spice mixes to prepare these types of meals.
- Always read food labels to check for added sodium and potassium salts and MSG in the list of ingredients, as MSG is widely added to processed food.

foods, salty snacks and salt added during the preparation of food. The average intake of salt in the UK is 12 g/day; optimally, this should be decreased to 6 g/day (100 mmol Na$^+$ per day).[18] Treatment with diuretics and salt restriction are routinely used in patients with hypertension with or without renal disease. An additional indication for the use of diuretics in patients with renal damage is fluid retention.

However, there are patients with kidney disease who have salt-losing nephropathy and require sodium supplementation. Restricting the intake of salt is also important to control thirst in dialysis patients with excessive interdialytic weight gains. Thirst is regulated by changes in plasma osmolality, mainly due to changes in serum sodium concentration, changes in body fluid volume and pressure, and angiotensin II. The hyperglycaemic diabetic patient may suffer from thirst due to an increase in plasma osmolality. Finally, lowering the dialysate sodium concentration in haemodialysis and peritoneal dialysis, in addition to dietary salt and fluid restriction, can improve hypertension, excessive interdialytic weight gain (IDWG) and fluid overload in dialysis patients.[19]

*Prevention of excessive IDWG and chronic fluid overload in dialysis patients (Table 19.11).* Excessive IDWG may not always be due to non-compliance with fluid intake. Solid food contains fluid and contributes to about 500–750 ml/day. Patients with a good appetite may thus gain excessive weight between haemodialysis treatments, due to both dry weight and excess fluid. This can be established by dietary assessment indicating a high protein and energy intake.[20] In spite of the fact that hyperglycaemia contributes to thirst, there appear to be no differences in IDWG between diabetic and non-diabetic kidney patients on haemodialysis.[21] Patients on haemodialysis should be advised to restrict their fluid intake so as not to gain more than 500 g in body weight per day. This generally means restricting intake to 500 ml in addition to urine volume of the previous day. In patients on peritoneal dialysis, the same principle applies, but they may be allowed more fluid depending on urine output and fluid removal during treatment. Fluid intake must be adjusted according to climate, season and ambient temperature.

*Potassium\* and hyperkalaemia (Table 19.12).* \*K$^+$ 1 mmol = 39 mg K$^+$

Hyperkalaemia is frequently found in patients with progressive kidney disease. Severe hyperkalaemia can be life-threatening if not treated immediately. The use of medications such as angiotensin-converting enzyme inhibitors (ACEI), beta-blockers, aldosterone inhibitors and non-steroidal anti-inflammatory drugs may contribute to the development of hyperkalaemia. Metabolic acidosis and hyperglycaemia in diabetic patients also contribute to hyperkalemia. Thus, foods with a high potassium content should be avoided, and the treatment regimen should be adjusted accordingly. The acceptability of the diet will be affected if the potassium restriction is excessive. Restriction to an intake of 60–70 mmol K$^+$/day or 1 mmol/kg per day will be enough to maintain acceptable serum potassium levels below 6.0 mmol/l in anuric haemodialysis patients. Once patients commence dialysis treatment and become progressively anuric, potassium restriction will become mandatory. Patients on peritoneal dialysis may not need a restricted potassium diet due to continuous potassium removal.

---

**Table 19.11   Hints for fluid control in dialysis patients.**

- Restrict salt intake
- Measure fluid allowance in a measuring jug and remove the amount taken during the day
- Always divide the allowance evenly during the day
- Use a small cup or glass instead of a large mug or large cup
- Drink only $\frac{1}{2}$ cup of fluid on each occasion
- Ice cubes quench thirst, but each cube contains 30 ml fluid and should thus be used with discretion
- Suck a lemon, lime or grapefruit wedge to stimulate the production of saliva or use chewing gum
- Take medicines at meal times unless contraindicated
- Save part of the fluid allowance when going out
- Daily measurement of weight is the best indicator of fluid intake in haemodialysis patients

**Table 19.12  Causes of hyperkalaemia.**

- Reduced renal function
- Metabolic acidosis, hyperglycaemia
- Increased catabolism
- Endocrine abnormalities
- Medications such as potassium supplements, potassium-sparing diuretics, ACE inhibitors, beta-blockers and non-steroidal anti-inflammatory drugs
- Constipation
- Excessive exercise, heatstroke, rhabdomyolysis

Ion-exchange resins may be used to treat hyperkalaemia or prevent it when patients are expected to take more potassium, as, for instance, at Christmas. However, ion-exchange resins may cause severe constipation and should be recommended for temporary use. Most foods contain potassium, but some types of fruit and vegetables contain more than others. Staple foods such as potatoes, as well as sweet potatoes, green bananas, plantains and other ethnic foods, may need to be included in the diet, but quantities can be restricted. Potassium salts such as dipotassium phosphate are food additives, but the quantity used is very small. Salt substitutes contain potassium, and foods containing salt substitutes, such as salt-reduced bread, need to be used with caution or should be avoided. Patients need to consult their dietitian for appropriate advice regarding the potassium content of specific foods, and which foods can be taken in moderate quantities and which should be avoided.

If potassium is removed by leaching (boiling in plenty of water), the loss of water-soluble vitamins will be greater. Vegetables cooked by steaming, stir-frying or microwave still contain as much potassium as the raw product.

Investigation of hyperkalaemia should include both dietary compliance and other possible causes.

*Calcium,* * *phosphorus and renal osteodystrophy.* *$Ca^{2+}$ 1 mmol = 40 mg, $P^{2+}$ 1 mmol = 31 mg
Deposition of calcium-phosphate salts in bone is essential to maintaining normal bone strength and growth. Normal calcium-phosphate metabolism, consisting of intestinal absorption, renal excretion and deposition in bone, is dependent on the interaction between the active form of vitamin D, calcitriol, and parathyroid hormone, as well as other factors.

'Renal osteodystrophy' is a term applied to several types of bone abnormalities that are commonly found in patients with impaired renal function. Calcitriol is produced in the kidney, by the 1-hydroxylation of 25-hydroxy-cholecalciferol. Reduction in the formation of calcitriol in the damaged kidney leads to decreased intestinal absorption of calcium and thus to hypocalcaemia. Moreover, with reduction in renal function, phosphorus is retained, leading to hyperphosphataemia and, together with hypocalcaemia, to hyperparathyroidism. Other factors include bone resistance to the action of parathyroid hormone in the presence of the uraemic state. In an attempt to reduce the intestinal absorption of phosphate, use has been made of phosphate binders, which are taken with food, bind to phosphate and thus prevent absorption. Unfortunately, most of these binders contain calcium, which may be absorbed, especially in patients receiving exogenous calcitriol. This will then lead to a high calcium-phosphate product in the serum and promote deposition of calcium salts in blood vessels, cardiac tissue, joints and periarticular tissues, lungs and skin.

This soft-tissue calcification is a major cause of morbidity and mortality and requires treatment and prevention early in the development of CKD.[22] During the predialysis phase of treatment, phosphate levels need to be controlled by lowering dietary phosphorus; by the use of phosphate binders, preferably non-calcium-containing products; and by dialysis once RRT is implemented. Phosphate binders should be taken shortly before or with food, particularly with main meals and with snacks that contain phosphorus and with milk-based nutritional supplements. Phosphate binders may be less effective when used with $H_2$-receptor antagonists to treat gastric and duodenal disorders. It has been reported that hyperphosphataemia may occur when ranitidine is prescribed in renal patients on phosphate-binding agents.[23]

Selevamer hydrochloride (Renagel) is a new phosphate binder that does not contain calcium. It binds the phosphorus in the food in a similar manner to calcium-based products but without the risk of hypercalcaemia, especially when calcitriol is prescribed to suppress parathyroid hormone production. Selevamer hydrochloride also lowers serum cholesterol, thereby having a beneficial effect on the lipid profile of kidney patients.[24]

Foods with a high protein content are mostly high in phosphorus and calcium. Examples of foods with a high phosphorus intake that can be restricted or avoided without affecting the quality of dietary intake are milk, yoghurt, cheese, fish with edible bones, offal, pulses/legumes, chocolate and nuts.

Normalizing a high protein intake or reducing dietary protein will reduce phosphorus intake. This may be beneficial during the predialysis phase, but patients on dialysis require a higher protein intake with a corresponding increase in the phosphorus intake. Phosphate binders will therefore continue to play an important role in the treatment and prevention of hyperphosphataemia.

The recommended calcium intake for predialysis patients is 1000–1500 mg/day, but phosphorus restriction may lead to a reduction in calcium intake. Calcium supplementation may be needed to correct hypocalcaemia. These supplements should be given between meals in order to prevent their binding to the phosphate binders and preferably at bedtime to maximize calcium absorption.

### Magnesium*. *$Mg^{2+}$ 1 mmol = 24 mg

Loss of renal function is associated with retention of magnesium. Magnesium-containing antacids are often used to relieve gastrointestinal problems and are potent phosphate binders. Moreover, in addition to side-effects secondary to the retention of magnesium salts, they can cause diarrhoea. They should thus be used sparingly if at all.

### Iron*. *Fe 1 mmol = 56 mg

Dietary iron is reduced when foods with a high iron content, such as meat, offal, pulses and green vegetables, are restricted. Most patients receiving recombinant human erythropoietin (EPO) as treatment for anaemia require iron supplements in order to maximize response to treatment. In order to prevent drug interactions, oral iron supplements should not be taken with phosphate binders but can be taken between meals. Many patients do not effectively absorb oral iron, and thus intravenous iron is often prescribed.

### Zinc

Meat, fish, pulses and wheat products are rich in zinc, and the recommended intake for adults is 1 mg elemental Zn/kg per day. Zinc deficiency is a well-known complication of uraemia and may be due to inadequate dietary protein intake or excessive losses of protein. Symptoms include impaired taste acuity, a metallic taste and impaired wound healing. Renal patients with established zinc deficiency may benefit from supplements taken between meals to enhance absorption.

### Vitamins

Vitamins regulate the metabolic pathways of protein, carbohydrate and fat. Chronic uraemia alters serum levels, body stores and function. Vitamin deficiency can occur with a restricted or an inadequate dietary intake. During dialysis, small molecules such as water-soluble vitamins, are removed. The fat-soluble vitamin A is a larger molecule, and its metabolites are more difficult to remove; therefore, accumulation could lead to toxicity.

Drug interactions may affect the activity of vitamin $B_6$, folic acid and vitamin $B_{12}$. These vitamins are important for the erythropoietic response in dialysis patients. Requirements for these vitamins may be high in order to reduce the high serum levels of homocysteine, which is thought to contribute to cardio-, cerebro- and peripheral vascular disease. At the present time, there is no definite evidence as to the therapeutic benefit of treatment of ESRD patients with hyperhomocysteinaemia.[25]

During each haemodialysis session, up to 125 mg vitamin C may be lost. Supplements may be needed in dialysis patients with a poor dietary intake. High-dose vitamin C supplements should be avoided in order to prevent hyperoxalosis leading to oxalate deposits in soft tissues.

There is as yet no agreement on recommendations of individual vitamin requirements, despite the fact that these are important nutrients for dialysis patients. Routine supplementation of water-soluble vitamins will probably outweigh the risk of deficiency, especially in patients who are nutritionally at risk due to chronic illness, depression and old age. Water-soluble vitamins should be taken after haemodialysis sessions.[26]

## REFERENCES

1. Daly AE, Obesity, diet and diabetes. Conference Report, 61st Scientific Session of the ADA, *Prac Diab Int* (2001) **18**:256.
2. Praga M, Obesity—a neglected culprit in renal disease, *Nephrol Dial Transplant* (2002) **17**:1157–9.
3. Ha TKK, Lean MEJ, Recommendations for the nutritional management of patients with diabetes mellitus, *Eur J Clin Nutr* (1998) **52**:467–81.
4. Mann L, Lean M, Toeller M et al, Recommendations for the nutritional management of patients with diabetes mellitus. The Diabetes and Nutrition Study Group (DNSG) of the European Association for the Study of Diabetes (EASD) 1999, *Eur J Clin Nutr* (2000) **54**:353–5.
5. Franz MJ, Bantle JP, Beebe CA, et al, Evidence-based nutrition principles and recommendations for the treatment and prevention of diabetes and related complications, *Diabetes Care* (2002) **25**:202–12.

6. Paisey RB, Frost J, Harvey P, et al, Five year results of a prospective very low calorie diet or conventional weight loss programme in type 2 diabetes, *J Hum Nutr Dietet* (2000) **15**:121–7.

7. Toeller M, Buyken AE, Protein intake—new evidence for its role in diabetic nephropathy, *Nephrol Dial Transplant* (1998) **13**:1926–7

8. Definition and classification of stages of chronic kidney disease (Part 4). In: *K/DOQI Clinical Practice Guidelines for Chronic Kidney Disease: Evaluation, Classification and Stratification, Am J Kidney Dis* (2002) **39** Suppl 1:S46–S75.

9. Pijls LTJ, de Vries H, Donker AJM, et al, The effect of protein restriction on albuminuria in patients with type 2 diabetes mellitus: a randomized trial, *Nephrol Dial Transplant* (1999) **14**:1445–53.

10. Kopple JD, Wolfson M, Chertow GM, et al, *KDOQI Clinical Guidelines for Nutrition in Chronic Renal Failure, Am J Kidney Dis* (2000) **35** Suppl 2.

11. Waugh NR, Robertson AM, Protein restriction for diabetic renal disease (Cochrane Review). Cochrane Library, 4 (Update Software: Oxford 2000).

12. Ikizler TA, Greene JH, Wingard RL, Spontaneous dietary protein intake during progression of chronic renal failure, *J Am Soc Nephrol* (1995) **6**:1386–91.

13. Pagenkemper JJ, Burke KI, Roderick SL, Nutritional management of the adult renal transplant patient, *J Renal Nutr* (1994) **4**:119–24.

14. Churchill DN, Taylor DW, Kesehaviah PR, Adequacy of dialysis and nutrition in continuous peritoneal dialysis: association with clinical outcomes, *J Am Soc Nephrol* (1996) **7**:198–207.

15. Jones CH, Serum albumin—a marker of fluid overload in dialysis patients?, *J Renal Nutr* (2001) **11**:59–61.

16. Green CJ on behalf of the Council of the British Association for Parenteral and Enteral Nutrition (BAPEN), Existence, causes and consequences of disease-related malnutrition in the hospital and community, and clinical and financial benefits of nutritional intervention, *Clin Nutr* (1999) **18** Suppl 2:3–28.

17. Churchill D, Adequacy of dialysis and nutrition in continuous peritoneal dialysis: association with clinical outcomes. *J Am Soc Nephrol* (1996) **2**:198–207.

18. MacGregor GA, Blood pressure: importance of the kidney and the need to reduce salt intake, *Am J Kidney Dis* (2001) **37** Suppl 2:S34–8.

19. Tomson CRV, Advising dialysis patients to restrict fluid intake without restricting sodium intake is not based on evidence and is a waste of time, *Nephrol Dial Transplant* (2001) **16**:1538–42.

20. Sherman RA, Cody RF, Rogers ME, Inter-dialysis weight gain and nutritional parameters in chronic dialysis patients, *Am J Kidney Dis* (1995) **25**:579–83.

21. Halverson NA, Wilkens KG, Worthington-Roberts B, Interdialytic fluid gains in diabetic patients receiving hemodialysis treatment, *J Renal Nutr* (1993) **3**:23–9.

22. Cannata-Andia J, Passlick-Deetjen J, Ritz E, Management of the renal patient: experts' recommendations and clinical algorithms on renal osteodystrophy and cardiovascular risk factors, *Nephrol Dial Transplant* (2000) **15** Suppl 5: S130–1.

23. Tan CC, Harden PN, Rodger RSC et al, Ranitidine reduces phosphate binding in dialysis patients receiving calcium carbonate, *Nephrol Dial Transplant* (1996) **11**:851–3.

24. Chertow GM, Burke KS, Dillon MA, et al, Long-term effects of sevelamer hydrochloride on the calcium phosphate product and lipid profile of haemodialysis patients. *Nephrol Dial Transplant* (1999) **14**:2907–14.

25. Shemin D, Bostom AG, Selhub J, Treatment of hyperhomocysteinemia in end-stage renal disease: a review, *Am J Kidney Dis* (2001) **38** Suppl 1:S91–4.

26. Makoff R, Vitamin replacement therapy in renal failure patients, *Miner Electrolyte Metab* (1999) **25**:75–8.

27. Stenvinkel P, Lonnqvist F, Schalling M, Molecular studies of leptin: implications for renal disease, *Nephrol Dial Transplant* (1999) **14**:1103–12.

28. Wright MJ, Woodrow JD, Young G, et al, Biocompatible dialysis membranes do not reduce plasma leptin levels. *Nephrol Dial Transplant* (2000) **15**:925–6.

# 20

# The use of transplantation in the patient with end-stage renal disease

Elizabeth Kendrick and Gabriel Danovitch

Diabetes mellitus (DM) has become the most common cause of renal failure in the US, and accounts for 45% of patients presenting for treatment of end-stage renal disease (ESRD).[1] The proportion of patients presenting with ESRD secondary to DM in other parts of the world is variable,[2,3] but it also appears that the increasing incidence, especially of type II DM, is having a significant impact on the demographics of ESRD in many other countries. As a result, DM is becoming the most common cause of ESRD in patients referred for renal transplantation. This chapter examines the impact of renal transplantation in diabetics with ESRD in general, as well as the role of pancreas transplantation in patients with DM.

## KIDNEY TRANSPLANTATION IN DM

In the 1970s and early 1980s, many transplant programs excluded diabetics from consideration for renal transplantation. The poor prognosis of these patients on dialysis; the poor rehabilitation potential associated with the comorbidities of retinopathy, neuropathy, and cardiovascular disease; and the increased risk of transplant-related complications were cited as reasons that these patients should not be considered for renal transplantation.[4,5] In centers that did perform transplants in diabetics during this period, survival exceeded that of diabetic patients remaining on dialysis. This, along with improved management of diabetic and uremic complications, has made transplantation a routinely accepted form of treatment for these patients.[6]

## Survival

Recent reports of patient survival in renal transplantation show a 94.8% 1-year and an 81.8% 5-year survival for recipients of cadaveric grafts, and a 97.6% 1-year and 91% 5-year survival for those receiving living donor transplants.[7] Patient survival in diabetic renal transplant recipients is 10–20% less than that of patients with other causes of renal disease at 3–5 years after a transplant in many series.[8,9] Death from cardiovascular disease is the major cause of mortality in these patients. It has been suggested that mortality after transplantation is higher in patients with type II DM than type I,[10] an outcome which may be a function of older age and a higher incidence of comorbidities in the former group of patients. Annual death rates of transplant recipients are approximately one-third those of diabetic patients remaining on dialysis,[11] a finding which may reflect the selection of healthier patients for transplantation. But when diabetic patients who had been transplanted were compared with patients remaining on the transplant list, presumably with similar comorbidities, patient survival was significantly better in transplant recipients.[11,12] Mortality was 38% less in transplanted patients than in those remaining on the transplant list. There does not appear to be any difference in renal-graft survival, when censored for death, between patients with DM and those with other causes of renal failure;[1,10] 5-year renal-graft survival is equivalent at 57.3% for DM and 59% for non-DM recipients.

## POST-TRANSPLANT COMPLICATIONS

### Surgical and urologic complications

Complications after renal transplantation are similar to those seen in recipients with ESRD due to other causes; however, there may be special considerations regarding presentation and management in the diabetic renal transplant recipient. Wound infections do not appear to be more common in diabetic renal transplant recipients as a group,[13] although the concurrent presence of obesity may increase the risk of this complication.[14] Urinary tract infections are common after renal transplantation, and they appear to be more common in diabetics and may require hospitalization for septicemia.[15] Infections with enteric bacteria are the most common etiology, but infections with fungal pathogens, such as *Candida*, may also occur. Bladder dysfunction due to autonomic neuropathy causing urinary reflux or retention contributes to the increased risk of this complication in conjunction with the use of immunosuppressive drugs, indwelling catheters and surgical changes in the anatomy of the urinary tract. Hyperglycemia and glucosuria can contribute to the increased risk of candiduria.[16] Urinary tract infections are more commonly seen in the early months after renal transplantation, but in some patients they may be a recurring problem. Diabetic patients with identified bladder dysfunction may be required to perform intermittent self-catheterization to reduce the risk of recurrent urinary tract infections. Sometimes, significant bladder dysfunction as a potential exacerbating factor may not be identified, and affected patients may benefit by long-term prophylactic antibiotics.

### Complications of immunosuppression

Transplant recipients are at increased risk of opportunistic infections with organisms such as *Pneumocystis carinii* and *Aspergillus* or other fungal organisms, as well as primary or reactivated infections with latent viruses, such as cytomegalovirus and herpes simplex, due to immunosuppression.[17] Overall, diabetic renal transplant patients do not appear to be at increased risk for the majority of these types of infectious complications compared to nondiabetic renal transplant patients, although, in some isolated case reports, diabetes is identified as a risk factor for infections with some fungal organisms such as *Mucor* and *Nocardia*.[18–21] This mirrors the increased frequency of some fungal infections in diabetics in general, such as cutaneous and rhinocere-bral zygomycosis and oral and vulvovaginal candidiasis.[22]

Long-term immunosuppression in renal transplantation increases the risk of some types of cancers, including nonmelanomatous skin cancers, Kaposi's sarcoma, and post-transplant lymphoproliferative disorder.[23] Recent evidence suggests there may also be an increased risk of renal cell carcinoma,[24] which may be related to acquired cystic disease. Other types of neoplasia can occur, but do not appear to be more common than in the general population. Diabetic transplant patients do not appear to be at increased risk of cancer; in fact, one study demonstrated a lower risk for type I DM patients with renal disease,[25] possibly related to the increased risk of death from cardiovascular disease.

### Cardiovascular disease

Forty percent of deaths in renal transplant recipients are secondary to cardiovascular events such as myocardial infarction and stroke,[26] and DM is one of the major risk factors for these events.[27] Diabetic renal transplant recipients have been shown to have three times the risk of events related to ischemic heart disease than the general population.[28] Female diabetic patients appear to be at particularly high risk. Other traditional risk factors for ischemic heart disease, such as age, hypertension, smoking, hypercholesterolemia and obesity, may also be present in these patients, contributing to their overall risk. Factors associated with ESRD and dialytic therapy present before transplantation, such as left-ventricular hypertrophy due to chronic volume overload, oxidation of lipids, vascular calcifications due to abnormalities in calcium and phosphorous metabolism, hyperhomocysteinemia, and increase in thrombogenic factor, can contribute to increased cardiovascular risk.[29,30] Some of these factors, such as volume overload and abnormalities in calcium and phosphorus metabolism, can improve after renal transplantation. However, the use of corticosteroids and the calcineurin inhibitors cyclosporine and tacrolimus for immunosuppression can cause lipid abnormalities to persist. High homocysteine levels may continue to be present, especially if graft function is impaired.[31]

Complications of peripheral vascular disease leading to amputation are the most common adverse event in diabetic kidney transplant patients and have been reported to occur in 13–25% of patients. Myocardial infarctions occur in 14–22% of patients, and up to 19% of patients have cerebrovascular events.[32] Not surprisingly, patients with evidence of pre-existing vascular disease are at higher risk of these complications.[33,34] This risk was further defined by Manske et al,[35] who showed that diabetic renal transplant candidates demonstrating one or more coronary artery stenoses on angiogram of greater than or equal to 75% had a sevenfold risk of amputation and a fourfold risk of myocardial infarction within 3 years after transplantation.

The importance of identifying the extent of pre-existing vascular disease, particularly coronary artery disease, in diabetic kidney transplant candidates cannot be overemphasized. Most transplant centers require noninvasive cardiac testing. A recent survey of renal transplant programs in the USA reported that 59% of programs screened diabetic transplant candidates with some type of noninvasive modality, such as nuclear perfusion scanning, exercise thallium testing or dobutamine echocardiography.[36] One program using thallium-201 myocardial perfusion scintigraphy found a low incidence of subsequent cardiac events in those patients with negative studies.[37,38] Those with positive studies underwent coronary angiograms with intervention for significant coronary lesions. Some centers, however, recommend initial evaluation of the diabetic renal transplant candidate by angiogram, given the high incidence of significant coronary artery disease in asymptomatic patients,[35,39] as well as in all patients with a known history of coronary artery disease. When significant coronary disease is found, myocardial revascularization, either by coronary artery bypass grafting or angioplasty, has acceptable short- and long-term results,[40,41] although early morbidity is high, as would be expected in these high-risk patients.

Given the impact of cardiovascular disease in diabetics with kidney disease, modifications of risk factors in order to decrease risk of progression and development of cardiovascular disease is important. Unfortunately, there are no prospective studies addressing the impact of specific intervention in kidney transplantation in general or diabetic recipients. Apart from assessing the extent of cardiovascular disease present prior to transplantation, periodic reassessment with noninvasive studies in asymptomatic, high-risk patients to help define any progression of coronary disease should be performed. The majority of centers ask for noninvasive testing on an annual basis in this high-risk group. New cardiac symptoms or events in patients waiting for a transplant clearly require urgent cardiologic evaluation and reassessment as to whether they remain suitable for a transplant.

## Recurrent nephropathy

In registry data, kidney-graft survival in diabetics does not appear to differ from those patients with other causes of ESRD. They do not appear to be at higher risk of immunologic graft loss from acute or chronic rejection.[1] However, renal lesions consistent with diabetic nephropathy have been reported to occur in the transplanted kidney as early as 2–3 years after transplant, the earliest lesion being arteriolar hyalinosis.[42] A low reported incidence of recurrent diabetic nephropathy and low risk of graft failure were reported in one registry study,[43] perhaps reflecting the lack of a systematic approach to renal transplant biopsy to assess renal abnormalities in this group of patients and the relatively short duration of follow-up. Conversely, a series with longer follow-up and a more systematic approach to performing biopsies of the renal transplant in diabetic transplant patients with renal dysfunction or proteinuria showed a high rate of graft failure, with development of diabetic nephropathy in the renal allograft.[44]

## Bone disease

Metabolic bone disease is common in patients with ESRD, in part due to secondary hyperparathyroidism.[45] That other factors can contribute to bone disease in the dialysis patient is evidenced by the high incidence of mixed-pattern and low-bone-turnover lesions that are seen in addition to the high-bone-turnover lesion typically associated with hyperparathyroidism. Long-term immunosuppression by corticosteroids can cause significant bone loss after transplantation, leading to osteoporosis, and may increase the risk of fractures.[46] Bone density can decrease by as much as one-third in the first 6 months after transplantation; this effect is associated with the higher doses of steroids used in this early period after transplantation. Bone density as measured by DEXA scan generally stabilizes or may actually improve with maintenance steroid doses of 7.5 mg/day or less. A few animal studies suggest that cyclosporine can contribute to bone loss as well;[47,48] this effect is not consistently seen in human studies. Diabetic transplant recipients seem to be at particularly high risk of fractures associated with low bone density, with an incidence of up to 40–49% in some studies.[49–51] Diabetes has been associated with low bone turnover and cortical osteopenia, whereas steroid-related bone loss generally affects cancellous bone. Most fractures appear to be appendicular, including ankles and feet, unlike the usual pattern of steroid-related osteoporotic fractures occurring in the axial skeleton. A number of recent studies have shown stabilization or even increases in bone mineral density with various treatment regimens in renal transplant patients in general—most consistently, in studies using vitamin D and calcium with or without bisphosphonates.[52] However, reduction of fracture risk has not consistently been used as an endpoint in these studies. The question of whether similar treatment would benefit bone disease in diabetic renal transplant patients as a specific group, given the differences in patterns of bone loss and fractures, has not yet been explored.

## Impact on secondary complications

Diabetics are at higher risk of cataract formation,[53] and the use of corticosteroids for immunosuppression can increase the risk of cataract progression in transplant recipients.[6,54] Diabetic transplant recipients should continue to have regular ophthamologic follow-up for this reason, as well as to monitor the progression of retinopathy. In general, however, renal transplantation seems to have little impact on whether retinopathy will improve or progress.[55] Some patients may have some improvement in symptoms of peripheral neuropathy or gastropathy after renal transplantation, but this appears to be related to resolution of the uremic state rather than to improvement in diabetic neuropathy per se.

Diabetic renal transplant recipients often require additional treatment for glycemic control after transplantation, due both to corticosteroid use and increased insulin clearance from a functioning renal transplant. Many patients whose diabetes had been controlled with diet or oral agents while on dialysis will need to be placed on insulin for adequate blood-sugar control after transplantation, and they should be notified of this prior to transplant.

## Post-transplant diabetes (PTDM)

Long-term use of steroids for immunosuppression can be associated with post-transplant diabetes (PTDM) in as many as 5–10% of renal transplant patients who were not diabetic prior to transplantation,[56] and this incidence may increase over time. There is evidence that both cyclosporine and tacrolimus have diabetogenic effects and may be contributing to the recently increasing incidence of this problem. Older age, higher body weight, and African-American race are additional risk factors for development of post-transplant diabetes. Patients who develop PTDM have been shown to develop secondary complications of DM such as retinopathy, neuropathy or nephropathy in the same time course that would be expected for pre-existing DM.[57]

## PANCREAS TRANSPLANTATION

Early attempts at whole organ pancreas transplantation in the 1970s had a high failure rate due to graft losses as a result of technical complications as well as a high rate of rejection in the era before the availability of cyclosporine.[58] Over time, both patient and graft survival has greatly improved with changes in surgical technique as well as advances in immunosuppressive therapy.

Pioneering work in whole organ pancreas transplantation was carried out at the University of Minnesota in the late 1960s and 1970s. These procedures were performed as pancreas transplant alone (PTA) or as pancreas transplant after kidney transplant (PAK) by a variety of techniques for duct management of exocrine secretions, including enteric drainage, open-duct drainage into the peritoneum and duct injection. Early experience was marred by a high rate of graft loss due to acute rejection in the era of corticosteroid- and azathioprine-based immune suppression. Technical complications leading to graft loss were common, including graft thrombosis, infection and anastomotic leak. With the introduction of cyclosporine in the 1980s, immunologic graft survival improved. The rate of acute rejection was still as high as 75%,[59] but by that time antilymphocytic antibodies had become available for treatment of steroid-resistant rejection.[60] In addition, the technique of bladder drainage of the pancreas allograft, in which the donor duodenal segment is anastomosed to the dome of the bladder, became the standard method for handling the exocrine secretions of the graft, and allowed for the measurement of urinary amylase as a marker of acute rejection. Graft loss due to technical complications was reduced by this method as well. In the early 1990s, tacrolimus became available and later mycophenolate mofetil. The use of these newer agents in pancreas transplantation has demonstrated lower rates of rejection and less steroid-resistant rejection than older agents.[60,61] Moreover, the use of tacrolimus-based immune suppression markedly improved the outcome in pancreas transplant alone.[62] More recently, the newer anti-interleukin-2 monoclonal antibodies, basiliximab and daclizumab, have been used as induction therapy in pancreas transplantation, with results that appear to be on a par with those using older antilymphocytic drug therapy, and do not seem to have the same increased risk of opportunistic infections.

Throughout the mid-1990s, the vast majority of pancreas transplants used bladder drainage for duct management of the graft. However, there are significant complications associated with this method (see surgical complications below). There has been a shift towards primary enteric drainage of the pancreas graft, such that, in 1998, 60% of transplants were performed in this way. The decrease in the rate of technical failure of enteric-drained grafts has also driven this change.[63] Venous drainage of enteric-drained pancreas grafts was accomplished by portal venous drainage in 20% of cases.

## Survival: simultaneous pancreas, kidney grafts

Almost 13 000 pancreas transplants were reported to the International Pancreas Transplant Registry from 1966 through September 1999, three-quarters of them performed in the USA.[24] Over 1000 pancreas transplants were reported in the USA in 1998. Outcomes reported to the United Network of Organ Sharing (UNOS) have shown a significant improvement in both patient and graft survival over time. The majority of pancreas transplants in the USA have been combined kidney-pancreas transplants (SPK). One-year patient survival has improved from 90% for 1987–8 cases to 95% for 1996–7. In addition, pancreas graft survival has improved from 74% to 85% at 1-year for the same time period; kidney graft survival improved from 83% to 91%. This improvement in outcome has come about despite the fact that recipients of pancreas transplants are becoming older: UNOS registry data show an increase in recipients older than 44 years of age from less than 5% in 1988 to greater than 20% in 1998–99.

## Survival: solitary pancreas grafts

Solitary pancreas transplants, either PTA or PAK, have made up only a small proportion of the total pancreas transplants in the USA. More recently, the proportion of PAK transplants performed has increased to more than 10% per year.[24] Concern over the surgical morbidity and the risk of immunosuppression in a nonuremic diabetic patient who does not also require a kidney transplant seems to account for the small number of patients in this group. Patient survival rates for solitary pancreas trans-

plants are comparable to those of SPK. Graft survival of PTA and PAK has been significantly worse, but registry data has shown improvement in more recent years. One-year graft survival for PTA has increased from 50% in 1987–8 to 69% in 1996–7; that for PAK from 56% to 74%. The use of newer immunosuppressive regimens in part accounts for this improvement. Technical graft loss due to thrombosis is higher in enteric-drained solitary grafts than in SPK recipients; the rate of other etiologies of technical graft failure, such as bleeding, anastomotic leak and infection, are no different.

The University of Minnesota recently reported their large experience in solitary pancreas transplantation (over 400 PAK and over 200 PTA patients).[62,64] They demonstrated excellent patient survival and survival of the pancreas graft approaching that of SPK transplant using tacrolimus-based immunosuppression. Survival of the kidney graft after PAK did not appear to be jeopardized by subsequent pancreas transplant.[64] Nonuremic patients with insulin-dependent DM (IDDM) were selected for PTA if they have very labile blood-sugar control despite intensive therapy, severe autonomic dysfunction including hypoglycemic unawareness, and well-maintained renal function.[62] In early experience, patients with a creatinine clearance of less than 80 ml/min were found to have a higher risk of eventual need for dialysis or renal transplantation after PTA, in part due to use of calcineurin inhibitors.

## Complications of pancreas transplantation

### Surgical

Pancreas transplantation has a higher complication rate than kidney transplantation alone. Surgical complications led to relaparotomy in 32% of patients in one series,[65] although a more recent study showed this incidence to be decreasing.[66] In particular, the need for relaparotomy for graft thrombosis or drainage of intra-abdominal infection was shown to decrease from 10% to 5.6% and 12% to 3.8%, respectively. This improved outcome has been attributed to better prophylactic regimens for prevention of graft thrombosis and infection, refinement in surgical technique and improved immunosuppression. Nevertheless, vascular thrombosis has a reported incidence of 10–35% and accounts for the majority of nonimmunologic graft failures.[66]

Other surgical complications requiring reoperation include bleeding and anastomotic leaks.[67] While overall graft survival appears to be no different between bladder-drained and enteric-drained pancreas grafts in combined SPK, enteric drainage is associated with a higher rate of intra-abdominal infections and graft thrombosis. Older donor age and recipient obesity have also been associated with increased risk of surgical complications.

## Urologic

Bladder drainage of pancreas allografts has a higher rate of complications overall. As many as 50–60% of patients have some type of urologic complication related to this method of exocrine drainage.[68,69] Conversion from bladder drainage to enteric drainage of the graft may be required in up to 10–20% of patients for complications related to bladder drainage.[59] Gross hematuria and recurrent urinary tract infections are the most common, with a reported incidence of 30% or more. Causes of hematuria include duodenitis of the allograft; infection; bladder calculi formed on retained sutures or staples, or bleeding from these areas; acute rejection; necrosis of the duodenal allograft; and arteriovenous fistula. Cystoscopy is necessary for definitive diagnosis, and sometimes the problem can be managed in this fashion. Prolonged catheter drainage, alterations in urinary pH due to pancreatic exocrine drainage, and impaired vesical mucosal integrity in the setting of bladder dysfunction that may already be present as a result of autonomic neuropathy can contribute to the occurrence of urinary-tract infection (UTI) in patients with bladder-drained grafts. Bacteremia has a urinary cause in greater than 50% of SPK recipients,[70] not solely in patients with bladder-drained grafts.

Reflux pancreatitis of the allograft associated with hyperamylasemia and pain over the graft has a reported incidence of 11–17%. This problem resolves quickly with temporary catheter drainage of the bladder, but needs to be distinguished from more serious problems such as an anastomotic leak or abscess. Reflux pancreatitis can occur at any time after transplantation and is thought to be the result of the reflux of urine into the pancreatic duct during micturition.

Other urologic complications can include urethral disruption, strictures, and penile complications in men. Dysuria not related to infection or other identifiable cause can also occur and is thought to be caused by irritation of the urothelium by pancreatic secretions and change in urine pH.

Bladder-drained pancreas allografts can also cause symptomatic volume depletion and metabolic acidosis as a result of the loss of bicarbonate-containing pancreatic exocrine secretions. Sodium bicarbonate supplements are usually required to correct metabolic acidosis, and symptomatic orthostatic hypotension may require additional sodium supplements, florinef or sympathomimetic agents to raise blood pressure.[71] Although fluid loss in bladder-drained pancreas grafts appears to contribute to orthostasis, this complication can also be seen in recipients of enteric-drained pancreas grafts, presumably due to autonomic dysfunction and resolution of chronic volume overload state in ESRD.

## Acute rejection

SPK patients have a higher risk of acute rejection than patients who have received only a kidney transplant (KTA).[72,73] Synchronous rejection in both organs occurs the vast majority of the time,[74] although acute rejection in the kidney graft can occur with normal renal function.[75] Acute rejection in the pancreas graft alone is uncommon and was shown to occur in only 3% of biopsies in one series.[74] Monitoring of serum creatinine and biopsy of the renal allograft are often used to diagnose acute rejection in double organ transplant patients. Other noninvasive means for early diagnosis of pancreas allograft rejection have been found to be useful, including measurement of urinary amylase in bladder-drained pancreas grafts,[76] and measurement of serum amylase and lipase,[77,78] although these tests lack specificity. Elevation in serum glucose is a rather late finding associated with advanced rejection and therefore much less helpful in the early detection and treatment of acute rejection of the pancreas.

Needle biopsy of the pancreas allograft done either cystoscopically, in the case of bladder-drained pancreas grafts, or percutaneously with radiologic guidance in enteric- or bladder-drained grafts, is the reference standard for diagnosis of acute rejection. Noninvasive studies may raise suspicion of acute rejection and can act as a guide to determine which patients may benefit from a biopsy. This approach has been shown to avoid unnecessary treatment for acute rejection in approximately 40% of patients.[79] The risks of significant complications due to this procedure appear to be low—biopsy-related pancreatitis and bleeding complications are the most common. If acute rejection in the pancreas graft is detected and treated early, long-term metabolic function of the graft appears to be unaffected.[80]

## Recurrent disease

Recurrence of diabetes due to recurrent autoimmune disease has been reported in pancreas transplant recipients.[81] This occurs despite continuance of immunosuppression. The diagnosis of recurrent disease versus other causes of graft failure (such as chronic rejection) depends on the findings of selective beta-cell loss on biopsy and the presence of markers of humoral autoimmunity, such as insulin antibodies.

## BENEFITS OF PANCREAS TRANSPLANTATION

### Metabolic

The most documented benefit of pancreas transplantation is sustained normoglycemia and freedom from the need for exogenous insulin.[82–86] Fasting blood sugars and HgbA1c have been shown to be maintained in the normal range in the majority of patients over the long term.[82,84] The majority of pancreas grafts have systemic venous drainage, and, as such, peripheral hyperinsulinemia is generally seen in transplant recipients because the first-pass extraction of insulin by the liver is lacking. Portal venous drainage of the pancreas allograft might be expected to abrogate peripheral hyperinsulinemia. A decrease in fasting serum insulin levels has been found by some,[87] but not by other investigators,[88,89] when comparing patients with portal versus systemic drainage of the pancreas graft, and the method of venous drainage did not seem to affect glucose metabolism. Denervation of the pancreas graft, negating tonic inhibition of insulin secretion, may also contribute.[90] However, most studies show normal C-peptide levels, indicating that the primary reason for hyperinsulinemia is decreased metabolism of insulin, and not increased secretion. Serum blood sugars after an oral glucose load have been shown to be slightly higher in pancreas transplant recipients than controls, and this, in conjunction with peripheral hyperinsulinemia, appears to define a state of insulin resistance in these patients. Corticosteroids used for immunosuppression are thought to contribute to the abnormality, and insulin resistance appears to improve with time 1 year after transplantation when the patient is on lower doses.[91] However, it may also be that insulin resistance is an appropriate response to hyperinsulinemia that exists for the aforementioned reasons.

There is evidence that pancreas transplantation improves defective glucose counterregulation resulting from prior episodes of hypoglycemia. The responses of epinephrine,[92] glucagon and growth hormone,[93] have been shown to improve in response to hypoglycemia as well as recognition of hypoglycemia.[92] Postprandial hypoglycemia has been reported to occur in a few pancreas transplant recipients, but it appears to be mild and usually not symptomatic.[94] Fasting hypoglycemia does not appear to be a problem in these patients.

### Recurrent nephropathy

Pancreas transplantation has clearly been shown to prevent the recurrence of diabetic nephropathy in the renal allograft in patients receiving SPK transplants,[95] and to prevent the progression of mild nephropathy in patients who have received a prior renal transplant.[96] In addition, reversal of established lesions of diabetic nephropathy has been documented in the native kidneys of nonuremic type I diabetic patients receiving a pancreas transplant alone, but only after 10 years.[97] Lesions of diabetic nephropathy were still present, but had not progressed at 5 years after transplantation; native renal function remained stable despite the use of cyclosporine.

### Retinopathy

Microvascular disease leading to retinopathy is common in pancreas transplant recipients, but evidence that this will improve after a pancreas transplant is mixed. Several small studies have shown stabilization of retinopathy in the majority of patients,[98–101] or improvement in a small number of patients,[102,103] while others have not. Ramsay et al[102] found that retinopathy did not progress during a 3-year period in pancreas transplant patients with continued graft function, as compared to progression of retinopathy in 70% of those patients whose grafts did not function. Lack of clear improvement in retinopathy after transplantation is probably related to the high percentage of patients presenting with severe retinal lesions or even blindness—lesions that are likely irreversible. One study demonstrating improvement in microangiopathy, as measured in the conjunctival circulation after pancreas transplantation,[104] gives promise that patients may benefit if transplanted at an earlier stage.

### Neuropathy

A few small studies are available documenting the course of diabetic neuropathy in pancreas transplant recipients. In one study of 10 patients, no improvement in lower extremity nerve conduction was seen 9 months after a pancreas transplant, although there was some improvement in subjective sensory symptoms,[105] perhaps related to improvement in overall sense of well-being. With longer follow-up, Kennedy et al noted no change in measures of peripheral and autonomic neuropathy at 42 months after pancreas transplantation, while the control group of nonuremic diabetic patients had progressive neuropathy.[106] Tyden et al[107] demonstrated improvement in nerve conduction and parasympathetic autonomic dysfunction after 2 years in SPK transplant patients, but this was also seen in patients who received a kidney transplant alone. A rapid initial improvement of conduction velocity within 1 year after transplantation, with subsequent stabilization of neuropathy, was noted by Nankivell et al.[108] Navarro et al[109] demonstrated that patients with a functioning pancreas transplant had early and sustained improvement in peripheral neuropathy, as compared to worsening symptoms in patients whose grafts had failed. Improvement in neuropathy was associated with less severe findings at the outset, again underscoring that patients with less severe pathology at the time of transplant may have greater benefit as a result of a pancreas transplant.

## Impact on cardiovascular disease

Correction of the diabetic state after pancreas transplantation may have beneficial effects on metabolic abnormalities that have been associated with increased risk of progression of cardiovascular disease. Despite the presence of systemic hyperinsulinemia and the use of immunosuppressive drugs, which can have an adverse effect on lipids, pancreas transplantation can result in normal or near normal lipid and lipoprotein concentration.[110,111] Pancreas transplant recipients have also been shown to have improved postprandial triglycerides, compared to diabetic patients who receive a kidney transplant alone[112] or nontransplanted IDDM patients, as well as higher high-density lipoprotein (HDL) levels, which may confer benefits in terms of cardiovascular risk. Pancreas transplantation has also been shown to normalize free fatty-acid metabolism when compared to uremic IDDM patients.[113] Others have found no obvious impact of pancreas transplantation on lipoprotein metabolism when compared to kidney transplant alone.[111] Portal drainage of the pancreas graft may confer some benefit in terms of lipid profile. While some investigators have noted no difference in total cholesterol and triglycerides when patients with systemic venous drainage of the pancreas graft were compared with those with portal venous drainage,[88,89] others have noted improvement in lipid profile and metabolism. Reduced very-low-density lipoprotein (VLDL), intermediate-density lipoprotein (IDL) and low-density lipoprotein (LDL) particles and improved HDL were noted

by Hughes et al;[114] activation of cholesterol ester transfer linked to peripheral hyperinsulinemia was present in patients with systemically drained pancreas grafts, but not in those with portal venous drainage,[115] suggesting a potential benefit of this technique in improving the cardiovascular risk profile.

Measures of endothelial dysfunction (endothelial-dependent dilation) and prothrombotic state have been shown to be improved in pancreas transplant recipients, and intimal media thickness of the carotid artery to be lower than in patients receiving a kidney transplant alone (KTA),[116] possibly decreasing cardiovascular risk. The incidence of hypertension has been shown to be less in pancreas transplant recipients than in KTA patients,[117,118] although Hricik et al[117] noted that this benefit was seen primarily in patients with a bladder-drained pancreas, and it is possible the effect is mediated by chronic volume depletion.

Despite evidence that pancreas transplantation appears to have a positive influence on several risk factors for atherosclerosis, studies looking at clinical outcomes related to cardiovascular disease have been mixed. Extensive carotid-wall abnormalities have been shown to persist despite pancreas transplantation.[119] Biesenbach et al[120] showed that pancreas transplantation failed to halt the progression of macrovascular disease; Morrissey et al[121] showed that pancreas transplant recipients had a higher incidence of peripheral vascular complications, including the need for amputation and lower extremity bypass graft surgery, than patients with KTA despite comparable rates of these complications prior to transplantation. Conversely, reversal of diastolic dysfunction[122] and improvements in left-ventricular function and geometry, as measured by echocardiography,[123] have been seen in patients receiving SPK versus KTA.

## Impact on patient survival

Some studies have shown an increased risk of death in short-term follow-up of SPK patients, compared to diabetic patients who received a KTA,[124,125] as a consequence of cardiovascular, infectious, and surgical complications that have already been discussed. However, several recent studies that have followed patients for as long as 5–10 years after transplantation have demonstrated a significant survival advantage of patients receiving a double organ transplant.[72,107,125–128] Ojo et al[125] estimated that SPK recipients can be expected to live 15 years longer than diabetic patients on the transplant list, and 10 years longer than those who have received a cadaveric kidney transplant. This improvement in survival did not manifest itself until 5 years after transplantation, demonstrating the impact of early mortality. A rather striking improvement in long-term survival in SPK recipients was also shown by Tyden et al[127] in a study in which 10-year survival was 60%, as compared to 37% for diabetics who had received a kidney transplant alone and 33% for SPK recipients whose pancreas graft functioned less than 2 years. The 10-year survival for SPK recipients was comparable to that of nondiabetic KTA recipients. Moreover, despite the higher upfront financial costs of SPK transplantation and the added costs related to early surgical and medical morbidity, a recent decision analysis model showed that, over the long term, SPK transplant was cost-effective when compared to both living-donor and cadaveric renal transplantation, and the expected cost per quality-adjusted year was approximately one-third what was expected for long-term dialysis.[129]

## Quality of life

SPK and KTA recipients report health-related quality of life below that of the general population, but similar to patients with other chronic diseases.[130] While several studies have demonstrated that both SPK and KTA patients with successful grafts report better health and quality of life after transplantation,[131] the addition of a pancreas graft can have a greater positive impact in this area, SPK recipients reporting greater improvement in physical health and perceived benefits in terms of secondary complications of diabetes.[131–133]

## CHOICE OF TRANSPLANTATION IN DIABETICS

Transplantation is the treatment of choice for diabetic patients with ESRD, given their improved survival compared to remaining on dialysis, and this group of patients should be referred to a transplant center to assess their candidacy. In addition, pancreas transplantation has ceased to be an experimental procedure and has come to represent a viable treatment option for type I diabetic patients. Absolute contraindications to transplantation include severe uncorrectable cardiac or pulmonary disease, unresolved chronic infections, significant chronic liver disease, metastatic/untreatable cancers and significant psychiatric disease.[17]

As discussed previously, treated or correctable cardiovascular disease is not a contraindication to transplantation, but patients need to be carefully evaluated for this before proceeding. Many transplant centers do not have an absolute age ceiling in considering someone for transplantation, and many successful transplants have been performed in the elderly, but advanced age does increase the risks of transplantation, and if the patient has significant comorbidity in addition, especially cardiovascular disease, the benefits of transplantation may be outweighed by the increased risk of mortality. The anticipated waiting time for a cadaveric organ if the patient has no potential living donors may compound the problem. A rule of thumb is that patients may be considered for transplantation if they are felt to have a life expectancy of at least 5 years. With the shortage of cadaveric donor organs, waiting times on the renal transplant list have become progressively longer, as much as 6 years or more in some areas; identification of a living donor can greatly expedite the process, and the patient also benefits by improved graft and patient survival. Potential living related donors for diabetic patients with ESRD require careful assessment of potential increased risk of developing diabetes in the future. Factors that can help quantitate future risk of diabetes and renal disease include family history of diabetes, renal disease and hypertension; ethnicity; history of gestational diabetes; an impaired glucose tolerance test; hyperlipidemia; and measurement of insulin levels and islet cell antibodies in some cases.[134]

Patients with type I diabetes and ESRD have several options for transplantation: they may be candidates for KTA, SPK or pancreas transplant after kidney transplantation (usually a living donor kidney). While a few centers have performed pancreas transplants without regard to C-peptide status in type II diabetes achieving glycemic control equal to that of type I DM SPK recipients,[135] this approach is not widely accepted. Significant underlying medical problems may limit the patient's option to KTA if the transplant center feels the risk is too great for the patient to undergo a pancreas transplant.[136] Most centers will not consider patients over age 55 for pancreas transplantation because of the lack of survival benefit in this group of patients.[125] Patients with pre-existing coronary artery disease, even if corrected, are at much higher risk of coronary events after transplantation. The potential benefits of SPK need to be weighed carefully against this risk: some transplant centers may recommend these patients for kidney transplant alone. Patients with severe peripheral vascular disease are unlikely to benefit from pancreas transplantation with respect to this complication. Significant aortoiliac disease may be felt to prohibitively increase the potential for technical complications and early graft loss due to thrombosis. Most patients with IDDM without a potential living kidney donor will opt for SPK transplantation if they are felt to be acceptable candidates despite the potential for increased complications, since the wait for a double organ transplant is much less than that for a cadaveric renal graft, as well as in view of the anticipated beneficial effects of the pancreas graft. If a patient has a potential living kidney donor, he can receive a live donor kidney transplant with the option of a pancreas transplant from a cadaveric donor at a later time. Some centers would advocate SPK, citing the fact that long-term patient and graft survival approaches that of patients receiving living donor transplants, as well as the cost-effectiveness of this approach[137] and the need for two separate surgeries with a sequential approach. Others might recommend living donor kidney transplant (especially if a related donor is available), with the option of a pancreas transplant afterwards, given the lower complication rate of KTA, excellent long-term results of living related kidney transplantation, and the lengthening waiting time for SPK transplantation, as well as the improved results of solitary pancreas transplantation. A pancreas transplant can be performed safely very soon after a kidney transplant.[138] A few centers perform living donor kidney transplants simultaneously with a cadaveric pancreas transplant, but this obviously requires a highly coordinated protocol.

The role of pancreas transplantation alone in nonuremic type I diabetics is not as straightforward as for patients with ESRD who also require a kidney transplant. It is somewhat less clear whether the risks of surgery and immunosuppression are outweighed by the potential avoidance or retardation of secondary complications of diabetes in patients who do not require a kidney transplant. Ideal candidates for PTA would be younger patients with low cardiac risk and secondary complications that are not so far advanced that there could be the expectation that pancreas transplantation may prevent progression and disability. The extent of any renal disease needs to be carefully assessed, measuring renal function, presence and extent of proteinuria, and possibly renal biopsy, since the nephrotoxic effect of calcineurin inhibitors can add to the future risk of progression of renal impairment.

## PANCREATIC ISLET TRANSPLANTATION

Early attempts at clinical pancreatic islet transplantation in type I DM patients in the 1970s showed poor results[139] and led to whole organ pancreas transplantation becoming a successful and accepted treatment for type I diabetes in patients with significant secondary complications. The major cause of failure was attributed to rejection. However, with the availability of more potent immunosuppressive drugs, such as antilymphocytic preparations and cyclosporine in the late 1980s, better results of islet cell transplants began to be reported in a few patients. Although only a minority of patients are insulin independent, continuing graft function could be demonstrated by a decrease in insulin requirements and by measurable C-peptide levels. Improvements in islet isolation techniques have also led to better results. The International Islet Transplant Registry has collected information on clinical islet transplants performed in 51 centers worldwide from 1990 to the present time, as well as historical data.[144] Of the 493 adult islet allografts reported to the registry in 1990–2000, only 11% were reported to be insulin independent at 1 year, with 41% graft survival as defined by basal C-peptide levels of greater than or equal to 0.5 ng/ml. There appears to be a trend towards increasing rates of insulin independence in more recent years compared to earlier in the decade, probably due to improved techniques in transplantation. The longest reported period of insulin independence after an islet cell allograft is 5 years and 10 months. The overwhelming majority of islet allotransplants have been performed in type I diabetics with ESRD, either after a renal transplant or as a simultaneous islet-kidney transplant. Because of concern over the risks of immunosuppression in nonuremic type I diabetics who would otherwise not be receiving a transplant, this patient group had usually not been considered candidates for islet transplantation until recently. A few patients with type II DM have received islet cell transplants in conjunction with a liver transplant for end-stage liver disease, with mixed results.[145,146]

### Technique of transplantation

Islets for transplantation are obtained from pancreata from cadaveric donors after selective digestion by bacteria-derived collagenases injected into the pancreatic duct.[147] Further purification of islets from exocrine tissue is achieved by cell separation based on density gradients. From there, techniques in different centers may vary as to the extent of purification of islets and whether they are infused into the recipient immediately or cultured for some period of time before use. In general, the purity of islet grafts does not seem to affect graft survival or insulin independence,[144,148] and, in fact, the purification of islets may actually be detrimental in causing insulin release and therefore decreased islet cell insulin.[149]

The majority of islet transplants are performed by intraportal infusion; however, other sites have been used in both human and animal studies, including subcutaneous placement of the graft, placement in the renal subcapsular space, the spleen, intrathymic, intraperitoneal, and even intrapancreatic sites. The intraportal site is preferable in terms of documented graft survival,[144] but some centers have felt a subcutaneous site of implantation could potentially make it easier to monitor the graft for rejection.[150] Intraportal infusion is performed under local anesthesia with radiologic guidance and, as such, has a much lower morbidity than whole organ pancreas transplantation. Complications of intraportal infusion of islets have included bleeding from the puncture site,[151] portal vein thrombosis,[152] disseminated intravascular coagulation,[153] and splenic infarct, as well as the side effects of immunosuppression.[154] In general, however, the complication rate for this procedure appears to be low.

## Barriers to success

There are several barriers to successful pancreatic islet allotransplantation. Immune-mediated mechanisms are felt to account for most graft loss; however, the experience with islet autotransplantation in non-diabetic patients after pancreatectomy suggests non-immune causes of graft loss as well: just 29% of patients undergoing autotransplantation of islets are insulin dependent at 1 year despite transplantation of an adequate number of islets.[144]

Nonspecific inflammation from release of proinflammatory cytokines by macrophages infiltrating the graft may cause destruction of islets.[147,155] Administration of deoxyspergualin, which blocks macrophage function, and antioxidants may abrogate this effect. Lack of engraftment and anoxia from decreased blood supply to the graft may be improved by pentoxifylline.[155] Endotoxin, which may be present in bacteria-derived collagenase, may increase the risk of graft nonfunction due to islet cell apoptosis.[156] Immune-mediated mechanisms are a significant cause of failure of islet allotransplants—both alloimmunity and recurrence of autoimmunity. Selective loss of insulin-staining cells in an islet allograft, suggesting recurrence of autoimmunity, has been reported,[157] and the presence or recrudescence of islet cell autoantibodies or glutamine acid decarboxylase antibody is associated with islet graft failure.[158,159] In addition, strong measures of alloreactivity are associated with graft failure.[159]

Recognition of acute rejection in islet allografts is problematic due to lack of clinically useful markers. Hyperglycemia and decreasing C-peptide levels are rather late events and so are less useful in preventing graft loss. One advantage of a simultaneous islet kidney (SIK) is that the kidney can be used as a marker for diagnosing and treating acute rejection. Forearm implantation of islets makes monitoring for acute rejection easier than portal implantation,[150] but, overall, this site is less successful for engraftment. The apparent improved outcome of islet cell transplants with antithymocyte globulin for induction immunosuppression suggests that this protocol may decrease acute rejection episodes.[144]

Several animal studies have addressed the issue of graft loss due to rejection and have shown success in inducing tolerance of islet transplants with protocols using donor-specific bone-marrow transplant,[160] blockade of costimulatory pathways[161] a decrease in rejection episodes by use of antibodies blocking leukocyte adhesion molecules.[162] In theory, microencapsulation of islets would prevent access to islet cells, thereby preventing immune recognition, but allow diffusion of glucose and insulin. This approach has enjoyed some success in animal studies,[163–165] but, to date, has had limited success in humans.[165,166]

Evidence for 'islet cell exhaustion' due to excessive stimulation from hyperglycemia after islet transplant, as well as a direct toxic effect of hyperglycemia on islet cells, is felt to have an impact on islet graft function. As a result, some centers use an intravenous insulin protocol after engraftment to avoid this problem.

Immunosuppressive drugs themselves may be a barrier to the optimum function of islet grafts. Conventional immunosuppression, including steroids and calcineurin inhibitors, is known to be diabetogenic, and this may be a factor in determining whether a recipient becomes insulin independent. Both cyclosporine and tacrolimus can impair insulin secretion,[167] but the effect of tacrolimus may be greater in this regard.[168]

Several factors have been associated with improved outcome after islet cell transplant.[144] A higher rate of insulin independence was seen if the cold ischemic time of the pancreas was less than 8 hr, if at least 6000 islet equivalents per kilogram body weight were engrafted into the patient, if induction immunosuppression by monoclonal or polyclonal antibodies was used, and if islet engraftment was performed via portal vein infusion. In fact, if all four of the criteria were present, 1-year graft survival, as defined by basal C-peptide level greater than or equal to 0.5 ng/ml was 87% (versus 68% in those without all criteria), and insulin independence at 1 year was 31% (versus 10%).

A breakthrough in clinical islet transplantation was recently reported by the Edmonton Islet Transplant Center; in this report, all seven consecutive patients who received islet transplants had sustained insulin independence at 4–15 months of follow-up.[154] This was achieved through a steroid-free protocol using an interleukin-2 blocking monoclonal antibody for induction and maintenance immunosuppression with sirolimus and low-dose tacrolimus. All patients required islet transplants from at least two sequential cadaveric donors to achieve insulin independence and at least 9000 islet equivalents per kilogram of body weight. This experience was recently extended, so that, at the most recent report, a total of 12 patients have received islet transplants, of whom 11 are insulin independent at a mean follow-up of 10 months.[169] These promising results have led to the initiation of a multicenter trial using this protocol in hope of replicating these results.[170]

## REFERENCES

1. United States Renal Data System (USRDS) Annual Data Report. Vol. 2001: National Institute of Diabetes and Digestive and Kidney Diseases (2000).
2. Rodriguez JA, Cleries M, Vela E, Diabetic patients on renal replacement therapy: analysis of Catalan Registry data, *Nephrol Dial Transplant* (1997) **12:** 2501–9.
3. Bergrem H, Leivestad T, Diabetic nephropathy and end-stage renal failure: the Norwegian story, *Adv Ren Replace Ther* (2001) **8:** 4–12.
4. Najarian J, Kjellstrand C, Simmons R et al, Renal transplantation for diabetic glomerulosclerosis. *Ann Surg* (1973) **178:** 477–84.
5. Kjellstrand C, Simmons R, Goetz F et al, Renal transplantation in patients with insulin-dependent diabetes, *Lancet* (1973) **2:** 4–8.
6. Veenstra D, Best J, Hornberger J et al, Incidence and long-term cost of steroid-related side effects after renal transplantation, *Am J Kidney Dis* (1999) **33:** 829–39.
7. 2000 Scientific Registry and Organ Procurement and Transplantation Network Annual Report. Vol. 2001: United Network of Organ Sharing (UNOS) (2001).
8. Munson J, Bennett W, Barry J et al, A case control study of renal transplantation in patients with type I diabetes, *Clin Transplant* (1992) **6:** 306–11.
9. Bleyer A, Donaldson L, McIntosh M et al, Relationship between underlying renal disease and renal transplantation outcome, *Am J Kidney Dis* (2001) **37:** 1152–61.
10. Kronson J, Gillingham K, Sutherland D et al, Renal transplantation for type II diabetic patients compared with type I diabetic patients and patients over 50 years old: a single center experience, *Clin Transplant* (2000) **14:** 226–34.
11. Wolfe R, Ashby V, Milford E et al. Comparison of mortality in all patients on dialysis, patients on dialysis awaiting transplantation, and recipients of a first cadaveric transplant, *N Engl J Med* (1999) **341:** 1725–30.
12. Meier-Kriesche H, Ojo A, Port F et al, Survival improvement among patients with end-stage renal disease: trends over time for transplant recipients and wait-listed patients, *J Am Soc Nephrol* (2001) **12:** 1293–6.
13. Stephan R, Munschauer C, Kumar M, Surgical wound infection in renal transplantation: outcome data of 102 consecutive patients without perioperative systemic antibiotic coverage, *Arch Surg* (1997) **132:** 1315–18.
14. Drafts H, Anjum M, Wynn J et al, The impact of pre-transplant obesity on renal transplant outcome, *Clin Transplant* (1997) **11:** 493–6.
15. Abbott K, Oliver JD 3rd, Hypolite I et al, Hospitalizations for bacterial septicemia after renal transplantation in the United States, *Am J Nephrol* (2001) **21:** 120–7.
16. Tolkoff-Rubin N, Rubin R, The infectious disease problems of the diabetic renal transplant recipient, *Infect Dis Clin North Am* (1995) 9:117–29.
17. Danovitch G, *Handbook of Kidney Transplantation* (Baltimore: Lippincott, Williams and Wilkins: 2001).
18. Latif S, Saffarian N, Bellovich K et al, Pulmonary mucormycosis in diabetic renal allograft recipients, *Am J Kidney Dis* (1997) **29:** 462–4.
19. Demirag A, Elkhammas E, Henry M et al, Pulmonary *Rhizopus* infection in a diabetic renal transplant recipient, *Clin Transpl* (2000) **14:** 8–10.
20. Magee C, Halligan R, Milford E et al, Nocardial infection in a renal transplant recipient on tacrolimus and mycophenolate mofetil, *Clin Nephrol* (1999) **52:** 44–6.
21. Reddy S, Holley J, Nocardiosis in a recently transplanted renal patient, *Clin Nephrol* (1998) **50:** 123–7.
22. Vasquez J, Sobel J, Fungal infections in diabetes, *Infect Dis Clin North Am* (1995) **9:** 97–116.
23. Penn I, Cancers in renal transplant recipients, *Adv Ren Replace Ther* (2000) **7:** 147–56.
24. International Pancreas Transplant Registry Year-End Update October 2000. Vol. 2001: University of Minnesota Department of Surgery (2000).
25. Danpanich E, Kasiske B, Risk factors for cancer in renal transplant recipients, *Transplantation* (1999) **68:** 1859–64.
26. Ojo A, Hanson J, Wolfe R et al, Long-term survival in renal transplant recipients with graft function, *Kidney Int* (2000) **57:** 307–13.
27. Arend S, Mallat M, Westendorp R et al, Patient survival after renal transplantation; more than 25 years' follow-up, *Nephrol Dial Transplant* (1997) **12:** 1672–79.
28. Kasiske B, Chakkera H, Roel J, Explained and unexplained ischemic heart disease risk after renal transplantation. *J Am Soc Nephrol* (2000) **11:** 1735–43.
29. Rostand S, Coronary heart disease in chronic renal insufficiency—some management considerations, *J Am Soc Nephrol* (2000) **11:** 1948–56.
30. Van Guldener C, Robinson K, Homocysteine and renal disease, *Semin Thromb Hemost* (2000) **26:** 313–24.
31. Stein G, Muller A, Busch M et al, Homocysteine, its metabolites, and B-group vitamins in renal transplant patients, *Kidney Int* (2001) **78:** s262–5.

32. Sung R, Althoen M, Howell T et al, Peripheral vascular occlusive disease in renal transplant recipients: risk factors and impact on kidney allograft survival, *Transplantation* (2000) **70:** 1049–54.

33. Rao K, Andersen R, The impact of diabetes on vascular complications following cadaver renal transplantation, *Transplantation* (1987) **43:** 193–7.

34. Carlstrom J, Norden G, Mjornstedt L et al, Increasing prevalence of cardiovascular disease in kidney transplant patients with type I diabetes, *Transpl Int* (1999) **12:** 176–81.

35. Manske C, Wilson R, Wang Y et al, Atherosclerotic vascular complications in diabetic transplant candidates, *Am J Kidney Dis* (1997) **29:** 601–7.

36. Danovitch G, Hariharan S, Pirsch J et al, Management of the waiting list for cadaveric kidney transplants: report of a survey and recommendations by the Clinical Practice Guidelines Committee of the American Society of Transplantation (2001).

37. Iqbal A, Gibbons R, McGoon M et al, Noninvasive assessment of cardiac risk in insulin-dependent diabetic patients being evaluated for pancreatic transplantation using thallium-201 myocardial perfusion scintigraphy, *Clin Transplant* (1991) **5:** 13–19.

38. Mistry B, Bastani B, Solomon H et al, Prognostic value of dipyridamole thallium-201 screening to minimize perioperative cardiac complications in diabetics undergoing kidney or kidney-pancreas transplantation, *Clin Transplant* (1998) **12:** 130–5.

39. Humar A, Kerr S, Ramcharan T et al, Peri-operative cardiac morbidity in kidney transplant recipients: incidence and risk factors, *Clin Transplant* (2001) **15:** 154–8.

40. Ferguson E, Hudson S, Diethelm A et al, Outcome after myocardial revascularization and renal transplantation: a 25-year single-institution experience, *Ann Surg* (1999) **230:** 232–41.

41. Manske C, Nelluri S, Thomas W et al, Outcome of coronary artery bypass graft surgery in diabetic transplant candidates, *Clin Transplant* (1998) **12:** 73–9.

42. Mauer S, Barbosa J, Vernier R et al, Development of diabetic vascular lesions in normal kidneys transplanted into patients with diabetes mellitus, *N Engl J Med* (1976) **295:** 916–20.

43. Hariharan S, Adams M, Brennan D et al, Recurrent and de novo glomerular disease after renal transplantation, *Transplantation* (1999) **68:** 635–41.

44. Hariharan S, Smith R, Viero R et al, Diabetic nephropathy after renal transplantation, *Transplantation* (1996) **62:** 632–35.

45. Lee D, Goodman W, Coburn J, Renal osteodystrophy: some new questions on an old disorder, *Am J Kidney Dis* (1988) **11:** 365–76.

46. Leidig-Bruckner G, Hosch S, Dodidou P et al, Frequency and prediction of osteoporotic fractures after cardiac or liver transplant: a follow-up study, *Lancet* (2001) **357:** 342–7.

47. Abdelhadi M, Ericzon B, Hultenby K et al, Structural skeletal impairment induced by immunosuppressive treatment in rats: cyclosporine versus tacrolimus, *Transpl Int* (2002) **15:** 180–7.

48. Inoue T, Kawamura I, Matsuo M et al, Lesser reduction in bone mineral density by the immunosuppressant FK506 compared with cyclosporine in rats, *Transplantation* (2000) **70:** 774–9.

49. Nisbeth U, Lindh E, Ljunghall S et al, Increased fracture rate in diabetes mellitus and females after renal transplantation, *Transplantation* (1999) **67:** 1218–22.

50. Chiu M, Sprague S, Bruce D et al, Analysis of fracture prevalence in kidney-pancreas allograft recipients, *J Am Soc Nephrol* (1998) **9:** 677–83.

51. Smets Y, van der Pijl J, de Fijter J et al, Low bone mass and high incidence of fractures after successful simultaneous pancreas-kidney transplantation, *Nephrol Dial Transplant* (1998) **13:** 1250–5.

52. Moe S, The treatment of steroid induced bone loss, *Curr Opin Nephrol Hypertens* (1997) **6:** 544–9.

53. Hutnik C, Nichols B, Cataracts in systemic diseases and syndromes, *Curr Opin Ophthalmol* (1998) **9:** 14–19.

54. Pai R, Mitchell P, Chow V et al, Posttransplant cataract: lessons from kidney-pancreas transplantation, *Transplantation* (2000) **69:** 1108–14.

55. Ekstrand A, Groop L, Pettersson E et al, Metabolic control and progression of complications in insulin-dependent diabetic patients after kidney transplantation, *J Int Med* (1992) **232:** 253–61.

56. Cosio F, Pesavento T, Osei K et al, Post-transplant diabetes mellitus: increasing incidence in renal allograft recipients transplanted in recent years, *Kidney Int* (2001) **59:** 732–7.

57. Markell M, Post-transplant diabetes: incidence, relationship to choice of immune drugs and treatment protocol, *Adv Ren Replace Ther* (2001) **8:** 64–9.

58. Sutherland D, Gruessner R, Dunn D et al, Lessons learned from more than 1,000 pancreas transplants at a single institution, *Ann Surg* (2001) **233:** 463–501.

59. Sollinger H, Odorico J, Knechtle S et al, Experience with 500 simultaneous pancreas-kidney transplants, *Ann Surg* (1998) **228:** 284–96.

60. Stratta R, Review of immunosuppressive usage in pancreas transplantation. *Clin Transplant* (1999) **13:** 1–12.

61. Gruessner R, Sutherland D, Drangstveit M et al, Mycophenolate mofetil in pancreas transplantation, *Transplantation* (1998) **66:** 318–23.

62. Gruessner R, Sutherland D, Najarian J et al, Solitary pancreas transplantation for nonuremic patients with labile insulin-dependent diabetes mellitus, *Transplantation* (1997) **64:** 1572–7.

63. Gruessner A, Sutherland D, Analyses of pancreas transplant outcomes for United States cases reported to the United Network for Organ Sharing (UNOS) and non-US cases reported to the International Pancreas Transplant Registry (IPTR). In: Terasaki A, ed. *Clinical Transplants* (Los Angeles, CA: UCLA Immunogenetics Center, 1999) 51–68.

64. Gruessner A, Sutherland D, Dunn D et al, Pancreas after kidney transplants in posturemic patients with type I diabetes mellitus, *J Am Soc Nephrol* (2001) **12:** 2490–9.

65. Gruessner R, Sutherland D, Troppmann C et al, The surgical risk of pancreas transplantation in the cyclosporine era: an overview, *J Am Coll Surg* (1997) **185:** 128–44.

66. Humar A, Kandaswamy R, Granger D et al, Decreased surgical risks of pancreas transplantation in the modern era, *Ann Surg* (2000) **231:** 269–75.

67. Feitosa Tajra L, Dawhara M, Benchaib M et al, Effect of the surgical technique on long-term outcome of pancreas transplantation, *Transpl Int* (1998) **11:** 295–300.

68. Hickey D, Bakthavatsalam R, Bannon C et al, Urologic complications of pancreatic transplantation, *J Urol* (1997) **157:** 2042–8.

69. Del Pizzo JJ, Jacobs S, Bartlett S et al, Urologic complications of bladder-drained pancreatic allografts, *Br J Urol* (1998) **81:** 543–7.

70. Smets Y, van der Pijl J, van Dissel J et al, Infectious disease complications of simultaneous pancreas kidney transplantation, *Nephrol Dial Transplant* (1997) **12:** 764–71.

71. Hurst G, Somerville K, Alloway R et al, Preliminary experience with midodrine in kidney-pancreas transplant patients with orthostatic hypotension, *Clin Transpl* (2000) **14:** 42–7.

72. Rayhill S, D'Alessandro A, Odorico J et al, Simultaneous pancreas-kidney transplantation and living related donor renal transplantation in patients with diabetes: is there a difference in survival?, *Ann Surg* (2000) **231:** 417–23.

73. Douzdjian V, Abecassis M, Corry P et al, Simultaneous pancreas-kidney versus kidney alone transplantation in diabetics: increased risk of early cardiac death and acute rejection following pancreas transplantation, *Clin Transpl* (1994) **8:** 246–51.

74. Hawthorne W, Allen R, Greenberg M et al, Simultaneous pancreas and kidney transplant rejection, *Transplantation* (1997) **63:** 352–8.

75. Shapiro R, Jordan M, Scantlebury V et al, Renal allograft rejection with normal renal function In simultaneous kidney/pancreas recipients, *Transplantation* (2000) **69:** 440–1.

76. Prieto M, Sutherland D, Fernandez-Cruz L et al, Experimental and clinical experience with urine amylase monitoring for early diagnosis of rejection in pancreas transplantation. *Transplantation* (1987) **43:** 73–9.

77. Sugitani A, Egidi S, Gritsch H et al, Serum lipase as a marker for pancreatic allograft rejection, *Clin Transplant* (1998) **12:** 224–7.

78. Papadimitriou J, Drachenberg C, Wiland A et al, Histologic grading of acute allograft rejection in pancreas needle biopsy: correlation to serum enzymes, glycemia and response to immunosuppressive treatment, *Transplantation* (1998) **66:** 1741–5.

79. Laftari M, Gruessner A, Bland B et al, Diagnosis of pancreas rejection: cystoscopic transduodenal versus percutaneous computed tomography scan-guided biopsy, *Transplantation* (1998) **65:** 528–32.

80. Morel P, Brayman K, Goetz F et al, Long-term metabolic function of pancreas transplants and influence of rejection episodes, *Transplantation* (1991) **51:** 990–1000.

81. Petruzzo P, Andreelli F, McGregor B et al, Evidence of recurrent type I diabetes following HLA-mismatched pancreas transplantation, *Diabetes Metab* (2000) **26:** 215–18.

82. Sutherland D, Najarian J, Greenberg B et al, Hormonal and metabolic effects of a pancreatic endocrine graft, *Ann Intern Med* (1981) **95:** 537–41.

83. Katz H, Homan M, Velosa J et al, Effects of pancreas transplantation on postprandial glucose metabolism, *N Engl J Med* (1991) **325:** 1278–83.

84. Nankivell B, Chapman J, Bovington K et al, Clinical determinants of glucose homeostasis after pancreas transplantation, *Transplantation* (1996) **61:** 1705–11.

85. Fernandez Balsells M, Esmatjes E, Ricart M et al, Successful pancreas and kidney transplantation: a view of metabolic control, *Clin Transplant* (1998) **12:** 582–9.

86. Nathan D, Fogel H, Norman D et al, Long-term metabolic and quality of life results with pancreatic/renal transplantation in insulin-dependent diabetes mellitus, *Transplantation* (1991) **52:** 85–91.

87. Cattral M, Bigam D, Hemming A et al, Portal venous and enteric exocrine drainage versus systemic venous and bladder exocrine drainage of pancreas grafts: clinical outcome of 40 consecutive transplant recipients, *Ann Surg* (2000) **232:** 688–95.

88. Martin X, Petruzzo P, Dawahra M et al, Effects of portal versus systemic venous drainage in kidney-pancreas recipients, *Transpl Int* (2000) **13:** 64–8.

89. Petruzzo P, Da Silva M, Feitosa L et al, Simultaneous pancreas-kidney transplantation: portal versus systemic venous drainage of the pancreas allograft, *Clin Transplant* (2000) **14:** 287–91.

90. Elahi D, Clark B, McAloon-Dyke M et al, Islet cell responses to glucose in human transplanted pancreas, *Am J Physiol* (1991) **261:** E800–8.

91. Christiansen E, Vestergaard H, Tibell A et al, Impaired insulin-stimulated nonoxidative glucose metabolism in pancreas-kidney transplant recipients. Dose-response effects of insulin on glucose turnover, *Diabetes* (1996) **45:** 1267–75.

92. Kendall D, Rooney D, Smets Y et al, Pancreas transplantation restores epinephrine response and symptom recognition during hypoglycemia in patients with long-standing type I diabetes and autonomic neuropathy, *Diabetes* (1997) **46:** 249–57.

93. Bolinder J, Wahrenberg H, Persson A et al, Effect of pancreas transplantation on glucose counterregulation in insulin-dependent diabetic patients prone to severe hypoglycemia, *J Intern Med* (1991) **230:** 527–33.

94. Redmon J, Teuscher A, Robertson R, Hypoglycemia after pancreas transplantation, *Diabetes Care* (1998) **21:** 1944–50.

95. Bohman S, Wilczek H, Tyden G et al, Recurrent diabetic nephropathy in renal allografts placed in diabetic patients and protective effect of simultaneous pancreas transplant, *Transplant Proc* (1987) **19:** 2290–3.

96. Bilous R, Mauer S, Sutherland D et al, The effects of pancreas transplantation on the glomerular structure of renal allografts in patients with insulin-dependent diabetes, *N Engl J Med* (1989) **321:** 80–5.

97. Fioretto P, Steffes M, Sutherland D et al, Reversal of lesions of diabetic nephropathy after pancreas transplantation, *N Engl J Med* (1998) **339:** 69–75.

98. Pearce I, Ilango B, Sells R et al, Stabilisation of diabetic retinopathy following simultaneous pancreas and kidney transplant, *Br J Ophthalmol* (2000) **84:** 736–40.

99. Chow V, Pai R, Champman J et al, Diabetic retinopathy after combined kidney-pancreas transplantation, *Clin Transplant* (1999) **13:** 356–62.

100. Konigsrainer A, Miller K, Steurer W et al, Does pancreas transplantation influence the course of diabetic retinopathy? *Diabetologia* (1991) **34:** S86–8.

101. Koznarova R, Saudek F, Sosna T et al. Beneficial effect of pancreas and kidney transplantation on advanced diabetic retinopathy, *Cell Transplant* (2000) **9:** 903–8.

102. Ramsay R, Goetz F, Sutherland D et al. Progression of diabetic retinopathy after pancreas transplantation for insulin-dependent diabetes mellitus, *N Engl J Med* (1988) **318:** 208–14.

103. Petersen M, Vine A, Progression of diabetic retinopathy after pancreas transplantation, *Ophthalmology* (1990) **97:** 496–500.

104. Cheung A, Perez R, Chen P, Improvements in diabetic microangiopathy after successful simultaneous pancreas-kidney transplantation: a computer-assisted intravital microscopy study on the conjunctival microcirculation, *Transplantation* (1999) **68:** 927–32.

105. Bentley F, Jung S, Garrison R, Neuropathy and psychosocial adjustment after pancreas transplant in diabetics, *Transplant Proc* (1990) **22:** 691–5.

106. Kennedy W, Navarro X, Goetz F et al, Effects of pancreatic transplantation on diabetic neuropathy, *N Engl J Med* (1990) **322:** 1031–7.

107. Tyden G, Bolinder J, Solders G et al, Improved survival in patients with insulin-dependent diabetes mellitus and end-stage diabetic nephropathy 10 years after combined pancreas and kidney transplantation, *Transplantation* (1999) **67:** 645–8.

108. Nankivell B, Al-Harbi I, Morris J et al, Recovery of diabetic neuropathy after pancreas transplantation. *Transplant Proc* (1997) **29:** 658–9.

109. Navarro X, Sutherland D, Kennedy W, Long-term effects of pancreatic transplantation on diabetic neuropathy, *Ann Neurol* (1997) **42:** 727–36.

110. Katz H, Nguyen T, Velosa J et al, Effects of systemic delivery of insulin on plasma lipids and lipoprotein concentrations in pancreas transplant recipients, *Mayo Clin Proc* (1994) **69:** 231–6.

111. Hughes T, Gaber A, Amiri H et al, Lipoprotein composition in insulin-dependent diabetes mellitus with chronic renal failure: effect of kidney and pancreas transplantation, *Metabolism* (1994) **43:** 333–47.

112. Foger B, Konigsrainer A, Ritsch A et al, Pancreas transplantation modulates reverse cholesterol transport, *Transpl Int* (1999) **12:** 360–4.

113. Luzi L, Groop L, Perseghin G et al, Effect of pancreas transplantation on free fatty acid metabolism in uremic IDDM patients, *Diabetes* (1996) **45:** 354–60.

114. Hughes T, Gaber A, Amiri H et al, Kidney-pancreas transplantation. The effect of portal versus systemic venous drainage of the pancreas on the lipoprotein composition, *Transplantation* (1995) **60:** 1406–12.

115. Bagdade J, Ritter M, Kitabchi A et al, Differing effects of pancreas-kidney transplantation with systemic versus portal venous drainage on cholesteryl ester transfer in IDDM subjects, *Diabetes Care* (1996) **19:** 1108–12.

116. Fiorina P, La Rocca E, Venturini M et al, Effects of kidney-pancreas transplantation on atherosclerotic risk factors and endothelial function in patients with uremia and type I diabetes, *Diabetes* (2001) **50:** 496–501.

117. Hricik D, Chareandee C, Knauss T et al, Hypertension after pancreas-kidney transplantation: role of bladder versus enteric pancreatic drainage, *Transplantation* (2000) **70:** 494–6.

118. La Rocca E, Fiorina P, Astorri E et al, Patient survival and cardiovascular events after kidney-pancreas transplantation: comparison with kidney transplantation alone in uremic IDDM patients, *Cell Transplant* (2000) **9:** 929–32.

119. Nankivell B, Lau S, Chapman J et al, Progression of macrovascular disease after transplantation, *Transplantation* (2000) **69:** 574–81.

120. Biesenbach G, Margreiter R, Konigsrainer A et al, Comparison of progression of macrovascular diseases after kidney or pancreas and kidney transplantation in diabetic patients with end-stage renal disease, *Diabetologia* (2000) **43:** 231–4.

121. Morrissey P, Shaffer D, Monaco A et al, Peripheral vascular disease after kidney-pancreas transplantation in diabetic patients with end-stage renal disease, *Arch Surg* (1997) **132:** 358–61.

122. Fiorina P, La Rocca E, Astorri E et al, Reversal of left ventricular diastolic dysfunction after kidney-pancreas transplantation in type I diabetic uremic patients, *Diabetes Care* 2000; **23:** 1804–10.

123. Gaber A, Wicks M, Hathaway D et al, Sustained improvement in cardiac geometry and function following kidney-pancreas transplantation, *Cell Transplant* (2000) **9:** 913–18.

124. Manske C, Wang Y, Thomas W, Mortality of cadaveric kidney transplantation versus combined kidney-pancreas transplantation in diabetic patients, *Lancet* (1995) **346:** 1658–62.

125. Ojo A, Meier-Kriesche H, Hanson J et al, The impact of simultaneous pancreas-kidney transplantation on long-term patient survival. *Transplantation* (2001) **71:** 82–90.

126. Becker B, Brazy P, Becker Y et al, Simultaneous pancreas-kidney transplantation reduces excess mortality in type I diabetic patients with end-stage renal disease, *Kidney Int* (2000) **57:** 2129–35.

127. Tyden G, Tollemar J, Bolinder J, Combined pancreas and kidney transplantation improves survival in patients with end-stage diabetic nephropathy, *Clin Transplant* (2000) **14:** 505–8.

128. Smets Y, Westendorp R, van der Pijl J et al, Effect of simultaneous pancreas-kidney transplantation on mortality of patients with type-1 diabetes mellitus and end-stage renal failure, *Lancet* (1999) **353:** 1915–19.

129. Douzdijian V, Ferrara D, Silvestri G, Treatment strategies for insulin-dependent diabetics with ESRD: a cost-effectiveness decision analysis model. *Am J Kidney Dis* (1998) **31:** 794–802.

130. Matas A, McHugh L, Payne W et al, Long-term quality of life after kidney and simultaneous pancreas-kidney transplantation, *Clin Transpl* (1998) **12:** 233–42.

131. Gross C, Limwattananon C, Matthees B et al, Impact of transplantation on quality of life in patients with diabetes and renal dysfunction, *Transplantation* (2000) **70:** 1736–46.

132. Piehlmeier W, Bullinger M, Kirchberger I et al, Evaluation of the quality of life of patients with insulin-dependent diabetes mellitus before and after organ transplantation with the SF 36 Health Survey, *Eur J Surg* (1996) **162:** 933–40.

133. Corry R, Zehr P, Quality of life in diabetic recipients of kidney transplants is better with the addition of the pancreas, *Clin Transpl* (1990) **4:** 238–41.

134. Simmons D, Searle M, Risk of diabetic nephropathy in potential living related kidney donors, *BMJ* (1998) **316:** 846–8.

135. Light JA, Sasaki TM, Currier CB et al, Successful long-term kidney-pancreas transplants regardless of c-peptide status or race, *Transplantation* (2001) **71:** 152–54.

136. Becker B, Odorico J, Becker Y et al, Simultaneous pancreas-kidney and pancreas transplantation, *J Am Soc Nephrol* (2001) **12:** 2517–27.

137. Douzdijian V, Escobar F, Kupin W et al, Cost-utility analysis of living-donor kidney transplantation followed by pancreas transplantation versus simultaneous pancreas-kidney transplantation, *Clin Transplant* (1999) **13:** 51–8.

138. Humar A, Sutherland D, Ramcharan T et al, Optimal timing for a pancreas transplant after a successful kidney transplant, *Transplantation* (2000) **70:** 1247–50.

139. Sutherland D, Report of International Human Pancreas and Islet Transplantation Registry cases through 1981, *Diabetes* (1982) **31** (Suppl 4): 112–16.

140. Warnock G, Kneteman N, Ryan E et al, Normoglycaemia after transplantation of freshly isolated and cryopreserved pancreatic islets in type 1 (insulin-dependent) diabetes mellitus, *Diabetologia* (1991) **34:** 55–8.

141. Scharp D, Lacy P, Santiago J et al, Insulin independence after islet transplantation into type I diabetic patient, *Diabetes* (1990) **39:** 515–18.

142. Ricordi C, Tzakis A, Carroll P et al, Human islet isolation and allotransplantation in 22 consecutive cases, *Transplantation* (1992) **53:** 407–14.

143. Warnock G, Kneteman N, Ryan E et al, Long-term follow-up after transplantation of insulin-producing pancreatic islets into patients with type 1 (insulin-dependent) diabetes mellitus, *Diabetologia* (1992) **35:** 89–95.

144. International Islet Transplant Registry. Vol. 2002: University Medical Center of Giessen, Germany (2002).

145. Ricordi C, Alejandro R, Angelico M et al, Human islet allografts in patients with type 2 diabetes undergoing liver transplantation, *Transplantation* (1997) **63:** 473–5.

146. Merenda R, Gerunda G, Neri D et al, Combined liver and islet transplant, *Transpl Int* (1997) **10:** 164–6.

147. Titus T, Badet L, Gray D, Islet cell transplantation for insulin-dependent diabetes mellitus: perspectives from the present and prospects for the future. Vol. 2001: *Expert Rev Mol Med* (2000).

148. Gores P, Sutherland D, Pancreatic islet transplantation: is purification necessary?, *Am J Surg* (1993) **166:** 538–42.

149. Brandhorst H, Brandhorst D, Brendel M et al, Assessment of intracellular insulin content during all steps of human islet isolation procedure, *Cell Transplant* (1998) **7:** 489–95.

150. Stegall M, Monitoring human islet allografts using a forearm biopsy site, *Ann Transplant* (1997) **2:** 8–11.

151. Secchi A, Socci C, Maffi P et al, Islet transplantation in IDDM patients, *Diabetologia* (1997) **40:** 225–31.

152. Oberholzer J, Triponez F, Mage R et al, Human islet transplantation: lessons from 13 autologous and 13 allogeneic transplantations, *Transplantation* (2000) **69:** 1115–23.

153. Froberg M, Leone J, Jesurun J et al, Fatal disseminated

intravascular coagulation after autologous islet transplantation, *Hum Pathol* (1997) **28**: 1295–8.

154. Shapiro A, Lakey J, Ryan E et al, Islet transplantation in seven patients with type I diabetes mellitus using a glucocorticoid-free immunosuppressive regimen. *N Engl J Med* (2000) **343**: 230–8.

155. Juang J, Bonner-Weir S, Wu Y et al, Beneficial influence of glycemic control upon the growth and function of transplanted islets, *Diabetes* (1994) **43**: 1334–9.

156. Berney T, Molano R, Cattan P et al, Endotoxin-mediated delayed islet graft function is associated with increased intra-islet cytokine production and islet cell apoptosis, *Transplantation* (2001) **71**: 125–32.

157. Stegall M, Lafferty K, Kam I et al, Evidence of recurrent autoimmunity in human allogeneic islet transplantation, *Transplantation* (1996) **61**: 1272–4.

158. Jaeger C, Brendel M, Hering B et al, Progressive islet graft failure occurs significantly earlier in autoantibody-positive than in autoantibody-negative IDDM recipients of intrahepatic islet allografts, *Diabetes* (1997) **46**: 1907–10.

159. Roep B, Stobbe I, Duinkerken G et al, Auto- and alloimmune reactivity to human islet allografts transplanted into type 1 diabetic patients, *Diabetes* (1999) **48**: 484–90.

160. Horton P, Hawthorne W, Walters S et al, Induction of allogenic islet tolerance in a large-animal model, *Cell Transplant* (2000) **9**: 877–87.

161. Inverardi L, Ricordi C, Tolerance and pancreatic islet transplantation, *Philos Trans R Soc Lond* (2001) **356**: 759–65.

162. Socha-Urbanek K, Urbanek K, Fiedor P, The role of adhesion molecules in allotransplanted islet cells rejection. Prolongation of islet cells allograft survival by antiadhesion treatment, *Ann Transplant* (1998) **3**: 5–9.

163. Mullen Y, Maruyama M, Smith C, Current progress and perspectives in immunoisolated islet transplantation, *J Hepatobiliary Pancreat Surg* (2000) **7**: 347–57.

164. Jain K, Yang H, Cai B et al, Retrievable, replaceable, macroencapsulated pancreatic islet xenografts. Long-term engraftment without immunosuppression, *Transplantation* (1995) **59**: 319–24.

165. Calafiore R, Transplantation of microencapsulated pancreatic human islets for therapy of diabetes mellitus. A preliminary report, *ASAIO J* (1992) **38**: 34–7.

166. Soon-Shiong P, Heintz R, Merideth N et al, Insulin independence in a type I diabetic after encapsulated islet transplantation, *Lancet* (1994) **343**: 950–1.

167. Tamura K, Fujimura T, Tsutsumi T et al, Transcriptional inhibition of insulin by FK506 and possible involvement of FK506 binding protein-12 in pancreatic beta-cell, *Transplantation* (1995) **59**: 1606–13.

168. Pirsch J, Miller J, Deierhoi M et al, A comparison of tacrolimus (FK506) and cyclosporine for immunosuppression after cadaveric renal transplantation. FK506 Kidney Transplant Study Group, *Transplantation* (1997) **63**: 977–83.

169. Ryan E, Lakey J, Rajotte R et al, Clinical outcomes and insulin secretion after islet transplantation with the Edmonton Protocol, *Diabetes* (2001) **50**: 710–19.

170. Bluestone J, Matthews J, Krensky A, The immune tolerance network: the 'Holy Grail' comes to the clinic, *J Am Soc Nephrol* (2000) **11**: 2141–6.

# 21

# Summary of the therapeutic approach to the patient with diabetic nephropathy

Geoffrey Boner and Mark E Cooper

Diabetes mellitus and its complications, which directly affect the vasculature throughout the body, are one of the scourges of the modern world. The annual incidence of both type 1 and type 2 diabetes is increasing, especially among populations with a previously reported low incidence of diabetes.[1] In type 2 diabetes, the dramatic increase in incidence has been defined as an epidemic related to sedentary lifestyle and excess nutrition, with certain ethnic groups having a genetic susceptibility.[2] Of particular importance is the involvement of the kidney, which is associated with substantial morbidity and mortality and with high treatment cost in both types of diabetes. The various authors contributing to this book have emphasized different aspects of diabetic renal disease. In this summary, we will highlight the important features of diabetic nephropathy and the measures for prevention and treatment of this condition.

Fourlanos and Kay (Chapter 2ii) have described the pathogenesis, clinical presentation and treatment of type 1 diabetes. They concluded their chapter with the hope that the investigation of different methods of preventing diabetes will provide us with a specific means for the prevention of this disease, and also for the treatment of the disease in its early stages. Moreover, the dramatic improvement in the transplantation of islet cells will provide a solution for some of the insulin-dependent patients, while others will have to wait for newer techniques, such as differentiated stem cells or xenotransplants.

Bennett and Nelson (Chapter 2i) have described the pathogenesis, epidemiology and clinical presentation of type 2 diabetes. The authors stressed the exponential growth in the number of patients presenting with this disease, especially in the less developed countries. It should be realized that the present increase in the incidence and prevalence of type 2

diabetes mellitus will result in a concomitant increase in the number of complications, with added morbidity and mortality over the next 20–30 years. This will present the governments of most countries with a substantial or even insurmountable financial burden.

The actual subject of this book, diabetic nephropathy, has been introduced by Jerums, Panagiotopoulos and MacIsaac (Chapter 3). In defining diabetic nephropathy, they have not only used a histologic definition, but have also stressed the importance of an increase in urinary protein excretion and, more specifically, the significance of the relatively small increase in the excretion of albumin, defined as microalbuminuria (30–300 mg/day), in the diagnosis of early renal involvement. They have also described the various theoretical factors promoting renal disease, and have followed the clinical presentation with a short description of the various therapeutic options.

The development and progression of diabetic nephropathy vary in different groups of patients and in different individuals. Genetic modifiers seem to play a role in determining at least part of this variation. Thomas (Chapter 4) has described the inherited susceptibility to diabetic nephropathy. He has described the familial aggregation of diabetic nephropathy, the ethnic variability and the influence of gender as supporting the role of genetic involvement. He has also suggested various avenues for genetic influence on diabetic nephropathy, including genetic hypertension, and genetic determinants of serum lipids, insulin sensitivity, the renin-angiotensin system, aldose reductase, the sodium/hydrogen exchanger and erythrocyte $Na^+/Li^+$ countertransport, among others. In addition, various metabolic byproducts and pathways, growth factors and hormones have been postulated to play a role in the progression of diabetic nephropathy. Schrijvers, De Vriese and Flyvbjerg (Chapter 5) have critically examined these different factors and have suggested possible therapeutic mechanisms for preventing or slowing progression.

## THE THERAPEUTIC APPROACH TO THE PATIENT WITH DIABETIC NEPHROPATHY

The therapeutic approach to patients with diabetic nephropathy is based mainly on strict control of hyperglycemia, antihypertensive treatment and low-protein diet. The lowering of serum lipids may also be advantageous in preventing progression of renal disease. There are also several potential therapeutic agents, which may play a role in the future. Moreover, with progression of diabetic nephropathy, efforts must be made to prevent and treat several comorbid conditions. In this section the approach to the diabetic patient with renal involvement is summarized (see Table 21.1 for a summary of the therapeutic approach).

---

**Table 21.1 Summary of the therapeutic approach to diabetic nephropathy.**

1. **Strict control of blood glucose**
   a. Beneficial in both type 1 and 2 diabetes
   b. Delays onset of microalbuminuria
   c. May not be as effective at slowing progression of overt renal disease
   d. Of importance in preventing other comorbid conditions such as retinopathy

2. **Treatment of hypertension**
   a. Lowering of blood pressure is the most important element in preventing progression of diabetic nephropathy
   b. The goals for treatment should be a blood pressure of 130/80 mmHg or less in all diabetic patients and 125/75 mmHg or less in patients with proteinuria greater than 1 g/day
   c. Nonpharmacologic therapeutic regimens
      i. Of major importance
         1. Physical activity
         2. Weight maintenance
      ii. Of moderate importance
         1. Sodium restriction and potassium supplementation
         2. Decreased protein diet
         3. Reduction in alcohol intake
   d. Pharmacologic agents
      i. Angiotensin-converting enzyme inhibitor or angiotensin II receptor blocker—first choice
      ii. Diuretic—preferably of the thiazide group—in small dosage
      iii. Calcium-channel blocker—dihydropyridines are more effective in reducing blood pressure, while nondihydropyridines may have some specific antiproteinuric effect
      iv. Beta-blockers are mainly indicated to suppress tachycardia induced by other drugs or when a specific indication is present such as cardiovascular disease
      v. Alpha-receptor blockers are useful in reducing blood pressure

3. **Low-protein diet**
   a. A low-protein diet (about 0.8 g/kg body weight per day of high biologic value) may have a modest effect on progression of the renal disease
   b. Patients must be closely followed to prevent protein malnutrition

**Table 21.1** *continued*

4. **Control of serum lipids**

   Hyperlipidemia should be treated in order to prevent cardiovascular complications and possibly to slow progression of renal disease

5. **Management of the patient with mild to moderate renal involvement**
   a. Define stage of renal disease
   b. Strict glycemic control (see 1)
   c. Antihypertensive treatment (see 2)
   d. Lifestyle modification

6. **Management of the patient with advanced renal involvement**
   a. Antihypertensive treatment (see 2)
   b. Metabolic control of hyperglycemia (see 1)
   c. Stop smoking
   d. Restrict dietary protein intake (see 3)
   e. Treat anemia
   f. Treat and prevent cardiovascular disease
   g. Treat hyperlipidemia
   h. Investigate and treat renal osteodystrophy
   i. Treat metabolic acidosis
   j. Adjust dosages of medications according to renal function
   k. Prepare for renal replacement therapy

7. **Treatment of patients with end-stage renal disease by dialysis**
   a. Use multidisciplinary team
   b. Decide on the mode of dialysis (hemodialysis or peritoneal dialysis)
   c. Prepare access (a–v fistula for hemodialysis or peritoneal catheter for peritoneal dialysis)
   d. Continue treating the patient as outlined in the previous section
   e. Institute dialytic therapy when the GFR is 10–15 ml/min
   f. Optimize quantity of dialysis and treat to avoid complications

8. **Treatment of patients with end-stage renal disease by transplantation**
   a. Renal transplantation
      i. Better survival than using dialysis
      ii. Living donor or cadaver donor
      iii. Early assessment for possibility of living donor
      iv. Early registration on cadaver kidney transplant waiting list
   b. Simultaneous renal and pancreas transplantation
      i. Reasonable success in type 1 diabetes
      ii. May not require insulin or may require reduced dosage
   c. Isolated pancreas transplantation
      i. Indicated in patients with brittle diabetes mellitus who have difficulty in control with insulin
   d. Pancreas islet cell transplantation
      i. Clinical trials are being conducted
      ii. Recent improvement in results
      iii. Hope for treatment of patients with type 1 diabetes

## Strict glucose control (Chapter 6)

Thomas, Krimholz and Viberti (Chapter 6) have examined the effects of strict glucose control. The hyperfiltration that is found early in both type 1 and type 2 diabetes may be reversed by strict glucose control.[3,4] However, the evidence as to the effect on renal hypertrophy is not as convincing. Two large studies have demonstrated that strict glucose control prevents the development of microalbuminuria in type 1 and proteinuria in type 2 diabetes.[5,6] However, it is still not clear whether intensified glycemic control can prevent the progression from microalbuminuria to overt nephropathy, and whether it can affect the decline in glomerular filtration rate (GFR). Of importance is the observation that normalizing blood-glucose levels following pancreas transplantation resulted in improvement in the histologic changes in the kidney 10 years after transplantation, but not after 5 years.[7]

Strict control of glucose is thus of cardinal importance in prevention of overt diabetic nephropathy in patients who have signs of early renal involvement (hyperfiltration and/or microalbuminuria) (see Chapter 13). However, there is no good evidence as to the effect of glucose control on the progression of renal disease in patients who have advanced nephropathy (see Chapter 14). Nevertheless, it is important even at these latter stages of the disease to maintain as near to normal blood glucose as possible in order to prevent other complications such as ketoacidosis, retinopathy, neuropathy, peripheral vascular and cardiovascular disease.[8]

## Antihypertensive treatment (Chapter 7)

Hypertension is often a concomitant finding in patients with diabetes. In patients with type 1 diabetes, the appearance of hypertension is linked to the appearance of microalbuminuria, whereas in type 2 diabetes, hypertension often antedates the diagnosis of diabetes. Not only is the presence of hypertension a risk factor for the development and progression of diabetic nephropathy, but it is an important risk factor for overall mortality.[9,10] Many studies have shown that reducing blood pressure can prevent the appearance of comorbid conditions and slow the progression of diabetic nephropathy. In fact, the treatment of hypertension is now considered to be the most important element in slowing progression. It has been suggested that the target values for the treatment of hypertension in diabetic patients should be 130/80 mmHg, and in patients with proteinuria greater than 1 g/day, the target should be 125/75 mmHg.[11]

The initial treatment of hypertension in diabetic patients, as described by Ravid and Rachmani in Chapter 7, like that in nondiabetic patients, should be nonpharmacological. Physical activity and maintenance of a normal body weight are of primary importance in reducing blood pressure. Salt restriction and potassium supplementation, reduced protein diet and reduced alcohol intake may have a modest effect in reducing blood pressure (see discussion in Chapter 7).

A few major well-controlled studies have shown that angiotensin-converting enzyme inhibitors (ACE-I) and angiotensin II receptor blockers (AIIR) not only reduce blood pressure, but also have additional renoprotective effects in both type 1 (ACE-I) and type 2 (AIIR) diabetic nephropathy.[12–14] It is now well established that interruption of the renin-angiotensin system with either ACE-I or AIIR should be the first-line agent for the treatment of hypertension in the diabetic patient.

Both thiazide and loop diuretics may be used as ancillary drugs in the treatment of hypertension in the diabetic patient. Calcium-channel blockers, especially of the dihydropyridine group, are especially effective in reducing blood pressure, but do not reduce proteinuria and probably do not have a specific renoprotective effect.[14] However, the members of the nondihydropyridine group of calcium-channel blockers may cause a reduction in proteinuria and are effective in combination with ACE-I.[15,16] Beta-blockers and alpha-receptor blockers are additional agents that may be used in the treatment of hypertension. Thus, we think that all diabetic patients with raised blood pressure should be treated initially with ACE-I or AIIR in an attempt to reach the treatment goals mentioned above. Low-dose diuretics, calcium-channel blockers, beta-blockers and alpha-receptor blockers may be subsequently added in order to achieve these goals.

## Low-protein diet (Chapter 8)

The effects of protein restriction on the progression of renal involvement have been investigated in both type 1 and type 2 diabetes. However, most studies were small and for a limited period of time. Waugh and Robertson have reviewed the results of the studies meeting specific criteria. Their conclusion is that protein restriction seems to have a significant, albeit small, effect on progression. We suggest that a low-protein diet may be used on condition that the diet is strictly controlled in order to prevent protein malnutrition. The role of the dietitian in planning the specific diet for each patient and monitoring patient compliance is discussed by Vennegoor (Chapter 19).

## Control of hyperlipidemia (Chapter 9)

Many of the studies reported by Jandeleit-Dahm and Bonnet in Chapter 9, demonstrate a significant correlation between the levels of serum lipids and progression of diabetic nephropathy in both type 1 and type 2 diabetes. However, interventional studies using HMG CoA reductase inhibitors have not always resulted in an improvement in progression. A recently published meta-analysis, indicated that lipid-lowering therapy was associated with diminished progression of renal disease.[17] Moreover, dyslipidemia in diabetic patients has been clearly demonstrated to be an important risk factor for cardiovascular and other vascular diseases. We are thus of the opinion that hyperlipidemia in the presence of diabetes mellitus, especially in the context of associated renal disease, should be treated both by diet and pharmacologically.

## Treatment of cardiac complications

Candido and Srivastava (Chapter 10) have described the important cardiac complications in diabetic patients, particularly if they have concomitant renal disease. Diabetes is associated with accelerated atherosclerosis and increased risk of coronary heart disease, congestive cardiac failure and sudden cardiac death. Indeed, it is postulated that there may be a specific cardiomyopathy in diabetes, independent of ischemic heart disease. This issue is controversial and unresolved. However, the high prevalence of cardiac dysfunction in diabetes and potential treatments for this condition have stimulated increasing basic and clinical research in this area. There is no doubt that patients with diabetic nephropathy, especially those with other risk factors, should be carefully monitored for cardiac complications and should receive prophylactic treatment.

## Treatment of acid–base and electrolyte disorders (Chapter 11)

Pollock (Chapter 11) has described the pathophysiology of the many electrolyte disturbances that may occur in patients with diabetic nephropathy. The most important is hyperkalemia, which may be a result of insulin deficiency, hyporeninemic hypoaldosteronism and hyperosmolality. This problem may be further exacerbated by concomitant treatments, including agents which interrupt the renin-angiotensin-aldosterone system, such as ACE-I, AIIR and spironolactone. There may also be derangements in sodium, calcium, magnesium and phosphate metabolism. Metabolic acidosis may occur even in diabetic patients with good glucose control and reasonably good renal function. This may be secondary to hyperkalemia, hypoaldosteronism or a primary tubular defect. The chapter includes an important discussion of acid–base or electrolyte disorders in diabetic patients secondary to the use of certain medications. These include lactic acidosis secondary to the use of metformin and hyperkalemia due to an array of medications, which are listed in Table 11.2. There is a discussion of water homeostasis and a description of the abnormalities in diabetic ketoacidosis. The role of the dietitian in preventing and treating some of these disorders may be found in Chapter 19. Physicians treating patients with diabetic nephropathy should be aware of these possible derangements in acid–base and electrolyte metabolism and treat them appropriately.

## Summary of management of the patient with mild to moderate renal involvement (Chapter 13)

The diabetic patient with mild to moderate renal involvement may be defined as the patient with signs of renal involvement (microalbuminuria to overt proteinuria) and/or reduced renal function (GFR of 30–90 ml/min). Bilous and Jones (Chapter 13) have described the diagnosis of microalbuminuria and the clinical diagnosis of diabetic nephropathy.

Good glycemic control is important during this stage of the disease. Maintenance of HbA$_{1c}$ below a value of 7% may reduce the rate of appearance of microalbuminuria in patients with normoalbuminuria. However, Bilous and Jones were not of the opinion that strict glycemic control had been shown to prevent the progression from microalbuminuria to overt proteinuria. Nevertheless, they suggested that strict control should be applied to prevent the progression of other microvascular complications, such as retinopathy. Similarly, there is little evidence to show that metabolic control may prevent or slow the decline in renal function. On the basis of one observational study,[18] they suggest that strict control should be instituted if $HbA_{1c}$ is greater than 8%.

Antihypertensive treatment, primarily with ACE-I, has not been shown reliably to prevent the development of microalbuminuria in patients with type 1 diabetes. Most of these patients are normotensive at the early stages of diabetes. However, patients with type 2 diabetes are often hypertensive at presentation, and early antihypertensive treatment may play a role in the primary prevention of microalbuminuria. Earlier in this chapter (under the heading 'Antihypertensive treatment'), the important role of treatment of hypertension with ACE-I and AIIR in the prevention of progression from microalbuminuria to overt proteinuria and in slowing progression of the disease was emphasized. Bilous and Jones stress the importance of treating the patients with microalbuminuria and/or hypertension with these agents, the aim being to reduce blood pressure to targets, as mentioned earlier under 'Antihypertensive treatment'.

The authors suggest that dietary protein restriction should be reserved for patients with declining renal function. Additional factors in the treatment of these patients include cessation of smoking, careful monitoring of renal function, early referral to a nephrologist, and management of cardiovascular risk factors and cardiovascular disease. Their recommendations are summarized in Table 13.3.

## Summary of management of the patient with advanced renal involvement (Chapter 14)

In advanced renal disease (GFR less than 30 ml/min or nephrotic range proteinuria), treatment is aimed at slowing the rate of progression of the renal disease, preventing or treating comorbid conditions, and preparing the patient for renal replacement therapy (RRT). At this stage, it is imperative that the patients are followed in a clinic specializing in the treatment of renal failure.

van Dijk and Boner have described the importance of control of hypertension in slowing progression of renal disease. Moreover, two recent large studies in patients with type 2 diabetes and moderate to advanced renal disease have show the beneficial effects of treatment with AIIR.[13,14] The treatment of hypertension is also important in the prevention and treatment of comorbid conditions such as cardiovascular disease. It must be remembered that patients with advanced renal disease are likely to require several antihypertensive agents in order to control blood pressure adequately. The various medications may be associated with complications such as increased serum creatinine or hyperkalemia in patients with severely reduced renal function, and the patients must thus be closely monitored.

Strict diabetic control has not been shown to be effective in slowing progression of renal disease at this stage. However, glycemic control should be maintained in order to prevent and treat other micro- and macrovascular complications. Smoking has been shown to be associated with accelerated progression in type 2 diabetes; thus, patients should be advised to stop smoking in order potentially to retard progression and to prevent comorbid conditions.[19] In spite of the fact that dietary protein restriction has been shown to slow the progression of renal disease, the documented effect in these studies has been rather small. Nevertheless, there is a role for protein restriction, but care must be taken that the patient does not develop protein malnutrition.

Anemia is an important complication of advanced renal disease. The degree of anemia tends to be greater in diabetic than in nondiabetic patients for the same degree of renal impairment. Anemia is one of the major factors in the clinical symptomatology of patients with renal failure and generally responds to treatment with human recombinant erythropoietin. Patients receiving erythropoietin must be closely followed and given iron supplementation according to need. The importance of hyperlipidemia and cardiovascular involvement, and their treatment in these patients has been fully described in Chapters 9 and 10. It thus imperative that all patients with advanced disease be checked for cardiovascular disease and hyperlipidemia and treated accordingly. Another possible complication of advanced renal disease is metabolic acidosis. This has been discussed by van Dijk and Boner (Chapter 14) and by Pollock (Chapter 11).

Renal osteodystrophy is found in almost all patients with advanced renal disease and requires specific diagnostic and therapeutic measures.

As renal function decreases, the doses of medications, especially those excreted by the kidney, have to be modified in order to prevent high blood levels and drug–drug interactions.

Patients with advanced renal involvement should thus be carefully followed and treated with all the therapeutic measures that have been described above (Table 21.1). Furthermore, these individuals should be referred to the treatment team responsible for preparing them for RRT.

## The use of dialysis in the treatment of diabetic patients with end-stage renal disease (ESRD) (Chapter 16)

The various options for RRT have been summarized by Woredekal and Friedman in Table 16.1. Briefly, the options include hemodialysis, peritoneal dialysis and transplantation. The decision as to the most suitable treatment for each patient will depend on many factors (Table 16.2). It is important that the patients with ESRD are seen and treated by a multidisciplinary team, which should include an endocrinologist, a nephrologist, a cardiologist, an ophthalmologist, a social worker, a dietitian and a specialist nurse. Patients whose GFR is less than 30 ml/min should be advised of the various options, and as soon as a decision is made of the preferred option, preparation for RRT should be started. For instance, an arteriovenous fistula should be established in patients who will be undergoing hemodialysis, and a peritoneal catheter should be inserted in those who will be treated with peritoneal dialysis. The various therapeutic modalities mentioned in the previous section on advanced renal disease will be continued at this stage. It is generally accepted that when the GFR of a diabetic patient with ESRD is in the range of 10–15 ml/min, RRT will be initiated. It should be remembered that both hemodialysis and peritoneal dialysis have specific complications, which are discussed in Chapter 16. The overall mortality and morbidity of diabetic patients receiving RRT are significantly greater than those of nondiabetic patients. Woredekal and Friedman have suggested that increasing the amount of delivered dialysis may improve the results. Thus, diabetic patients receiving dialytic therapy should be closely followed, and the quantity of dialysis should be adjusted.

## The use of transplantation in the treatment of diabetic patients ESRD (Chapter 20)

Danovitch and Kendrick (Chapter 20) have described a striking improvement in the results of kidney transplantation over the last few years.[20,21] In spite of the fact that diabetic patients tend to fare less well after transplantation than nondiabetic patients, the survival of diabetic subjects who receive a kidney transplant is better than on dialysis.[20,21] This is true in spite of the fact that kidney transplantation is associated with many complications as a result of the surgical procedure, the immunosuppressive therapy and the primary disease. Thus, kidney transplantation, using either a cadaver donor or living donor, is the preferred mode of treatment of ESRD due to diabetic nephropathy. Therefore, all suitable patients should be counseled about this option.

Early attempts to transplant a pancreas into diabetic patients were initially associated with a high complication rate and a low success rate. Improvement in surgical technique and in the immunosuppressive therapy has made this an acceptable form of treatment. Cadaver donor pancreas transplantation can be performed simultaneously with a kidney transplant in diabetic ESRD patients, or as a solitary graft in patients who still have remnant kidney function but have brittle diabetes. The survival rates and various complications of pancreas transplantation can be found in Chapter 20.

An exciting avenue of treatment is the transplantation of pancreatic islets. Until the last few years, the success rate was very low. However, Shapiro et al reported in 2000 a series of successful islet transplantations using a steroid-free regimen.[22] It remains to be determined how applicable this approach will be at other centers.

## FUTURE STRATEGIES FOR THE TREATMENT OF DIABETIC NEPHROPATHY (Chapter 12)

Langham et al (Chapter 12) have described many novel approaches in the treatment of diabetic nephropathy. Most of these strategies are based on various pathogenetic pathways of the disease. Some of them are in the development stage, whereas others have reached the stage of clinical trials. However, there is as yet no clinical proof of the beneficial effects of these agents.

### Advanced glycation end products (AGEs)

AGEs are thought to play an important role in the development of diabetic nephropathy. The putative therapeutic strategies are prevention of the formation of AGEs, the use of cross-link breakers that can break down AGEs, and substances which block the receptors for AGEs. All these approaches to interrupt AGE-dependent pathways are under current investigation.

### Protein kinase C (PKC)

Protein kinase C (PKC), an important intracellular enzyme, is activated in the presence of hyperglycemia. PKC may activate a myriad of growth factors that may be pathogenetic in diabetic nephropathy. Several PKC inhibitors have been generated and are being investigated. In particular, an inhibitor of the $\beta_2$ isoform of PKC is under intensive clinical investigation.

## Newer treatments for hypertension

Various new inhibitors of vasoactive hormone formation are being developed and tested. One example is omapatrilat, a dual inhibitor of ACE and neutral endopeptidase. It is postulated that inhibiting these vasoactive pathways will lead not only to better blood pressure control but also superior renoprotection.

None of these newer strategies has been approved for widespread clinical use.

## TREATMENT OF COMORBID CONDITIONS ASSOCIATED WITH DIABETES MELLITUS AND KIDNEY INVOLVEMENT

There are many complications of diabetes mellitus that are aggravated by the presence of diabetic nephropathy and the associated hypertension and cardiovascular disease. In this book, we have attempted to discuss the treatment of some of these conditions.

## Pregnancy in the patient with diabetic nephropathy

Ferrier and Gallery (Chapter 15) have described the effects of diabetes on pregnancy and fetal outcome. They have then discussed the effects of pregnancy on diabetes and renal disease in patients with diabetic nephropathy. These authors stress the need for early counseling of the diabetic female patient and careful monitoring of the pregnancy by a multidisciplinary team. Optimization of pregnancy outcome requires strict control of blood glucose; strict control of hypertension; avoiding medications, such as ACE-I and AIIR, that are contraindicated in pregnancy; regular monitoring of pregnancy; and planned delivery.

## Retinopathy

Retinopathy is a ubiquitous complication of diabetic nephropathy and a leading cause of blindness. Axer-

Siegel and Dotan (Chapter 17) have listed the risk factors for diabetic retinopathy as duration of disease, quality of metabolic control, hyperlipidemia, presence of hypertension and degree of renal involvement. The importance of careful treatment of diabetic patients on dialysis is stressed. All patients with diabetic nephropathy should be examined by an ophthalmologist annually. Treatment of hypertension, especially with ACE-I, and metabolic control are emphasized. Laser photocoagulation is indicated in patients with significant macular edema and proliferative retinopathy. Vitrectomy may need to be performed in patients showing progressive retinopathy with macular hemorrhage and retinal detachment.

## Diabetic foot and peripheral vascular disease

Most patients with diabetic nephropathy have some evidence of neuropathy and vascular disease. The clinical manifestations of these complications, especially in the limbs, are an important cause of morbidity. McNally and London (Chapter 18) have described the epidemiology, clinical manifestations and treatment of these conditions.

The important clinical manifestations are ulceration and ischemic vascular disease of the limbs. The authors have shown other factors, such as neuropathy, foot deformity, arterial disease and infections, to be associated with diabetic foot problems. They have provided important techniques for the clinical assessment of peripheral neuropathy, vascular disease and infection. Patients with diabetic nephropathy should be assessed frequently for the presence of diseases of the feet. Prevention and treatment include protection of the foot by appropriate footwear, careful foot care, optimizing vascular supply to the leg and optimizing control of vascular risk factors and diabetes. The importance of preventing and treating diabetic complications must be a major priority in all clinics attended by diabetic patients. These patients should be regularly examined by specialist nurses who have received special training in the care of the diabetic foot. It is highly desirable that all dialysis nurses receive similar training and regularly assess their patients. Once again, early treatment of diabetic lesions in the foot requires a multidisciplinary team with diabetologists, vascular surgeons, podiatrists, and orthopedic and general surgeons.

## CONCLUDING REMARKS

Diabetes mellitus is undoubtedly one of the most important health hazards in the twenty-first century. The many serious complications of diabetes make it a leading cause of morbidity and mortality. This book has been devoted mainly to the description of diabetic nephropathy. Involvement of the kidney in diabetes is generally associated with other comorbid conditions as well as a progressive loss of renal function. The extremely high cost of treating the patient with ESRD has made this one of the major components in the health expenditure of most developed countries. It is not clear how the governments of these countries will be able to deal with the ever-increasing burden of diabetic patients requiring RRT. Prevention of diabetes, renal involvement and the other comorbid conditions appears to be the optimal approach to be taken. This, however, requires a concerted effort and cooperation by the various government agencies, diabetologists, family practitioners, nephrologists, cardiologists, ophthalmologists, podiatrists, dietitians and specialist nurses. We hope that this book provides guidelines for the directions which may contribute to improving the current prevention and management of diabetic nephropathy and comorbid conditions.

## REFERENCES

1. Onkamo P, Väänänen S, Karvonen M et al, Worldwide increase in incidence of type I diabetes—the analysis of the data on published incidence trends, *Diabetologia* (1999) **12**: 1395–403.
2. Zimmet P, Albert KGMM, Shaw J, Global and social implications of the diabetes epidemic, *Nature* (2001) **414**: 782–7.
3. Wiseman MJ, Saunders AJ, Keen H et al, Effect of blood glucose control on increased glomerular filtration rate and kidney size in insulin-dependent diabetes, *N Engl J Med* (1985) **312**: 617–21.
4. Vora JP, Dolben J, Williams JD et al, Impact of initial treatment on renal function in newly-diagnosed type 2 (non-insulin-dependent) diabetes mellitus, *Diabetologia* (1993) **36**: 734–40.
5. Diabetes Control and Complications (DCCT) Research Group, Effect of intensive therapy on the development and progression of diabetic nephropathy in the Diabetes Control and Complications Trial, *Kidney Int* (1995) **47**: 1703–20.
6. UK Prospective Diabetes Study (UKPDS) Group, Intensive blood-glucose control with sulphonylureas or insulin compared with conventional treatment and risk of complications in patients with type 2 diabetes (UKPDS 33), *Lancet* (1998) **352**: 837–53.
7. Fioretto P, Steffes MW, Sutherland DE et al, Reversal of lesions of diabetic nephropathy after pancreas transplantation, *N Engl J Med* (1998) **339**: 69–75.
8. Mogensen CE. Microalbuminuria, blood pressure and diabetic renal disease: origin and development of ideas. *Diabetologia* (1999) **42**: 263–85.
9. Stamler J, Vaccaro O, Neaton JD et al, Diabetes, other risk factors, and 12-yr cardiovascular mortality for men screened in the Multiple Risk Factor Intervention Trial, *Diabetes Care* (1993) **16**: 434–44.
10. Bakris GL, Williams M, Dworkin L, Preserving renal function in adults with hypertension and diabetes: a consensus approach. National Kidney Foundation Hypertension and Diabetes Executive Committees Working Group, *Am J Kidney Dis* (2000) **36**: 646–61.
11. Lewis EJ, Huniscker LG, Bain RP et al, The effect of angiotensin-converting-enzyme inhibition on diabetic nephropathy, *N Engl J Med* (1993) **329**: 1456–62.
12. Brenner BM, Cooper ME, de Zeeuw D et al, Effects of losartan on renal and cardiovascular outcomes in patients with type 2 diabetes and nephropathy, *N Engl J Med* (2001) **345**: 861–9.
13. Lewis EJ, Hunsicker LG, Clarke WR et al, Renoprotective effects of the angiotensin-receptor antagonist irbesartan in patients with nephropathy due to type 2 diabetes. *N Engl J Med* (2001) **345**: 851–60.
14. Parving HH, Lehnert H, Brochner-Mortensen J et al, The effect of irbesartan on the development of diabetic nephropathy in patients with type 2 diabetes, *N Engl J Med* (2001) **345**: 870–8.
15. Bakris G, White D, Effects of an ACE inhibitor combined with a calcium channel blocker on progression of diabetic nephropathy, *J Hum Hypertens* (1997) **11**: 35–8.
16. Bakris GL, Weir MR, De Quattro V et al, Effects of an ACE inhibitor/calcium antagonist combination on proteinuria in diabetic nephropathy, *Kidney Int* (1998) **54**: 1283–9.
17. Fried LF, Orchard TJ, Kasiske BL, Effect of lipid reduction on the progression of renal disease: a meta-analysis, *Kidney Int* (2001) **59**: 260–9.
18. Mulec H, Blohme G, Grande B et al, The effect of metabolic control on rate of decline in renal function in insulin-dependent diabetes mellitus and microalbuminuria, *Nephrol Dial Transplant* (1998) **13**: 651–5.
19. Chuahirun T, Wesson DE, Cigarette smoking predicts faster progression of type 2 established diabetic nephropathy despite ACE inhibition, *Am J Kidney Dis* (2002) **39**: 376–82.
20. Wolfe RA, Ashby VB, Milford EL, Ojo AO et al, Comparison of mortality in all patients on dialysis, patients on dialysis awaiting transplantation, and recipients of a first cadaveric transplant, *N Engl J Med* (1999) **341**: 1725–30.
21. Meier-Kriesche HU, Ojo OA, Port FK et al, Survival improvement among patients with end-stage renal disease: trends over time for transplant recipients and wait-listed patients. *J Am Soc Nephrol* (2001) **12**: 1293–6.
22. Shapiro AMJ, Lakey JRT, Ryan EA et al, Islet transplantation in seven patients with type I diabetes mellitus using a glucocorticoid-free immunosuppressive regimen. *N Engl J Med* (2000) **343**: 230–8.

# Index

Note: Page numbers in **bold** refer to figures in the text; those in *italics* to tables or boxed material